Medical Library Service

College of Physicians and Surgeons of
British Columbia

MASTER TECHNIQUES IN ORTHOPAEDIC SURGERY™
THE HIP

MASTER TECHNIQUES IN ORTHOPAEDIC SURGERY™

Series Editor
Roby C. Thompson, Jr., M.D.

Volume Editors

THE FOOT AND ANKLE
Kenneth A. Johnson, M.D.

RECONSTRUCTIVE KNEE SURGERY
Douglas W. Jackson, M.D.

KNEE ARTHROPLASTY
Paul A. Lotke, M.D.

THE HIP
Clement B. Sledge, M.D.

THE SPINE
David S. Bradford, M.D.

THE SHOULDER
Edward V. Craig, M.D.

THE ELBOW
Bernard F. Morrey, M.D.

THE WRIST
Richard H. Gelberman, M.D.

THE HAND
James W. Strickland, M.D.

FRACTURES
Donald A. Wiss, M.D.

THE HIP

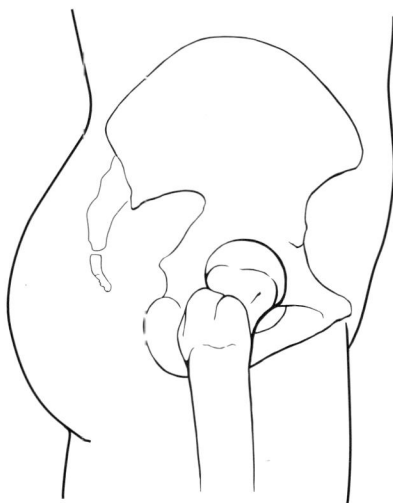

Editor

CLEMENT B. SLEDGE, M.D.
Professor of Orthopedic Surgery
Harvard Medical School
Department of Orthopedics
Brigham and Women's Hospital
Boston, Massachusetts

Illustrator

Hugh Thomas
New York, New York

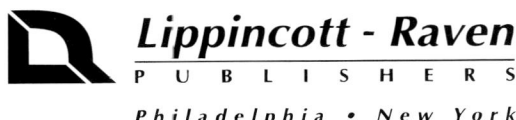

Philadelphia • New York

Acquisitions Editor: Kathey Alexander
Development Editor: Anne M. Sydor
Manufacturing Manager: Dennis Teston
Production Manager: Laurence Bernstein
Production Editor: Janice Lochansky
Cover Designer: Jeane Norton
Indexer: Lynne Mahan
Compositor: Maryland Composition
Printer: Worzalla

© 1998, by Lippincott—Raven Publishers. All rights reserved. This book is protected by copyright. No part of it may be reproduced, stored in a retrieval system, or transmitted, in any form or by any means—electronic, mechanical, photocopy, recording, or otherwise—without the prior written consent of the publisher, except for brief quotations embodied in critical articles and reviews. For information write **Lippincott-Raven Publishers, 227 East Washington Square, Philadelphia, PA 19106-3780.**

Materials appearing in this book prepared by individuals as part of their official duties as U.S. Government employees are not covered by the above-mentioned copyright.

Printed in the United States of America

9 8 7 6 5 4 3 2 1

Library of Congress Cataloging-in-Publication Data
The hip / edited by Clement B. Sledge; illustrator, Hugh Thomas.
    p.   cm.—(Master techniques in orthopaedic surgery ™ : v. 9)
  Includes bibliographical references and index.
  ISBN 0-7817-0034-5
  1. Hip joint—Surgery. I. Sledge, Clement B., 1930–
II. Series.
    [DNLM: 1. Hip Joint—surgery. 2. Hip Fractures—surgery. 3. Hip
Prosthesis—methods. WE 168 M423 1997 v.9]
RD549.H49   1997
617.5´81059—dc21
DNLM/DLC
for Library of Congress

Care has been taken to confirm the accuracy of the information presented and to describe generally accepted practices. However, the authors, editors, and publisher are not responsible for errors or omissions or for any consequences from application of the information in this book and make no warranty, express or implied, with respect to the contents of the publication.

The authors, editors, and publisher have exerted every effort to ensure that drug selection and dosage set forth in this text are in accordance with current recommendations and practice at the time of publication. However, in view of ongoing research, changes in government regulations, and the constant flow of information relating to drug therapy and drug reactions, the reader is urged to check the package insert for each drug for any change in indications and dosage and for added warnings and precautions. This is particularly important when the recommended agent is a new or infrequently employed drug.

Some drugs and medical devices presented in this publication have Food and Drug Administration (FDA) clearance for limited use in restricted research settings. It is the responsibility of the health care provider to ascertain the FDA status of each drug or device planned for use in their clinical practice.

To John Charnley, who made it all possible
by virtue of his foresight and single-minded devotion
to the task of solving the problem of the arthritic hip

CONTENTS

Contributors xi

Acknowledgments xiii

Series Preface xv

Preface xvii

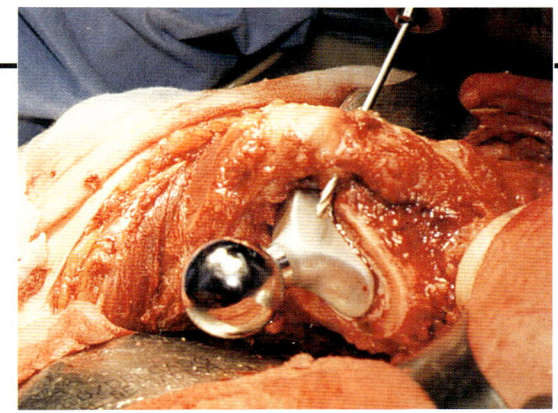

PART I   SURGICAL APPROACHES

Chapter 1
Posterior Approach   3
Thomas P. Sculco

Chapter 2
Direct Lateral Approach   15
Roby C. Thompson, Jr. and Kevin Hardinge

Chapter 3
Transtrochanteric Approach   33
Harlan C. Amstutz and Joseph Yao

Chapter 4
Anterior Lateral Approach   51
Paul J.P. Pongor and Maurice E. Müeller

PART II   FRACTURES

Chapter 5
Acetabular Fractures: Surgical Approaches and Technique   73
David L. Helfet, Arthur L. Malkani, and Craig S. Bartlett

Chapter 6
Surgical Management of Intertrochanteric Fractures   109
James F. Kellam

Chapter 7
Young Patients with Femoral Head Fractures   139
M. L. Chip Routt, Peter T. Simonian, and Sigvard T. Hansen

PART III ALTERNATIVES TO TOTAL HIP ARTHROPLASTY

Chapter 8
Reconstructive Osteotomies of the Pelvis for the Correction of Acetabular Dysplasia   157
Michael B. Millis

Chapter 9
The Intertrochanteric Osteotomy   183
Robert Poss and Alastair Younger

Chapter 10
Arthrodesis: The Vancouver Technique   197
Robert W. McGraw, Clive P. Duncan, and Christopher P. Beauchamp

PART IV PRIMARY TOTAL HIP ARTHROPLASTY

Chapter 11
Templating   211
Clement B. Sledge and John B. Sledge

Chapter 12
Cemented Primary Total Hip Arthroplasty   217
Chitranjan S. Ranawat, Michael J. Maynard, and Rajiv G. Deshmukh

Chapter 13
The Hybrid Total Hip Replacement   239
William H. Harris

Chapter 14
Cementless Primary Total Hip Arthroplasty   259
Ajai Cadambi and Charles A. Engh

PART V REVISION TOTAL HIP ARTHROPLASTY

Chapter 15
Secondary Total Hip Arthroplasty: After Infection   283
Eduardo A. Salvati and Jay R. Lieberman

CONTENTS

Chapter 16
    Acetabular Revision 295
Clement B. Sledge and Hugh P. Chandler

Chapter 17
    Revision Total Hip Arthroplasty: The Femoral Stem 305
Aaron G. Rosenberg

    Chapter 17A
        Revision with Cemented Femoral Component 309
Craig G. Mohler and Dennis K. Collis

    Chapter 17B
        Revision with Cementless Stem Technique 325
Mark Barba and Wayne G. Paprosky

    Chapter 17C
        Impaction Grafting with Cement 335
W. E. Michael Mikhail and Lars Weidenhielm

    Chapter 17D
        Allograft-Prosthetic Composite Reconstruction 343
Michael J. Hejna

Subject Index 355

CONTRIBUTORS

Harlan C. Amstutz, M.D.
Medical Director, Joint Replacement Institute, Orthopaedic Hospital, 2400 S. Flower Street, Los Angeles, California 90007

Mark Barba, M.D.
Fellow, Adult Joint Reconstruction Fellowship Program, Central DuPage Hospital, 25 N. Winfield Road, Winfield, Illinois 60190

Craig S. Bartlett, M.D.
Fellow, Orthopaedic Trauma Service, Hospital for Special Surgery, 535 East 70th Street, New York, New York 10021

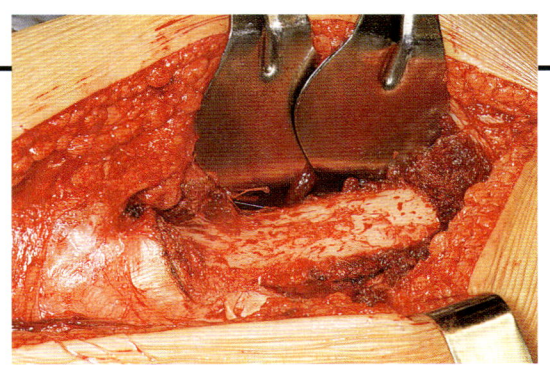

Christopher P. Beauchamp, M.D., F.R.C.S.C.
Department of Orthopaedics, Vancouver Hospital and Health Science Centre, 910 West 10th Avenue, Vancouver, British Columbia, Canada V5Z 4E3

Ajai Cadambi, M.D.
Clinical Instructor in Orthopaedic Surgery, John Peter Smith Orthopaedic Residency Program, Fort Worth, Texas 76104

Hugh P. Chandler, M.D.
Assistant Clinical Professor, Department of Orthopaedic Surgery, Harvard Medical School, 15 Parkman Street, Boston, Massachusetts 02114; and Visiting Orthopaedic Surgeon, Massachusetts General Hospital, 1126 Jackson Tower, Boston, Massachusetts 02114

Dennis K. Collis, M.D.
Associate Clinical Professor, Department of Orthopaedics and Rehabilitation, Oregon Health Sciences University, Portland, Oregon 97201

Rajiv G. Deshmukh, M.D.
Junior Assistant Attending Surgeon, Comprehensive Arthritis Service, Hospital for Special Surgery, 535 East 70th Street, New York, New York 10021

Clive P. Duncan, M.D., F.R.C.S.C.
Professor and Chairman, Department of Orthopaedics, University of British Columbia, 90 West 10th Avenue, Vancouver, British Columbia, Canada V5Z 4E3

Charles A. Engh, M.D.
Clinical Associate Professor, Department of Orthopaedics, University of Maryland School of Medicine, Baltimore, Maryland 21201; and Medical Director, Anderson Orthopaedic Research Institute, 2501 Parker's Lane, Alexandria, Virginia 22307; and Medical Director, Inova Center for Joint Relacement, Alexandria, Virginia 22307

Sigvard T. Hansen, M.D.
Professor, Department of Orthopaedics, Harborview Medical Center, 325 9th Avenue, Seattle, Washington 98104

Kevin Hardinge, M.Ch.Orth., F.R.C.S.
Hunterian Professor, Royal College of Surgeons of England, Centre for Hip Surgery, Wrightington Hospital, Appley Bridge, Wigan, United Kingdom WN6 9EP

William H. Harris, M.D.
Clinical Professor of Orthopaedic Surgery, Harvard Medical School, 15 Pearlman Street, Boston, Massachusetts 02114; and Chief, Hip and Implant Unit, Massachusetts General Hospital, 1126 Jackson Tower, Boston, Massachusetts 02114

Michael J. Hejna, M.D., Ph.D.
Assistant Professor, Department of Orthopaedic Surgery, Rush Medical College, 1725 W. Harrison Street, Chicago, Illinois 60612

David L. Helfet, M.D.
Associate Professor of Orthopaedic Surgery; and Director of The Combined Orthopaedic Trauma/Fracture Service, Hospital for Special Surgery, New York Hospital, 535 E. 70th Street, New York, New York 10021

James F. Kellam, M.D.
Department of Orthopedic Surgery, Carolinas Health Care System: Carolinas Medical Center, 1000 Blythe Boulevard, Charlotte, North Carolina 28232

Jay R. Lieberman, M.D.
Assistant Professor of Orthopaedic Surgery, Department of Orthopaedic Surgery, UCLA School of Medicine, Center for the Health Sciences, 10833 Le Conte Avenue, Los Angeles, California 90024

Arthur L. Malkani, M.D.
Department of Orthopedics, Hospital for Special Surgery, 535 E. 70th Street, New York, New York 10021

Michael J. Maynard, M.D.
Assistant Professor of Orthopedic Surgery, Hospital for Special Surgery/Cornell University Medical Center, 535 East 70th Street, New York, New York 10021

Robert W. McGraw, M.D., F.R.C.S.C.
Professor of Orthopaedics, Department of Orthopaedics, Vancouver Hospital and Health Science Centre, 910 West 10th Avenue, Vancouver, British Columbia V5Z 4E3

W. E. Michael Mikhail, M.D., F.A.C.S.
Clinical Professor of Orthopaedic Surgery, Medical College of Ohio, PO Box 10008, Toledo, Ohio 43699; and the McMaster/Gardner Professor of Orthopaedic Bioengineering Research, The University of Toledo, Toledo, Ohio 43699

Michael B. Millis, M.D.
Associate Professor of Clinical Orthopaedic Surgery, Harvard Medical School, 15 Parkman Street, Boston Massachusetts 02114, and Associate in Orthopaedic Surgery, The Children's Hospital, 300 Longwood Avenue, Boston, Massachusetts 02115

Craig G. Mohler, M.D.
Orthopedic Surgeon, Orthopedic and Fracture Clinic of Eugene, Eugene, Oregon 97401; and Clinical Instructor, Oregon Health Sciences University, Portland, Oregon 97201

Prof. Maurice E. Müeller
Lindenhof Hospital, Brengardent Strasse 117, CH-3001 Bern, Switzerland

Wayne G. Paprosky, M.D.
Associate Professor, Rush Medical College, 1725 W. Harrison Avenue, Chicago, Illinois 60612; and Staff Orthopaedic Surgeon, Department of Adult Reconstructive Surgery, Central DuPage Hospital, 25 N. Winfield Road, Winfield, Illinois 60190

Paul J.P. Pongor, M.D.
Instructor in Surgery, Director of Orthopaedic Registry, Department of Surgery, Beth Israel Deaconess Hospital/New England Baptist Hospital, 110 Francis Street, Boston Massachusetts 02215

Robert Poss, M.D.
Professor of Orthopedic Surgery, Harvard Medical School, 15 Parkman Street, Boston, Massachusetts 02114, Department of Orthopedics, Brigham and Women's Hospital, 75 Francis Street, Boston, Massachusetts 02115

Chitranjan S. Ranawat, M.D.
Clinical Professor of Orthopedic Surgery, Department of Orthopedic Surgery, Cornell University Medical Center, Lenox Hill Hospital, 130 E. 77 Street, New York, New York 10021

Aaron G. Rosenberg, M.D.
Professor of Orthopedic Surgery, Department of Orthopedic Surgery, Rush Medical College, 1725 W. Harrison Avenue, Suite 1063, Chicago, Illinois 60612

M. L. Chip Routt, M.D.
Associate Professor, Department of Orthopaedics, University of Washington, Harborview Medical Center, 325 9th Avenue, Seattle, Washington 98104

Eduardo A. Salvati, M.D.
Professor of Orthopedic Surgery, Cornell University Medical College, Hospital for Special Surgery, 535 East 70th Street, New York, New York 10021

Thomas P. Sculco, M.D.
Professor of Surgery, Department of Orthopedics, Cornell University Medical Center, Hospital for Special Surgery, 535 East 70th Street, New York, New York 10021

Peter T. Simonian, M.D.
Associate Professor, Department of Orthopedic Surgery, University of Washington Medical Center, Seattle, Washington 98195

Clement B. Sledge, M.D.
Professor of Orthopedic Surgery, Harvard Medical School, 15 Parkman Street, Boston, Massachusetts 02114, and Department of Orthopedics, Brigham and Women's Hospital, 75 Francis Street, Boston, Massachusetts 02115

John B. Sledge, M.D.
Department of Orthopedics, Boston University Medical Center, 818 Harrison Avenue, Boston, Massachusetts 02118

Roby C. Thompson, Jr., M.D.
Professor of Orthopaedic Surgery, Department of Orthopaedic Surgery, University of Minnesota, 420 Delaware Street, SE, Minneapolis, Minnesota 55455

Lars Weidenhielm, M.D.
Associate Professor, Karolinska Institute, Department of Orthopaedics, St. Goran Hospital, P.O. Box 12500, S-11281 Stockholm, Sweden

Joseph Yao, M.D.
1521 N. Tenth Street, Blytheville, Arkansas 72315

Alastair Younger
Fellow, Department of Orthopedics, Brigham and Women's Hospital, 75 Francis Street, Boston Massachusetts 02115

ACKNOWLEDGMENTS

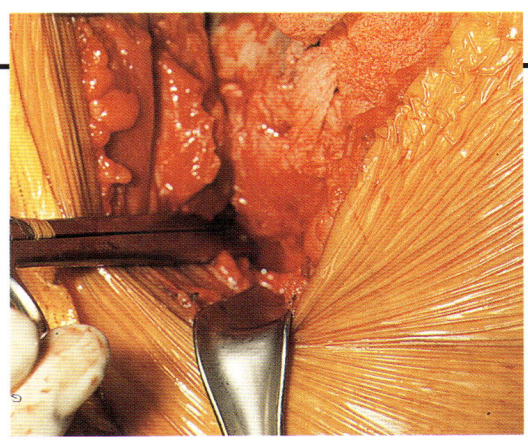

It takes many people and much effort to produce a book. When that book is truly a work of art, as this book is, everyone must be a perfectionist. First and clearly most important, are the authors; they have done an outstanding job, sometimes under extreme deadline pressure. I thank them all. Kathey Alexander and her crew at Lippincott-Raven are truly outstanding professionals who will accept nothing but the highest quality. The illustrator, Hugh Thomas, has produced beautiful examples of his craft, reinforcing the well-known fact that drawings are often much more informative than photographs. As always with an effort like this, it is family time that is sacrificed; I thank my wife, Georgia Sledge.

SERIES PREFACE

Master Techniques in Orthopaedic Surgery is a ten-volume series of operative atlases designed to provide in-depth descriptions of surgical techniques that are preferred by surgeons recognized by their peers as master surgeons in their area of specialization.

The ten volume editors, all recognized leaders based on their research and educational contributions, have advanced the surgical state of the art in our field. The chapter authors were selected for their experience and skills, and were asked to present their material in a personal manner, highlighting their unique perspectives and observations for the reader.

These atlases are designed to help the practitioner deal with the difficult but common problems encountered in daily practice. Surgical procedures that are in the developmental phase, such as vascularized fibular grafting for osteonecrosis, or procedures largely restricted to referral centers, such as reconstruction for limb salvage following tumor resection, have not been covered since procedures such as these are rarely performed by the orthopaedic practitioner. Likewise, the common, straightforward procedures that offer few complications and little difficulty have also been avoided.

These books take you into the operating room and let you peer over the shoulder of the surgeon at work. The color

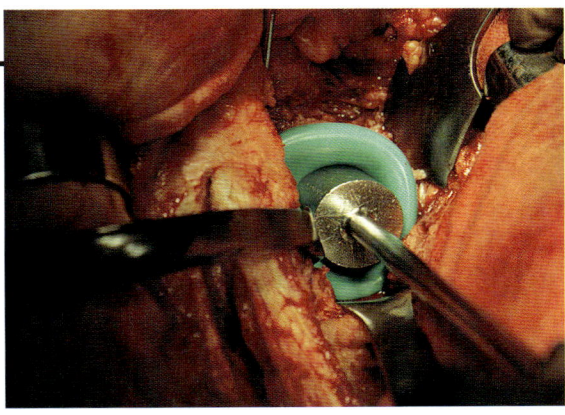

photographs and accompanying drawings guides the orthopaedist step-by-step through a procedure. The commentary, organized in a standard format throughout the series, offers one specific technical advice, as well as tips and pearls gained through the surgeon's years of experience.

The shared knowledge and expertise found in these pages are presented to enable the surgeon to undertake surgical procedures with greater confidence and improved proficiency.

Roby C. Thompson, Jr., M.D.
Series Editor

PREFACE

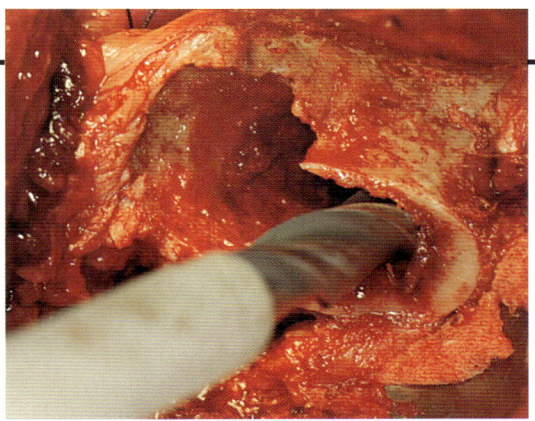

This book is a collection of descriptions of operations as performed by acknowledged "masters". There is no attempt to be comprehensive or all-inclusive. Instead, common operative procedures have been selected and the preferred operative approach of the author is illustrated and described.

A major strength of the volume is the quality of the illustrations. Uniformity of this quality is assured by having the same artist illustrate the entire book. In addition, a single uniform format has been adopted so the reader can easily become familiar with the style as successive chapters are read.

The best way to use this book is to read a chapter that pertains to a particular patient and operation that you are planning. Add your own experience and preferences, but remember that the procedures described have served the authors in numerous instances. I can guarantee that you will find each chapter useful and informative.

Clement B. Sledge, M.D.

MASTER TECHNIQUES IN ORTHOPAEDIC SURGERY™
THE HIP

PART I

Surgical Approaches

1
Posterior Approach

Thomas P. Sculco

INDICATIONS/CONTRAINDICATIONS

The posterior approach in primary total hip arthroplasty is now commonly utilized with a high rate of success. There are a number of reasons for its use and these include, (1) ease of dissection and relative atraumatic soft tissue exposure, (2) reduced blood loss because of minimal dissection, (3) wide exposure for acetabular and femoral reaming and prosthetic insertion, (4) ability to reconstruct the posterior soft tissues in most patients after implant insertion, (5) rapid rehabilitation. Almost all patients undergoing total hip arthroplasty are suitable candidates for the posterior approach except for those who have bony ankylosis or severe ectopic periarticular bone where trochanteric osteotomy is necessary for mobilization of the hip. The hip in patients with severe congenital hip dysplasia and high-riding femoral heads dislocated from the true acetabulum also is best exposed by trochanteric osteotomy. The abductor mechanism in these patients must be mobilized as the limb is lengthened, and an osteotomy facilitates this. The posterior approach is also useful for revision total hip replacement; repair of the posterior soft tissues that have been reflected from the femur and posterior acetabulum may be undertaken at the conclusion of the revision procedure.

Concern exists regarding higher dislocation rates following arthroplasty with the posterior approach when compared to the anterolateral and transtrochanteric approaches (4,6,9,10,13). The postulated reasons for an increased risk of dislocation include, (1) improper acetabular component positioning as a result of inadequate exposure obtained during the posterior approach, (2) lack of a lateral check rein as compared to that provided by trochanteric advancement with the transtrochanteric approach, and (3) loss of posterior capsular and musculotendinous stabilizing structures as a result of the surgical release. To address the loss of posterior soft tissue stability in this setting, I have utilized a technique of posterior capsulorrhaphy in conjunction with the reattachment of the external rotators, specifically the piriformis tendon and conjoined tendon, to the region of the posterior aspect of the greater trochanter and proximal femur. Those patients in whom this reconstruc-

---

T. P. Sculco, M.D.: Department of Orthopedics, Cornell University Medical Center, Hospital for Special Surgery, New York, New York 10021.

tion may be difficult or not possible are patients with severe protusio deformity or marked external rotation contractures. In both of these conditions the posterior structures are contracted, and the capsule cannot be approximated to the femur after hip reconstruction.

Surgical repair of the posterior structures in total hip arthroplasty has received relatively little attention in the literature. The posterior approach as first described by Von Langenbeck in 1874 contained no mention of this topic, and most descriptions over the next century, including those of Kocher, Gibson, and Moore did not include posterior repair as part of the surgical closure (2,8). Some descriptions of its use in total hip replacement either favored no posterior repair or did not comment on the subject (3,4). In fact, complete posterior capsulectomy has been advocated (4).

Posterior soft tissue repair has been mentioned briefly but without elaboration of technical details (1,5,7,12). Methods described include repair of the external rotators with and without capsular reattachment. They also include repairs with and without bony fixation of sutures.

I advocate repair of both external rotators and capsule. The theoretical result of repairing both structures is a dynamic and passive resistance to internal rotation. One might postulate that the capsular reattachment could lead to an undesirable external rotation contracture. This, however, has not been my experience.

PREOPERATIVE PLANNING

The hip should be templated for proper sizing preoperatively to ensure proper implant selection and restoration of leg length. Using the center of rotation of the femoral head as a landmark and drawing a line to the top of the lesser trochanter on the nonaffected side will give an accurate measurement of the femoral length. This measurement (taken with a ruler that allows for x-ray magnification) can be verified at surgery if there is not significant distortion of the femoral head/neck. The center of rotation of the prosthetic femoral head to the top of the lesser trochanter should approximate this measurement to ensure restoration of femoral length.

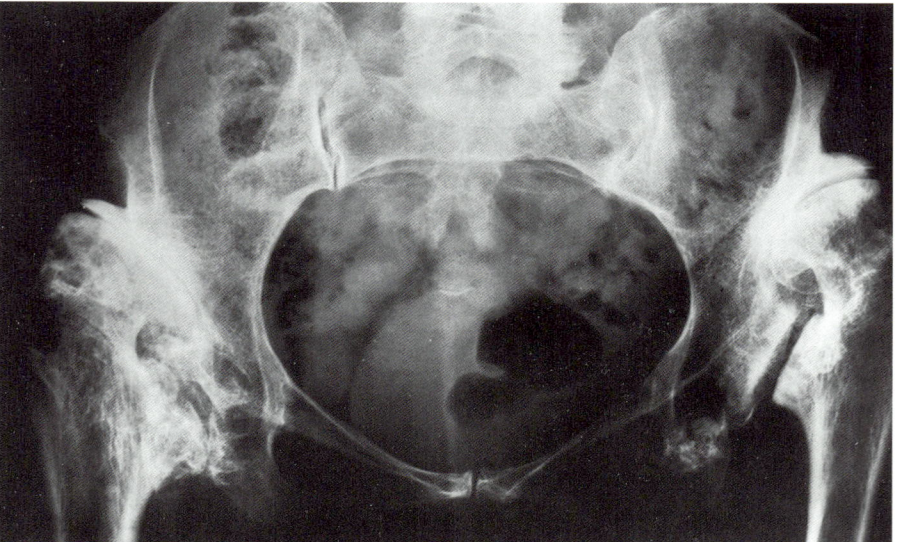

Figure 1. Osteoarthritis secondary to congenital hip dysplasia with complete lack of continuity between femoral head and acetabulum. Trochanteric osteotomy recommended due to contracted and shortened abductor mechanism.

Standard anteroposterior pelvic and lateral hip and proximal radiographs are obtained. These films will clarify the extent of ectopic bone or ankylosis in a stiff hip. Additionally the extent of hip dysplasia and femoral head/acetabular contact can be identified. If there is complete dislocation of the femoral head with superior migration, trochanteric osteotomy will be necessary. Osteotomy facilitates exposure in these ankylosed and dysplastic hips and allows for adjustment of the abductor mechanism (Fig. 1).

Clinical examination of the hip is carried out in the usual fashion and range of motion and hip muscle power should be recorded.

SURGERY

The patient is positioned in the lateral decubitus position on a fracture table. Anterior and posterior supporting pads are used to fix the pelvis in the true lateral position. A scapular padded support is used. A double arm board is used with the axillae and shoulders well protected. A vertical laminar flow room with plastic panels is used to create an enclosed operating area. Battery-powered body-exhaust systems are routinely used. The limb is draped free to allow mobilization of the leg during the operative procedure.

A posterolateral incision is used (Fig. 2). This extends from approximately 4 cm below the greater trochanter proximally for a total length of about 12 to 15 cm. The fascial incision should be made directly over the greater trochanter, and it is important that this incision remain in the plane of the lateral femur to avoid incising into the gluteus maximus, as this leads to increased bleeding and makes dissection more complex. The tendon of the gluteus maximus is partially released several millimeters from its insertion into the gluteal crest of the femur. It is particularly important to release this tendon adequately to allow mo-

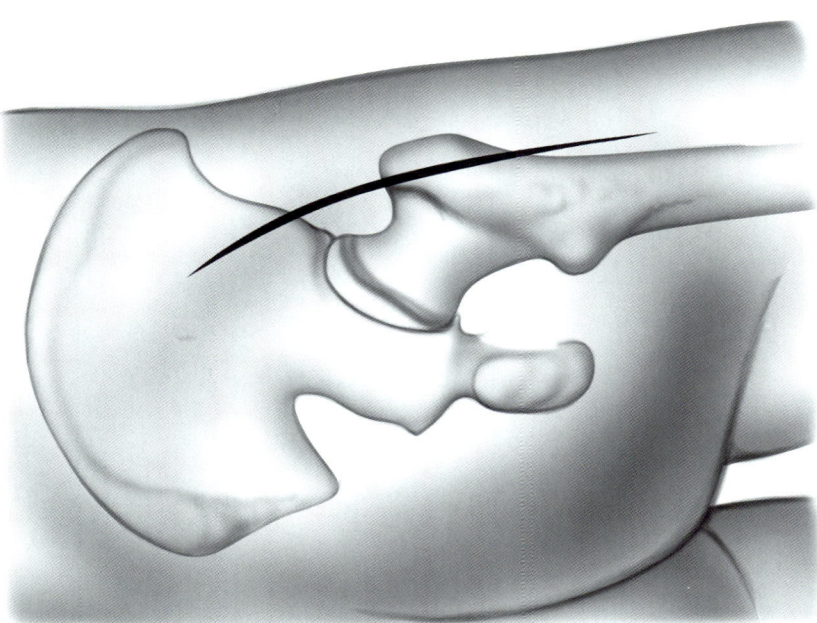

Figure 2. Posterolateral incision is utilized.

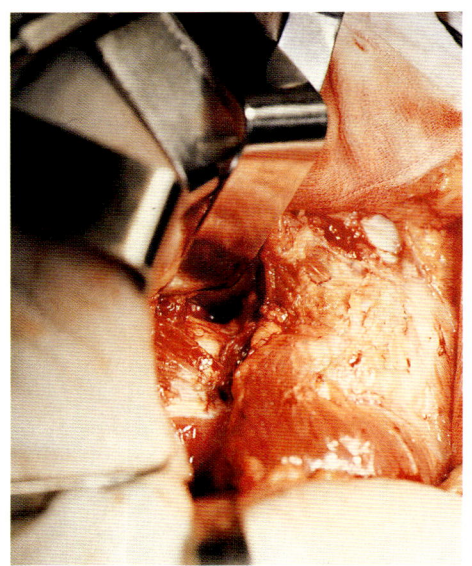
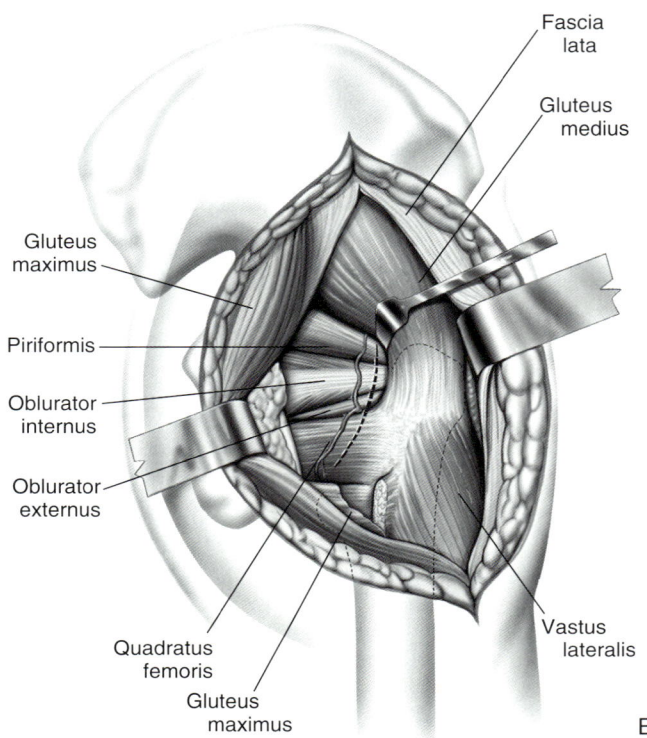

Figure 3 A, B. Posterior exposure of the external rotators.

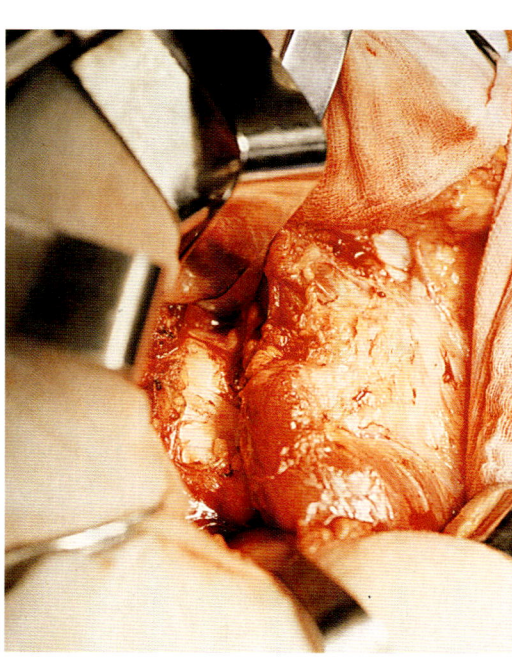

Figure 4. External rotators have been released from the posterior capsule.

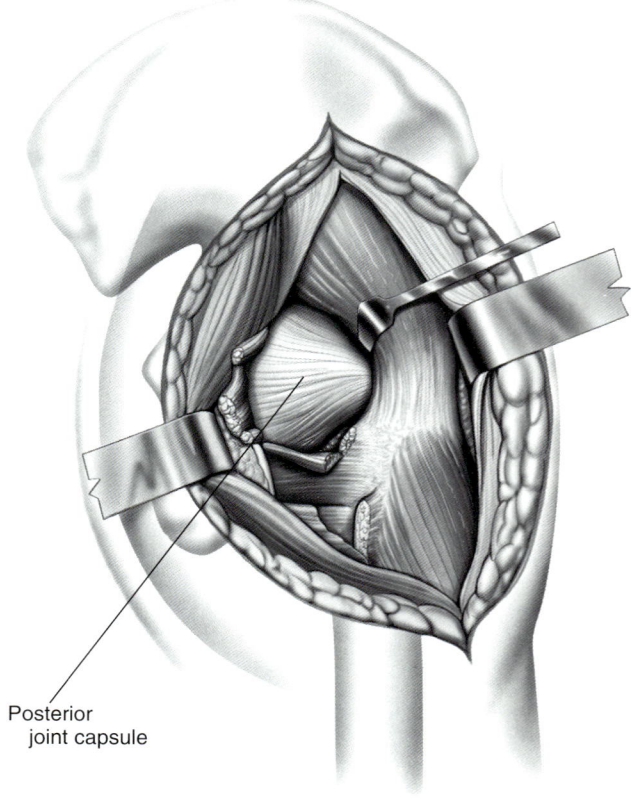

Figure 5. The conjoined tendon and piriformis tendon are released from their insertion into the posterior greater trochanter.

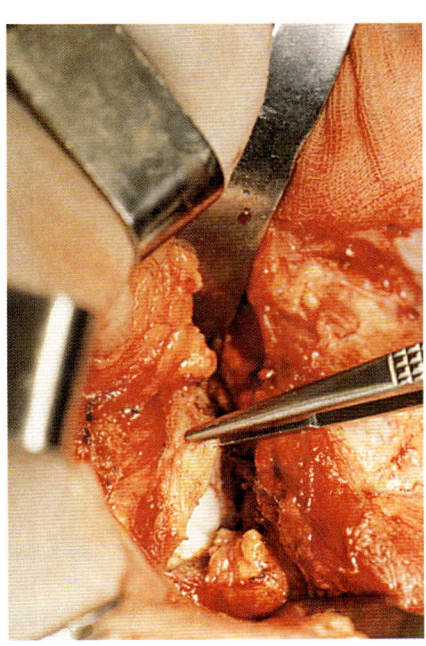

Figure 6. Capsulotomy has been performed with a wide and long posteromedial flap of capsule.

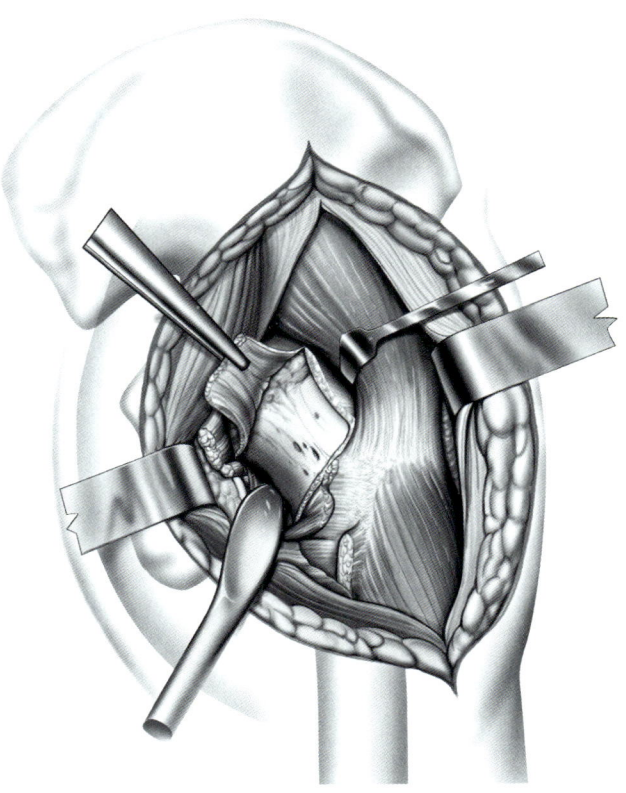

Figure 7. Trapezoidal posteriorly broad based capsular flap is created.

bilization of the femur into full internal rotation when exposure of the femur is being performed. In thin patients with preserved range of motion, exposure may be possible without release of any of the gluteus tendon. Exposure of the external rotators (Fig. 3) is provided by placing a right-angled narrow Hohmann retractor under the gluteus medius and minimus to retract these muscles anteriorly. Inferiorly, an Aufranc retractor is inserted above the quadratus femoris muscle. This will isolate the insertion of the external rotator tendons. The tendons are released at the site of their insertion into the posterior greater trochanter (Fig. 4). Care is taken not to enter the posterior hip capsule. The tendons will retract posteromedially as internal rotation of the femur is performed but are easily found after implantation of the prosthesis (Fig. 5).

The entire posterior capsule is now exposed and a posteriorly based flap is created from this capsule. Using electrocautery, the capsule is incised along the base of the neck. This capsulotomy is continued posterosuperiorly and posteroinferiorly to the acetabular labrum (Figs. 6,7). It is important to diverge with these capsular incisions to keep the posteromedial aspect of the flap as wide as possible. Additionally, incising the capsule along its intertrochanteric attachment allows the flap to be of sufficient length to allow its closure at the conclusion of the procedure. The femoral neck and head will now be visible (Fig. 8). The capsule is dissected from the inferior neck of the femur, and the insertion of the upper half of the quadratus femoris is released. Dislocation of the hip is now possible.

Exposure of the acetabulum is effected by using a C-shaped, long Hohmann retractor, which is placed over the anterior wall of the acetabulum. A Steinman pin is inserted superiorly under the gluteus minimus for superior exposure. A broad Hohmann retractor, which is at a right angle, is used posteriorly and is inserted into the ischium. Inferiorly an Aufranc retractor is used just below the inferior transverse acetabular ligament. The anterior capsule is released to allow the anterior Hohmann retractor to mobilize the femur anteriorly and for better positioning of this retractor. Global exposure is now accomplished, and further resection of the acetabular labrum and reaming can commence (Fig. 9).

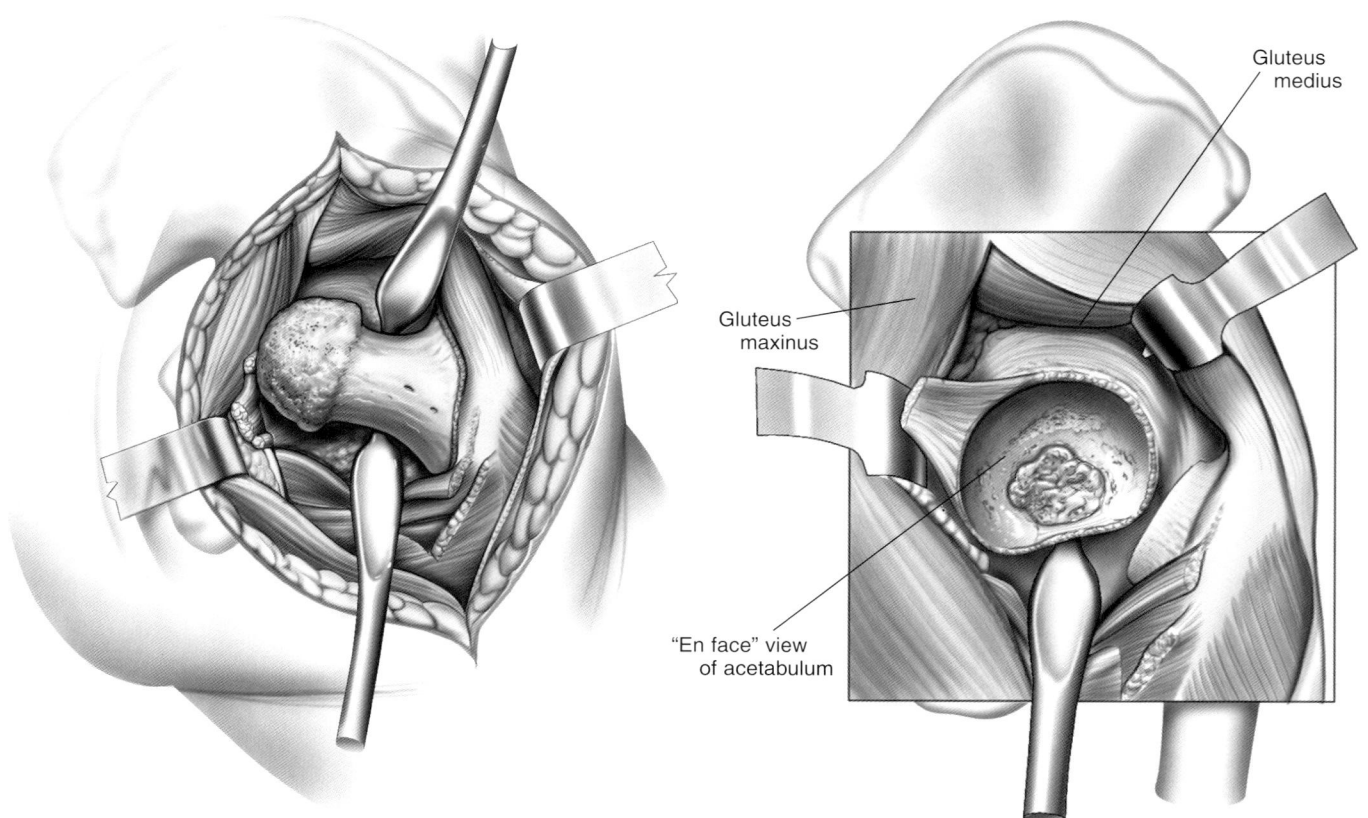

Figure 8. The hip is dislocated and retractor used to isolate the femoral neck.

Figure 9. After periacetabular soft-tissue release, global exposure of the acetabulum by appropriate retractors is possible.

After the acetabular component has been inserted, femoral exposure is facilitated by a broad, toothed retractor, which is placed under the anterior femoral neck and levers the femur anteriorly into the wound. There must be adequate release of the soft tissues about the upper femur to allow full internal rotation, flexion, and adduction of the femur. An Aufranc retractor is placed under the anterior femoral retractor and also is used to lift the femur into the wound. A standard right-angled Hohmann retractor can be used above the greater trochanter to reflect the abductor superiorly. The femur is then reamed, and the femoral component inserted.

Following placement of the acetabular and femoral prosthesis, preparation is made for the posterior soft-tissue repair. Two drill holes are made in the proximal femur with a one-eighth-inch drill bit (Fig. 10). Keith needles with loop sutures are inserted into these holes so that the loop end of the suture is posterior (Figs. 11, 12).

After reduction of the hip, the posterior capsule and external rotators are repaired using two #1 nonabsorbable sutures. The first nonabsorbable suture is placed into the superior capsule entering on the inner side of the capsule and exiting posteriorly. The suture is continued as a mattress suture through the piriformis tendon. The suture is then brought through the capsule so that both free ends of the suture are now inside the capsule. A second suture is passed in a similar fashion inferiorly into the capsule and the conjoined tendon, which is affixed as the piriformis tendon had been superiorly.

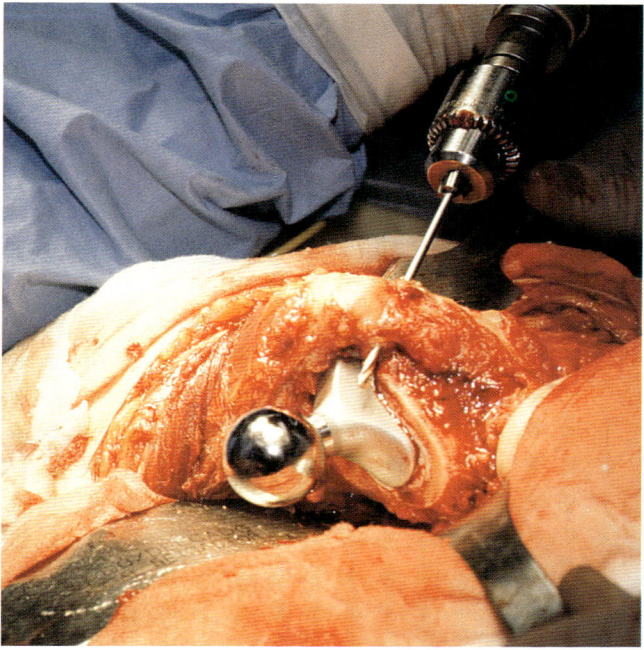

Figure 10. Drill hole being made through the greater trochanter.

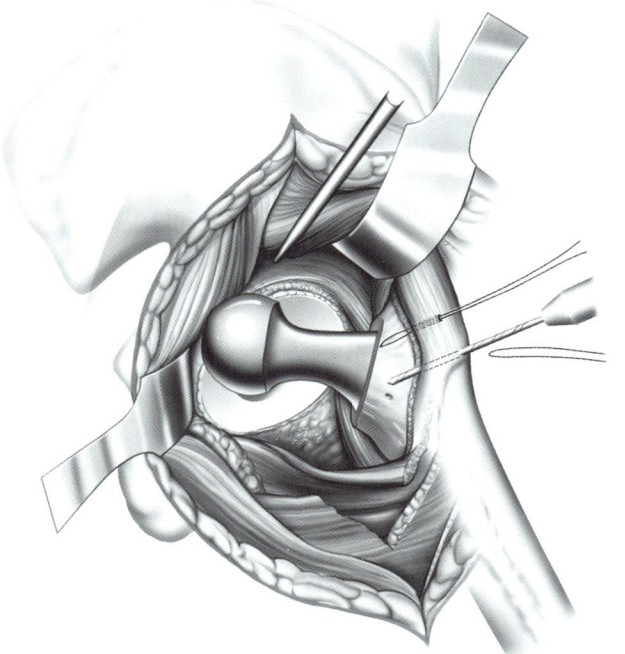

Figure 11. Two drill holes are placed through the greater trochanter exiting posteriorly. Loop sutures are then placed through these drill holes.

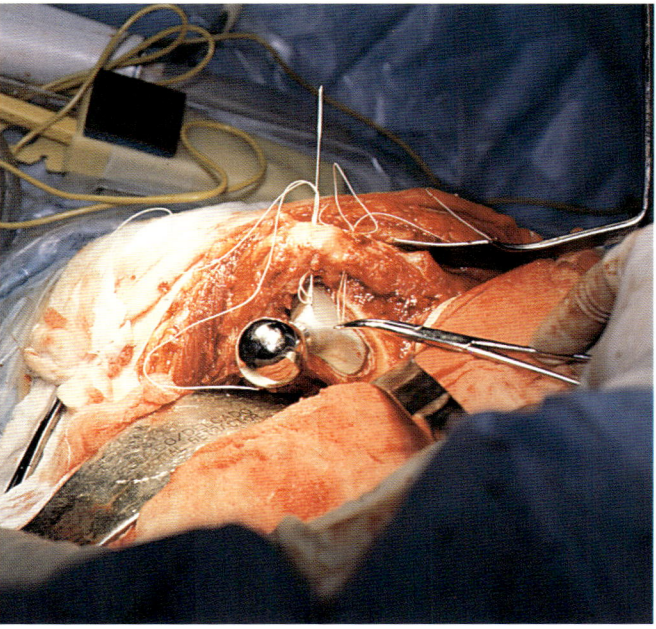

Figure 12. Two loop sutures are placed through the trochanteric drill holes.

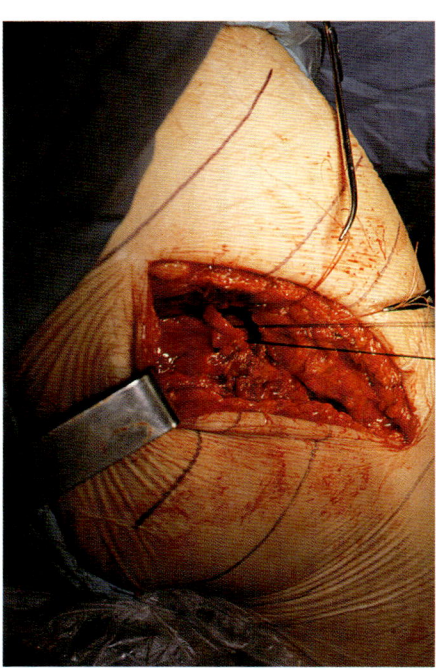 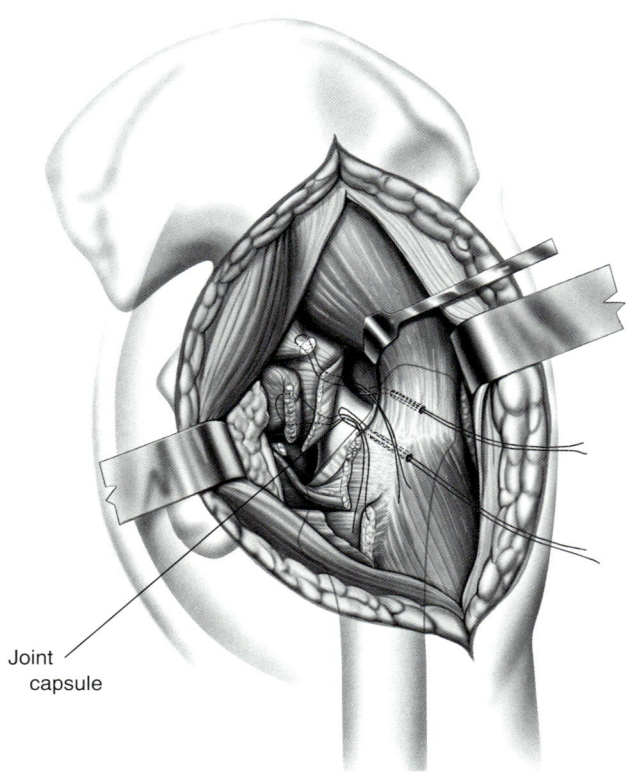

Figure 13. Sutures are placed through the capsule and external rotators and passed through the two holes in the greater trochanter.

Figure 14. Sutures have been placed into the capsule and external pyriformis (second suture will be placed into conjoined tendon and capsule).

The two ends of the upper suture are placed into the loop of the upper trochanteric suture and brought through the trochanteric hole by pulling the nonabsorbable suture through the trochanteric loop suture (Figs. 13, 14). The inferior nonabsorbable suture is passed through the trochanter in a similar fashion. By externally rotating the leg and tying these sutures together under maximal tension, the posterior capsular flap with the external rotator tendons will be approximated to the posterior trochanter, thereby closing the posterior aspect of the hip joint (Figs. 15, 16). Fascial, subcutaneous, and skin closure is effected in the usual manner. A compressive dressing is applied to the limb and suction drains are used routinely.

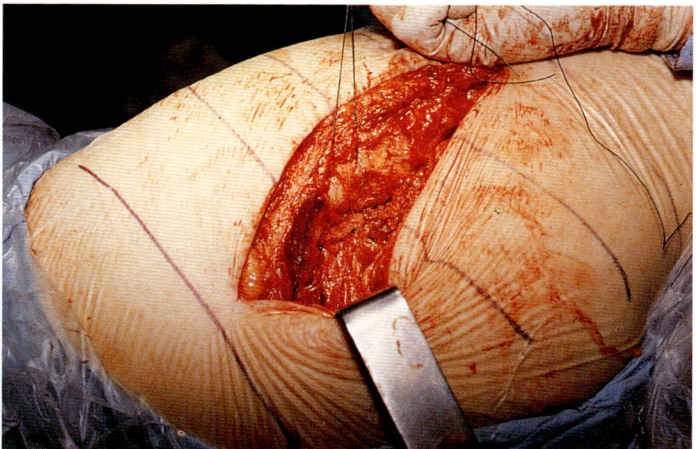

Figure 15. Sutures are tied under tension, thereby reconstituting the posterior capsule and external rotators.

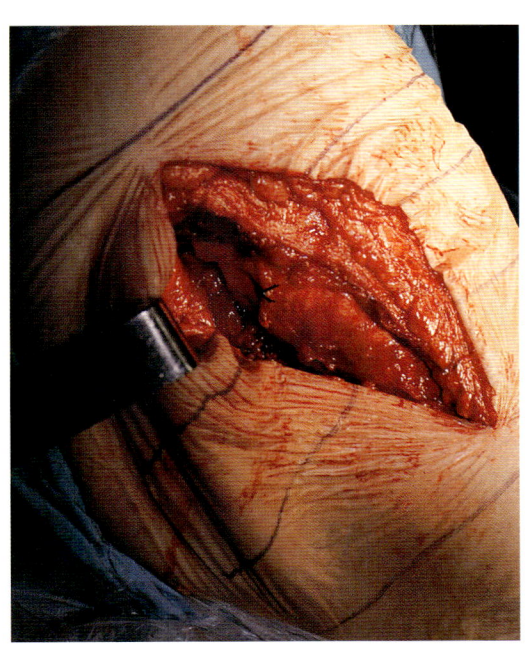 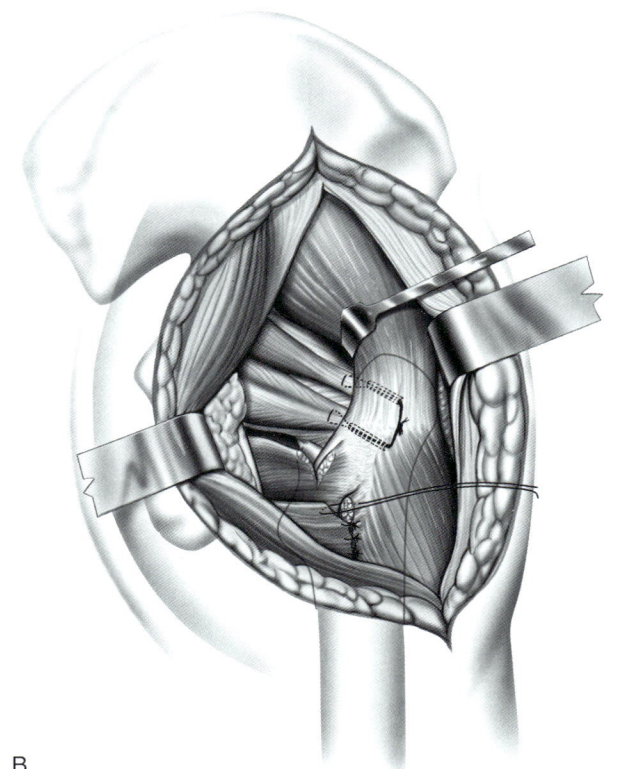

Figure 16 A, B. The sutures are tied to repair the posterior capsule and external rotators.

POSTOPERATIVE MANAGEMENT

Postoperatively, patients are maintained in suspension slings with the legs abducted. Ambulation begins on postoperative day 1 or 2, depending on amount of wound swelling or drainage or degree of pain. A walker is used initially, and patients are advanced to a single cane prior to discharge. They must be independent in transferring in and out of bed, able to walk with a cane, and able to ascend and descend stairs. This usually requires a week postoperatively. At discharge the patients are instructed in activities to be avoided: sitting in low chairs, excessive hip flexion and internal rotation, lying on the operated hip. On a return visit five to six weeks postoperative, most patients are ambulating without external support, and all precautions are removed at this time. Abductor exercises are begun at this time. Use of a cane is encouraged in patients who have a continued abductor tilt.

Patients treated with this approach recover significantly faster than those with trochanteric osteotomy; they become independent in ambulation more quickly, have less pain, and sustain less intraoperative blood loss. Additionally there is no danger of trochanteric nonunion or need to remove painful hardware at a later date.

COMPLICATIONS

The chief complication cited for the posterior hip approach is the increase in posterior dislocation of the prosthetic hip. Utilizing a posterior repair as outlined, the incidence of hip dislocation should be reduced to the one- to two-percent range. In a review of 543 Charnley low-friction arthroplasties performed by the author utilizing this posterior tenocapsullorraphy there were seven dislocations for a rate just above one per cent (11). A second potential complication of the posterior approach to the hip is communication between the hip joint and the skin with absent soft tissues posteriorly. Theoretically, should hip drainage persist, open access from the exterior through the wound could contaminate the hip joint. This is another reason that repair of the posterior capsule and the external rotators is important. This repair provides an additional layer of soft tissue covering the posterior aspect of the hip joint. Contamination is thus reduced, and communication into the joint is impeded.

Care must be taken during the posterior exposure to avoid injury to the sciatic nerve, which may travel close to the external rotator tendons. Additionally, when the femoral canal is reamed and the femoral component inserted, the sciatic nerve may be under increased tension due to the need to maximally internally rotate, flex, and adduct the limb. In heavy patients with a thick fat layer, considerable levering force may be exerted posteriorly to expose the femur, and this may also compromise the sciatic nerve and compress it. It is important to be sure the soft-tissue release is extensive enough in these patients to allow full mobilization of the femur without undue stretch or compression on the sciatic nerve. This includes release of the entire gluteus maximus tendon, if necessary, from its insertion into the femur. Full limb positioning for femoral reaming must be possible without undue force.

Repair of the posterior capsule and external rotator tendons may be technically not possible when there is significant contracture with shortening of the posterior capsule. Also, when the limb is lengthened to accomodate leg length inequality, the capsule may not be long enough to allow secure closure. In these instances, the remaining posterior capsule and external rotators should be repaired, even if there remains a gap posteriorly. Although not ideal, this reconstruction will provide some posterior closure and a check-rein effect to internal rotation in the immediate postoperative period.

A further criticism of the posterior approach has been that there is chance of contamination of the skin by bowel organisms and increased risk for wound infection. To avoid this complication, the skin incision is not reflected posteriorly into the buttock. A gently curved lateral incision is used, which passes mildly posterior when the incision is superior to the greater trochanter.

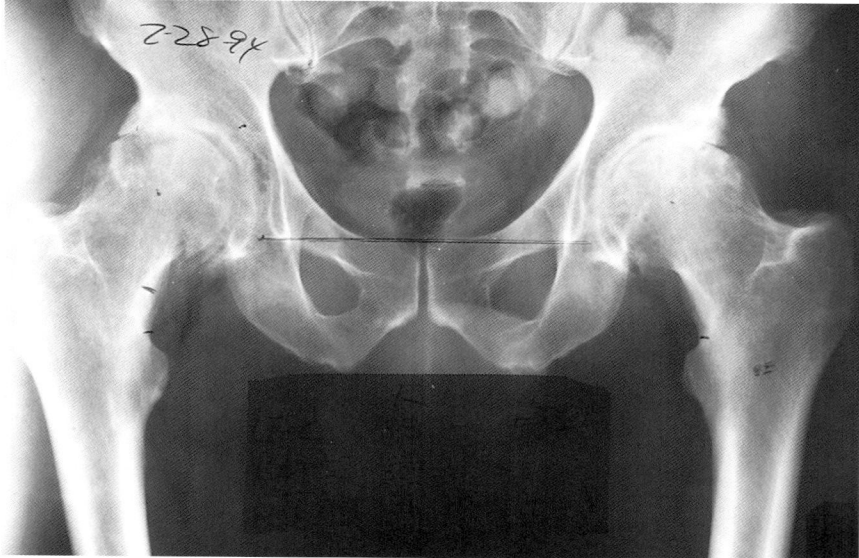

Figure 17. Radiograph demonstrating advanced osteoarthritis of the hip in this 70-year-old patient.

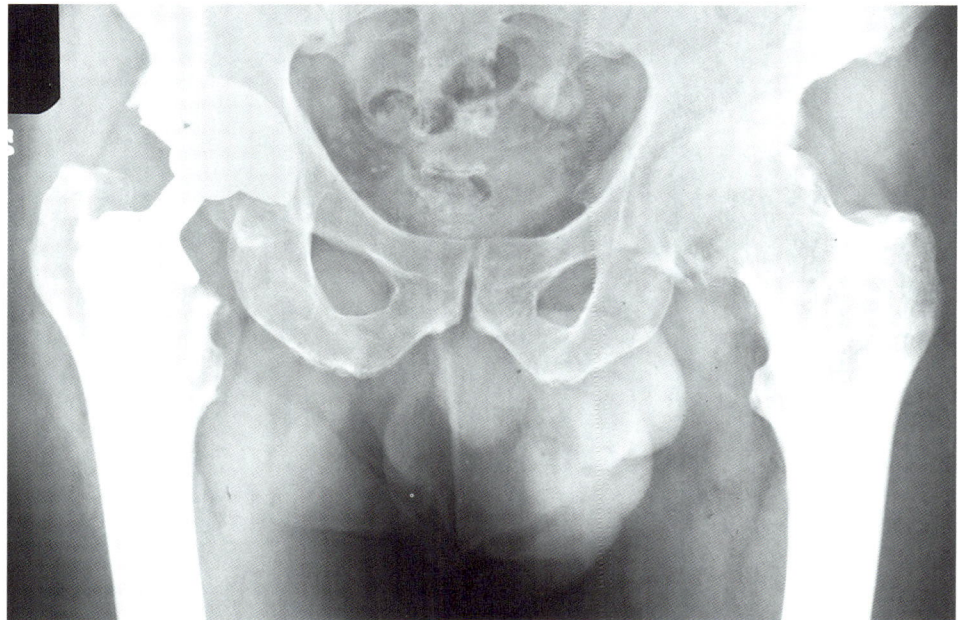

Figure 18. Postoperative radiograph after capsulorrhaphy.

ILLUSTRATIVE CASE

M. J. is a 70-year-old male with osteoarthritis of the hip. He became increasingly disabled and now almost always ambulated with a cane when outdoors. He noted stairclimbing had become limited, and he had to descend stairs one step at a time. Night pain was also present. Nonsteroidal medications were tried by his rheumatologist but without improvement in his symptoms. On examination, he walked with a coxalgic gait and had severe limitation of hip motion, particularly rotation. Radiographs demonstrated obliteration of the joint space with a medial acetabular osteophyte (Fig. 17). With the patient's severe pain and disability from his hip arthritis, total hip replacement was recommended. The patient gave two units of autologous blood prior to surgery.

The patient underwent uncomplicated total hip replacement, utilizing an hybrid technique under epidural anesthesia. The posterior approach was utilized with the capsule and external rotators repaired.

The patient stood on the first postoperative day and over the next three days was advanced to a cane. He was discharged on postoperative day 5 transferring and ambulating without difficulty (Fig. 18).

RECOMMENDED READING

1. Calandruccio, R. A.: Arthoplasty of the hip. In: Crenshaw, A. H., editor; *Campbell's Operative Orthopaedics*. The C. V. Mosby Co., St. Louis, 1987.
2. Gibson, A.: Posterior exposure of the hip joint. *J. Bone J. Surg.*, 32B:183–86, 1950.
3. Gore, D. R., Murray, M. P., Sepic, S. B., and Gardner, G. M.: Anterolateral compared to posterior approach in total hip arthroplasty. *Clin. Orthop. Rel. Res.*, 165:180–87, 1982.
4. Harris, W. H.: The porous total hip system: Surgical technique. In: Harris, W. H., editor. *Advanced Concepts in Total Hip Replacement*. Slack Inc., New Jersey, 1985.
5. Hunter, S. C.: Southern hip exposure. *Orthopaedics*, 9:1425–28, 1986.
6. Johnson, R., Hallin, E., Nordstrom, B., and Lidgren, L.: Modified technique in the dorsal approach in total hip arthroplasty. *Arch. Orthop. Traumat. Surg.*, 99:43–45, 1981.

7. Marcy, G. H., Fletcher, R. S.: Modification of the posterolateral approach to the hip for insertion of femoral head prosthesis, *J. Bone Joint Surg.*, 36A:142–43, 1954.
8. Moore, A. T.: The self locking metal prosthesis. *J. Bone J. Surg.*, 39A:811–27, 1957.
9. Roberts, D. A., Fu, F. H., McClain, E. J., and Ferguson, A. B.: A comparison of the posterolateral and anterolateral approaches to total hip arthroplasty. *Clin. Orthop. Rel. Res.*, 187:205–210, 1984.
10. Robinson, R. A., Robinson, H. J., and Salvati, E. A.: Comparison of the transtrochanteric and posterior approaches for total hip replacement. *Clin. Orthop. Rel. Res.*, 147:143–47, 1980.
11. Sculco, T. P., and Moran, M. C.: Posterior tenocapsulorrhaphy in primary total hip arthroplasty. Presented at the American Academy of Ortho. Surgeons, March 10, 1991, Anaheim.
12. Stillwell, W. T.: *The Art of Total Hip Arthoplasty*. Grune and Stratton, Orlando, FL, 1987.
13. Woo, R. Y. G., Morrey, B. F.: Dislocations after total hip arthroplasty. *J. Bone J. Surg.*, 64A:1295–1306, 1982.

2

Direct Lateral Approach

Roby C. Thompson, Jr. and Kevin Hardinge

INDICATIONS/CONTRAINDICATIONS

The lateral approach to the hip has become more popular in the past 15 years after the publication of Hardinge's "Direct lateral approach to the hip" (1). Others have described this approach or variations of it as the anterolateral approach (5), and the original description by McFarland and Osborne (4) was an extension of the posterior approach to the hip. For the sake of clarity, in this chapter, we will confine our nomenclature to the "direct lateral approach," where the posterior tendon of the gluteus medius is left attached to the trochanteric tubercle, anterior to the piriformis fossa. This is the Hardinge modification of the McFarland and Osborne approach, which separated the entire gluteus medius and vastus lateralis in continuity from the greater trochanter and reflected that muscular envelope anteriorly.

This is a useful approach in exposure of the hip joint for arthrotomy and uncomplicated arthroplasty. Additionally, with this extensile exposure, the vastus lateralis muscle can be reflected from the shaft of the femur to facilitate application of hardware or other requirements. The literature on joint replacement suggests that the incidence of dislocation is lower when the direct lateral approach is used than when the posterior approach is used (3,6,7). When early hip flexion is unavoidable, some consider this a relative indication for selection of this approach. However, the choice of approach is largely one of surgeon comfort. Familiarity with anatomic landmarks in any approach is essential to proper positioning of prosthetic components and avoidance of injury to vital structures.

The contraindications to this approach are largely self-evident, e.g., when exposure of the posterior aspect of the acetabulum is desired or demanded, such as the need to remove screws and/or plates from the posterior lip of the acetabulum. Relative contraindications include contractures, scar tissue, and other deformities that require a trochanteric osteotomy

---

R. C. Thompson, Jr. M.D.: Department of Orthopaedic Surgery, University of Minnesota, Minneapolis, Minnesota 55455.

K. Hardinge, M.CH. ORTH., F.R.C.S.: Centre for Hip Surgery, Wrightington Hospital, Apply Bridge, England WN6 9EP.

for exposure and mobilization of the soft tissues and extensive visualization of the femoral canal such as that needed for cement removal in revision hip surgery.

When approaching the hip joint, some surgeons find no advantage to extending the incision of the gluteus medius into the lateralis and have thus modified the original approach to remove the anterolateral section of the gluteus medius and gluteus minimus fibers in continuity.

An additional variable based on the surgeon's preference is the choice between the supine and the lateral decubitus positions of the patient. We will cover both of these positions in this chapter, as both provide the same exposure and require the same planning and postoperative care as well as shared advantages and complications.

PREOPERATIVE PLANNING

When selecting any approach for arthroplasty, it is important to measure leg lengths carefully and plan accordingly for desired adjustments as part of the surgery. The possible need for trochanteric osteotomy is also an important consideration when choosing the anterolateral approach. Detaching the anterior fibers of the gluteus medius may complicate the reattachment of the trochanter and certainly is unnecessary if an osteotomy is to be performed.

SURGERY

Supine Position

The direct lateral approach, with the patient lying in the supine position, offers excellent conditions for implant orientation, and using the bilateral bony landmarks of the anterior

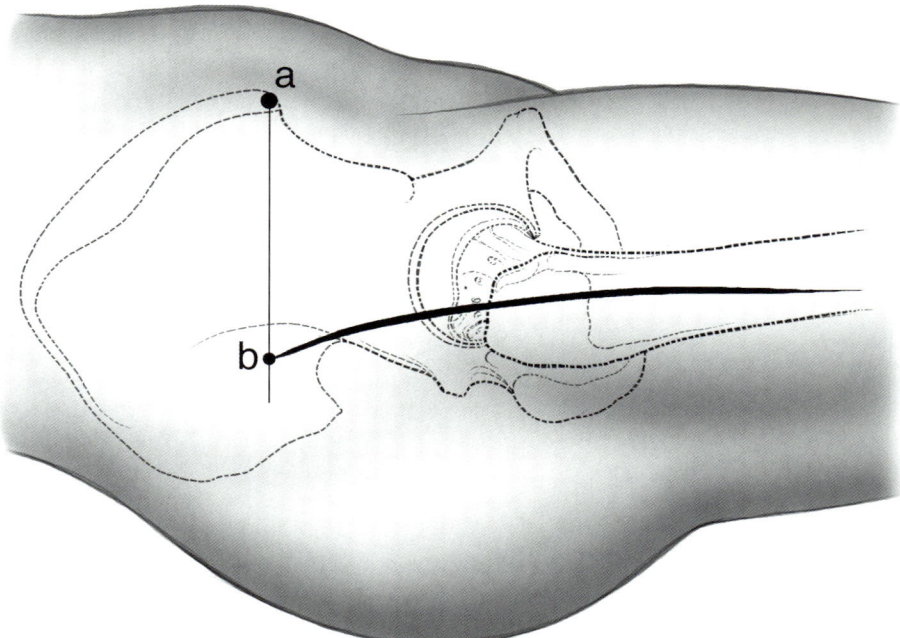

Figure 1. The skin incision centers on the vastus lateralis ridge of the greater trochanter, passes distally down the midlateral aspect of the femur and proximally curves posteriorly to reach the line (a–b) that passes vertically downward from the anterior superior iliac spine. The incision is typically 24 cm long.

superior iliac spine, patellae, and medial malleoli of the ankles, it allows for an accurate correction of leg-length discrepancy by direct comparison. It differs from the lateral decubitus position in that no attempt is made in the direct lateral approach to preserve the continuity of the gluteus medius and vastus lateralis. Access to the hip joint is facilitated by drawing the patient to the side of the operating table so that the ipsilateral greater trochanter lies just lateral to the table edge.

Initial Incision. The midpoint of the initial incision is formed by the greater trochanter, palpated through the subcutaneous tissue, and depending upon the amount of subcutaneous fat, will typically be 24 cm in length (Fig. 1), horizontal as it passes down the shaft of the femur, and gently curving as it passes posteriorly over the buttock muscles, and typically it stops at a line dropped vertically from the anterior superior iliac spine in a posterior direction.

Superficial Dissection. The skin incision opens up and presents the subcutaneous fat. Deep palpation at the midpoint of the incision will indicate the bony greater trochanter so that the sharp and blunt dissection of subcutaneous fat can be achieved to expose the greater trochanter, which is covered by the intact deep fascia. The deep fascia is incised over the middle of the greater trochanter, and, the tissue layers having been isolated, the deep fascia is incised distally to expose the bulging vastus lateralis (Fig. 2).

The deep fascia is incised along the midlateral line of the femur to the end of the skin incision. Proximally the incision of the deep fascia extends posteriorly in the direction of the fibers of the gluteus maximus (Fig. 2), so that it separates the fibers of the muscle. With the

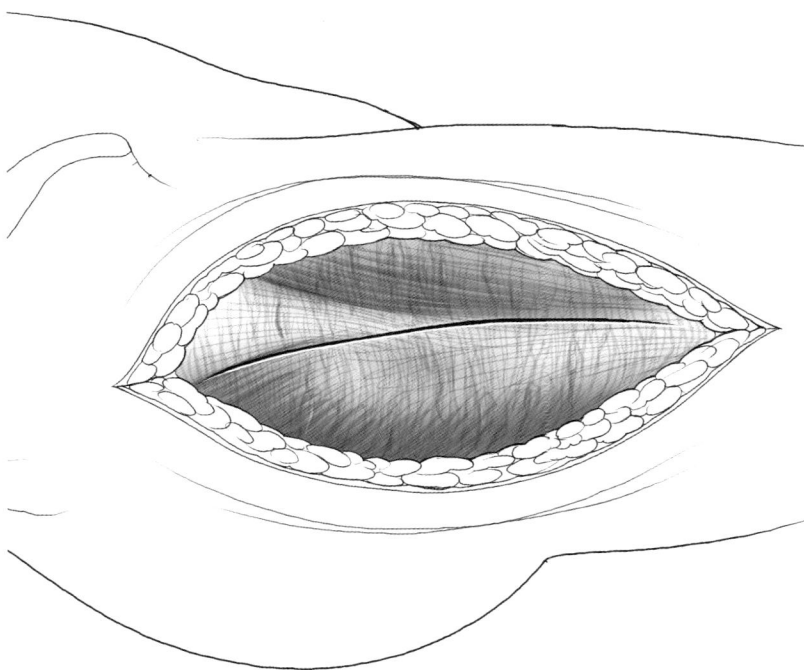

Figure 2. The incision of the deep fascia starts over the greater trochanter at its prominent, easily palpable midpoint and extends distally in the midlateral line of the femur to expose the bulging lateralis. Proximally, it curves posteriorly in the same direction as the fibers of the gluteus maximus so that the incision splits the muscle and does not cut across the fibers. In the distal and proximal extension, the incision of the deep fascia extends to the limits of the skin incision.

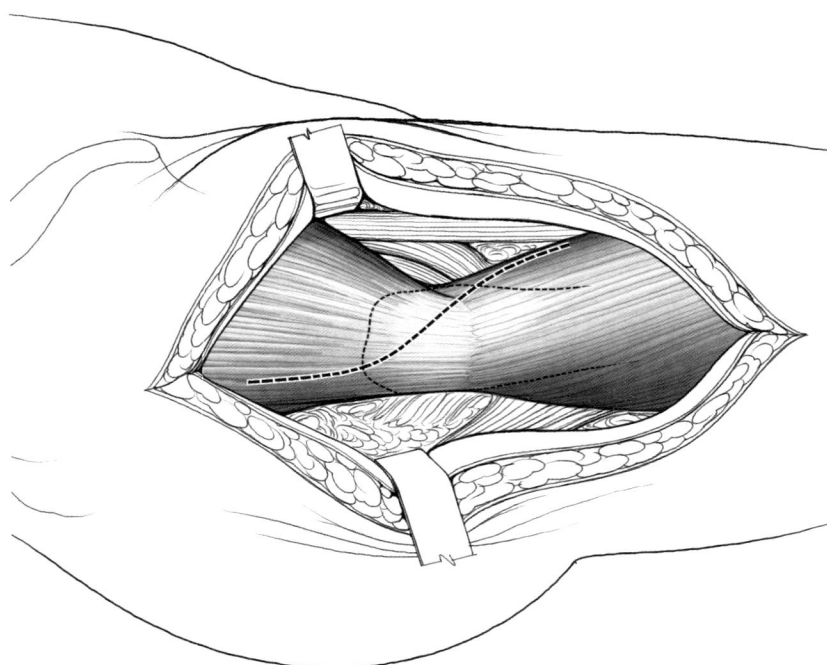

Figure 3. Incision of the tendon of the gluteus medius leaves a cuff of tendon on the greater trochanter for subsequent suture, extends distally into the vastus lateralis, and proximally extends from the apex of the greater trochanter in the direction of the fibers of the gluteus medius. It is a superficial splitting of the outer layer of the gluteus medius and stays away from the superior gluteal nerve, which is deep.

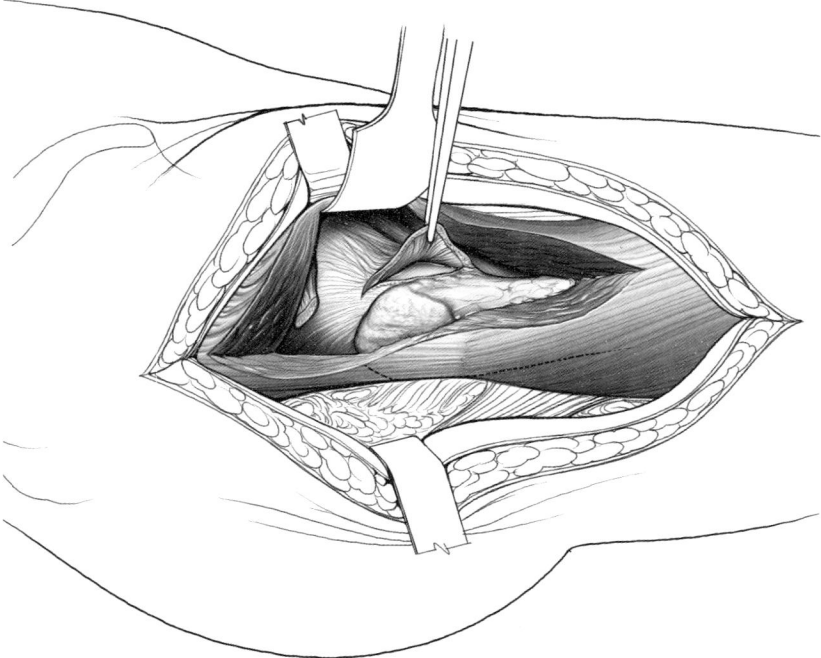

Figure 4. The space in front of the greater trochanter passing onto the front of the neck of the femur is developed by separating off the gluteus minimus muscle and the ligament of Bigelow insertions by use of the cutting diathermy. The bulging capsule of the hip joint is thus exposed, and arthrotomy is confirmed by release of joint fluid when the capsule is pierced. Adduction of the thigh across the contralateral extended legs moves the anterior border of the gluteus medius anteriorly so that additional anterior retraction is rarely necessary.

greater trochanter fully exposed (Fig. 3), the initial incision retractor is inserted with the anterior blade level with the anterior border of gluteus medius.

Deep Dissection. The gluteus medius has a tendinous insertion to the greater trochanter and the tendon of insertion can be demonstrated and moved on the bone by blunt forceps. This tendon of insertion is incised, leaving a cuff still attached to the trochanter for subsequent suture (Fig. 3). At the apex of the trochanter the gluteus medius is incised horizontally for 4 cm only. This incision must be superficial to avoid damage to the superior gluteal nerve (2). As the tendon is incised, the thigh is gently brought across the body by adduction so as to open up the space in front of the neck of the femur. It is not usual to need retraction by an assistant at this stage, as the gap opens up spontaneously.

As the femur is gently drawn across the body by adduction, the cutting diathermy detaches the tendon of the gluteus medius, gluteus minimus, and the ligament of Bigelow to expose the capsule of the hip joint (Fig. 4). When the capsule of the hip joint is incised, joint fluid is released that confirms that the hip joint has been entered. The capsule is lifted off the neck of the femur, and dislocation is helped by adduction and division of the capsule at the inferolateral aspect (in the four o'clock position in the case of the left hip and in the case of the right hip, in the eight o'clock position).

Dislocation. When dislocation of the hip is necessary or desirable, the thigh is gently adducted across the contralateral extended thigh by an assistant or "leg holder" who stands on the other side of the table (Fig. 5). No strong force is necessary, and if there is any obstruction to the adduction maneuver, it is important to ensure that there is no soft-tissue structure tethering the head and preventing dislocation.

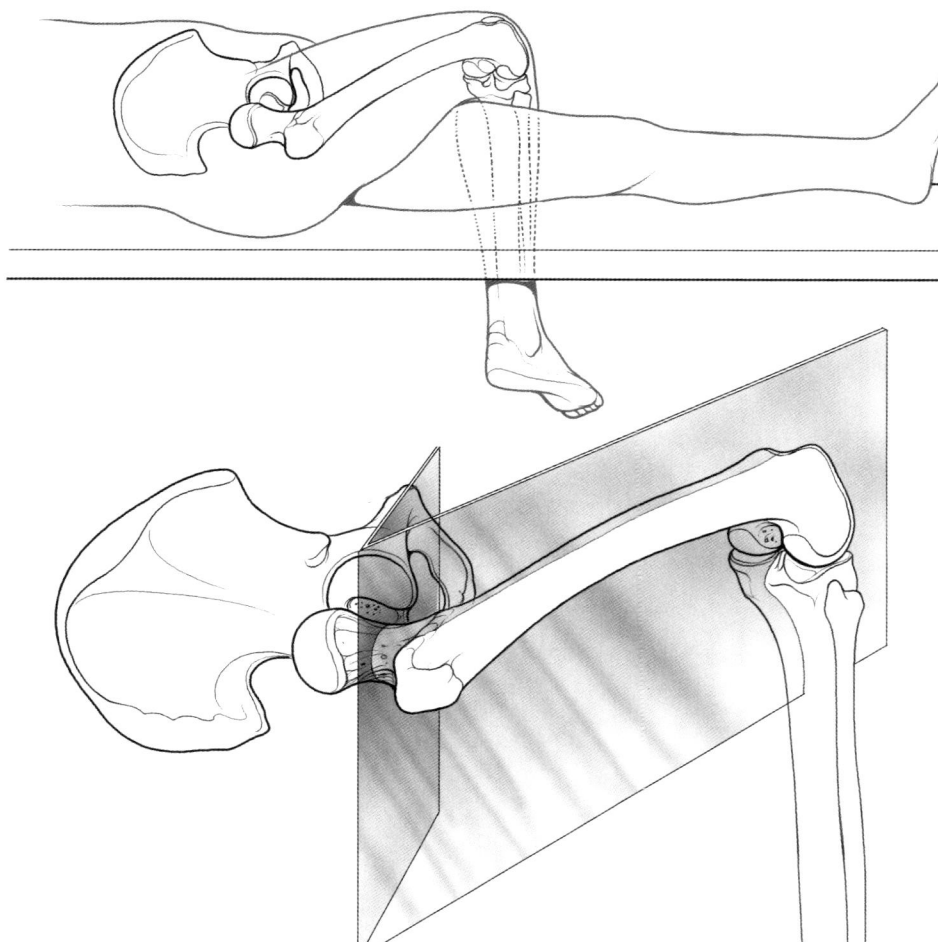

Figure 5. The key element of the direct lateral approach in the supine position is that it is possible to reference the vertical tibia of the operated leg once it has been adducted across the body and dislocation of the operated hip has occurred. It is then possible to position the femoral implants directly to allow an optimum range of motion without abutment.

Dislocation should occur as a result of gentle adduction and a little terminal external rotation. It will be accompanied by rupture of the ligamentum teres, if it is still present, but it is unusual to find that in degenerative arthrosis of the hip that it has been attenuated or destroyed by the degenerative process. It will occasionally be necessary to assist dislocation of the hip by applying leverage under the neck of the femur, and this is best performed using a curved cholecystectomy-type forceps placed beneath the neck to apply gentle leverage.

Additionally, the curved forceps can occasionally be used in lifting off adherent capsule from the front of the neck of the femur. In this way—with adduction, external rotation at the end of the range of adduction, and by adequate soft-tissue release around the front of the neck of the femur and also of the limbus in the four or eight o'clock position, respectively, for left and right hips—dislocation is achieved as a gentle procedure.

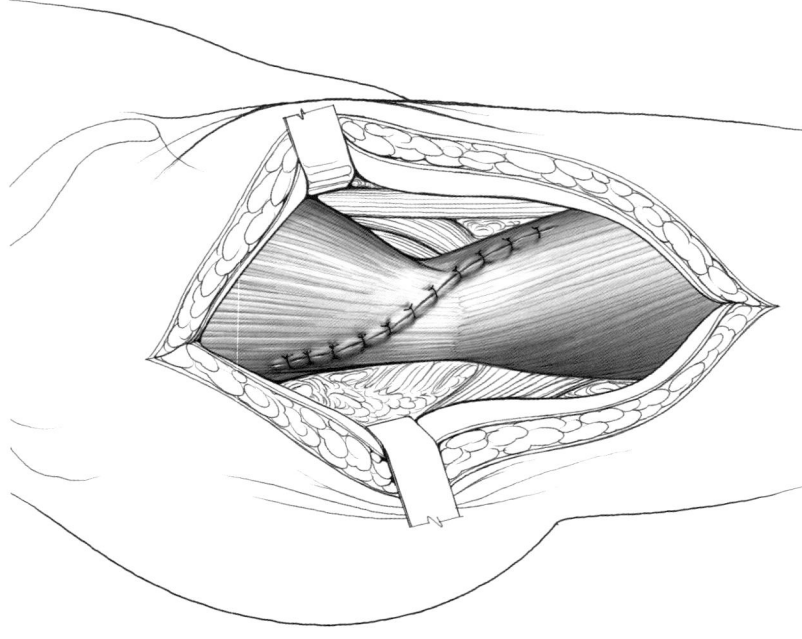

Figure 6. The repair of the gluteus medius is tendinous and uses interrupted nonabsorbable sutures.

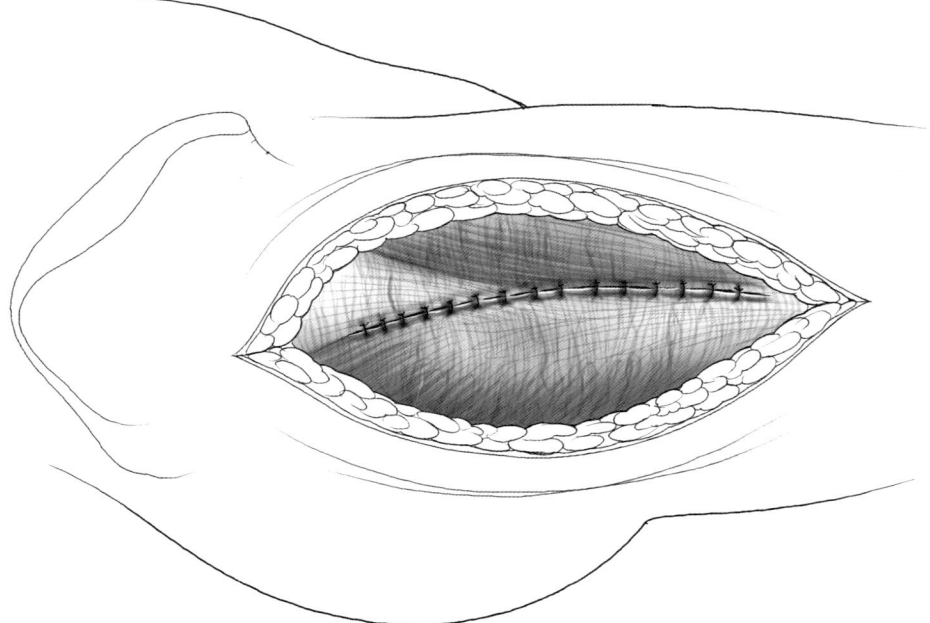

Figure 7. The deep fascia is closed with interrupted sutures of nonabsorbable material to permit early weight bearing.

Closure. The ligament of Bigelow and the gluteus minimus are reattached to their insertions. Closure of the gluteus medius is performed with a series of interrupted and nonabsorbable sutures. This is a tendinous closure and thus allows early mobilization (Fig. 6). The deep fascia is similarly closed with nonabsorbable interrupted sutures (Fig. 7). Two drains are inserted beneath the deep fascia and one subcutaneously. These are removed after 48 hours.

Lateral Decubitus Position

Some surgeons prefer this approach with the patient in the lateral decubitus position. When this position is used, care must be taken to stabilize the pelvis to avoid loss of orientation during the procedure (Fig. 8). An axillary roll is placed beneath the down axilla to protect the brachial plexus from impingement. All bony prominences are also carefully padded, including the peroneal nerve on the down leg and the olecranon and the medial epicondyle on the down arm.

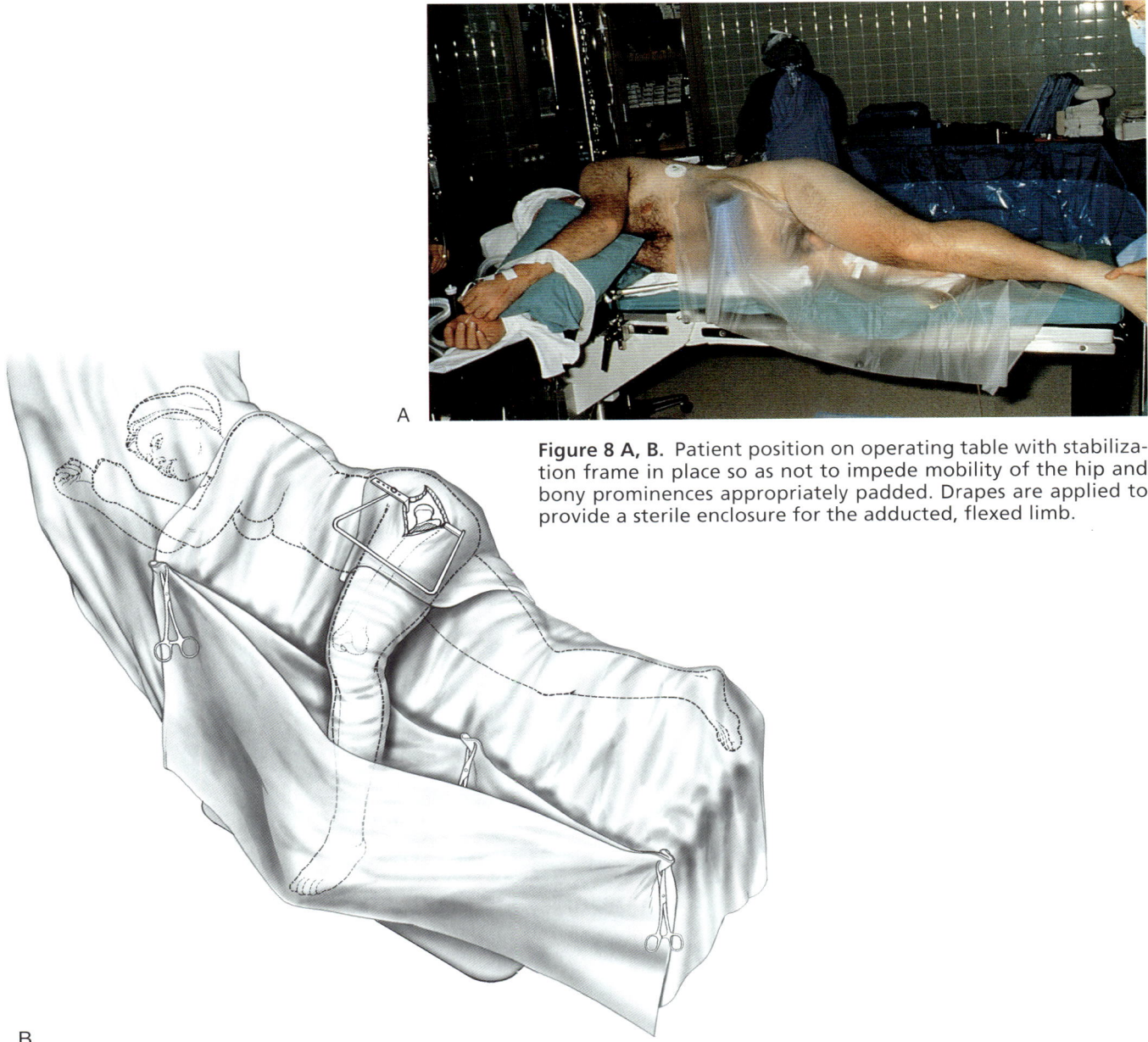

Figure 8 A, B. Patient position on operating table with stabilization frame in place so as not to impede mobility of the hip and bony prominences appropriately padded. Drapes are applied to provide a sterile enclosure for the adducted, flexed limb.

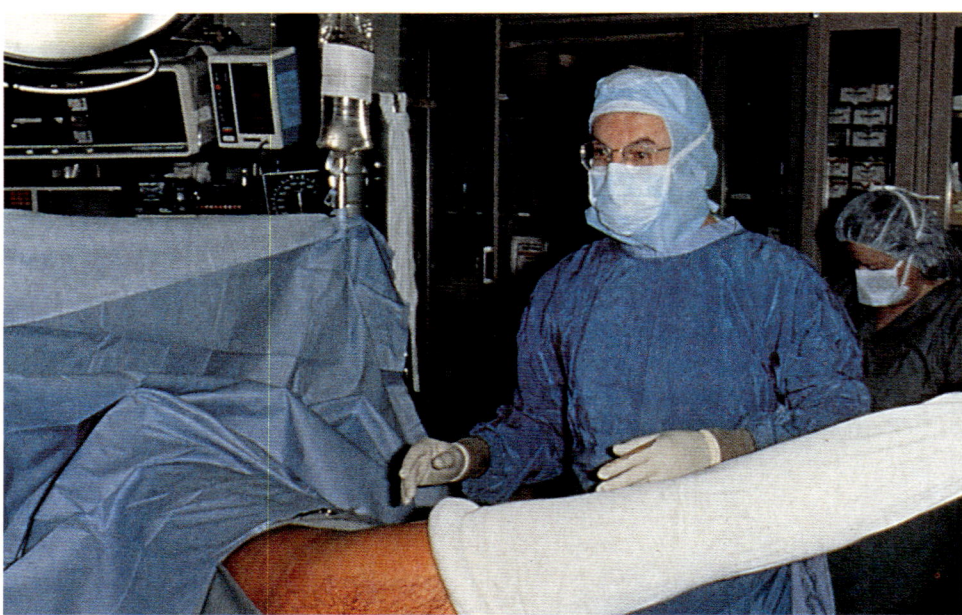

Figure 9. The entire limb has been prepped from toe to lower abdomen and is being draped free.

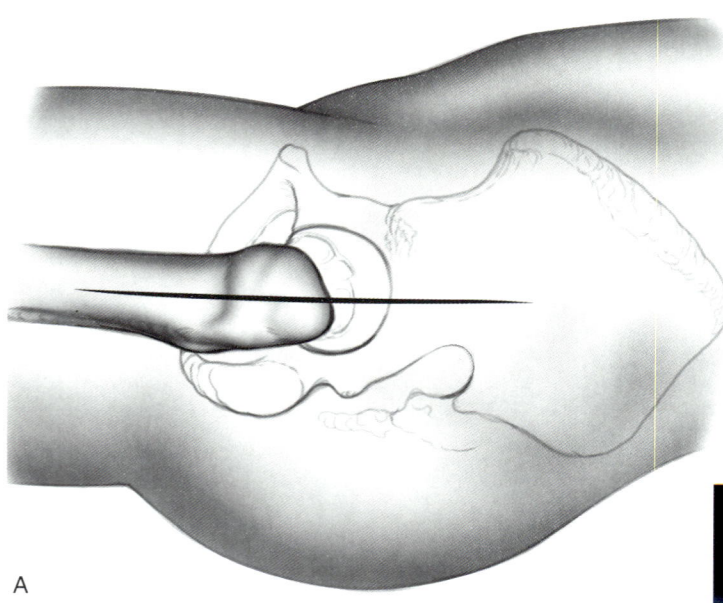

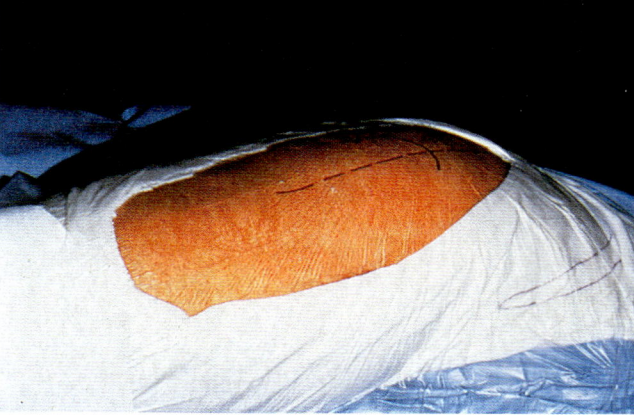

Figure 10 A, B. Intraoperative view of the incision. Iliac crest is to the left outlined on the waterproof barrier drape, and the site of the incision over the trochanter is outlined on the waterproof barrier drape.

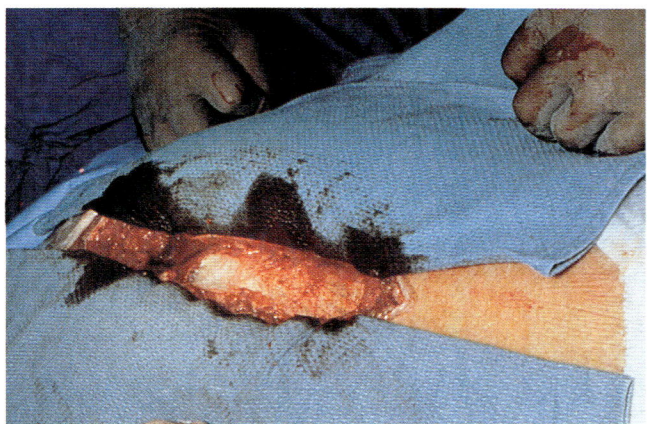

Figure 11. Intraoperative view of the incision. Skin and subcutaneous tissue have been incised down through the tensor fascia lata, and towels have been sewn to the tensor fascia lata and reflected.

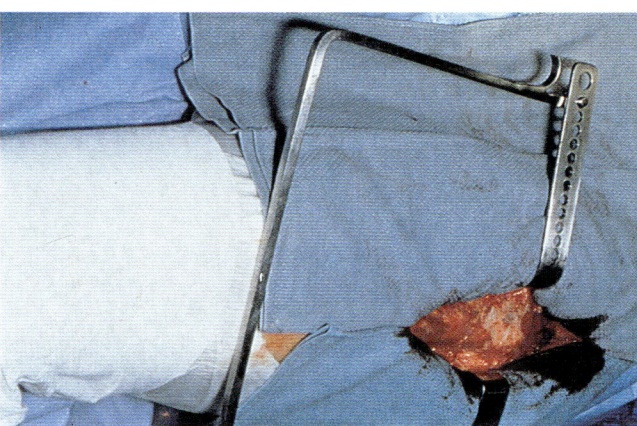

Figure 12. A Charnley self-retaining retractor is in place in the incision with the long limb of the retractor anterior.

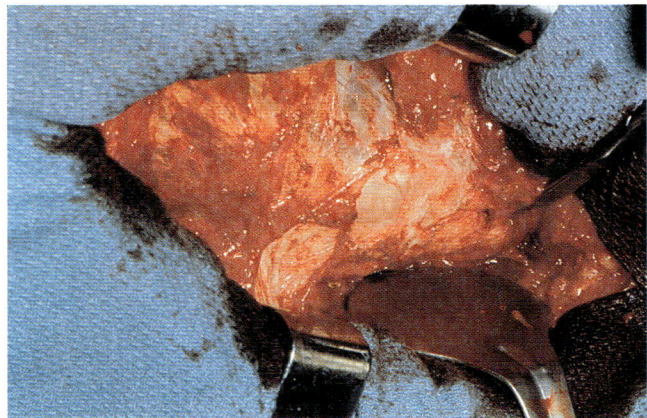

Figure 13. The trochanteric bursa has been excised and the greater trochanter is visualized. A Bennett retractor has been placed posterior to the greater trochanter to displace the tensor fascia behind the trochanter.

We prefer adjustable pelvic stabilization devices that fit the pneumatic fluoroscopic table. To allow flexion and adduction of the femur without impingement on the stabilization post, the anterior post must be positioned well above the anterior superior iliac spine. Waterproof drapes are used to isolate the extremity, and the entire extremity is prepared from well above the anterior superior iliac spine circumferentially to include the foot and ankle if joint replacement is to be performed (Fig. 9). The limb is then draped free, a stockinette rolled over the entire limb, and an opening made in the area of the stockinette overlying the site of surgery. The area for incision is then sealed with a waterproof barrier drape, and the site for incision is exposed from well above the anterior superior iliac spine on the lateral margin of the hip to midthigh or lower, if necessary (Fig. 10).

A midlateral incision is outlined over the center of the greater trochanter, and the incision is begun, exposing the tensor fascia lata distally first and then splitting the tensor fascia lata proximally over the greater trochanter. Towels are sewn to the tensor fascia and the towels are reflected to protect the subcutaneous tissue (Fig. 11). A self-retaining Charnley type of retractor is placed in the wound to expose the trochanter and the trochanteric bursa (Fig. 12). The thick fibrous tendon of the gluteus medius is identified at the posterior aspect of the trochanteric attachment, and the bursa is removed from the anterior aspect of the trochanter (Fig. 13). A cutting cautery is utilized to create a hockey stick incision in the fas-

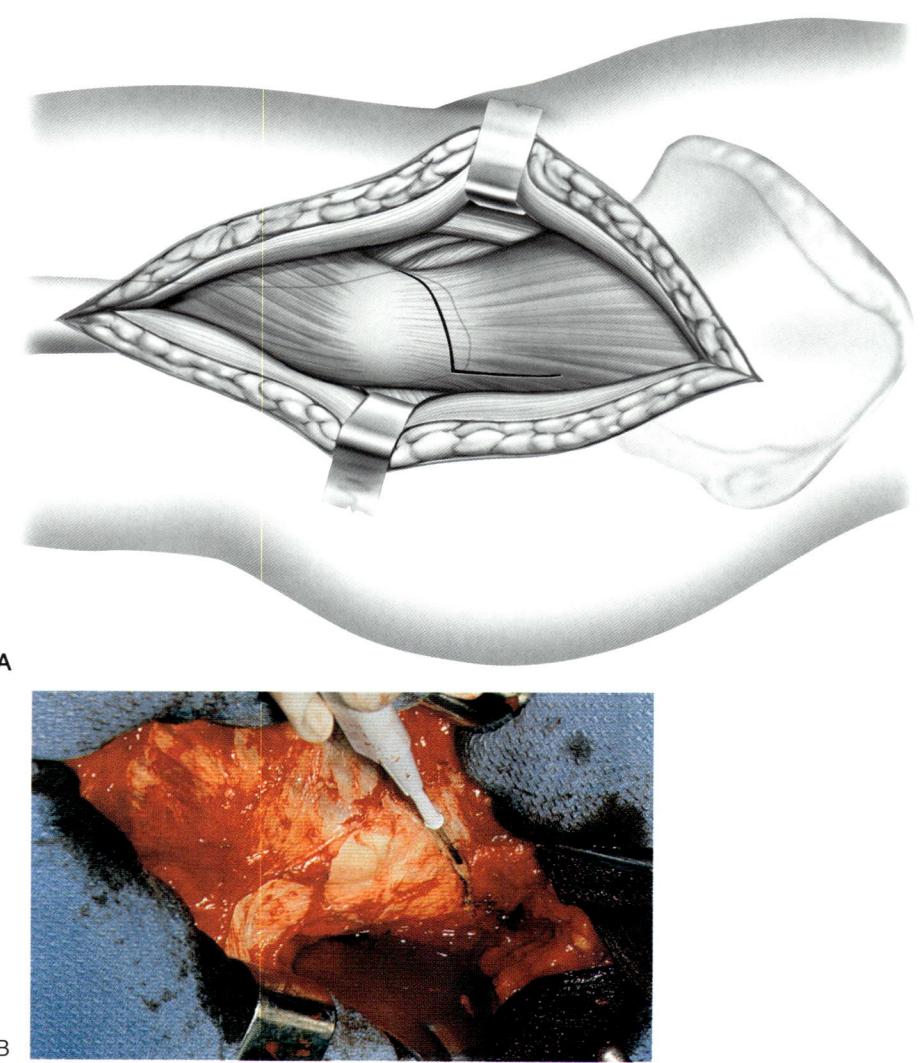

Figure 14. (A) The hockey stick incision begins just anterior to the tendon of the gluteus medius at its insertion into the trochanteric tubercle. (B) Cautery tip illustrates the line of division of the gluteus medius attachment into the trochanter.

cia of the gluteus medius with the posterior limb of the incision anterior to the gluteus medius tendon and extending no more than 2 cm into the external fascia of the gluteus medius (Fig. 14). Limiting the cephalad dissection into the gluteus medius fascia avoids inadvertent injury to the branch of the superior gluteal nerve supplying the gluteus medius anteriorly. The remaining anterior limb of the "hockey stick" is carried distally along the trochanter. Gentle blunt dissection posteriorly along the initial interval is extended with scissors to avoid injury to the anterior fibers of the superior gluteal nerve and artery. The fibers of the gluteus medius and minimus are separated from the anterior fibers of the iliacus and the reflected head of the rectus (Figs. 15, 16). At this point, a Hohmann retractor is placed beneath the straight head of the rectus femoris, which can be palpated just below the anterior inferior iliac spine. A blunt cobra retractor may then be placed around the inferior medial aspect of the femoral neck (Fig. 17).

When a total hip replacement is to be performed, leg-length measurement is made in the predislocated condition by placing a drill hole in the greater trochanter and positioning a Meyerding-type retractor with drill bits into the pelvis (Fig. 18). Arrange the limb on the table in a reproducible fashion, and measure from a fixed position on the pelvis to the drill bit in the trochanter.

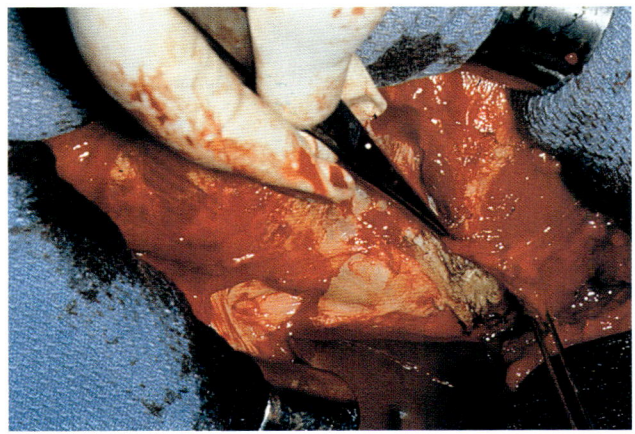

Figure 15. Intraoperative view of incision. The gluteus medius and minimus tendon are detached with the posterior and anterior limbs held in the forceps.

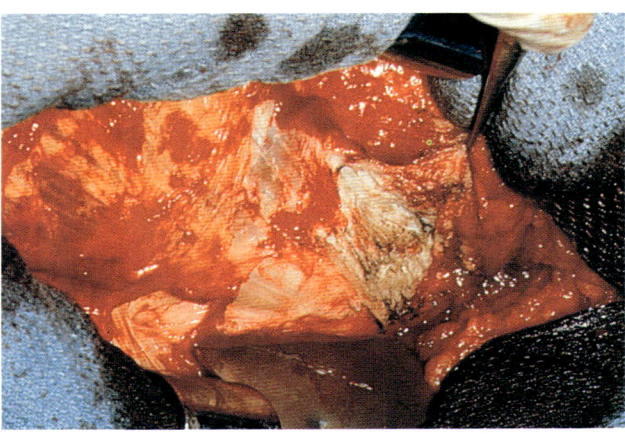

Figure 16. Intraoperative photograph showing the separation of the gluteus minimus muscle and the ligament of Bigelow. The gluteus medius and minimus are reflected superiorly, and the capsule of the hip joint is seen below the elevated muscle.

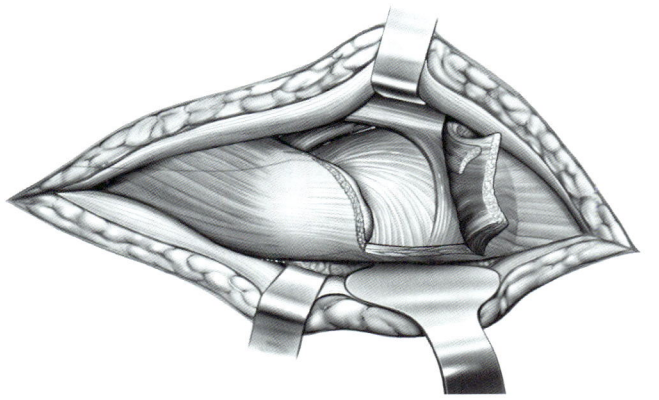
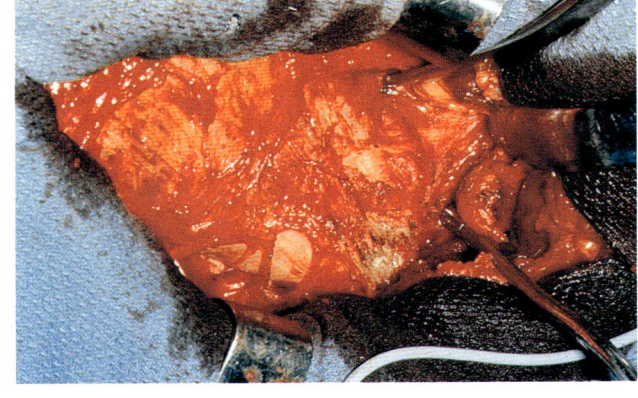

A   B

Figure 17. (A) A long, curved Hohmann retractor is placed under the straight head of the rectus femoris muscle and the fibers of the iliopsoas. (B) Intraoperative view of retraction of the rectus femoris muscle.

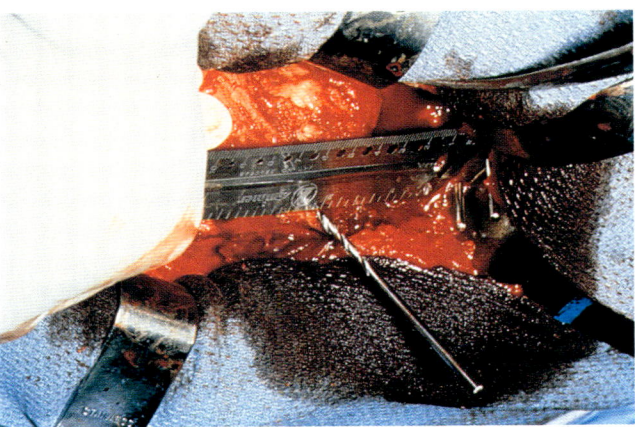

Figure 18. The Meyerding-type retractor is positioned on the ileum to hold the abductor muscles superiorly and is held in place with drill bits. From that fixed position on the pelvis, a measurement is made to a position on the greater trochanter, which is marked with another drill bit for leg-length measurements after dislocation.

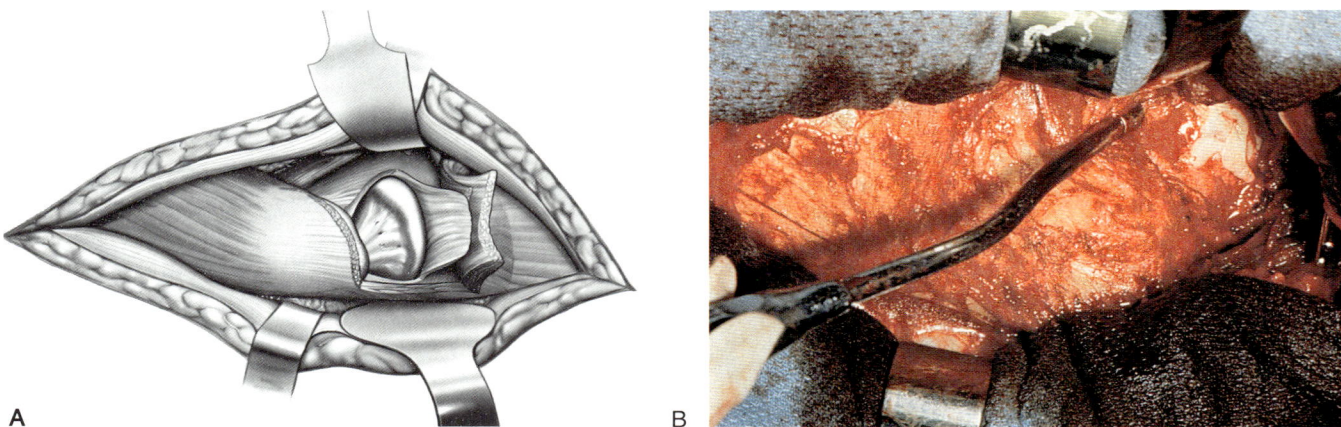

Figure 19. (A) The capsule of the hip joint is excised and the femoral head is exposed. (B) Intraoperative view showing exposure of the femoral head.

The capsule of the hip is excised in a U-shaped fashion (Fig. 19), and a sterile envelope is created from drapes, which are sealed at the bottom and top on the side of the drape (Figs. 8 and 20). Dislocate the femoral head using a Mueller skid by externally rotating and adducting the leg (Fig. 21). Place the limb in the bag and elevate the proximal femur with a large Bennett retractor behind the trochanter to displace the femur anterior to the tensor fascia lata (Fig. 22). If a total hip replacement is to be performed, the femoral head and neck cuts are made using the appropriate jigs. Expose the acetabulum by placing a medium Hohmann retractor in the ischial fossa on the posterior aspect of the acetabulum to displace the femur posteriorly (Figs. 23, 24). With the anterior Hohmann retractor beneath the straight head of the rectus, excellent exposure of the acetabulum is obtained. When a total hip replacement is performed, orientation of the acetabular component can be easily car-

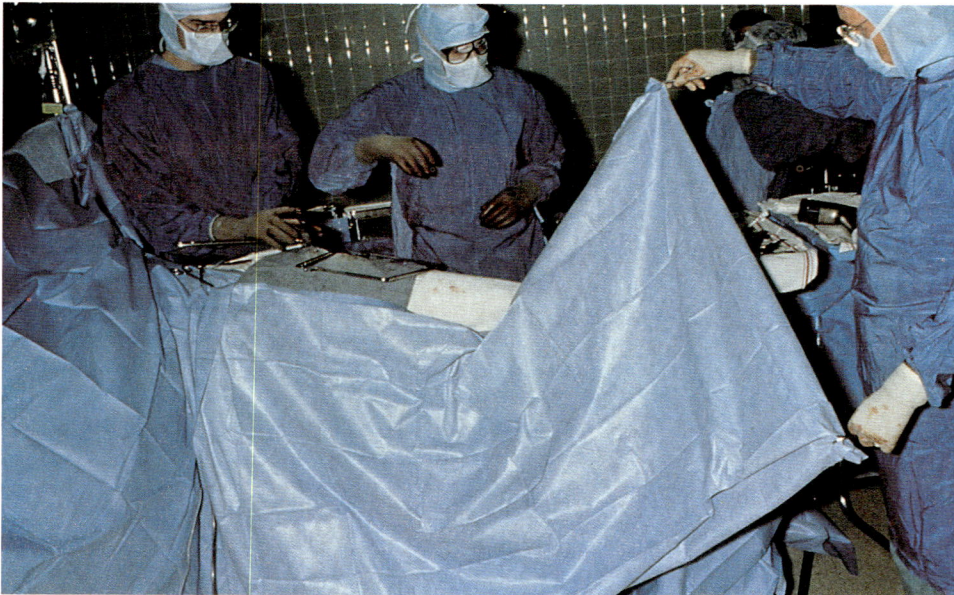

Figure 20. A sterile envelope in which to place the limb when it is dislocated has been prepared; the distal ends of the envelope are clipped to prevent contamination during the manipulation of the limb.

2 DIRECT LATERAL APPROACH

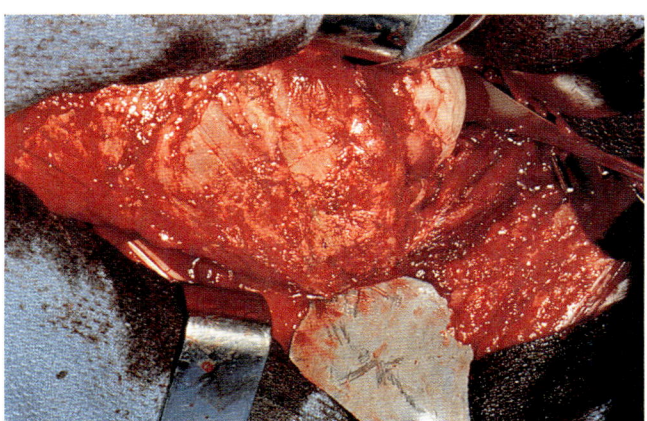

Figure 21. The femoral head is positioned for dislocation with the Muller hip skid in the upper right separating the femoral head from the acetabulum.

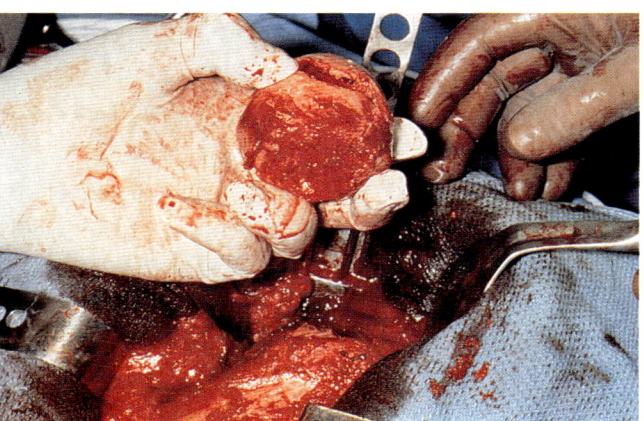

Figure 22. The hip has been dislocated and the limb has been adducted and flexed and positioned in the envelope for division of the femoral neck in preparation of the femoral canal. The femoral head has been osteotomized and removed.

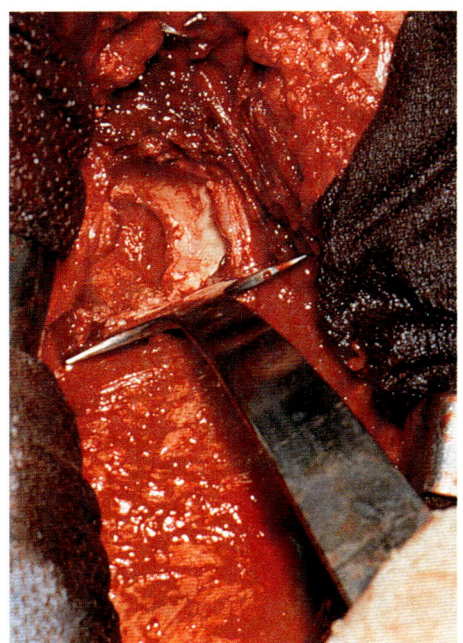

Figure 23. Additional capsule has been removed from the acetabulum, which is visualized in preparation for reaming. A broad Hohmann retractor is placed under the posterior lip of the acetabulum, and then holds the femoral shaft at the intertrochanteric region posterior to the acetabulum. The limb has been brought out of the envelope and back onto the operating table for the acetabular preparation.

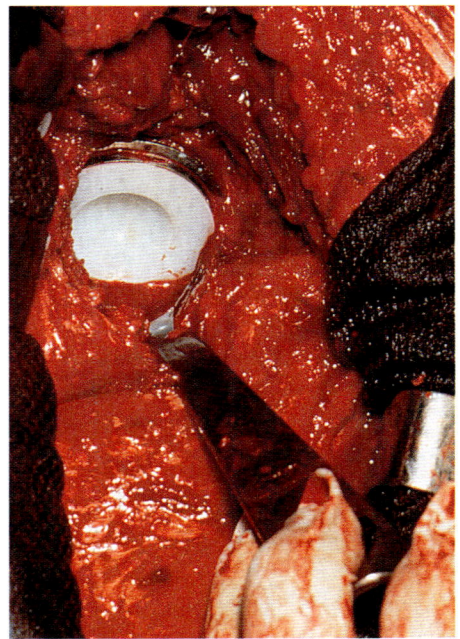

Figure 24. The view of the acetabulum after insertion of components shown here gives a good example of the acetabular exposure and orientation that is present with this approach.

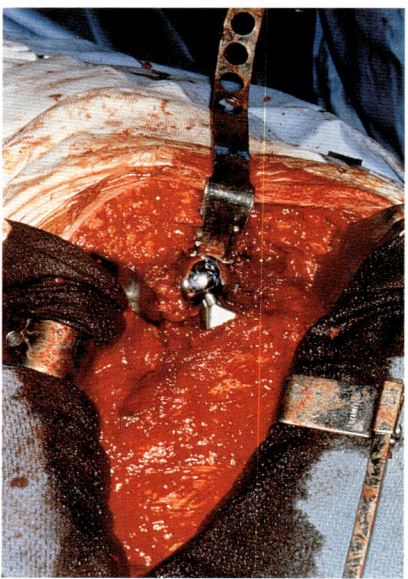

Figure 25. The femoral component has been placed in the femoral canal and is ready for reduction after appropriate sizing and length measurements had been established with trial components. The fixed pelvic retractor seen above the femoral head is the reference point for leg-length measurements in the trial reductions. Care must be taken to avoid injury to the femoral head from the metallic retractors during reduction.

ried out by confirming the position of the pelvis on the table during the reaming procedure and in the subsequent acetabular implantation. The proximal femur is broached using the appropriate instruments, the femoral component is inserted into position, and the trial reduction is carried out with measurements being simulated for lengthening or shortening based on the predislocation measurement (Fig. 25).

After the implanted retractors have been removed and the hip is reduced, careful attention must be devoted to reattachment of the abductor mechanism to the anterior portion of the trochanter. Our preference is to secure the gluteus tendons to the bone using three drill holes. The first is made at the apex of the posterior aspect of the reflection starting outside the incision in the gluteus fascia and passing from outside inward (Fig. 26). Pass a heavy suture through that drill hole and secure the first loop of a figure-eight

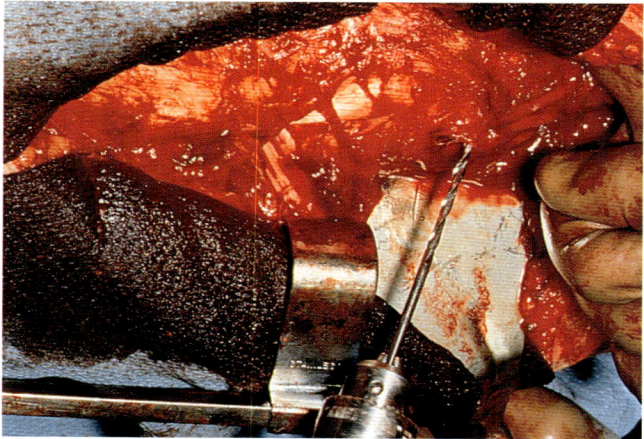

Figure 26. The first drill hole is being placed in the trochanter from posterior to anterior in the trochanter and outside of the line of division of the previous gluteus medius tendon.

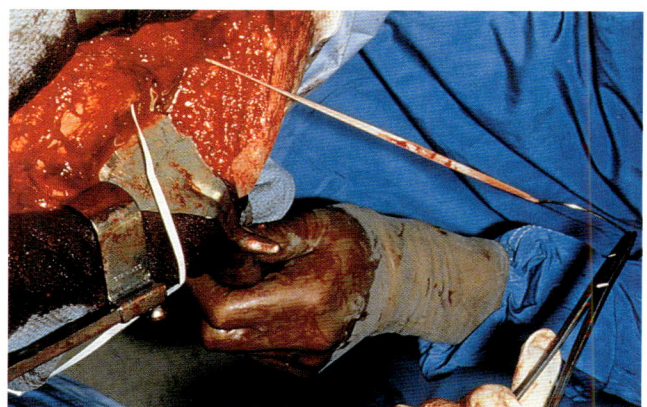

Figure 27. A 5-mm Mersilene suture is passed from the outside of the trochanter through the trochanter superior to the prosthetic device and up through the posterior aspect of the gluteus medius muscle, which had been detached at the level of the hockey stick detachment.

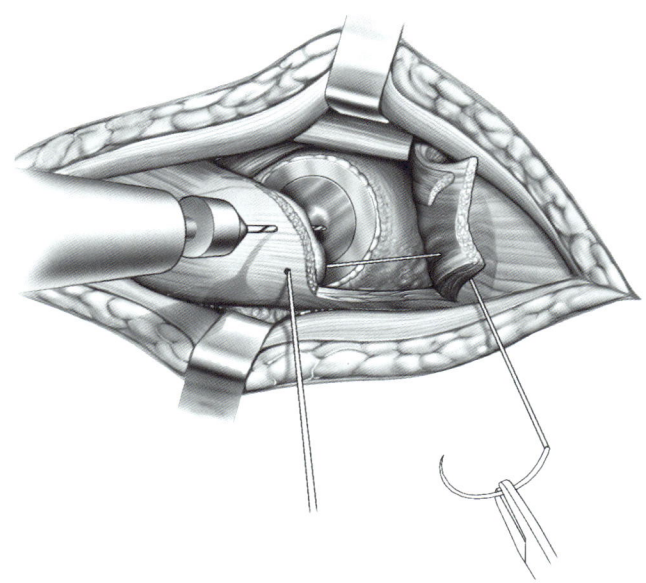

Figure 28. The first suture has been passed and the second drill hole is placed in the midportion of the greater trochanter.

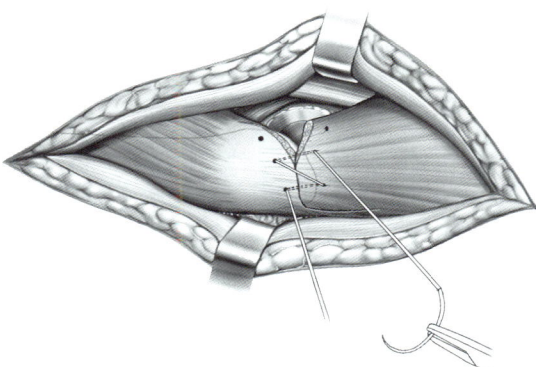

Figure 29. The first Mersilene suture has been passed through the second drill hole and out through the midportion of the gluteus medius tendon and is in position to be tied in a figure-of-eight fashion.

suture through the most posterior portion of the reflected gluteus (Figs. 27, 28). The second drill hole is made halfway between the posterior and the anterior margin, and the second limb of the figure-of-eight of the 5-mm Mersilene tape is passed back through the femur up through the gluteus medius fascia (Fig. 29). The third drill hole is made at the anteriormost limb of the detachment, and a similar figure-eight suture is passed with the second limb of the figure-of-eight (Fig. 30). As these sutures are snugged up, the abductor mechanism is brought back over the trochanter in a secure fashion, tied into position, and oversewn with a no. 1 nonabsorbable braided suture to reinforce the repair. Closure is carried out by continuous sutures in the tensor fascia lata with interrupted subcutaneous sutures and an intradermal skin suture.

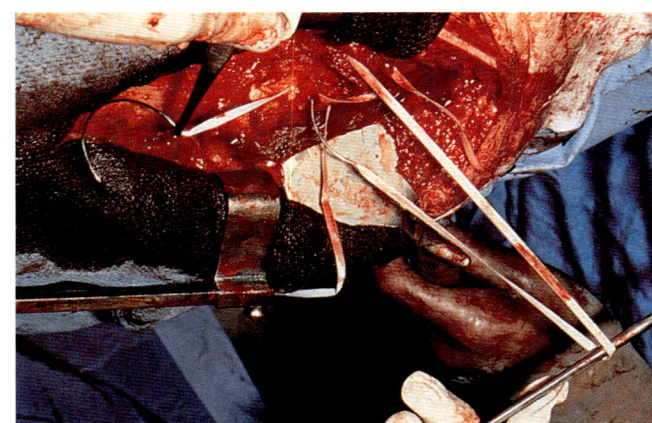

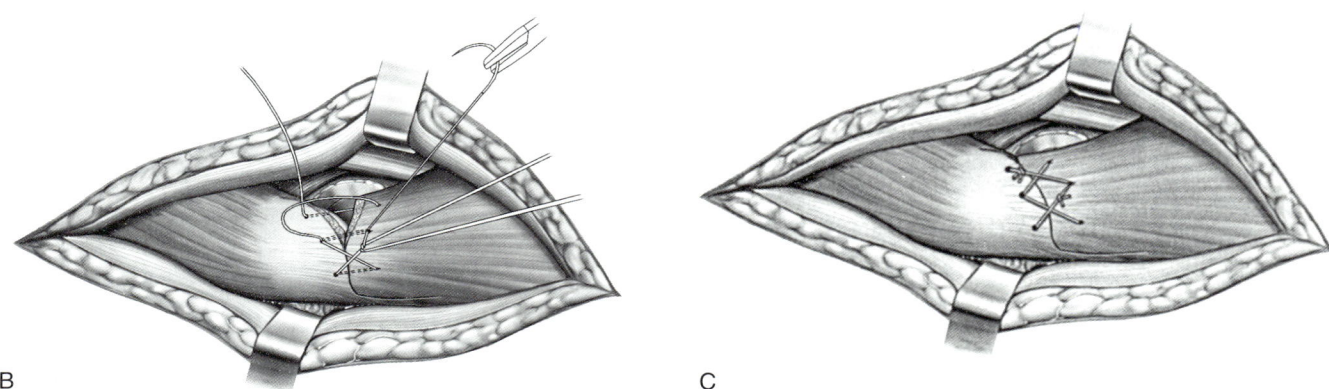

Figure 30. (A) The second Mersilene tape has been passed through the anterior drill hole in the trochanter up through the anterior fibers of the gluteus and back through the dentral drill hold, exiting through the midportion of the gluteus medius tendon. (B) The two Mersilene sutures in place with the first throw and the posterior suture being tied down. (C) The posterior suture has been secured and the anterior suture is now being secured in a figure-eight fashion giving secure fixation to the gluteus medius muscle and tendon.

POSTOPERATIVE MANAGEMENT

The patient usually has an abduction pillow applied before turning to a stretcher and is positioned supine with hip flexion as comfortable. As soon as the patient is recovered sufficiently from anesthesia, the head of the bed may be elevated as desired for respiratory assistance and dietary needs. When drains are used, we prefer silastic drains of 2 to 3 mm exiting from beneath the tensor fascia through the skin anterior and distal to the hip. When the suction drains are collecting less than 50 mL in eight hours, we remove the drains and allow the patient to sit.

We inform patients that they can expect to be in bed with a pillow between their knees for 24 hours after surgery. They can usually begin ambulating at that time with crutches or a walker, as deemed appropriate. For the uncomplicated arthroplasty, we anticipate discharge within 5 to 7 days and define the criteria for discharge as the ability to get in and out of bed unassisted, use toilet facilities unassisted, and dress without aid. We insist on the use of crutches for six weeks in order to protect the abductor repair and do not allow any resistive exercises during the first six weeks. Isometric quadriceps, hamstrings, and calf exercises are initiated in the first 48 hours and performed throughout the initial recovery. At 6 to 8 weeks after surgery resistive exercises for hip flexors and abductors are initiated, and when the patient is stable with contralateral support only, he progresses to a cane or single crutch. The continued use of a cane is urged until there is a negative Trendelenburg and the patient can lift the thigh in a lateral position against gravity, indicating good abductor function (generally 8 to 12 weeks).

COMPLICATIONS

The most common complication of this approach is loss of fixation of the abductors from the trochanter, which results in abductor lurch and puts the patient at risk for further complications such as implant failure. The technique described in this chapter for reattachment of the anterior fibers of the gluteus medius and minimus minimizes the chance that this complication will occur. Meticulous attention to detail in the closure is imperative to avoid avulsion of these muscles from the anterior portion of the greater trochanter.

The second most discussed complication is injury to the anterior branch of the superior gluteal nerve that innervates the anterior two-thirds of the abductors. This can be avoided by limiting cephalad extent of dissection in the muscles to 2 cm (Figs. 14, 15).

Heterotopic ossification is a common occurrence following this approach; however, it is usually mild, and it is less common than in the posterior approach. The incidence of this complication can be decreased by careful protection of the muscles during retraction and by protective padding with sponges when reaming the acetabulum or the femur to avoid seeding the pericapsular muscles with marrow elements.

Injury to the femoral nerve may occur if the anterior Hohmann retractor is positioned superior to the iliopsoas muscle rather than under the musculotendinous portion of the muscle when that retractor is positioned distal to the anteroinferior spine of the ilium (Fig. 17).

Other complications such as sciatic nerve damage and vascular injuries are not common or unique to this approach and can be avoided by careful attention to anatomic orientation during the exposure.

The literature relative to complications in the anterolateral approach has shown a lower incidence of dislocation of the hip compared with the posterior approach, and no substantial difference could be determined when comparing the anterolateral to posterior approach for the incidence of heterotopic ossification. Complications that have been reported with the anterolateral approach as described here include avulsion of the abductor musculature with resultant abductor weakness and injury to the anterior innervation of the gluteus medius and minimus by traction on the superior gluteal nerve anterior branch to these muscles.

RECOMMENDED READING

1. Hardinge K. E.: The direct lateral approach to the hip. *J. Bone Joint Surg.*, 64B:17–19, 1982.
2. Jacobs, L. G. H., and Buxton, R. A.: The course of the superior gluteal nerve in the lateral approach to the hip. *J. Bone Joint Surg.*, 71A:1239–1243, 1989.
3. McCollum, D. E., and Gray, W. J.: Dislocation after total hip arthroplasty. *Clin. Orthop. Rel. Res.*, 261:159, 1990.
4. McFarland, B., and Osborne, G.: *J. Bone Joint Surg.*, 36B:364–367, 1954.
5. Morrey, B. F., Adams, R. A., and Cabanella, M. E.: Comparison of heterotopic ossification after anterolateral, transtrochanteric, and posterior approach total hip arthroplasty. *Clin. Orthop. Rel. Res.*, 188:160–167, 1984.
6. Vicar, A. J., and Coleman, C. R.: A comparison of anterolateral transtrochanteric and posterior surgical approaches in primary total hip arthroplasty. *Clin. Orthop. Rel. Res.*, 188:152–159, 1984.
7. Woo, R., and Morrey, B.: Dislocation after total hip arthroplasty. *J. Bone Joint Surg.*, 64A:1295–1306, 1982.

3

Transtrochanteric Approach

Harlan C. Amstutz and Joseph Yao

INDICATIONS/CONTRAINDICATIONS

The transtrochanteric approach for total hip arthroplasty (THA) has a role in revision surgery, in difficult primary surface replacement cases of dislocation and where leg length is altered. Trochanteric osteotomy provides wide exposure facilitating component removal in revision THA and facilitates access to proximal femur.

While a grossly loose femoral component may be easily removed without the necessity of trochanteric osteotomy (depending on the component's geometry with respect to the femur), components that are more securely fixed are harder to remove. Porous-coated prostheses may be more easily removed after trochanteric osteotomy. Osteotomes or motorized cutting instruments can be brought in from lateral to medial through the osteotomy site and into the bone–prosthetic interface. This method is particularly useful when the femoral component has a large collar that extends anteriorly and posteriorly, blocking the passage of cement-removal instruments from above. Prostheses with a broad proximal-lateral shoulder can potentially fracture the greater trochanter during their extraction if care is not taken to excavate the medial aspect of the trochanter. This may leave only a cortical shell of trochanter. Trochanteric osteotomy in these cases may be desirable to prevent fracture related to component removal and in order to preserve bone and facilitate component extraction.

Hip stability and biomechanics can be enhanced by trochanteric advancement. Trochanteric reattachment in a more proximal or distal location can optimize abductor muscle tension in instances of leg shortening or lengthening, respectively.

There are no absolute contraindications for trochanter osteotomy. However, there are many risk factors that should be considered, which influence the ability to secure rigid fixation sufficient to secure a bony union such as osteopenia, bone-stock loss (reducing the size

---

H. C. Amstutz, M.D.: Joint Replacement Institute, Orthopaedic Hospital, Los Angeles, California 90007.

J. Yao, M.D.: 1521 North Tenth Street, Blytheville, Arkansas 72315.

of the greater trochanter), and inability of the patient to follow a postoperative regimen. Furthermore, there are now several new techniques available that make attractive options in selected situations such as trochanter slide, increasing the size distally and anteriorly. In this regard, the transfemoral approach of Wagner is especially useful in major revision surgery, greatly facilitating the removal of ingrowth components, cement, and distal osteolytic foci.

PREOPERATIVE PLANNING

Preoperative planning is helpful in deciding whether a trochanteric osteotomy will be necessary and what type of osteotomy to make. Assessment of the femoral component's shape helps in deciding whether a large or small trochanteric fragment will be optimal. Trochanteric osteotomy enhances visualization of the distal femoral canal, especially medially after the femoral component is removed, and facilitates safe distal cement removal. Abduction strength, hip stability, leg-length inequality, muscle bulk, and obesity are factors to assess on clinical examination of the patient. These factors will help to determine whether or not advancement of the trochanter will be desirable. Access can be improved in extremely muscular or obese patients.

Preoperative roentgenographic analysis should include an assessment of bone quality, the anticipated difficulty of extracting the current THA components, the type of components in place, and measurement of relative leg lengths. Bone quality can be estimated on roentgenograms, and it can be confirmed at surgery. Alternative methods of trochanteric fixation may be chosen when bone quality is poor.

SURGERY

We utilized trochanteric osteotomy in nearly all of our THAs and all our hemisurface and full-surface replacements from 1967 to 1985. Subsequently, trochanteric osteotomy has been used for some surface replacements and difficult primary and revision cases. Our goal has been to develop a secure and reliable trochanteric fixation technique that minimizes the size of the fixation materials. Our technique minimizes the incidence of trochanteric bursitis and allows the fixation materials to be removed when necessary under local anesthesia through a small incision. Our technique has evolved with time. Experimental work demonstrated the importance of using a combination of vertical and horizontal wires to resist forces that tend to displace the trochanteric fragment superiorly and anteriorly. We originally used a two-wire (Fig. 1) interlocking technique but later developed a three-wire interlocking technique (Fig. 2). This was used initially for cases requiring stronger fixation such as revision cases, those with marked osteopenia, cases scheduled to undergo postoperative radiation therapy for prophylaxis against heterotopic ossification, and in cases involving large, heavy males. Because of its improved results, this technique is now used routinely. The three-wire technique added a second vertical wire to share the superiorly directed forces between two wires. Another advantage of using three wires is the additional tension effect that occurs as the second throw of the knot in the horizontal wire is tightened around the two vertical wires, pulling them together. Most recently, four wires have been used in selected cases requiring maximum stability as in certain revision THA and in cases of trochanteric reattachment after a trochanteric nonunion. Two vertical wires are combined with two horizontal wires in this technique (Fig. 3). Dall-Miles cables have been used in some exceptionally difficult cases instead of our standard cobalt-chromium beaded wires. However, the wire fragmentation after fracture of these multi-filament cables is disconcerting, and we rarely use them now.

Our techniques of trochanteric fixation utilize wires placed under tension and square knots to prevent wire slippage. Others have designed methods that involve twisting wire ends for maintaining tension. In our experience there is a fine line between optimal wire tension and the tension at which wire breaks when it is twisted, and therefore we believe knotting the wire is safer.

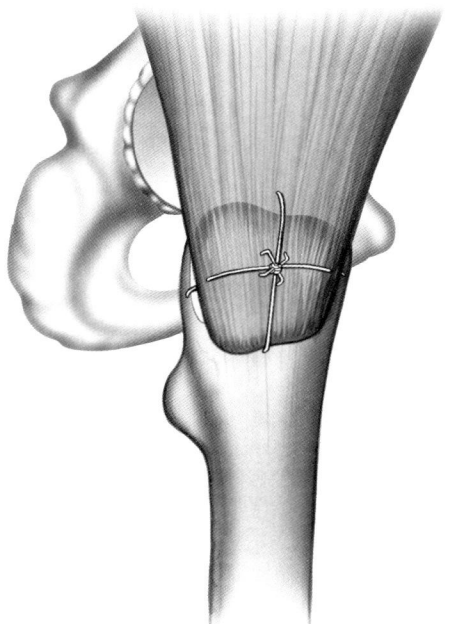

Figure 1. Two-wire trochanteric reattachment technique.

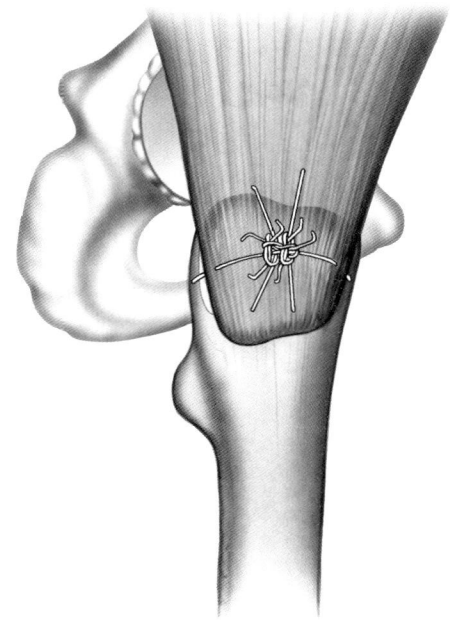

Figure 2. Three-wire trochanteric reattachment technique.

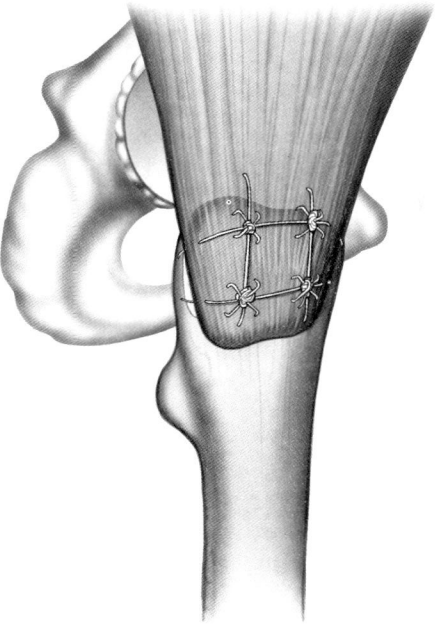

Figure 3. Four-wire technique. Note the two independent two-wire interlocking systems.

Technique

The patient is placed in the lateral decubitus position. Pubic and sacral supports are used to rigidly stabilize the pelvis. A lateral skin incision is made centered over the greater trochanter (Fig. 4). The proximal portion of the incision may be gently curved posteriorly. The fascia lata and fascia of the gluteus are split in line with their fibers. A Charnley retractor is used to retract the soft tissues anteriorly and posteriorly. The trochanteric bursa is either excised or reflected posteriorly. The gluteus maximus tendon is divided from its femoral insertion when it is tight or when wide exposure is desired. A tonsil clamp is placed deep to the tendon, and the tendon is divided with electrocautery. The leash of vessels located distally are localized, clamped, and cauterized. The gluteus maximus tendon should be divided close to the femur in order to protect the sciatic nerve, which is located posteriorly. The vastus lateralis tendon is divided transversely 1 cm distal to its origin on the vastus ridge of the femur. This leaves a cuff of tissue still attached to bone that can be used during reattachment.

The capsule is incised anteriorly and posteriorly, facilitated by externally and internally rotating the limb, respectively. A Gigli saw passer is inserted intracapsularly through these capsular incisions. The obturator is removed from the passer, and a Gigli saw is inserted (Fig. 5). The Gigli saw passer is removed, and the Gigli saw is used to make the osteotomy (Fig. 6). The location of the saw is palpated in the medial lateral plane to be sure the size of the trochanteric fragment will be appropriate. The trochanteric piece should generally be at least 3 cm long in order to provide a sufficient bony bed for reattachment. When the limb

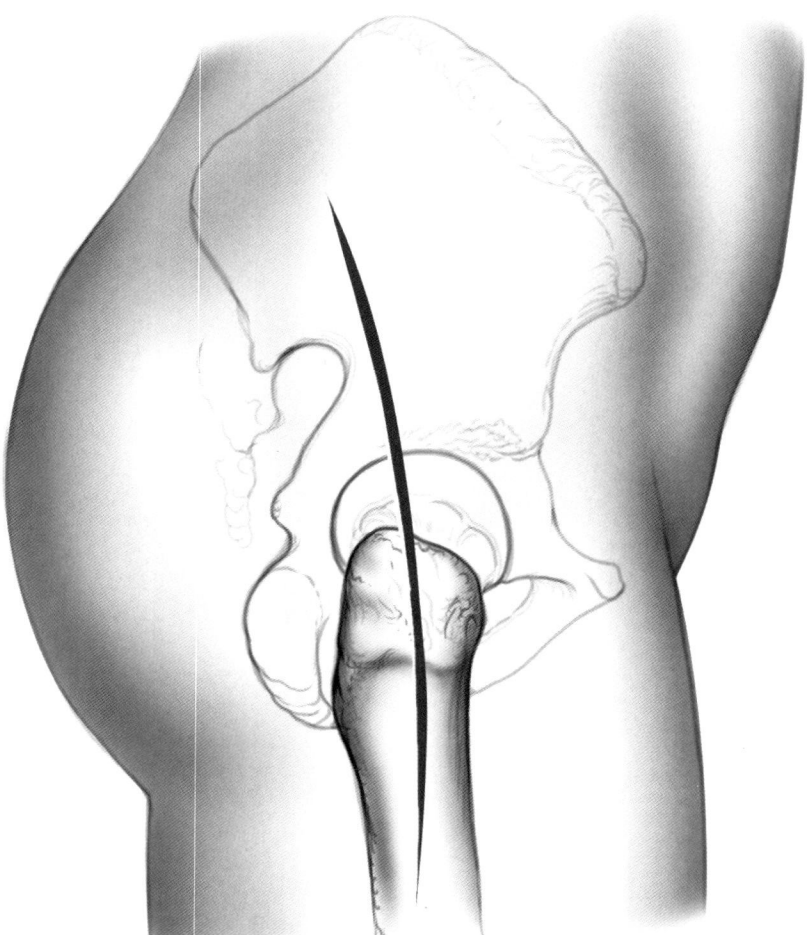

Figure 4. Lateral skin incision centered over the greater trochanter.

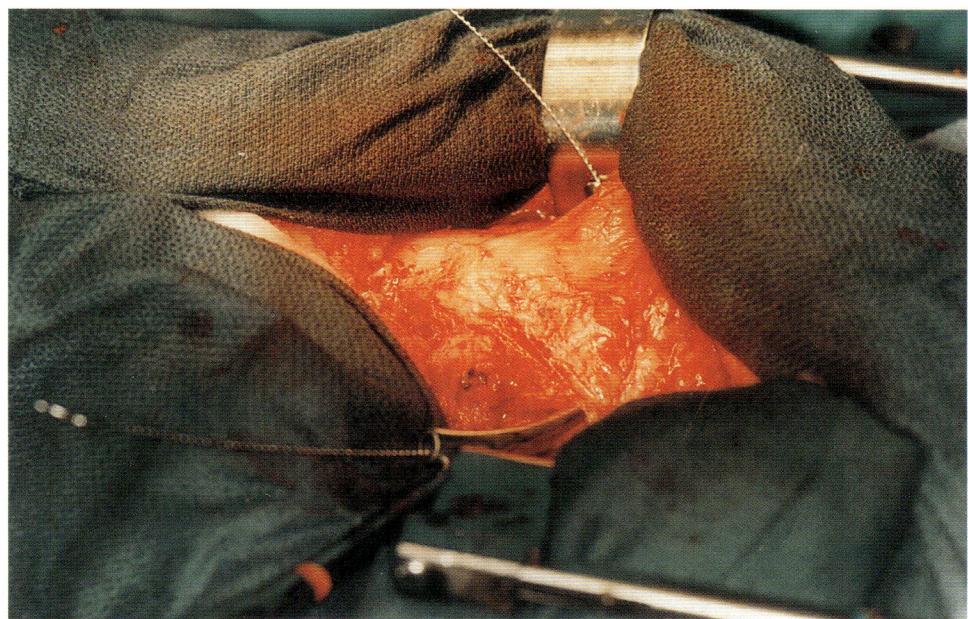

Figure 5. Gigli saw inserted through the Gigli saw passer after removal of the obturator.

is lengthened, as long a trochanteric piece as possible is made (more than 4 cm). The longer trochanteric fragment can then be reattached in a more proximal position to avoid excessive tension on the gluteus medius muscle. As the greater trochanter is located posteriorly, internally rotating the hip about 20 degrees places the plane of the osteotomy more nearly parallel to the floor when the patient is in the lateral decubitus position. The osteotomy should end distal to the vastus ridge. A smaller trochanteric fragment is desirable for hemisurface or full-surface replacements in order to avoid placing a stress riser near the

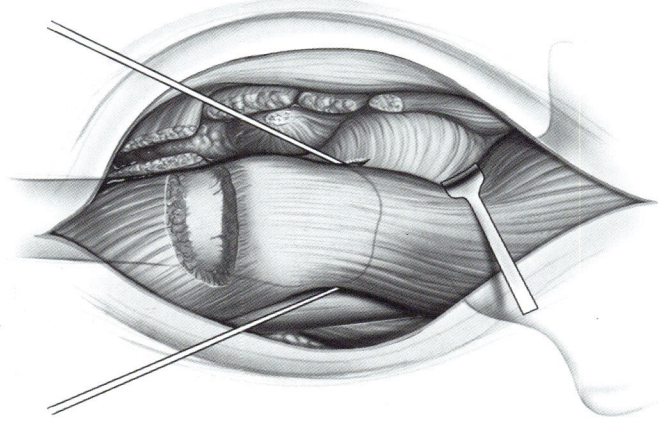

Figure 6. The Gigli saw is used to create the osteotomy after the Gigli saw passer has been removed.

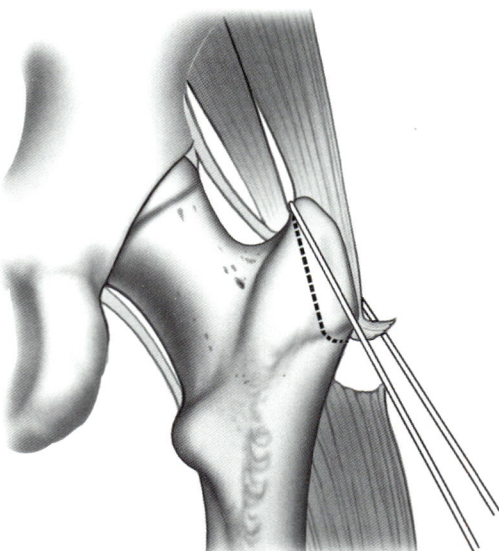

Figure 7. The Gigli saw is passed between the gluteus medius and minimus muscles in order to avoid creating a stress-riser near the femoral neck in surface replacements.

femoral neck. The Gigli saw is passed in the plane between the gluteus medius and the gluteus minimus tendons in these cases instead of the usual intracapsular position (Fig. 7).

The cut surface of the osteotomy is made as flat as possible to provide maximum bone contact for reattachment and to allow flexibility for proximal or distal placement of the fragment (Fig. 8). A 5-mm elevation, or "ski jump," is made at the distal portion of the osteotomy by raising the handles of the Gigli saw during the last 1 cm of the cut. The resultant bony prominence provides a place to impale the trochanteric piece and adds rotational stability when the piece is impacted prior to wire fixation. A special 5 cm wide, straight osteotome or oscillating saw may be used to make the osteotomy instead of the Gigli saw. The wide osteotome is especially useful in revision cases to avoid fragmentation of the trochanteric piece when the plane of the osteotomy passes through acrylic cement.

The trochanteric fragment is reflected proximally once the osteotomy is completed. Gelfoam is placed on the cut surfaces of the trochanter, and pressure is applied with a lap

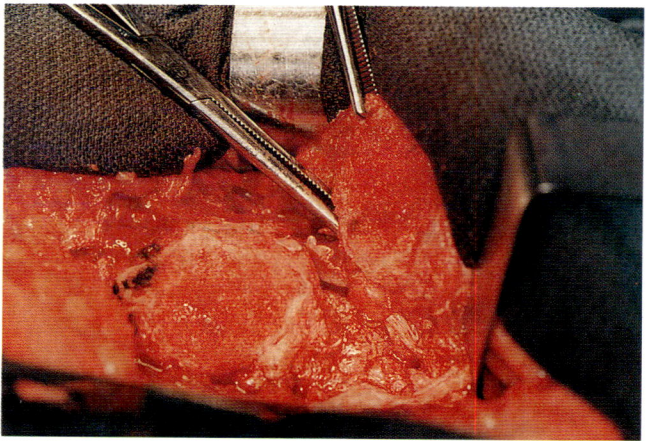

Figure 8. The osteotomy is made as flat as possible to maximize bone contact for reattachment.

sponge to achieve hemostasis. In cases where a small trochanteric piece is made, the gluteus minimus tendon is detached from the proximal femur and reflected proximally by elevating it from the underlying hip capsule. In routine cases, the larger trochanteric piece and its attached gluteus medius and minimus tendons are reflected proximally and held with three smooth one-eighth inch diameter Steinmann pins placed just distal to them (Fig. 9A, B). The Steinmann pins are driven with a mallet through the inner and outer tables of the ilium at least 1 cm proximal to the acetabular rim. The posterior pin is placed as far proximally as possible into the ilium in order to maximize space for femoral preparation. The pins are placed 2 to 3 cm apart and serve as retractors as well as reference points for intraoperative leg length measurements. Measurements are taken from the base of each Steinmann pin to the inferiormost point of the trochanteric bed which can be marked with electrocautery. The leg is placed in line with the patient's body so it will be in a reproducible position when measurements are taken. The measurements are recorded and compared with those taken at the end of the operation to confirm that the appropriate leg length has been achieved. Measurements performed from the three pins allows greater accuracy than those performed from one or two pins.

Capsulotomy is now performed at the base of the femoral neck. The hip can then be dislocated using flexion, abduction, and external rotation. The hip capsule is excised and femoral and acetabular preparation is performed as necessary for the particular prostheses.

Preliminary steps for trochanteric reattachment are performed prior to femoral component implantation. Holes are drilled in the proximal femur for wire placement. The vertical wire or wires are placed into the intramedullary canal when using cemented prostheses, so the wires can be anchored when the cement is inserted. The wires should exit through drill holes 1 to 2 cm distal to the vastus ridge, depending on the distance the trochanter will be advanced. The drill holes should be placed 1 cm apart. One vertical wire may be sufficient when there is good bone stock and when the trochanteric bed is composed largely of cancellous bone. However, we now routinely use two vertical wires and believe these are essential if the trochanter is osteoporotic, if the trochanteric bed is cortical bone or partially

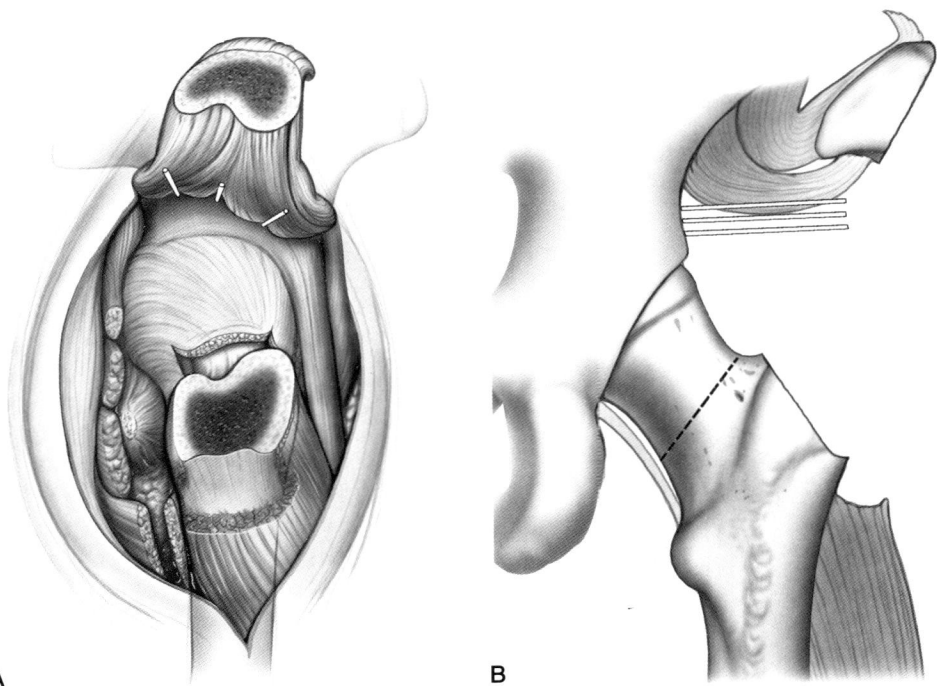

Figure 9. The hip viewed from the side (A) and from the front (B) showing the trochanteric fragment and attached gluteus medius and minimus tendons retracted proximally by three Steinmann pins placed through both tables of the ilium.

acrylic, or if postoperative radiation therapy is planned for prophylaxis against heterotopic ossification. The wire ends are manually pulled to be sure they will not cut out of the bone when they are tightened later. Beaded 18- or 19-gauge cobalt-chromium wire is recommended. We prefer to use 19-gauge wire because it is more flexible. A self-capturing drill/wire guide is helpful when making the holes and passing the wires through the bone (Fig. 10). The guide is held in place after the hole has been drilled. The distal portion of the guide has a notch that grasps the beaded end of the wire as it is passed through the proximal end of the guide and through the bone. The guide greatly simplifies wire passage and eliminates difficulties associated with finding the drill holes, which are often partially hidden by soft tissue.

Vertical wire placement technique is modified in the case of a cementless stemmed femoral component. The drill holes are placed in an intracortical location using the drill/wire guide in order to avoid contact between the wires and the femoral component. One wire is placed anterior and one is placed posterior to the trochanteric bed. The holes should be placed as far laterally as possible in cases of surface replacement in order to avoid creating stress risers with drill holes at the base of the femoral neck (Fig. 11).

A single transverse wire is placed through a drill hole 5 to 10 mm deep to the midportion of the trochanteric bed. The wire should be placed at least 10 mm deep when the bone is osteoporotic. The drill bit can potentially nick the previously placed vertical wires since its path passes across that of the vertical wires. Wire nicks can produce stress risers and subsequent wire fracture. The vertical wires are initially pulled only slightly through their holes. Once the transverse hole has been drilled and the transverse wire has been passed, the vertical wires are pulled through further so any potentially nicked areas of wire are

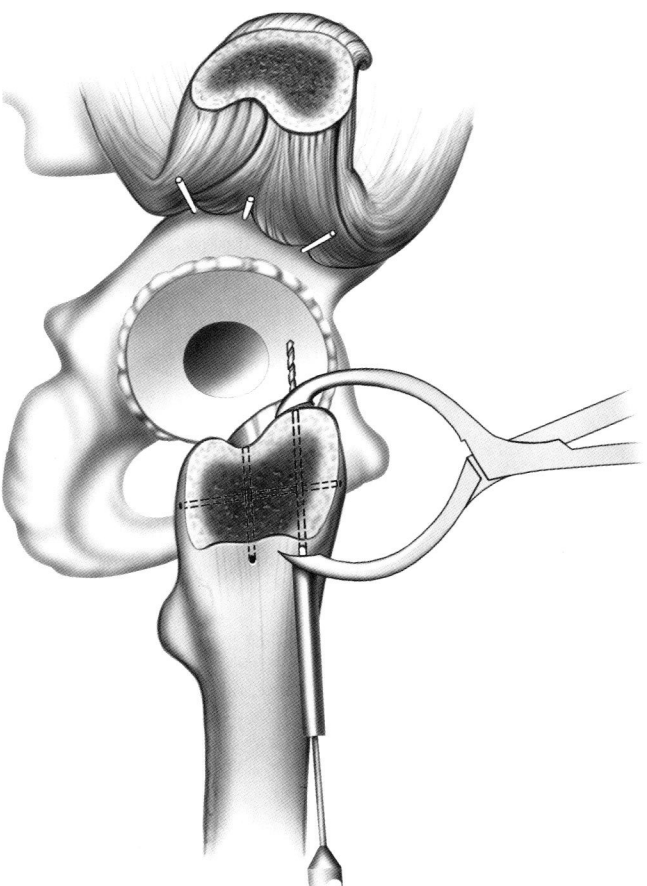

Figure 10. A self-capturing drill/wire guide assists drilling holes and passing wires through the proximal femur.

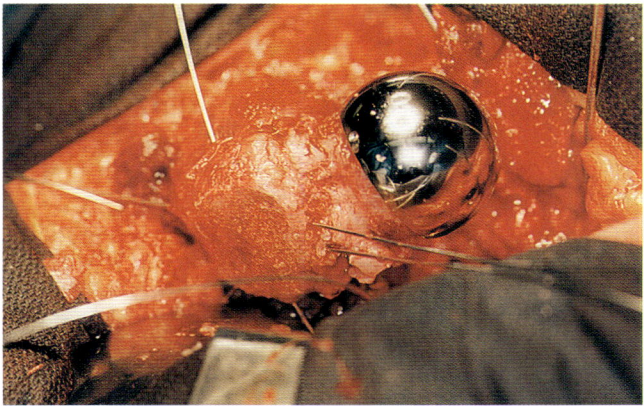

Figure 11. Drill holes for wire placement should be positioned as laterally as possible in the proximal femur in order to avoid creation or stress risers at the base of the femoral neck in surface replacements.

placed near the wire ends which will be cut off later (Fig. 12A, B). The transverse wire is placed in the intramedullary canal when acrylic is used to fix the femoral component, and it is placed in an intracortical location when a cementless stemmed femoral component is implanted. The ends of the individual wires are carefully tagged with different clamps (eg., wire pullers, Snowden pincers, curved Kelley or Kocher clamps) to aid in their identifica-

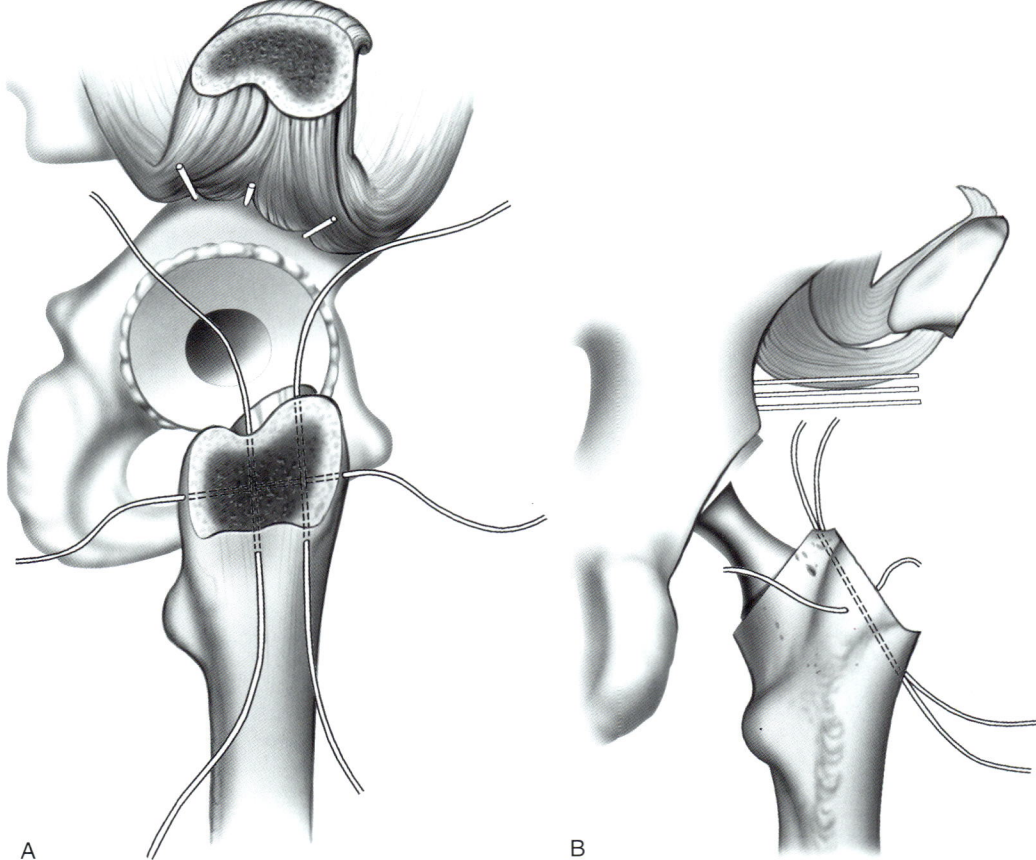

Figure 12. Side (A) and front (B) views of the hip showing wires passed deep to the trochanteric bed for a three-wire technique.

tion while tying them later. The femoral component is now implanted, once the wires have been inserted through their drill holes.

Leg-length measurements are made after trial prosthetic components have been placed. The bases of the three Steinmann pins and the distal aspect of the osteotomy are again used as reference points for measurement. These measurements are compared to those taken at the beginning of the operation, and intraoperative adjustments may be made as necessary to achieve the desired leg length.

The Steinmann pins are removed from the ilium, releasing the trochanteric fragment and the gluteus medius muscle. The gluteus minimus tendon is still attached to the trochanteric fragment in routine cases. The gluteus minimus tendon is released from the proximal femur in cases where a small trochanteric fragment is desired and the osteotomy plane falls between the gluteus medius and minimus tendons. In these cases, the gluteus minimus tendon is simply allowed to fall back into its natural position.

The trochanteric piece is held with a trochanteric holder, which also serves as a drill guide. The proximal ends of the vertical wires are first passed through the gluteus medius and minimus tendons over the superior pole of the trochanteric piece. The vertical wire should be passed over the midportion of the superior aspect of the trochanteric piece if only one vertical wire is used. The vertical wires should be separated by 1 to 2 cm if two vertical wires are used. A pointed-tip tonsil clamp facilitates the passage of the vertical wires through the tendinous tissue. The trochanteric holder is now used as a drill guide for the remaining wires (Fig. 13A, B), but it is important to place those holes as close as possible to the wires emanating from the trochanteric base in the advance position of the trochanter. Holes drilled for the transverse wire should be placed as peripherally as possible to keep

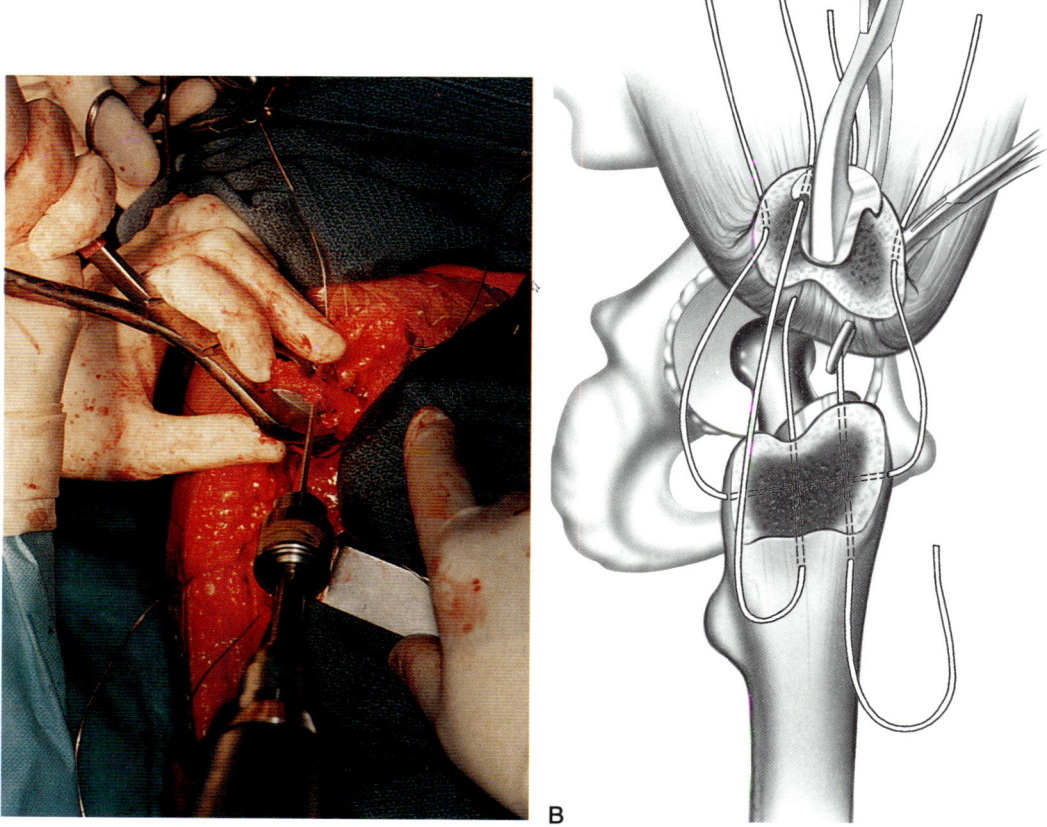

Figure 13 A, B. The trochanteric holder holds the trochanteric piece and assists with pulling it distally for reattachment. It also serves as a drill guide. A tonsil clamp facilitates passage of wires through tendon while the trochanteric holder secures the trochanteric piece.

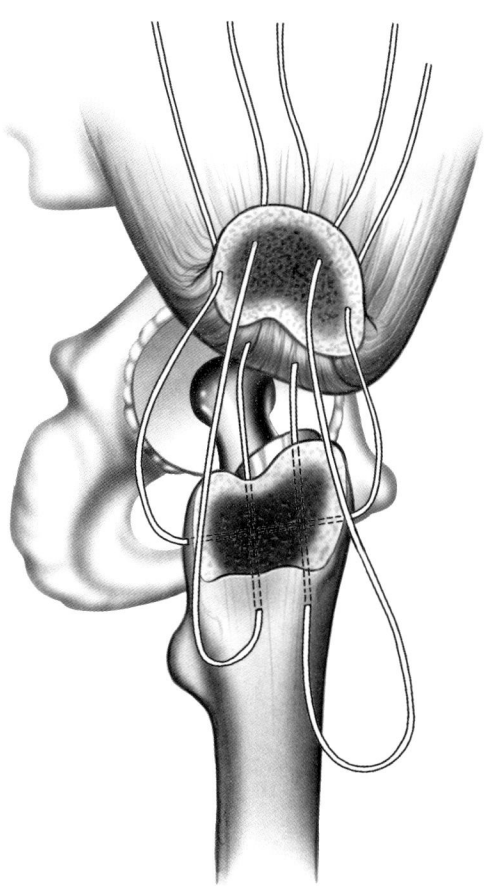 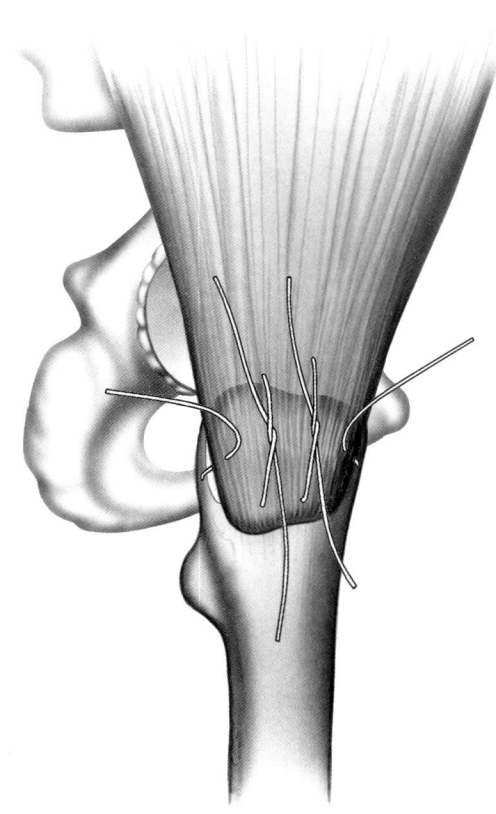

Figure 14. Wires have been passed through the trochanteric fragment. The proximal ends of the vertical wires are used to pull the fragment distally.

Figure 15. The vertical wires are placed about 1cm apart. The first throw of a square knot has been thrown in each of the vertical wires.

the wire out of the osteotomy interface, otherwise it will prevent the trochanteric piece from sitting flush on the trochanteric bed during reattachment. The distal holes are drilled 1 to 2 cm proximal to the distal tip of the trochanteric fragment, depending on the amount of trochanteric advancement desired.

The remaining wires are now passed through the trochanteric fragment (Fig. 14). The trochanter holder is released from the fragment, and the proximal ends of the vertical wires are used to pull the trochanteric fragment distally, providing the appropriate degree of advancement, generally 1 to 2 cm. The first throw of a square knot is placed in each of the vertical wires (Fig. 15). The wires are partially placed on tension with a traction-bow wire tightener. The trochanter is checked for proper rotational alignment. A lap sponge is placed over the trochanteric fragment, and a mallet is used to impact the fragment gently into the area of the trochanteric ridge (Fig. 16). The bony prominence of the distal vastus ridge acts like a "ski jump," and it adds greater stability when the trochanteric fragment is impacted onto it. The vertical wires are tightened further, and the wire tighteners are left attached to the wires as the trochanteric piece is checked for stability. Further tightening is done if necessary.

The first throw of a square knot is now placed in the transverse wire. The transverse wire must be placed perpendicular to the osteotomy plane in order to achieve maximum compressive forces. The transverse wire is tightened with another traction-bow wire tightener. The wire is palpated to be sure there are no loose wire loops and to ensure that the wires are not slipping, and their wire tighteners may be removed once the transverse wire has been tightened. The second throws of a square knot are placed into each of the vertical wires, and

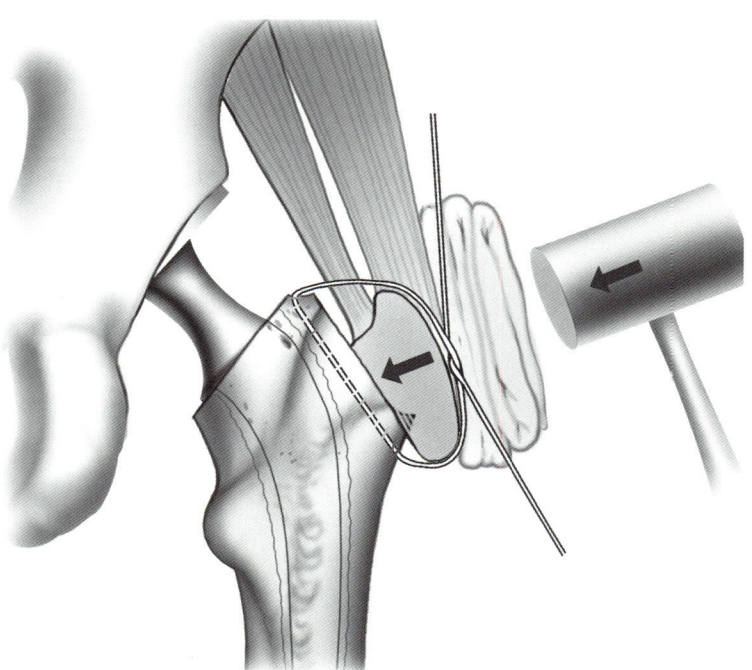

Figure 16. A lap sponge is placed over the trochanteric fragment and a mallet is used to impact the fragment gently into the area of the trochanteric ridge, providing greater stability.

they are tightened (Fig. 17). The wire tighteners are removed from the vertical wires, and the wire ends are cut. The square knots in the vertical wires pass around the transverse wire. The transverse wire is prevented from slipping once the knots are tied in the vertical wires. The wire tightener can be removed from the transverse wire, and the second throw of a square knot is placed into the transverse wire (Fig. 18). The first and second throws of the square knot in the transverse wire pass around both of the vertical wires. The two vertical wires are pulled closer together, tensioning them further when the second throw of the square knot in the transverse wire is tightened (Fig. 19). The wire ends are cut about 1 cm long and are bent to a right angle with Snowden wire pincers or needle-nose pliers. Each wire end is impacted into the trochanteric fragment in order to minimize potential soft tis-

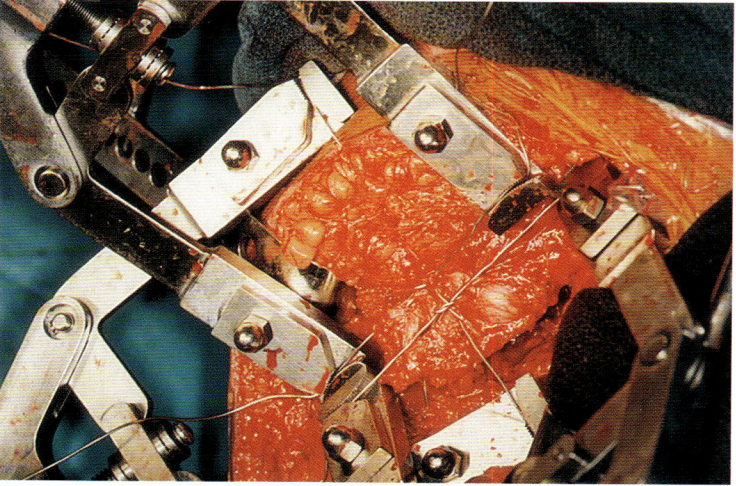

Figure 17. The second throw of a square knot is placed in each of the vertical wires, and they are tightened around the transverse wire, which has the first throw of a square knot in it. The square knots in the vertical wires prevent the transverse wire from slipping.

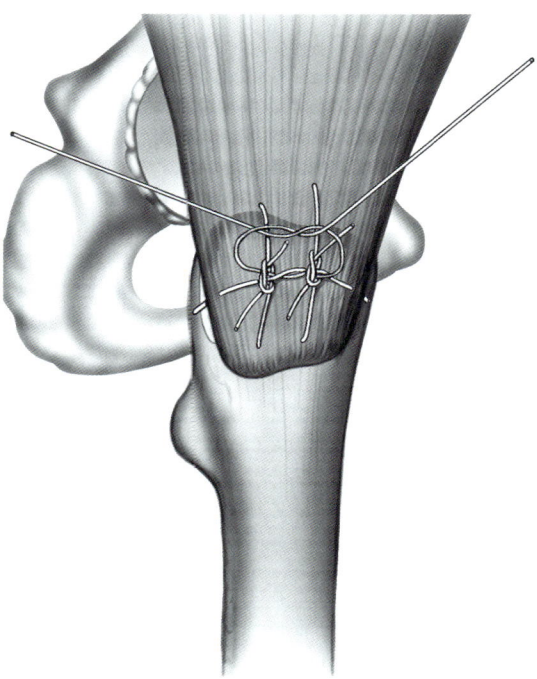

Figure 18. The second throw of a square knot is placed in the transverse wire as this wire passes around the two vertical wires.

sue irritation (Fig. 20). The vastus lateralis tendon is repaired with no. 1 or 0 absorbable suture to augment trochanteric fixation. The wound is then closed routinely in layers.

Several technical points are worthwhile noting. There is a learning curve associated with applying the appropriate amount of wire tension. The screw mechanism of standard traction-bow wire tighteners tends to gall with repeated use, making it necessary to apply more force to achieve the optimum degree of wire tension. This greatly lessens the ability of the surgeon to assess tension in the wire. We prefer an improved wire tightener with a screw

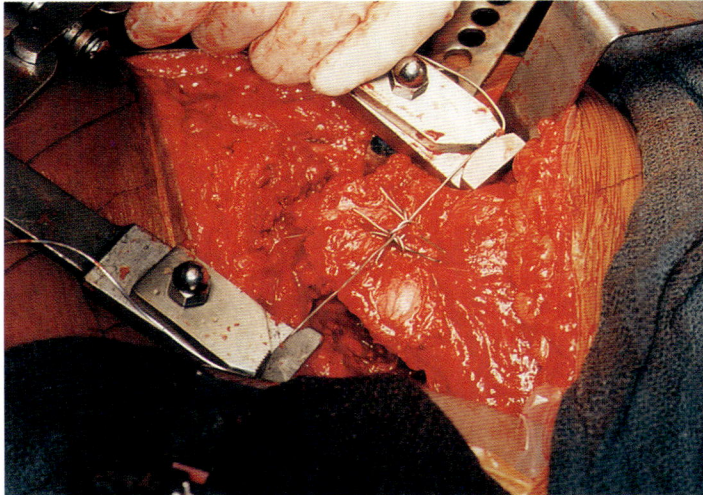

Figure 19. Tightening the second throw of the square knot in the transverse wire pulls the two vertical wires toward one another, tensioning them further.

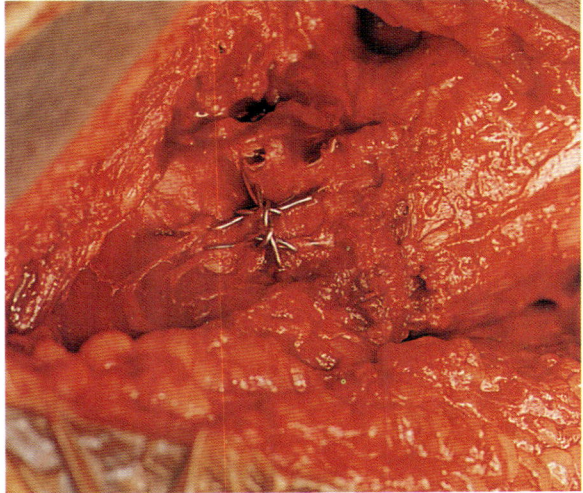

Figure 20. All wire ends are cut, bent 90 degrees, and impacted into the trochanteric fragment to minimize their prominence.

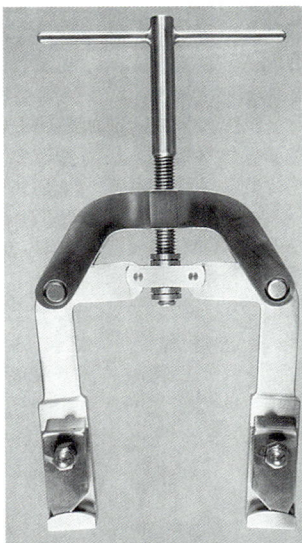

Figure 21. The improved wire tightener resists galling and allows smoother and more even application of wire tension.

mechanism fabricated from harder, more durable steel that resists galling and allows smoother and more even application of wire tension, DePuy #2069–85–001 (Fig. 21).

A long, vertical osteotomy is used in cases where leg lengthening is anticipated. Such cases include THA for congenital hip dysplasia or revision of a subsided femoral component. The longer trochanteric fragment allows more flexibility in the location of trochanteric fixation in order to maintain optimal abductor tension.

A poor trochanteric bed may be present, compromising reattachment of the trochanteric fragment. Poor quality bone is frequently present in revision cases. Cortical bone may be present in cases of significant trochanteric advancement beyond the cancellous trochanteric bed. Fish-scaling the lateral femoral cortex with an osteotome or a motorized burr is done if the reattachment site includes cortical bone. Cancellous bone from acetabular reamings can be used to graft the reattachment site if bone quality is poor or if there are defects in the trochanteric fragment.

It is important to assess stability between the trochanteric fragment and its bed and to determine whether any wire has been cut out of the trochanteric bed. This is detected by an abrupt loss in wire tension during wire tightening. All wires should be inspected in such an event, and they should be replaced with new wires if there is any question as to their integrity.

POSTOPERATIVE MANAGEMENT

Postoperatively, the trochanteric osteotomy is protected by toe-touch weight bearing for two months. A longer duration of protected weight bearing may be necessary if there are any risk factors for nonunion. Exercises including active hip flexion are encouraged if there is judged to be excellent rotational stability of the impacted trochanteric fragment to its bed. Active abduction is delayed until the osteotomy is healed as seen on followup roentgenograms. Abduction exercises and progressive weight bearing can generally begin at three months postoperatively if there is no evidence of trochanteric shift or wire breakage. Bony union of the osteotomy is difficult to assess unless the postoperative roentgenogram is directed tangentially to the osteotomy plane, and this requires that the extremity be internally rotated approximately 20 degrees. The decision to advance therapy and weight bearing is based on the absence of trochanteric migration, evaluation of and roentgenogram made tangential to the osteotomy, and the degree of bony apposition achieved at surgery. If there is any doubt about healing, avoid active abduction for four months. If there is any migration or wire breakage, delay active abduction until six months.

COMPLICATIONS

The most common serious complication associated with the transtrochanteric approach is trochanteric nonunion. Reported rates of nonunion range from 0% to 17.4%. Potential problems associated with nonunion include pain and abductor weakness. The most recent review of our experience with trochanteric osteotomy in cemented TR-28 THA's demonstrated nonunion rates of 4.9% (18 of 366) in primary cases and 7.1% (15 of 211) in revision cases. The majority of TR-28 trochanteric nonunions occurred in cases of osteoarthritis (38%) and failed THA (34%). The incidence of nonunion was lowest in cases of rheumatoid arthritis (3%) and congenital hip dysplasia (0%). Increased body weight was a risk factor for nonunion. Patient age, sex, and height were not associated with nonunion. Technical error in trochanteric reattachment was implicated in most cases of nonunion. Common technical errors included the presence of untensioned wire loops indicating inadequate wire tightening, superficial wire placement, and insufficient trochanteric impaction onto the vastus ridge. A less commonly encountered error included reattaching the trochanteric fragment in a tilted position, decreasing the surface contact between the fragment and the bed. Two cases of nonunion received postoperative radiation therapy (1000 and 2000 rads) for the prevention of heterotopic ossification. The trochanteric osteotomy was not shielded from the radiation field at that time, something that we now recommend.

Hip abduction strength and Trendelenburg status were not affected by trochanteric nonunion in our TR-28 THA series if the amount of separation between the trochanteric fragment and its bed was less than 10 mm (Grade I separation). These functional parameters decreased progressively with an increase in separation to Grade II (separation of 1 to 2 cm) and Grade III (>2 cm separation). There were no significant differences in UCLA hip scores for pain, walking, function, and activity level between nonunion cases and the overall series for either TR-28 or surface replacement groups.

Wire fracture is frequent after trochanteric osteotomy. We observed fractured wires in 53% of the TR-28 nonunion cases. Wire removal is generally unnecessary. Wire removal was performed in only two (4.5%) nonunion cases, a rate identical for the series as a whole (37 of 741 cases). Wires may be removed under local anesthesia after either the two- or three-wire techniques. The skin and subcutaneous tissues are infiltrated with local anesthesia and the wire knots are exposed through a small incision. Soft tissues that have grown into the knots are removed. Each wire is cut on one side of its knot. Each knot is grasped with pliers and the wires are removed with a vigorous jerk while an assistant applies downward pressure on the hip.

Trochanter reattachment should be considered if the trochanter migrates and there is abductor weakness. However, in our experience we have seen only one patient who had significant, related pain following trochanteric nonunion. In this patient, the trochanter separated for a distance of less than .5 cm, and a definite pseudoarthrosis developed with sclerosis of the opposing surfaces. The weakness was judged to be caused by the pain, and this was confirmed by Xylocaine injection. Fortunately, reattachment was accompanied by bony, union, pain relief, and increased abductor strength.

It is unusual that we recommend and carry out trochanteric reattachment for migration and weakness because, although the operation is modest, the postoperative management is not. In reattachment, the bone ends must be freshened with clean-cut bone surfaces. Initial stability must be achieved, and if the fragment is small and optimal bone is not present (which is often the case), stability will be difficult to maintain and union slow. Serious consideration should be given to spica immobilization to ensure that the patient will not overstress the wire fixation. Nonunion following an operation for a nonunion will have a considerably higher incidence than a primary reattachment.

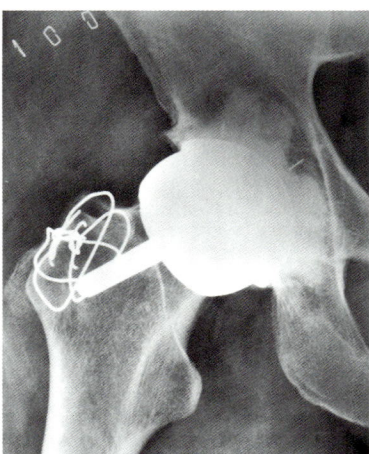

Figure 22. Immediate postoperative radiograph showing the position of the trochanter and wires.

ILLUSTRATIVE CASE FOR TECHNIQUE

G. S.: 44-year-old male who had steroid therapy for allergic rhinitis and developed avascular necrosis of the right femoral head. Patient underwent a right cemented surface replacement using the McMinn metal/metal bearing prosthesis on 11 November 1993. The trochanter was advanced 1 cm and reattached using the three-wire interlocking technique. The immediate postoperative radiograph (Fig. 22) was taken with the hip externally rotated so that the x-ray is not in the plane of the osteotomy and illustrates the position of the trochanter and the wires. Figure 23 shows the one-year followup film with the hip in neutral rotation. There is bony union of the trochanter in the advanced position.

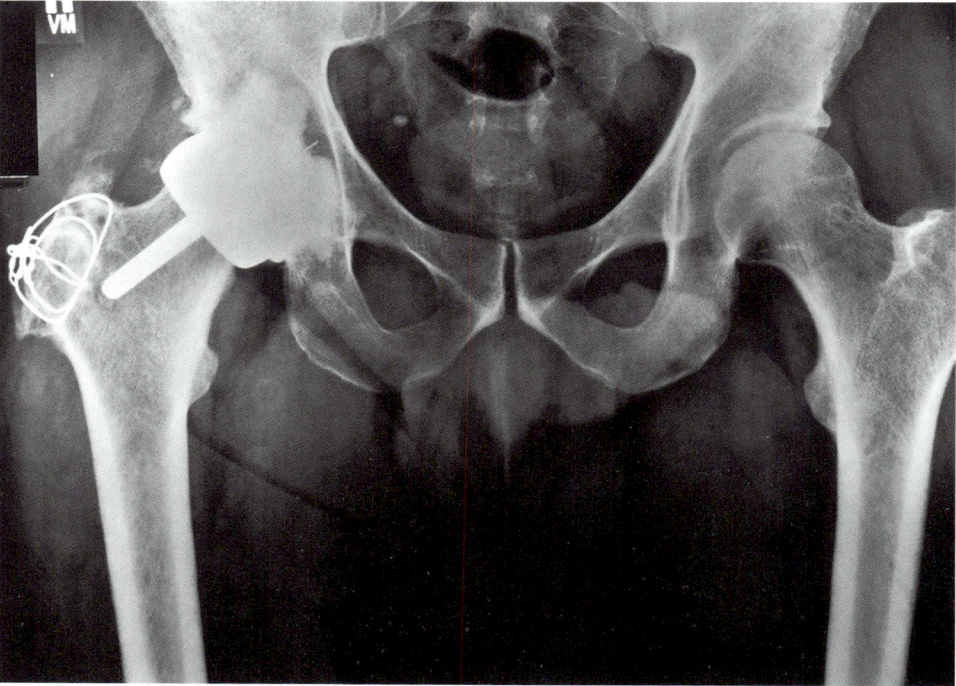

Figure 23. One-year postoperative radiograph shows bony union of the trochanter.

RECOMMENDED READING

1. Amstutz, H.C., Mai, L.L., and Schmidt, I.: Results of interlocking wire trochanteric reattachment and technique refinements to prevent complications following total hip arthroplasty. *Clin. Orthop.*, 183:82, 1984.
2. Amstutz, H.C., and Maki, S.: Complications of trochanteric osteotomy in total hip replacement. *J. Bone Joint Surg.*, 60A:214, 1978.
3. Amstutz, H.C., and Yao, J.: Trochanteric nonunion (ch. 33, pp. 457–468). In: *Hip Arthroplasty*. Churchill Livingstone, 1991.
4. Amstutz, H.C., Yao, J., and Leipzig, J.: Results of trochanteric osteotomy in total hip arthroplasty. Submitted.
5. Boardman, K.P., Bocco, F., and Charnley, J.: An evaluation of a method of trochanteric fixation using three wires in Charnley low-friction arthroplasty of the hip. *Clin. Orthop.*, 132:31, 1978.
6. Browne, A.O., and Sheehan J.M.: Trochanteric osteotomy in Charnley low-friction arthroplasty of the hip. *Clin. Orthop.*, 211:128, 1986.
7. Dall, D.M.: Cable techniques for trochanteric and femoral allograft fixation. *Techniques Orthop.*, 6(3):7, 1991.
8. Glassman, A.H.: Complications of trochanteric osteotomy. *Orthop. Clin. North Amer.*, 23(2):321, 1992.
9. Jensen, N.F., and Harris, W.H.: A system for trochanteric osteotomy and reattachment for total hip arthroplasty with ninety-nine percent union rate. *Clin. Orthop.*, 208:174, 1986.
10. Schutzer, S.F., and Harris, W.H.: Trochanteric osteotomy for revision total hip arthroplasty. *Clin. Orthop.*, 227:172, 1988.
11. Thomas, B., Amstutz, H.C., and Yao, J.: Surgical approaches to the hip joint (ch. 17, pp. 457–468). In: *Hip Arthroplasty*. Churchill Livingstone, 1991.
12. Wroblewski, B.M.: Reattachment of the greater trochanter after hip replacement. *J. Bone J.S.*, 67B:736, 1985.

4

Anterior Lateral Approach

Paul J. P. Pongor and Maurice E. Müeller

Originally described by Watson-Jones (8) the anterolateral approach allows for excellent exposure of the femoral neck and acetabulum without the need for a trochanteric osteotomy. By largely passing in front of the gluteus medius, the anterolateral approach limits damage to this important hip abductor. However, in order to obtain an adequate exposure, the more anterior fibers of the gluteus medius require division.

The anterolateral approach may be indicated for patients with scarring or otherwise inappropriate soft tissues for either direct, lateral, or posterior approach. It is particularly useful for patients in whom the risk of posterior dislocation is great or who have neurological conditions such as Parkinson's disease, spasticity, or severe flexion deformity. The anterolateral approach is particularly useful in patients undergoing bilateral simultaneous total hip arthroplasty in that the patient is operated on in a supine position making it unnecessary to reposition, reprep and redrape the patient. An assessment of leg length is facilitated by having the patient in the supine position with both lower extremities available for visual inspection.

Having the patient in the supine position improves airway access and control as well as pulmonary mechanics. This is a particular advantage in elderly patients and in patients with respiratory difficulties, particularly patients with ankylosing spondylitis, in whom limited chest expansion may be further compromised by the lateral decubitus position. The position of the acetabular component is easier to judge from the anterolateral approach than from lateral or posterior approaches, and the dislocation rate is very low, probably due to a combination of visualization of the acetabular component from this approach and the ability to judge its position more accurately. The incidence of heterotopic ossification is also very low. A particular advantage of the anterolateral approach is that the incidence of injury to the abductor muscles is extremely low, particularly when compared to the direct lateral approach.

The anterolateral approach is contraindicated in obese and/or heavily muscled patients, and the incision is not easily extended if wider exposure is needed—for example, if there are unexpected defects in the posterior rim of the acetabulum that need to be addressed.

P. J. P. Pongor, M.D.: Department of Surgery, Beth Israel Deaconess Hospital, Boston, Massachusetts 02215.
M. E. Müeller: Lindenhof Hospital, CH-3001 Bern, Switzerland.

PREOPERATIVE PLANNING

Careful preoperative planning is essential to ensure the expected operative outcome. Preoperative planning provides information about the appropriate prosthesis, depth of acetabular reaming, and the level of the femoral neck resection, as well as correct positioning and orientation of the components. The plan ensures that the surgeon has anticipated potential intraoperative difficulties such as the resection of osteophytes, acetabular bone grafting, or need for a trochanteric osteotomy. Significant leg length discrepancies are also addressed within the preoperative plan. A carefully prepared preoperative plan requires an anteroposterior (AP) radiograph of the pelvis including the proximal third of both femurs, component templates, tracing paper, a black pencil to silhouette the bones, and a red pencil to silhouette the implant.

After selecting the appropriate implant, three tracings are made of the preoperative AP radiograph. The first tracing (tracing A) follows the bony contours of the healthy hemipelvis, the greater and lesser trochanters, and the inner borders of the medullary canal. The second tracing (tracing B) follows the bony contours of the diseased hemipelvis. The last tracing (tracing C) is of the of the diseased femoral head and neck, greater trochanter, lesser trochanter, and medullary canal contours. The actual planning is a four-step process. (Fig. 1)

Step 1: Tracing A, the healthy hemipelvis, is superimposed on the template of the chosen implant. When the outer diameter of the acetabular component corresponds with the weight-bearing segment of the acetabular contour, the socket is outlined on the drawing. At the same time, the medial edge of the femoral stem has to touch the inner border of the medial femoral cortex. With offset reproduced, the trochanteric reference line (T), the femoral resection line (F), and the outlines of both trochanters and the femoral prosthesis are added to the tracing.

Step 2: Tracing B, the diseased hemipelvis, is now superimposed on an inverted tracing A. The pelvic silhouettes roughly coincide. The acetabular component is now copied at its anatomic locations. This helps determine the depth of acetabular reaming.

Step 3: Tracing C, the diseased femoral silhouette, is superimposed on the inverted tracing A in such a way that the trochanters are at the same level. The trochanteric reference line (T), and the resection line (R), as well as the silhouette of the chosen

Figure 1. Planning for the anterolateral approach is a four-step process.

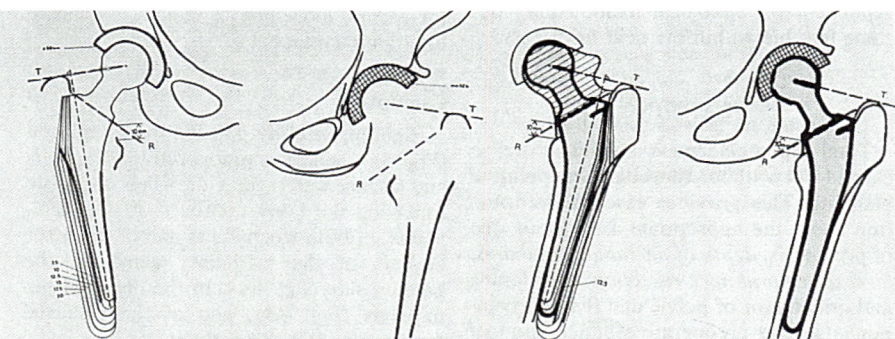

Fig. 8. Example 1 for preoperative planning. Healthy hip on the right, coxarthrosis on the left. Equal leg length is aimed for. Radiograph of healthy and diseased hemipelvis. (A) On the healthy side tracings of contours of pelvis, both trochanters, and inner borders of medullary canal. (B) On the diseased side tracings of pelvis; (C) and femur. (D) The template for the regular-stem prosthesis. (A') Tracing A superimposed on the template in such a way that the socket corresponds to the level of the acetabulum and the medial edge of the stem touches the medial border of the medullary canal. (Note: In some instances slight adjustments are necessary to compensate for variations in medialization/lateralization of the femoral shaft. By doing this, leg length must not be altered.) Socket and reference lines T and R are drawn in. The distances between tip of greater trochanter and T-line and lesser trochanter and R-line are measured and entered. Note: Use adapted ruler of the template. (B') Tracing B superimposed on turned tracing A'. The pelvic contours should be matched. The socket is drawn in. (C') Tracing C is first superimposed on tracing B'. Both trochanters should be matched. Enter the two reference lines. Now transfer tracing C over the template and move it in such a way that the medial edge of the prosthesis touches the inner border of the medial cortex while the reference lines coincide. Draw in the largest prosthesis. (D') The composite of B' and C' equals the prospective postoperative result.

femoral prosthesis are carefully drawn onto the tracing C. If the medullary canals do not match, the stem size may be adjusted with the aid of an appropriate femoral component template.

Step 4: Finally, tracing B, the diseased hemiplevis, is superimposed on tracing C, the diseased proximal femur, and the nonresected femoral portion and the chosen prosthesis are drawn in. The composite corresponds to the anticipated postoperative result.

Although the procedure at first may seem confusing, the four steps allow the surgeon to base the reconstruction on the healthy hip, helping to ensure the correction of the leg length discrepancies and reproducing appropriate biomechanical offset.

OPERATIVE TECHNIQUE

Patient Positioning

The procedure can be performed with the patient supine or in the lateral decubitus position using a modified Kocher approach. The supine position may be preferred with its advantage in facilitating correct positioning of the prosthetic components during the procedure. In addition to the standard instruments used for the insertion of a total replacement, special instruments, such as narrow-tipped retractors, greatly facilitate exposure and help avoid damage to surrounding neurovascular structures.

INITIAL INCISION AND SUPERFICIAL DISSECTION

Originally the incision was described as curved, 12 to 15 cm in length, and starting from the midpoint of a line joining the anterosuperior iliac spine to the tip of the greater trochanter. The distal part of the incision was to parallel the femoral shaft with the angle between these two arms of the incision approximately 130 degrees, its apex of the incision positioned just behind the greater trochanter (5). Correct position of the apex was felt to be important for allowing adequate access to the exposed femoral neck later in the procedure (Fig. 2). More recently, however, a straighter, less curved incision has been

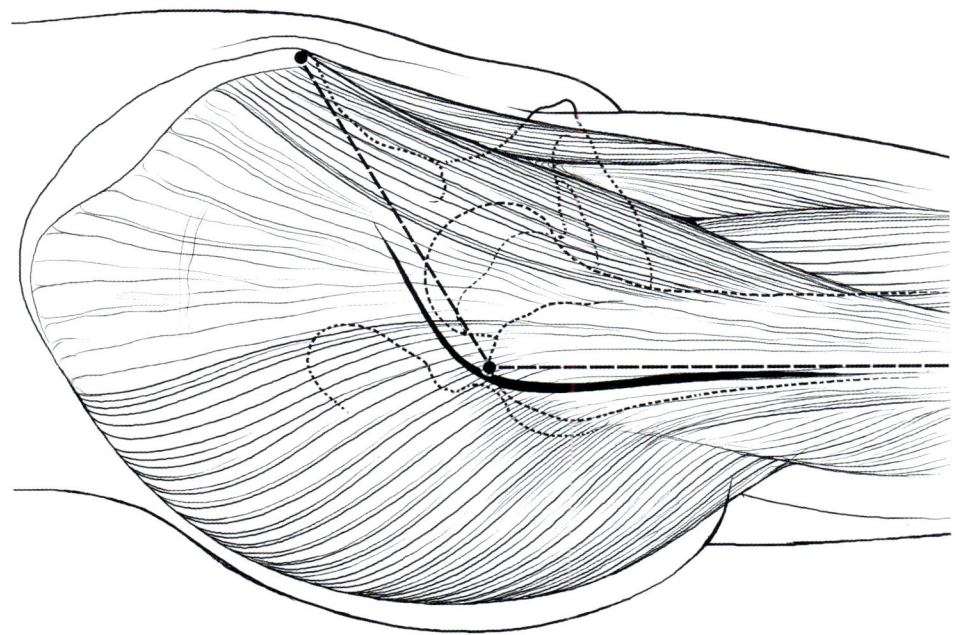

Figure 2. The incision as it was originally described is curved, 12 to 15 cm in length, and beginning at the midpoint of a line from the anterosuperior iliac spine to the tip of the greater trochanter. The distal portion is parallel to the femoral shaft with an angle of approximately 130 degrees between the two arms of the incision. The apex of the incision is positioned just behind the greater trochanter to allow adequate access to the femoral neck.

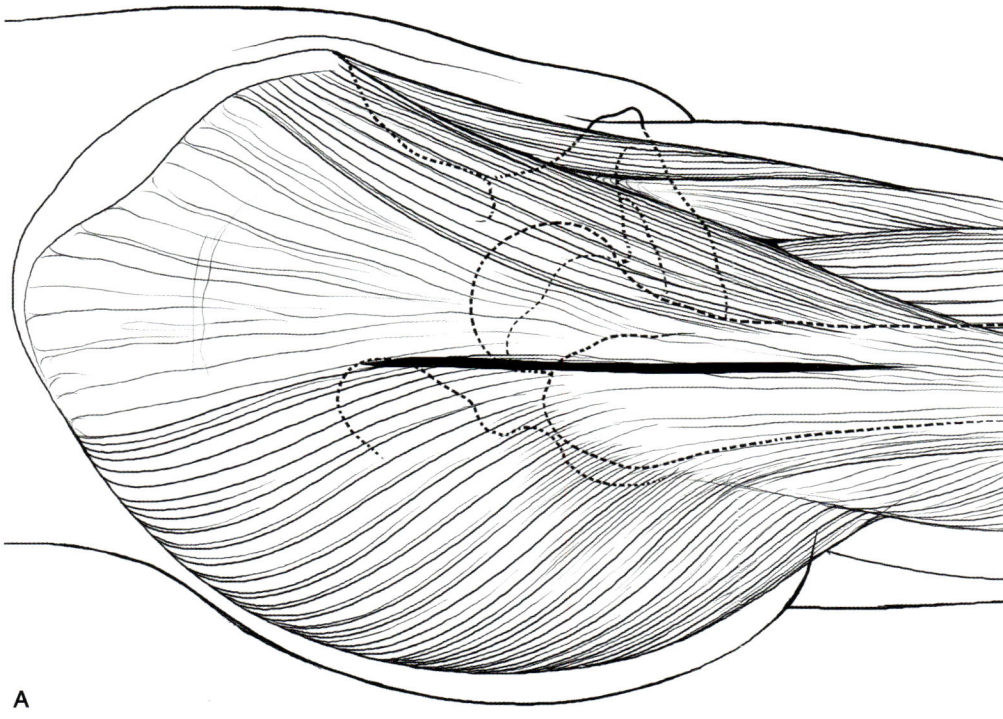

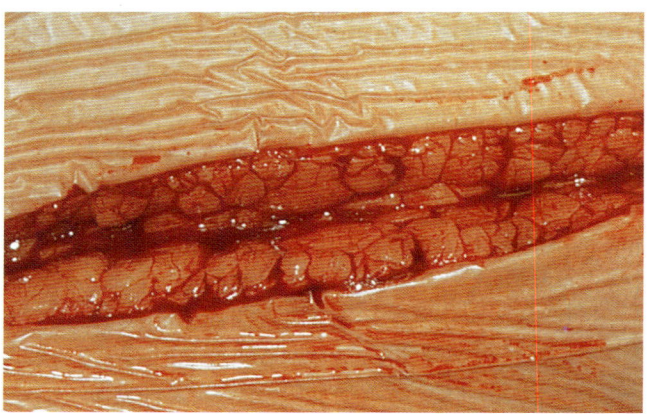

Figure 3 A, B. A less curved incision than described in Fig. 2 has also been described and should be used in obese patients.

advocated (Fig. 3). A similar incision is used to incise the underlying iliotibial band. In obese patients, the incision should be straight and longer in length.

Deep Dissection

The hip joint is approached in the interval between the tensor fascia lata and glutei, sparing the nerve to the tensor fascia lata (Fig. 4). The branch of the superior gluteal nerve to the tensor fasciae lies in this interval and should be carefully protected during this approach.

A transverse incision is used to release the anterior third of the distal attachment of the gluteus medius from the lateral aspect of the trochanter. Development of the interval between the gluteus medius and minimus may be aided by placing a bone hook around the

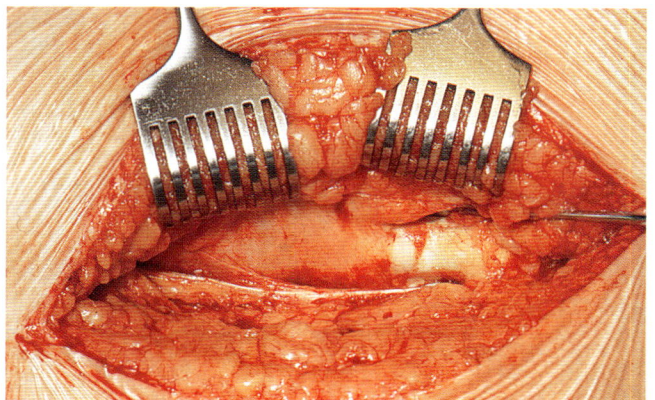

Figure 4. The tensor fascia lata and glutei are divided, being careful to spare the nerve to the tensor fascia lata.

gluteus medius, applying proximal tension, and then sharply dividing the anterior fibers of the medius until the bursa between the gluteus minimus and the greater trochanter is opened (Fig. 5). This will expose the gluteus minimus tendon underneath. The tendon of the gluteus minimus is cut approximately 1 cm from its attachment to the ventral aspect of the greater trochanter and tagged for later repair (Fig. 6b). If necessary, more of the gluteus medius may be released to avoid damaging the muscle during the procedure.

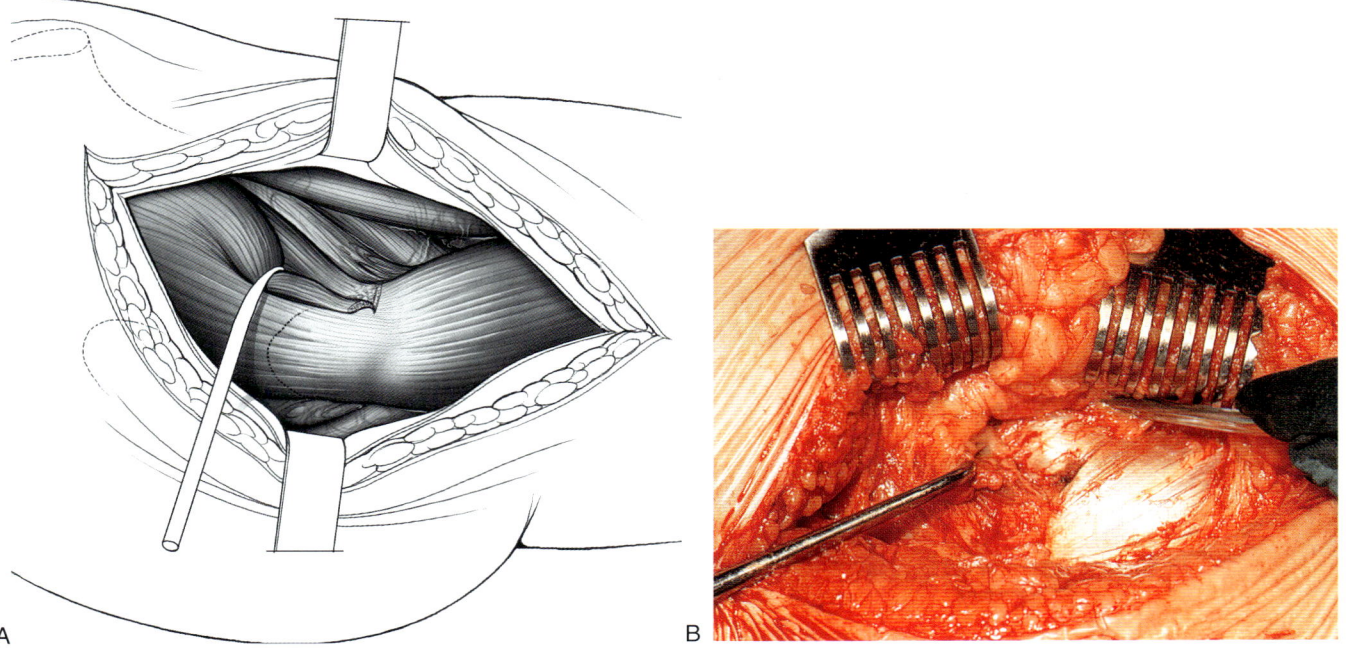

Figure 5. (A) The anterior third of the distal attachment of the gluteus maximus is released from the lateral aspect of the trochanter by means of a transverse incision. The interval between the gluteus medius and minimus is aided by placing a bone hook around the gluteus medius, applying proximal tension and sharply dividing the anterior fibers of the medius to open the bursa between the gluteus minimus and the greater trochanter. (B) Intraoperative photograph showing the division of the gluteus medius and minimus.

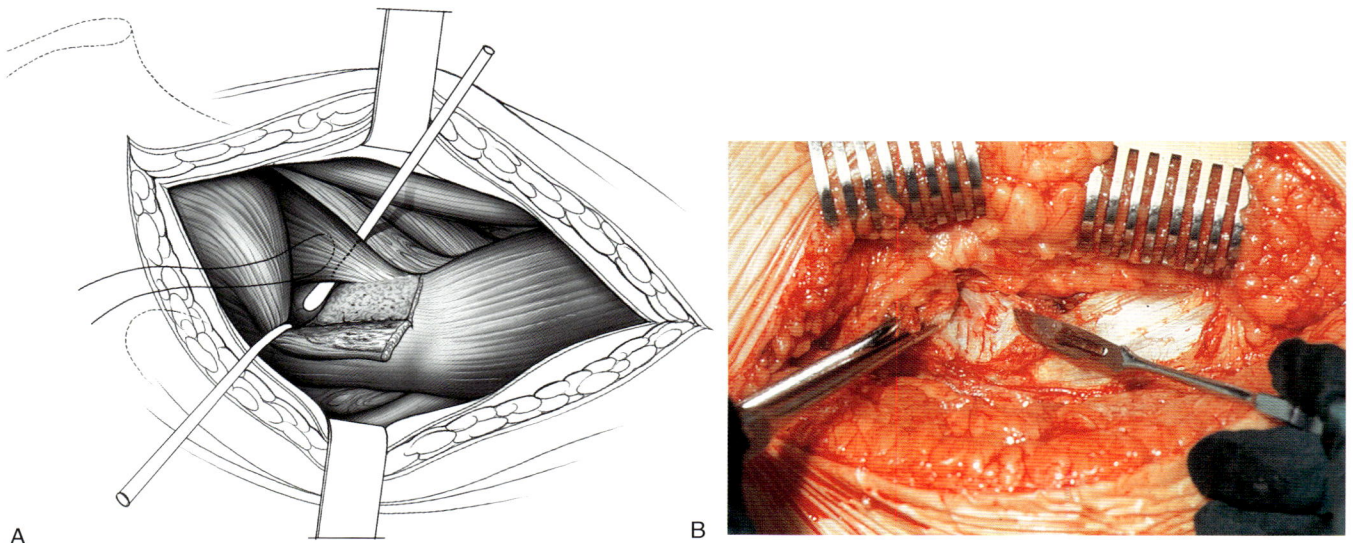

Figure 6 A, B. The tendon of the gluteus minimus is cut and tagged for later repair.

Joint Capsule Exposure

Three long, narrow-pointed lever-retractors are carefully positioned within the wound: Two are placed on the capsule on each side of the neck and the third behind the anterior rim of the acetabulum (Fig. 7). Great care must be taken to ensure that this last retractor is in contact with bone rather than slipping into the soft tissues anterior to the acetabular rim and damaging the femoral nerve (Fig. 5a). A large, T-shaped capsular incision is then made. On either side of the exposed femoral neck, two blunt-tipped retractors are placed between the neck and the joint capsule. These three retractors encircle the neck and protect the structures behind the joint (Fig. 8). Excision of the capsule should be as complete as possible in order to permit an easy dislocation of the stump of the neck. Often, especially with an external rotation contraction, the short external rotators require division during capsular excision (2).

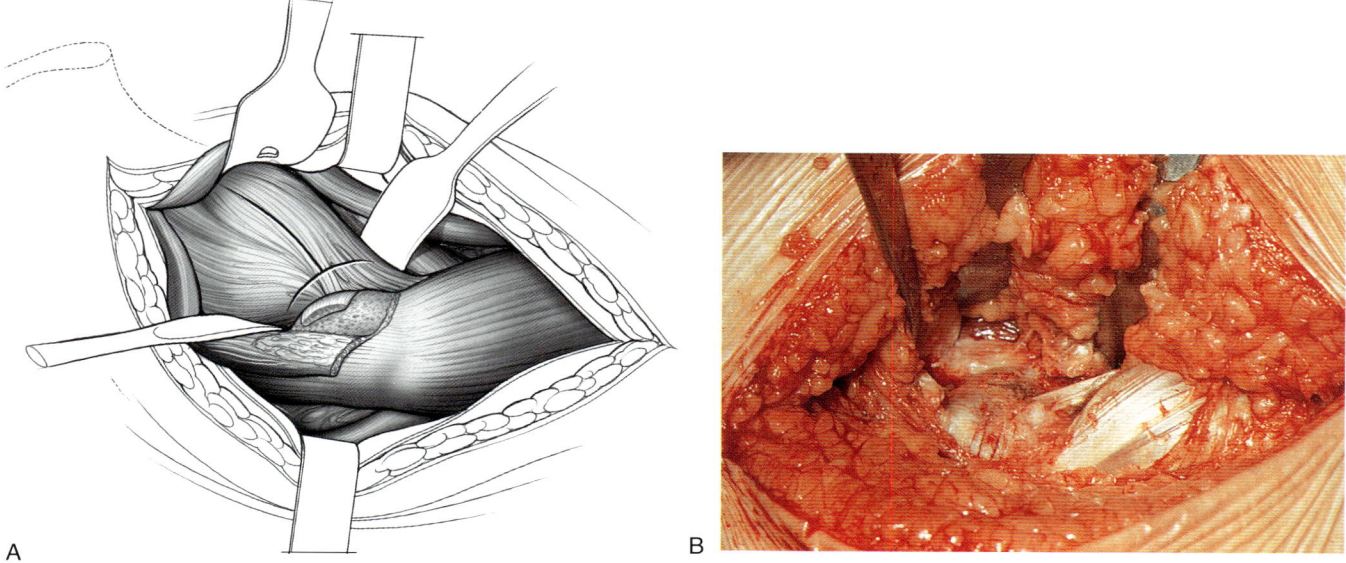

Figure 7 A, B. Two long, narrow-pointed retractors are placed on the capsule on each side of the neck, and a third long, narrow-pointed retractor is placed behind the rim of the acetabulum.

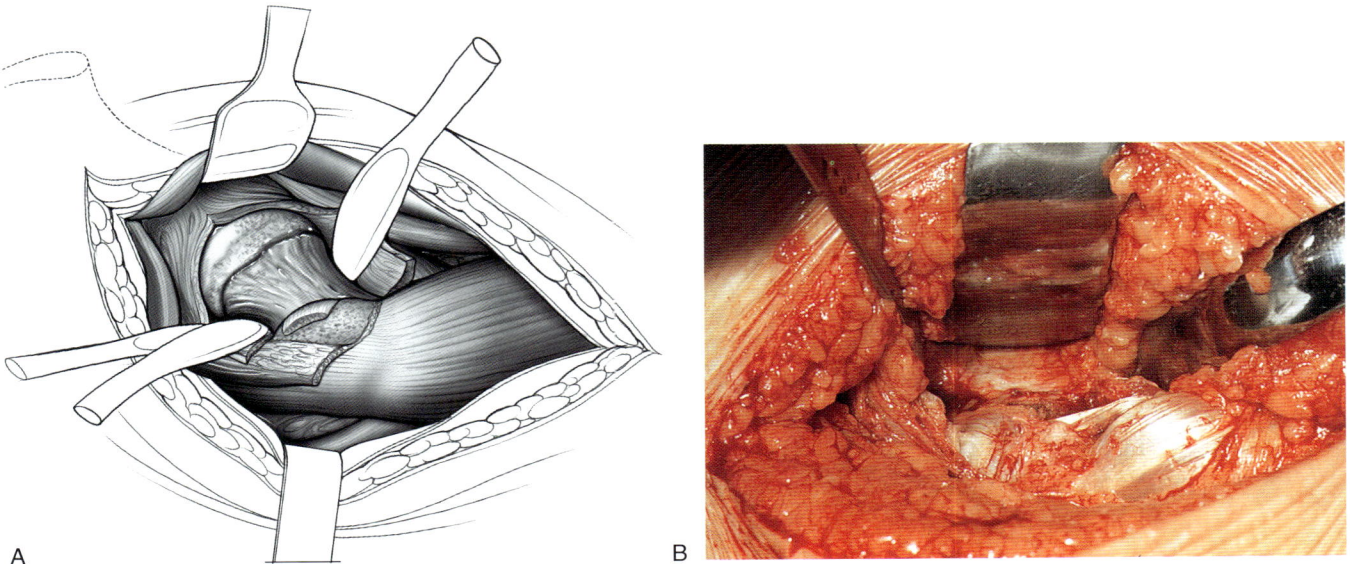

Figure 8 A, B. The three retractors are used to encircle the femoral neck and protect the structures behind the joint.

Femoral Neck Division and Femoral Head Removal

The femoral neck is now adequately exposed to allow for a safe, controlled division with the aid of an oscillating saw. A flat chisel is then introduced between the bony surfaces and is used to spread the osteotomy (Fig. 9). This helps ensure that the division of the femoral neck is complete. A corkscrew is deeply inserted into the femoral head with a lever introduced between the two articular surfaces to aid in dislocation of the resected femoral head (Fig. 10). If dislocation is not possible because of a severely deformed joint, fragmentation of the head with a chisel may be necessary (4).

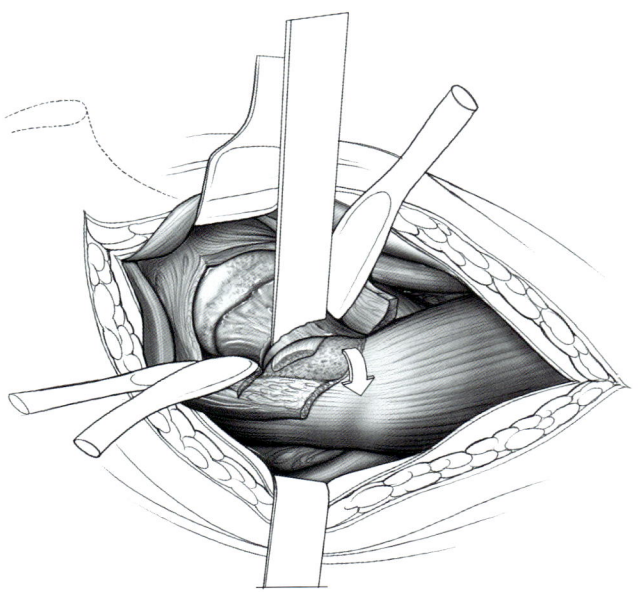

Figure 9. Use of a flat chisel to spread the osteotomy.

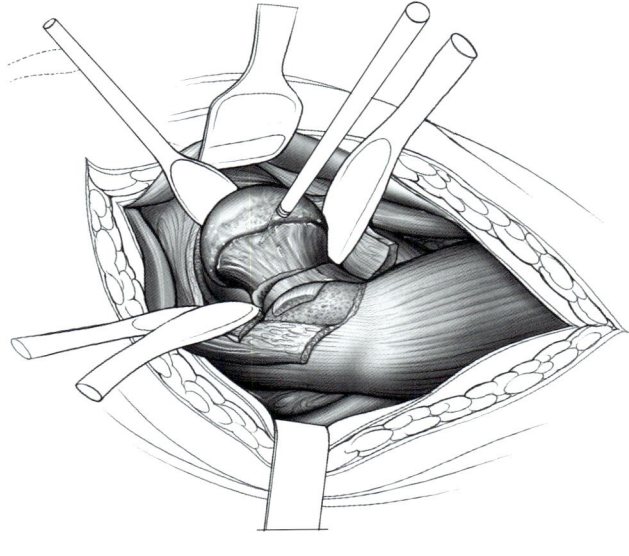

Figure 10. A corkscrew, deeply inserted into the femoral head, with a lever introduced between the articular surfaces, aids in dislocation of the femoral head.

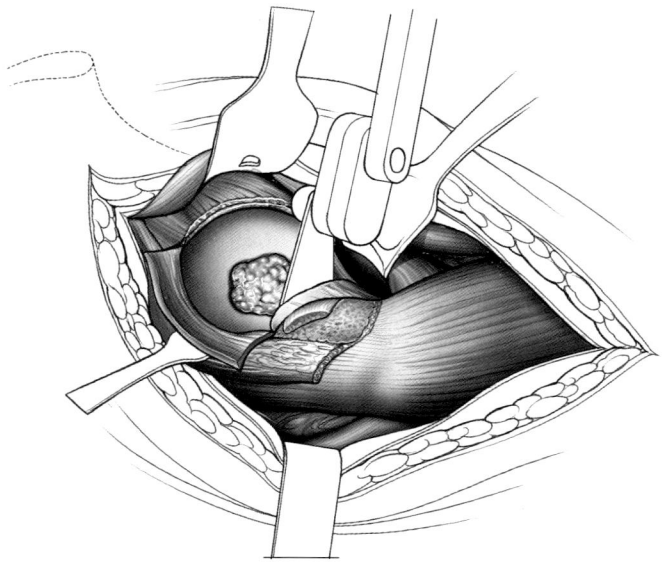

Figure 11. An oscillating saw is used to trim the femoral neck definitively.

Completion of the Femoral Neck Division

The leg is now gently externally rotated. With the oscillating saw, the femoral neck is definitively trimmed 1 or 2 cm above the lesser trochanter as previously calculated on the graphic preoperative plan (Fig. 11). The line of resection should be almost perpendicular to the bicondylar axis of the knee and should also form an angle of 45 degrees with the femoral diaphysis. With the knee orientation used as the point of reference, the goal of 10 degrees of femoral anteversion is also carefully considered during the trimming of the femoral neck.

Capsular Excision

The remainder of the anterior aspect of the capsule is excised along with the incision of the posterior aspect of the capsule to permit easy delivery of the femoral neck stump into the wound (Fig. 12). To protect the iliopsoas tendon, it is necessary to identify its course prior to incision of the capsule. One must also remain attentive to the course of the femoral nerve, the femoral artery, and the femoral veins running along the anteroinferior aspect of the capsule. A separate incision is occasionally necessary to repair these structures if they are inadvertently injured while the remainder of the capsule is addressed. With excessively thick capsules, it is occasionally difficult to incise the posterior capsule or excise the remainder of the anterior capsule. The use of a bone hook helps facilitate this step. Care should be taken to identify and coagulate all bleeding vessels exposed during capsular excision.

Positioning of Acetabular Retractors

In order to gain adequate exposure of the acetabulum, correct positioning of the acetabular retractors is essential. A long-handled curved retractor is inserted over the anterior lip of the acetabulum. The teeth of a second retractor are positioned around the posterior inferior acetabular rim and used to depress the proximal femur. In placing this femoral retractor, it is necessary slightly to abduct and flex the thigh. This will allow the teeth of the retractor to be placed underneath the posterior inferior acetabular rim. The femoral retractor

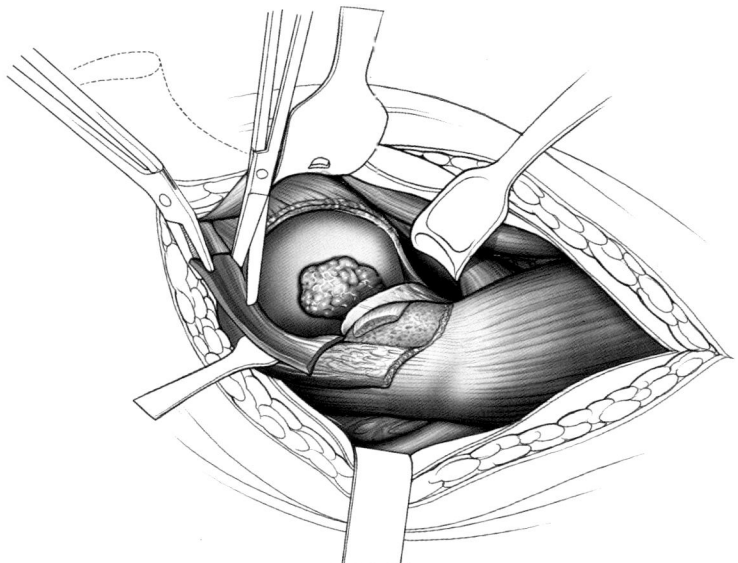

Figure 12. The anterior aspect of the capsule is excised to permit easy delivery of the femoral neck stump into the wound.

may then be fixed in place by hammering the points into the bone. Hooking a weight to the retractor and clamping it to the patient's thigh drape eliminates the necessity of manual retraction. Finally, a third, short-pointed retractor is placed into the superior rim of the acetabulum (Fig. 13). This should allow for full 360 degree exposure of the acetabulum. Again, care should be taken to ensure that the retractors are kept close to bone to avoid serious neurovascular complications.

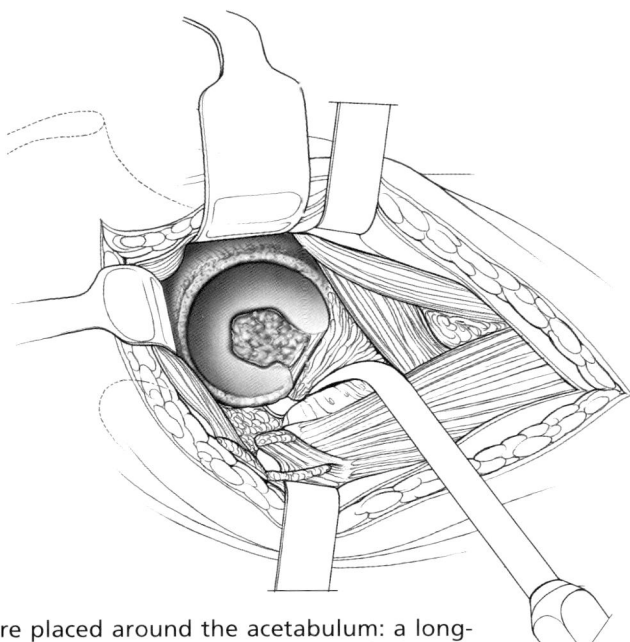

Figure 13. Three retractors are placed around the acetabulum: a long-handled curved retractor over the anterior lip of the acetabulum, a tooth retraced around the posterior inferior acetabular rim, and a short-pointed retractor into the superior rim of the acetabulum.

Preparation of the Acetabular Bed/Insertion of Component

The acetabulum is now optimally exposed to allow preparation of the bed for insertion of the component. Classically, the acetabulum is fashioned with flat and swan-neck chisels to first remove the osteophytes. Deepening of the acetabulum is performed with hand or power reaming. Care must be taken to avoid excessive weakening of the floor, which could eventually lead to fatigue fractures of the pelvis. The component may be inserted after adequate preparation of the bed. Proper orientation of the socket is essential. The aim is to achieve 42 to 45 degrees of inclination (Fig. 14) and 5 to 15 degrees of anteversion (Fig. 14B) in order to obtain a range of flexion of 110 degrees or more.

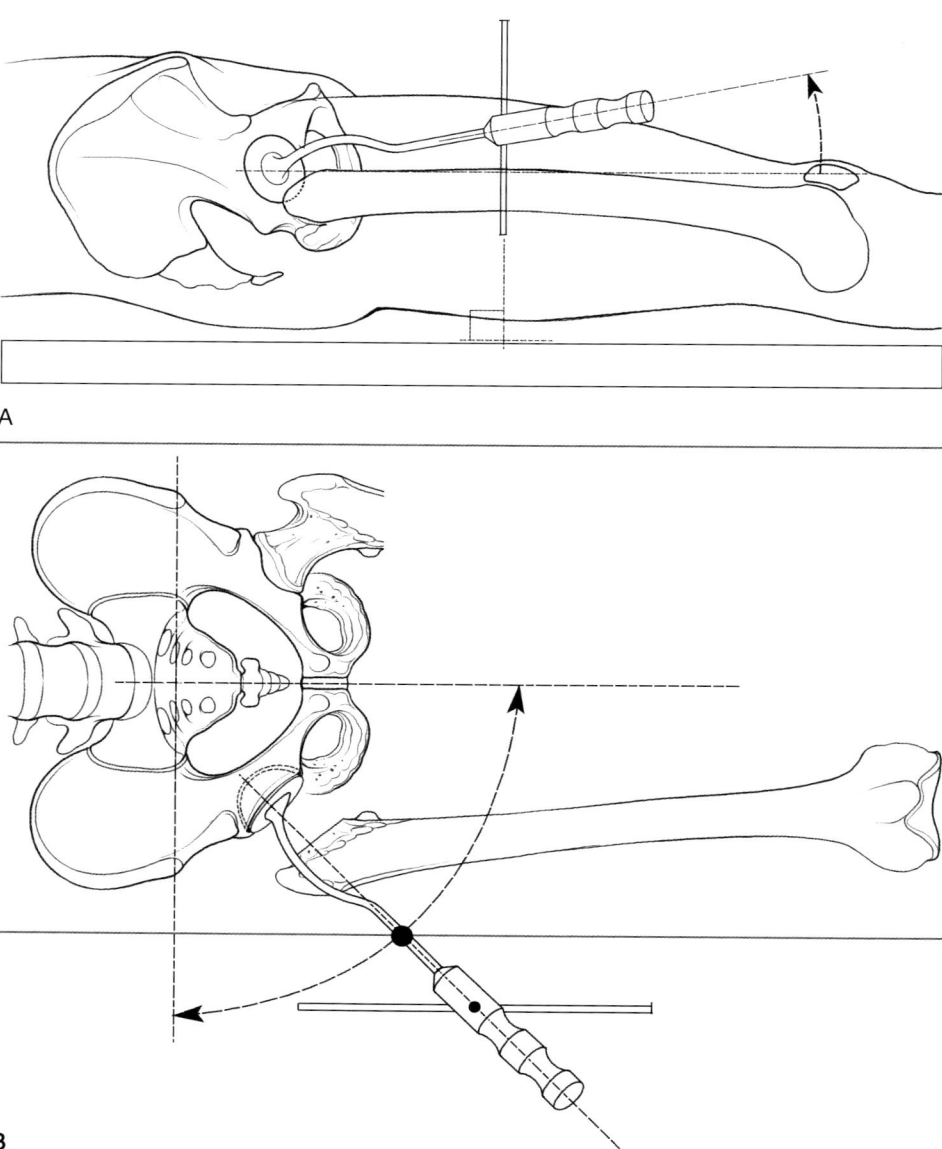

Figure 14. After preparation of the acetabular bed and insertion of the component, the socket is oriented with (A) an inclination of 42 to 45 degrees and (B) 5 to 15 degrees of anteversion in order to obtain a range of flexion of 110 degrees or more.

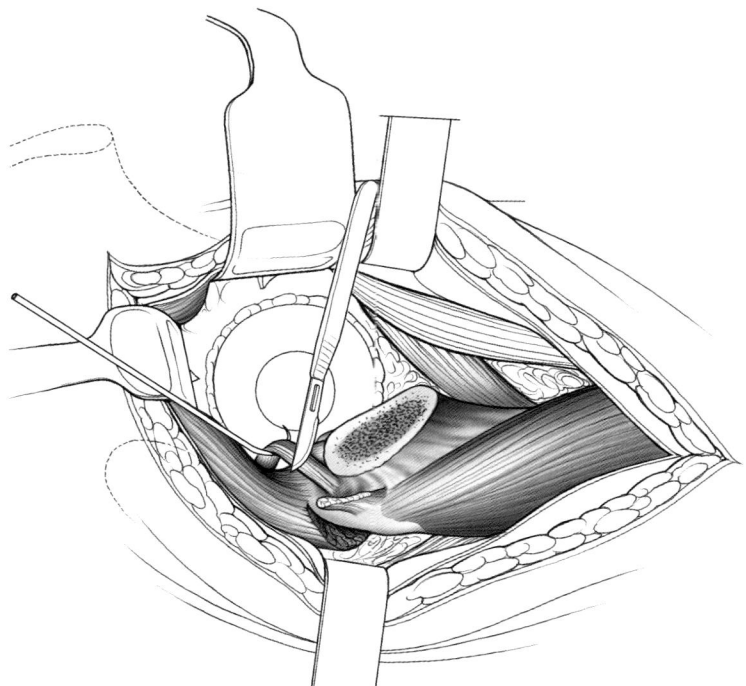

Figure 15. Dividing the piriformis near its insertion to the tip of the greater trochanter can be used to release excessive tension.

Periacetabular Soft-Tissue Examination

After completion of the insertion of the acetabular component, an examination of the soft tissue tension is in order. With preoperative external rotation deformities, division of the piriformis muscle may be required. This can be examined by placing the limb in internal rotation. If excessive tension is noted, the piriformis may be pulled forward with a bone hook and carefully divided near its insertion to the tip of the greater trochanter (Fig. 15). With very stiff hips, all external rotators may require division; however, the quadratus femoris should not be divided. Transection of the quadratous femoris with inadvertent division of its accompanying artery could lead to a serious postoperative hematoma. All sources of bleeding should be visualized and coagulated at this point.

Femoral Neck Exposure and Preparation

A wide self-retaining retractor is placed under the greater trochanter to aid in lifting the femur anteriorly. The leg is then pulled in external rotation and maximal flexion and adduction until the heel touches the contralateral shoulder (Fig. 16A). The glutei are protected by a second small retractor. A third small retractor is placed under the psoas (Fig. 16B). The distance between the division of the neck and the lesser trochanter is first palpated and then measured. This measurement is compared to the distance previously estimated on the preoperative plan, and the neck cut is adjusted as required. The base of the femoral neck is first prepared using a chisel to gouge out cancellous bone from the center of the neck (Fig. 16C).

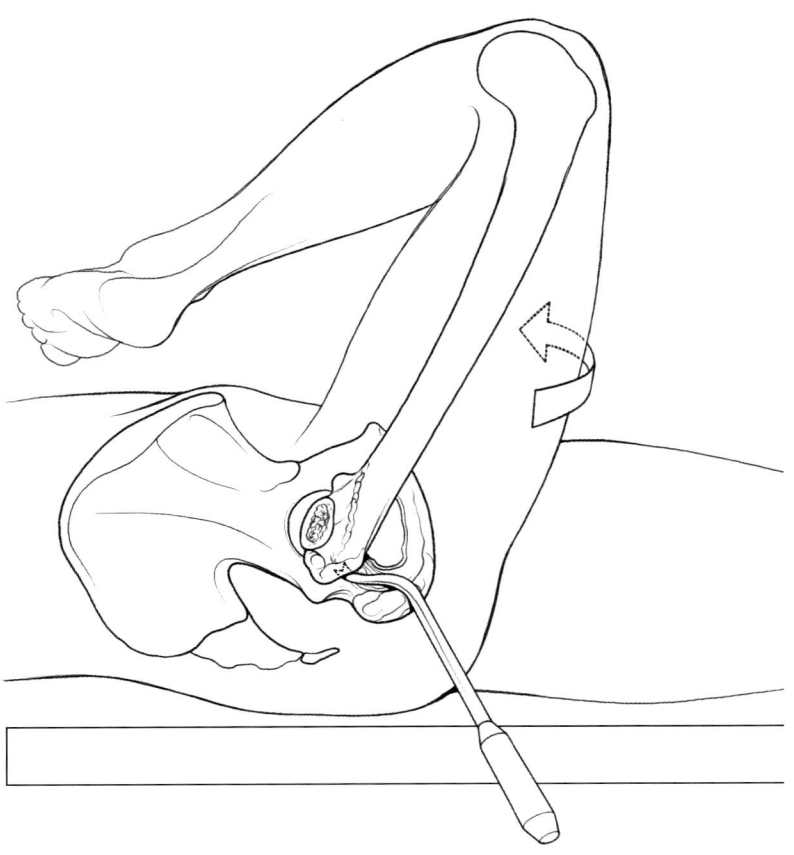
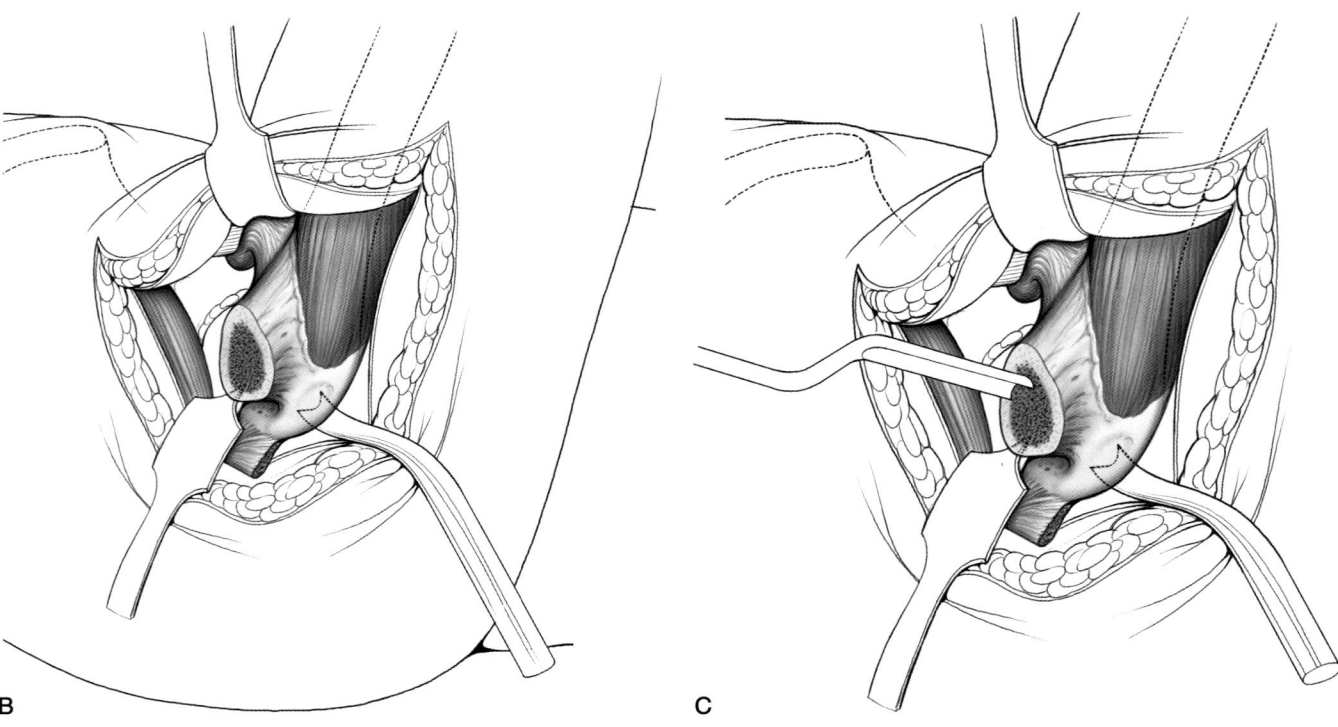

Figure 16. The femoral neck is exposed and prepared in three steps: (A) External rotation is used to achieve maximal flexion and adduction until the heel touches the contralateral shoulder. (B) the glutei and psoas muscles are retracted (C) a chisel is used to gouge out cancellous bone from the neck.

Femoral Medullary Canal Preparation

The femoral canal is explored using a long curette (Fig. 17). This exploration is essential; without a proper exploration, it is difficult to establish the exact direction of the canal and determine whether the cut surface of the neck is sufficiently clear for reaming. This step also helps avoid perforation of the cortex with the rasp. The neck must be perfectly visualized, and if it is not, adjust the position of the leg. The remainder of the medullary canal is prepared guided by the hip system chosen and its instrumentation (Fig. 18). Regardless of the system, care should be taken to ensure that the anteversion of the new canal is no more that 10 degrees. During preparation of the femur, the broaches must be inserted as laterally as possible to avoid damage or perforation of the femoral shaft.

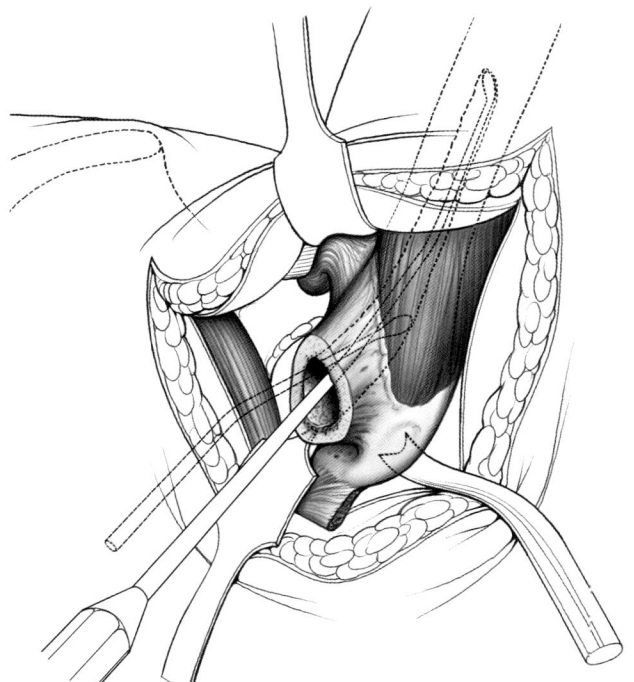

Figure 17. A long curette is used to explore the femoral canal.

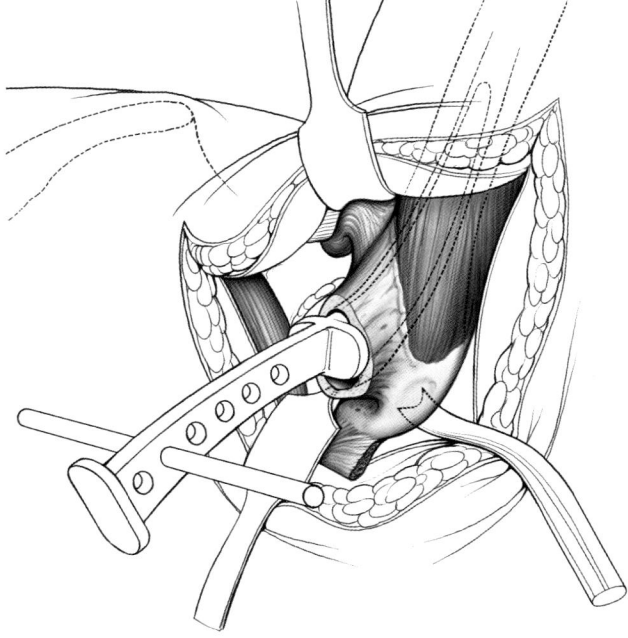

Figure 18. The remainder of the femoral canal is prepared using the hip system instrumentation.

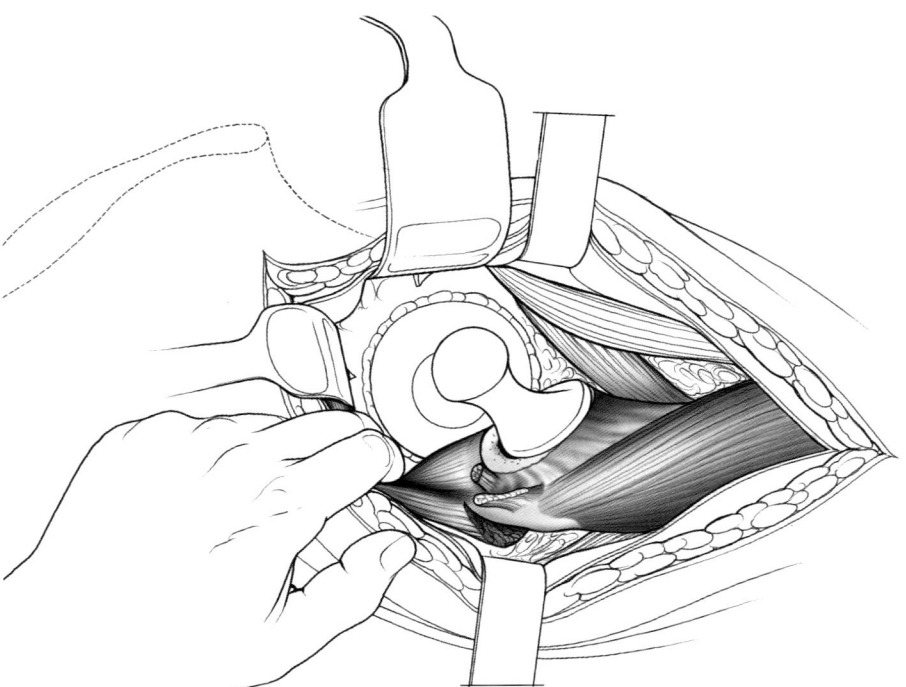

Figure 19. Two fingers are used to push the glutei aside and allow for prosthesis insertion.

Trial Prosthesis Insertion

The trial prosthesis is inserted after adequate canal preparation. The glutei are easily pushed aside with two fingers (Fig. 19). If a collared prosthesis is chosen and if the seat of the collar on the femoral cortex is not satisfactory, or if the distance between the lesser trochanter and the collar is not as previously calculated, the necessary corrections may be made with the oscillating saw. The hip is then gently reduced.

Assessing Component Orientation and Position

Once reduced, the orientation between the head and the cup can be carefully examined. Note the angle formed between the acetabular component and the base of the femoral head (Fig. 20); it is equal to the sum of the anteversion of the neck and the cup. This sum should measure approximately 20 to 30 degrees to allow for flexion of more than a right angle. Retracting the glutei with a right-angle retractor, a Kirschner wire is passed along the tip of the greater trochanter at right angles to the shaft, aiming toward the midline (Fig. 20). The distance between this Kirschner wire and the middle of the prosthetic femoral head can be measured and compared to the preoperative graphic plan. Again, adjustments in depth of insertion or orientation of the femoral component may be necessary. With hip in extension, the leg is rotated to bring patellar orientation in the sagittal plane to neutral. Anteversion of the femoral component in this position should measure approximately 10 to 15 degrees.

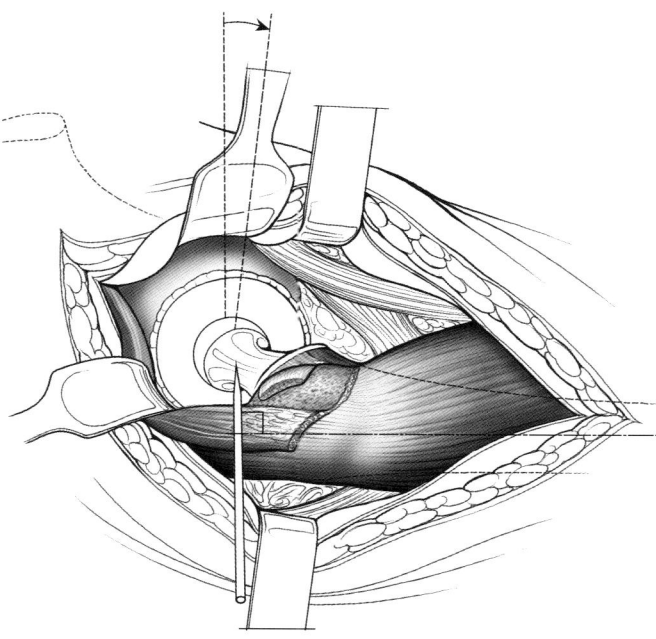

Figure 20. The angle between the acetabular component and the base of the femoral head is 20 to 30 degrees to allow for flexion of greater than 90 degrees.

Assessing Component Stability

The hip is next flexed to 90 degrees (Fig. 21). If internal rotation is restricted, further division of the posterior capsule and/or short external rotators may be necessary. Any tendency to dislocate should be assessed along with potential causes such as posterior impingement of the trochanter on residual posterior acetabular osteophytes. The prosthesis is

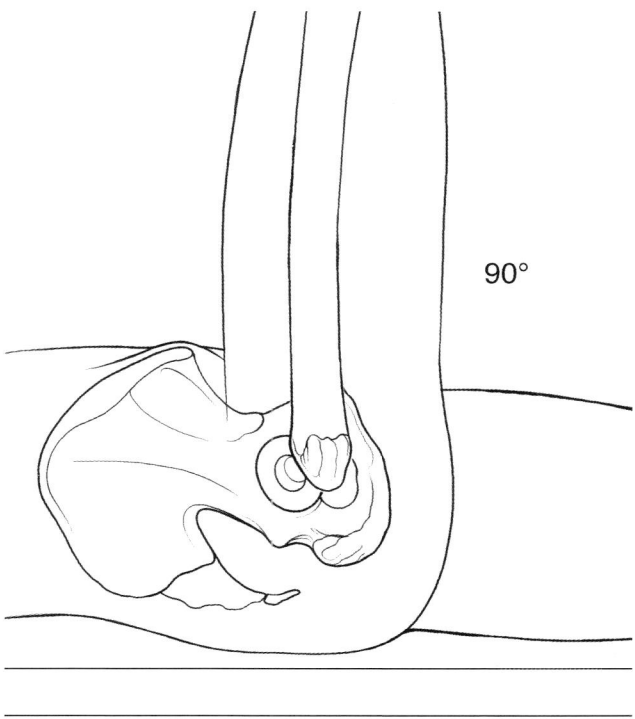

Figure 21. To assess component stability, the hip is flexed to 90 degrees.

then dislocated. The dislocation is aided by passing a hook around the neck of the prosthesis and applying traction to the leg in abduction and external rotation (Fig. 22).

Final Medullary Canal Preparation/Component Insertion

A sharp curette is used to remove all debris left during rasping of the canal (Fig. 23). If a cemented component is used, a medullary canal plug is placed and its depth carefully checked. A small suction tube is inserted into the medullary canal to the level of the canal plug to allow air and blood to escape during the pressurization and placement of the femoral component (Fig. 24).

After aggressive irrigation and antegrade insertion of cement using a cement gun fitted with a pressurization collar, the femoral prosthesis is inserted. Orientation of the prosthesis during insertion is important. Care must be taken to ensure that the prosthesis is introduced in a slightly valgus or neutral position.

During the last 2 cm of cement insertion, the suction tube is removed and the prosthesis is driven to its final position (Fig. 24B). Measurements are taken between the prosthesis and the lesser trochanter during insertion to ensure that the device has been precisely placed at its predetermined level. All excess cement and debris are removed while waiting for the cement to harden.

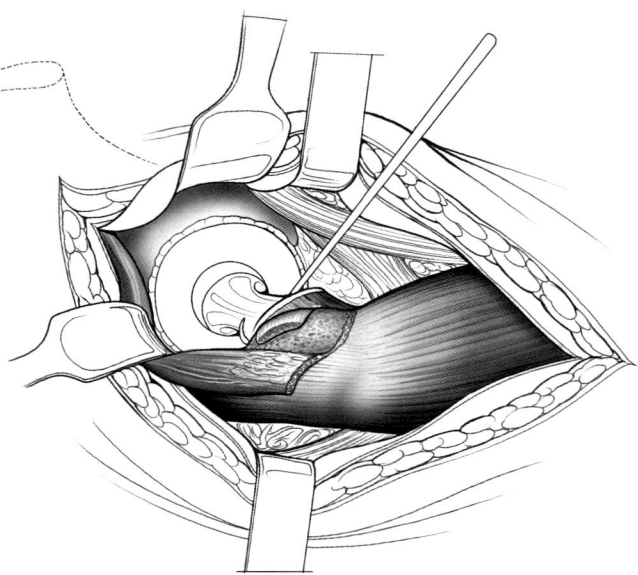

Figure 22. The prosthesis is dislocated by passing a hook around the neck of the prosthesis and applying traction to the abducted and externally rotated leg.

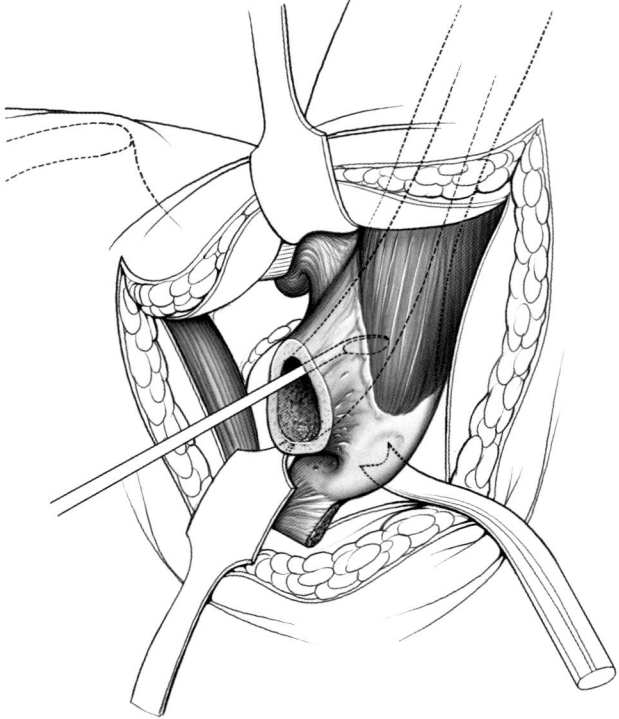

Figure 23. With a sharp curette, the femoral canal is cleaned of all debris left from rasping.

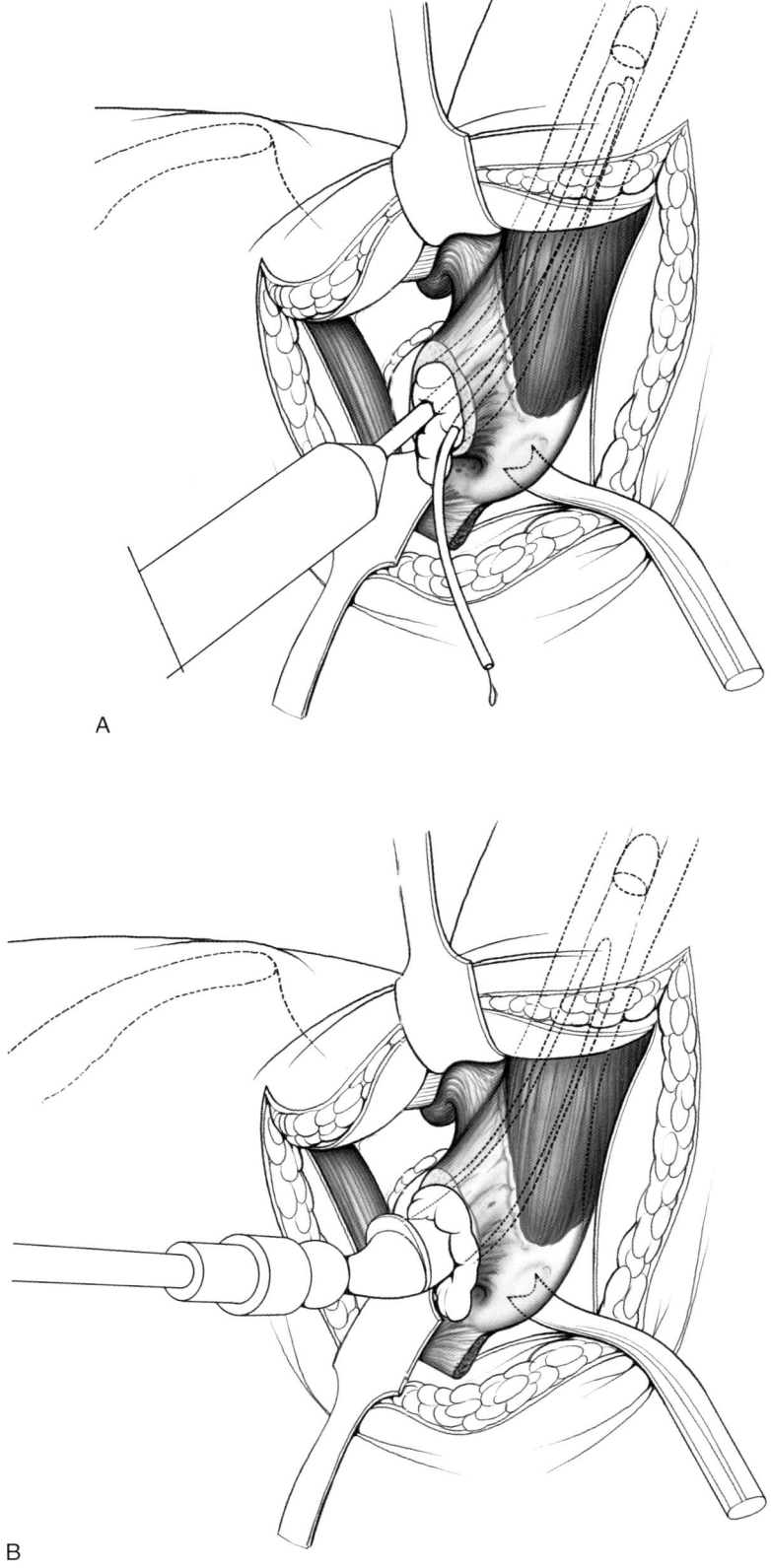

Figure 24. (A) A small suction tube, inserted into the medullary canal to the level of the cement plug, allows air and blood to escape during pressurization and insertion of the femoral prosthesis. (B) The tube is removed and the prosthesis is driven to its final position during the last two centimeters of cement insertion.

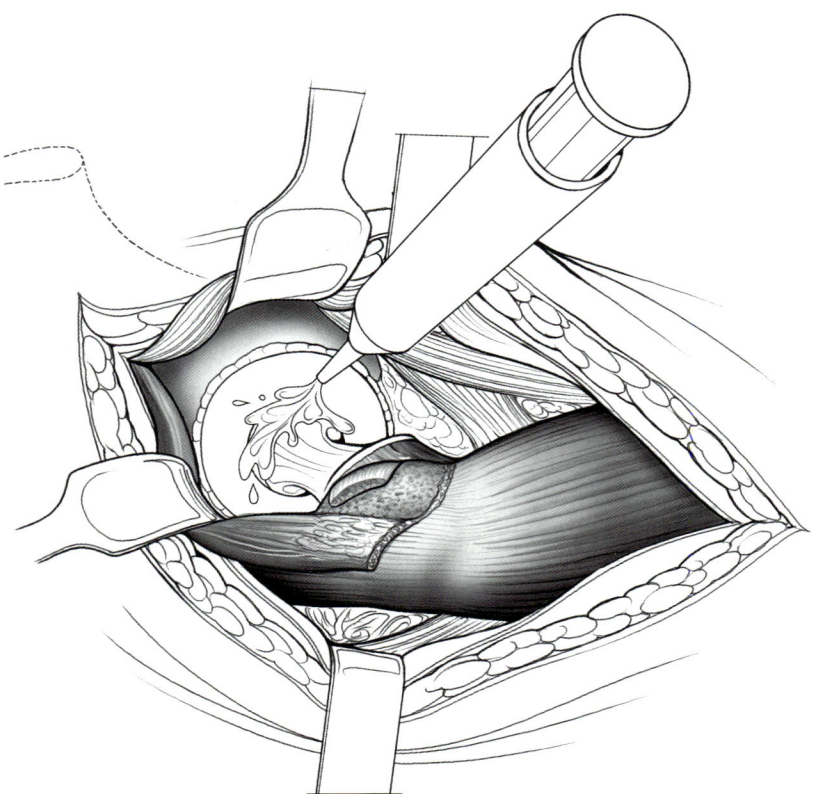

Figure 25. After reduction of the prosthesis, traction is applied to the leg, and the wound is copiously irrigated before closure.

Closure

The prosthesis is reduced. The distance between the lesser trochanter and femoral head as well as the distance between the perpendicular from the tip of the greater trochanter and the femoral head are remeasured and compared to the preoperative plan. Any evidence of posterior impingement may be addressed at this time. A careful check for bleeding, interposition of cement, bone debris, or soft tissue is carried out. With traction applied to the leg, the wound is copiously irrigated (Fig. 25).

The gluteus minimus tendon is sutured to its attachment. Also, the released anterior aspect of the gluteus medius is now sutured to the vastus lateralis. The soft tissue is carefully inspected for injured or crushed glutei and bony debris. If left behind, these may serve as a source of ectopic bone formation. Suction drains are placed, one at the level of the prosthesis and the second subcutaneously.

POSTOPERATIVE MANAGEMENT

Excessive soft tissue retraction, particularly when exposing the anterior aspect of the acetabulum can predispose to hetertrophic ossification. An excessive medius release with a poor repair may lead to a postoperative limp, another known complication of the anterolateral approach. Because of the concern with the abductor repair, ambulation is initiated with the aid of a cane on the contralateral extremity for the first six weeks. Once abductor strength is regained, full weight bearing may be allowed. Even with initiation of full weight bearing, abductor strengthening continues to be a focus of concentration.

COMPLICATIONS

As mentioned, major complications are less frequent with the anterolateral approach than with other approaches. Femoral nerve damage may occur either from improper placement of the anterior acetabular retractor with the tip not being kept on bone during insertion or by injury during coagulation of nearby vessels. The femoral nerve may also be damaged either directly during the process of drilling for acetabular fixation holes in the cemented use or by screw fixation in an uncemented acetabular component. In addition, if perforation occurs in the anterior acetabular shell and a cemented component is being used, cement extrusion may occur and damage the femoral nerve. Most injuries to the femoral nerve are transient and resolve spontaneously within 4 to 8 months.

Damage to the femoral artery and vein is also possible because of their proximity in this exposure. However, the portion of the operation during which these vascular structures are most vulnerable is during excision of the anterior capsule. With the anterolateral approach, the anterior capsule can be directly visualized, thus lessening the likelihood of injury to the anterior neurovascular structures.

ILLUSTRATIVE CASE

A 58-year-old female presented with pain in the right hip with limited function. Radiographs revealed advanced osteoarthritis of the right hip (Fig. 26). Because of her relative youth, a ceramic femoral head was chosen for her prosthesis (Fig. 27). She underwent replacement of the right hip without complications and at four years' follow-up, continued to function well without complaints (Fig. 28).

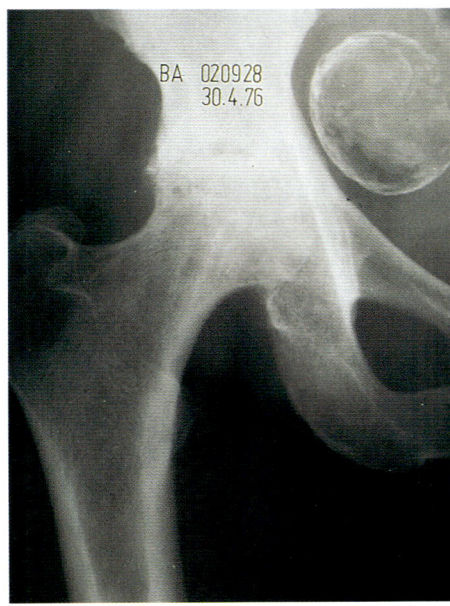

Figure 26. Preoperative radiograph shows primary arthrosis.

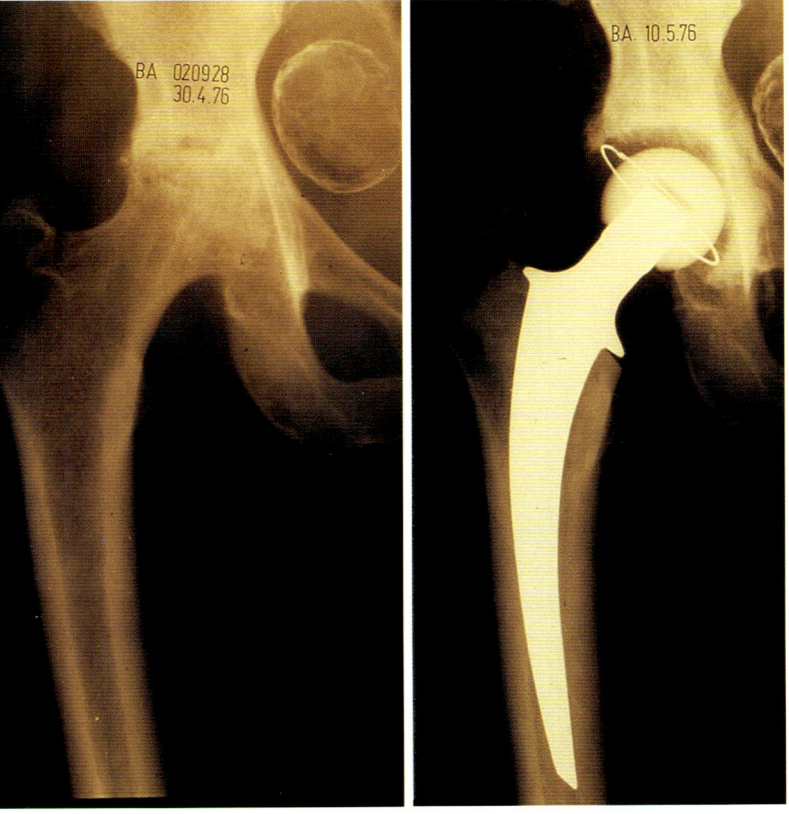

Figure 27. Anteropostero radiograph immediately after surgery shows implantation of a ceramic prosthesis.

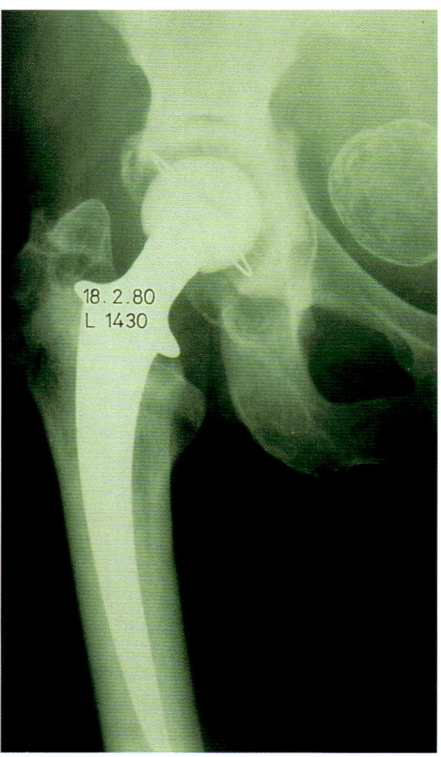

Figure 28. Anteropostero radiograph taken four years after surgery.

RECOMMENDED READING

1. Eftekhar, N. S.: Applied surgical approaches. In Eftekhar, N. S. (ed.): *Total Hip Arthroplasty*. Mosby, St. Louis 1993, p. 52.
2. Müller, M. E.: Total hip prostheses. *Clin. Orthop. Rel. Res.*, 72:46, 1970.
3. Müller, M. E.: Technique of total hip replacement. In Tronzo, R. G. (ed.): *Surgery of the Hip Joint*. Lea & Febiger, Philadelphia, 1973.
4. Müller, M. E.: Osteotomy of the greater trochanter. Part I: Total hip replacement without trochanteric osteotomy. In Harris, W. H. (ed.): *The Hip: Proceedings of the Second Open Scientific Meeting of the Hip Society, 1974*. Mosby, St Louis, 1974.
5. Müller, M. E.: Total hip replacement: Planning, technique, and complications. In Cruess, R. L., Mitchell, N. S. (eds.): *Surgical Management of Degerative Arthritis of the Lower Limb*. Philadelphia, Lea & Febiger, 1975, p. 91.
6. Müller, M. E.: Total Hip Reconstruction. In Evarts, C. M. (ed.): *Surgery of the Musculoskeletal System*. Edinborough, London, and New York, Churchill Livingstone, 1983, p. 223.
7. Nazarian, S., Tisserand, P. H., Brunet, C. H., Müller, M. E.: Anatomic basis of the transgluteal approach to the hip. *Surg. Radiol. Anat.*, 9:27, 1987.
8. Watson-Jones, R.: Fracture of the neck of the femur. *Brit. J. Surg.*, 23:787, 1935.

PART II

Fractures

5

Acetabular Fractures: Surgical Approaches and Technique

David L. Helfet, Arthur L. Malkani, and Craig S. Bartlett

INDICATIONS/CONTRAINDICATIONS

Current principles of acetabular fracture management have undergone some modifications but are largely based upon the classification scheme and surgical approaches initially described by Judet et al. (1,2) and altered slightly by Letournel et al. (3–6). Based upon their work, these authors have recommended operative fixation of all displaced acetabular fractures in order to restore the articular surface of the acetabulum and prevent posttraumatic arthritis.

The indications for operative fixation of acetabular fractures include displacement of the articular surface, incongruence of the joint, unacceptable roof arc measurements (7), incarceration of an intraarticular fragment within the joint, and any subluxation of the femoral head. The timing of surgery is dependent upon several factors including the availability of an experienced surgeon; stabilization of associated visceral, skeletal, and soft tissue injuries; and completion of all imaging studies necessary for preoperative planning. A femoral head dislocation or an incarcerated intraarticular fragment following closed reduction needs to be addressed promptly to minimize the incidence of femoral head avascular necrosis and posttraumatic arthritis.

PREOPERATIVE PLANNING

The preoperative evaluation begins with a thorough physical examination and appropriate trauma workup, including identification of all associated skeletal and visceral injuries. Patients with acetabular fractures often present with associated skeletal injuries to such

---

D. L. Helfet, M.D. and A. L. Malkani, M.D.: Department of Orthopaedics, Hospital for Special Surgery, New York, New York 10021.

C. S. Bartlett, M.D.: Orthopaedic Trauma Service, Hospital for Special Surgery, New York, New York 10021.

structures as the pelvis, femur, and ipsilateral knee. An accurate neurologic examination is mandatory as the incidence of preoperative, posttraumatic sciatic nerve compromise following acetabular fractures can range from 12% to 38% (6–15).

In addition, these patients are at high risk for developing a deep vein thrombosis (DVT), as are all individuals with lower extremity fractures (in some series reported as high as 60%) (16,17,28). Therefore, they should be screened for a DVT and prophylaxed if a delay in surgery is anticipated. Our preferred method of evaluation is magnetic resonance venography, which has proved extremely sensitive and reliable (18). Our preoperative anticoagulation regimen presently includes 5000 units of heparin subcutaneously every eight hours in conjunction with compression boots. Patients presenting with an increased risk of DVT or those with DVT documented preoperatively are managed with an inferior vena caual filter and intravenous heparin prior to surgery.

A thorough understanding of the complex pathoanatomy involved in the acetabular fracture is extremely important prior to operative fixation. An accurate diagnosis of the basic fracture pattern can be accomplished with three basic roentgenograms described by Judet et al. (1). An anterior-posterior (AP) view of the pelvis, an iliac oblique view of the acetabulum, and an obturator oblique view of the acetabulum. These three roentgenographic views provide the necessary information that allows the surgeon to map the fracture pattern on a pelvic model as part of the preoperative plan.

The addition of conventional computed tomography (CT) scans with axial cuts allows for better appreciation of the extent of injury to the acetabulum, especially the identification of posterior-wall fractures, rotation of the columns, and the presence of intraarticular fragments or femoral head fractures. Axial CT scans can also help identify associated injuries to the posterior aspect of the pelvis such as a sacroiliac joint disruption or sacral fracture.

Three-dimensional CT can help provide a better understanding of the spatial relationship of the fracture pattern relative to the pelvis as a whole. Although its role is not yet altogether defined, it can be useful when viewed real-time on a monitor that allows visualization of the fracture from various projections. Three-dimensional CT scans can be used in conjunction with plain roentgenograms, including Judet views, and axial CT scans for teaching and to facilitate preoperative planning, especially in late cases such as acetabular nonunions and malunions.

SURGICAL APPROACH

The most important factor associated with a good clinical outcome following an acetabular fracture appears to be anatomic restoration of the articular surface, but achieving such a reduction may be very difficult. Thus, the goal of the surgeon is to restore joint congruency with the least morbidity. The approach utilized depends upon the experience of the operating surgeon but should be one that has the greatest chance of a successful reduction (anatomic) and stabilization of the joint surface.

Mayo (19) has pointed to five major factors that affect this decision: the fracture pattern, the local soft-tissue conditions, the presence of associated major systemic injuries, the age and projected functional status of the patient, and the delay to surgery. Although elaborate, the Letournel-Judet classification system is clinically useful in this regard (4,6). Importantly, any injuries to the pelvic ring must also be considered when determining the proper approach.

Fracture patterns that strictly involve the posterior elements are best exposed through the Kocher-Langenbeck approach, whereas the ilioinguinal approach is better suited for fracture patterns that involve the anterior aspect of the acetabulum. However, the choice of the proper approach for more complex fracture patterns may not be as straightforward. Transverse fractures can be approached either posteriorly or anteriorly depending upon the direction of the major displacement and involvement of the acetabular wall. A **T**-type fracture pattern can pose a difficult problem with respect to the operative approach, and where both columns are separated, may require an extensile approach or simultaneous anterior and posterior exposures to obtain a reduction.

High transverse or **T**-type fracture patterns with involvement of the weight-bearing dome often require an extensile approach to gain adequate access to the roof of the acetabulum in order to anatomically reduce the articular surface. Associated both-column fractures are the most impressive for their involvement and displacement of both the anterior and posterior columns and their complete dissociation from the intact ilium and axial skeleton. In those fractures without posterior column comminution, a significant posterior-wall fracture, or sacroiliac joint involvement, an ilioinguinal approach is optimal, but alternatively an extensile approach is required.

Typically, extensile approaches are not the first choice for any fracture (6,12,19). However, they become a preferred alternative in situations that preclude other approaches. For example, infection rates with the ilioinguinal approach rise rapidly in the presence of nearby suprapubic catheters and colostomies (20), and delayed surgical treatment of the acetabular fractures after two to three weeks is difficult without significant exposure (6,12). After this time, the ability to obtain an anatomic reduction drops from 75% to 62% of cases (6) due to the increasingly difficult task of meticulously taking down varying amounts of callus.

In complex fracture patterns that involve the weight-bearing dome, an extended iliofemoral approach may be required. However, one must appreciate that this approach is associated with the highest incidence of heterotopic ossification and postoperative morbidity (6,12,22,23).

When addressing complex fracture patterns that involve displacement of both anterior and posterior structures, an alternative to the extensile approach is a simultaneous or sequential anterior and posterior approach.

Perhaps the most troubling finding when planning a posterior or extended approach is blunt trauma to the gluteal muscle mass and peritrochanteric region. Contusions and abrasions over this area may herald the presence of the Morel-Lavalle lesion. The area is usually fluctuant secondary to a large hematoma developing under the degloved skin and subcutaneous tissues. This lesion must be addressed separately with surgical decompression, debridement, and drainage (16). Another relative contraindication for a posterior or extensile approach is the presence of a closed-head injury, which has the potential in and of itself to lead to massive heterotopic ossification (24).

Surgical Technique

Operating Room Preparation. The patient is placed on a radiolucent operating table that allows intraoperative traction and fluoroscopy. All cases should be performed under general anesthesia with hypotension, if possible, to decrease blood loss. The addition of epidural catheterization is also beneficial due to reduced inhalation anesthetic requirement (19), reduced blood loss, and improved postoperative pain relief.

A Foley catheter is placed in the patient's bladder, and vascular access is obtained with two large-bore intravenous catheters. We also routinely use an intraoperative cell saver to minimize patient exposure to homologous blood. This permits recycling of about 20% to 30% of the effective blood loss (25).

In addition, we employ intraoperative sciatic-nerve monitoring using somato-sensory evoked potentials (SSEP) and spontaneous electromyography (EMG) for all cases (8,10,11). The entire extremity is prepped free, and sterile subdermal electrodes are inserted. The sensory electrodes are inserted adjacent to the common peroneal and posterior tibial nerves and the motor adjacent to the tibialis anterior, peroneous longus, and abductor hallicus. These techniques are important, especially in patients at risk for developing an iatrogenic sciatic-nerve injury, i.e., those already demonstrating preoperative nerve compromise and those with a fracture pattern that includes a posterior column or wall fracture.

KOCHER-LANGENBECK APPROACH

This approach allows direct access to the whole posterior column and wall of the acetabulum and digital access to the quadrilateral plate and pelvic brim. The patient is placed in the prone position on a radiolucent or fracture table with the hip extended and the knee flexed 90 degrees throughout the procedure to minimize the incidence of iatrogenic sciatic nerve injury (Fig. 1). The lateral decubitus position may be employed in isolated posterior-wall and/or column fractures. All bony prominences are well padded, and the patient is supported on a bean bag.

Prior to the surgical incision, all bony landmarks are outlined with a sterile marking pen. These landmarks include the postero-superior iliac spine, the greater trochanter, and the shaft of the femur. The incision for the Kocher-Langenbeck approach begins 5 cm distal to the posterior superior iliac spine, curves over the greater trochanter, and ends along the lateral aspect of the femoral shaft just distal to the insertion of the gluteus maximus tendon (Fig. 2). The iliotibial band is incised up to the greater trochanter until the fascia overlying the gluteus maximus muscle is encountered.

At this point, the fibers of the gluteus maximus muscle are bluntly separated with two fingers aiming towards the postero-superior iliac spine (Fig. 3). If the gluteus maximus muscle is divided too far medially, the inferior gluteal neurovascular bundle may be compromised. The superior gluteal neurovascular bundle is at risk with exposure of the greater sciatic notch and sciatic buttress and should be identified and protected with carefully placed retractors. Next the trochanteric bursa is incised and the gluteus maximus tendon tagged and released. It is imperative to identify the sciatic nerve at this point lying on the belly of the quadratus femoris muscle (Fig. 4). Fractures of the posterior wall or column of the acetabulum may have significant associated soft-tissue injuries, such as avulsion of the tendon of the piriformis muscle, that can distort normal anatomy and place the sciatic nerve at risk for an iatrogenic injury. Once the sciatic nerve has been identified, it should be followed to its pelvic exit at the greater sciatic notch.

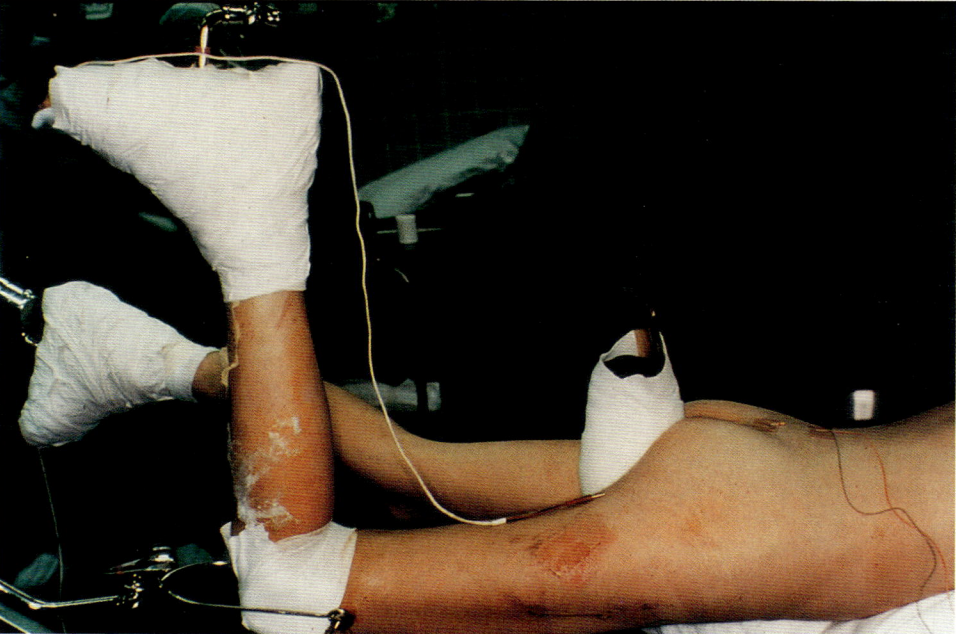

Figure 1. Patient prone on Judet fracture table with hip extended, knee flexed, and distal femoral skeletal traction in place.

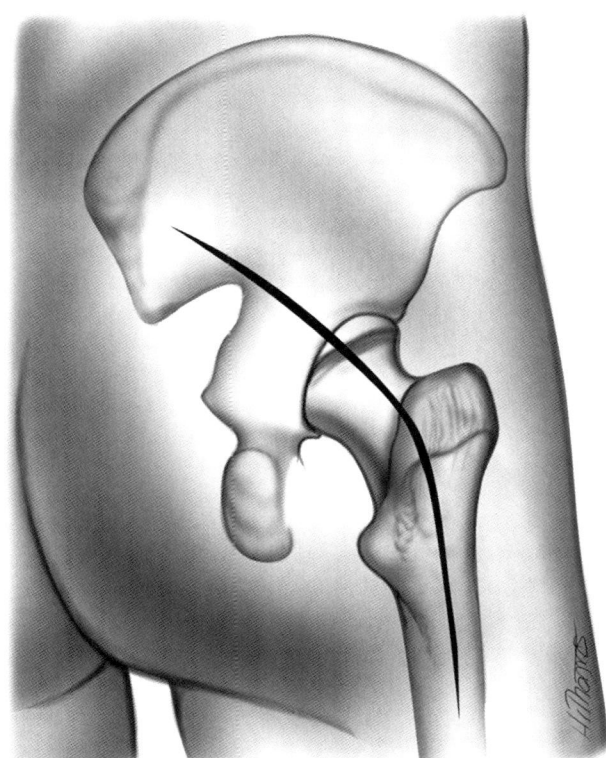

Figure 2. Surgical incision for the Kocher-Langenbeck approach, right side.

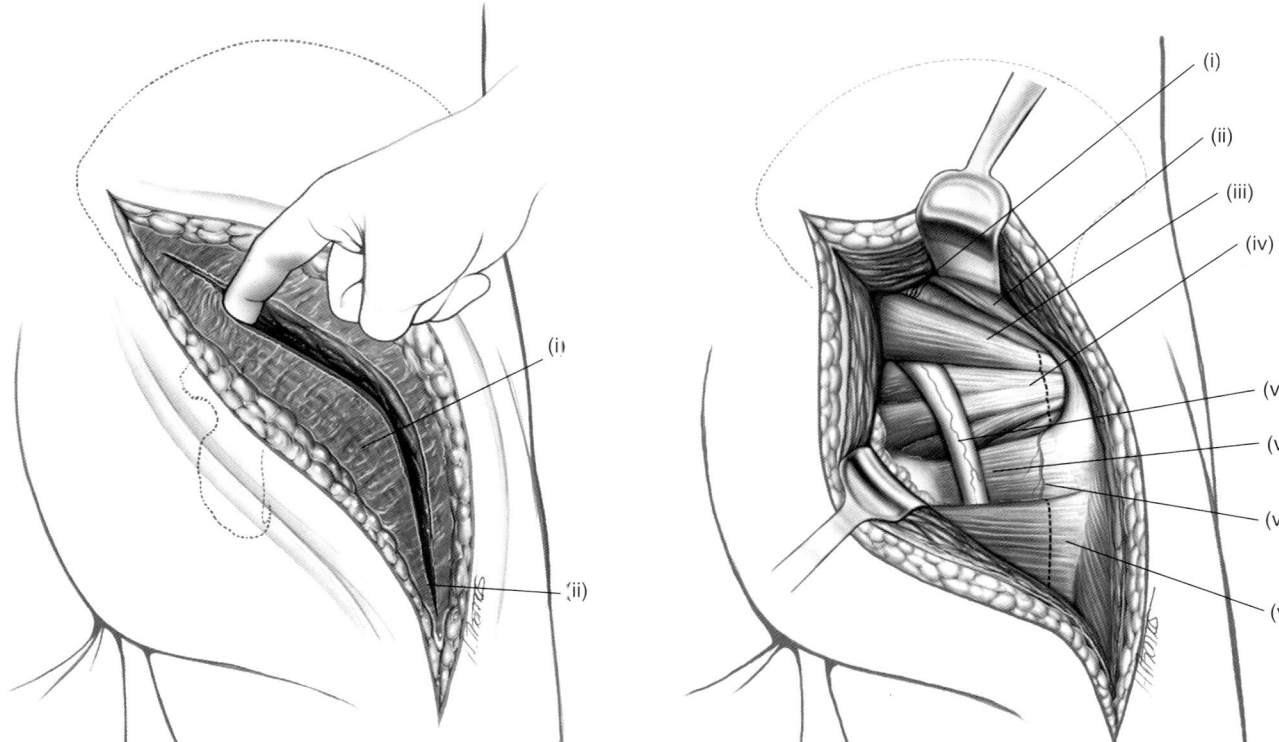

Figure 3. Finger splitting of the gluteus maximus proximal to the greater trochanter—this separates the upper one-third (blood supply: superior gluteal artery) from the lower two-thirds (blood supply: inferior gluteal artery), right side. (i) Fibers of gluteus maximus; (ii) Iliotibial band.

Figure 4. Posterior exposure of the sciatic nerve, tagging and incision of the piriformis and external rotators, right side. (i) Superior gluteal neurovascular bundle; (ii) Gluteus medius; (iii) Piriformis; (iv) External rotators: superior and inferior gemelli and obturator Internus; (v) Sciatic nerve; (vi) Quadratus femoris; (vii) Medial femoral circumflex artery; (viii) Tendonous femoral insertion of gluteus maximus.

The sciatic nerve is at constant risk during the Kocher-Langenbeck approach. It must be protected at all times during the operative procedure (Fig. 5). We routinely perform intraoperative sciatic-nerve monitoring using SSEPs and spontaneous EMGs. The neurotechnologist can detect sciatic-nerve compromise through intraoperative monitoring of EMG activity (immediately) or via significant unilateral changes in amplitude and latency of the SSEPs. A prompt response is required by the surgical team if nerve compromise is detected. Traction should be released and retractors that have been placed against the nerve removed until the EMG activity ceases or the potentials return to baseline.

The pudendal nerve is also at risk, as it exits the pelvis through the greater sciatic notch and reenters through the lesser sciatic notch. It can be injured through vigorous dissection or poorly placed retractors around the ischial spine. It can also be injured through excessive traction on a fracture table at the level of the perineal post.

Exposure of the posterior column of the acetabulum is performed in a stepwise manner from the greater sciatic notch to the ischial tuberosity, avoiding injury to the sciatic nerve. The medial femoral circumflex artery is at risk during exposure of the posterior column. Its branches are buried in the muscle of the quadratus femoris (Figs. 4 and 5) and can be injured if the quadratus femoris muscle is released at its insertion on the femur. The tendon of the piriformis muscle is tagged and released approximately 1.5 cm from its insertion on the greater trochanter. The piriformis muscle is retracted back towards the sciatic notch to gain exposure of the superior aspect of the posterior column of the acetabulum. Digital palpation of the quadrilateral space is possible through the greater sciatic notch. However, the superior gluteal neurovascular bundle exits here and is at risk from too vigorous a dissection, excessive retraction, or poorly placed retractors in the area of the greater sciatic notch or sciatic buttress (Fig. 5).

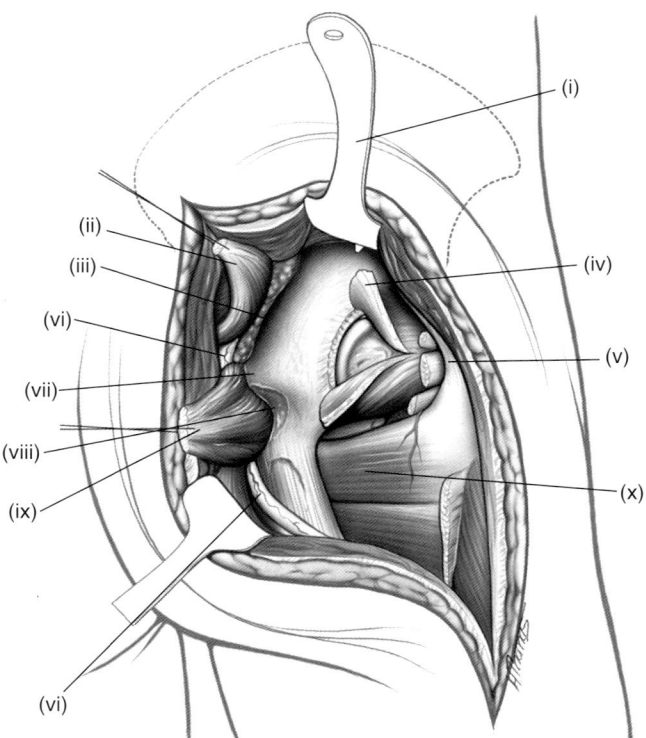

Figure 5. Completed exposure of the posterior column and wall and hip joint through the Kocher-Langenbeck approach, right side. (i) Hohmann retractor under the gluteus medius; (ii) Piriformis; (iii) Greater sciatic notch; (iv) Posterior hip capsulectomy; (v) Gluteus medius; (vi) Sciatic nerve; (vii) Ischial spine; (viii) Lesser sciatic notch; (ix) Obturator internus and gemelli; (x) Quadratus femoris.

Next, the conjoined tendons of the inferior and superior gemellus muscles and the tendon of the obturator internus muscle are tagged and transected. The obturator internus muscle is followed to the lesser sciatic notch where a blunt curved Hohmann or sciatic nerve retractor is carefully inserted. The obturator internus protects the pudendal neurovascular structures in addition to the sciatic nerve. The pudendal neurovascular bundle is at risk as it exits the pelvis through the greater sciatic notch and reenters through the lesser sciatic notch. If further exposure of the postero-inferior aspect of the acetabulum is required, the quadratus femoris muscle is released from its pelvic origin and not from its femoral insertion where the medial femoral circumflex artery is at risk. The bursa of the hamstrings overlying the ischial tuberosity is cleared with an elevator to expose the tendinous origin of the hamstring muscles.

At this point, the entire posterior column can be visualized from the greater sciatic notch to the ischial tuberosity. A Hohmann retractor can be inserted into the ilium under the tendon of the gluteus medius muscle to gain further exposure of the posterior-superior aspect of the acetabulum. The hip capsule throughout the exposure should be left intact to preserve the blood supply to the femoral head. Posterior-wall fragments are identified and their edges debrided sharply. Intraarticular fragments can be removed at this point through distraction of the hip joint via femoral traction with a fracture table (Fig. 1) or with a femoral distractor (Fig. 6).

In isolated posterior-wall fractures, after assuring that all intraarticular fragments have been removed from the joint, the reconstruction of the posterior wall is accomplished temporarily with Kirshner wires and then with lag screws and buttress plating with a 3.5-mm reconstruction plate. The plate has to be molded from the sciatic buttress across the posterior wall to the ischium.

In more than one-fourth of cases with posterior-wall involvement, there is marginal impaction of the articular surface (26). As the femoral head dislocates, it not only fractures the posterior wall, but implodes the articular surface. This is readily identified on the CT scan and has to be anatomically reduced at the time of surgery. Most often, when the articular surface is elevated in order to assure its congruency with the remainder of the acetabulum, there is a metaphyseal defect underlying the articular fragment. By creating a small window in the greater trochanter, cancellous bone can be obtained as needed to bone graft this defect.

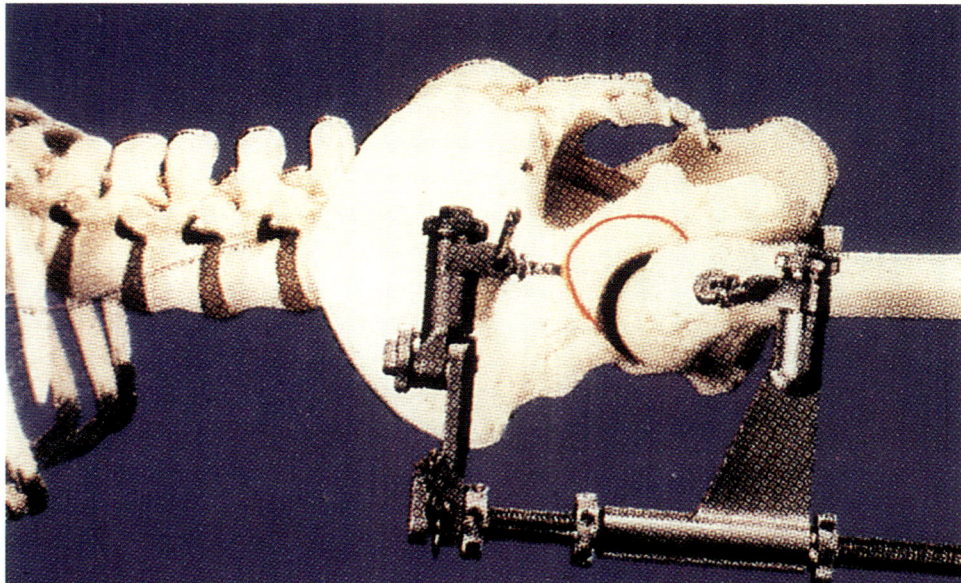

Figure 6. "Saw bones" pelvis in the prone position with femoral distractor applied to allow hip joint distraction. Note the Schanz screw in the sciatic buttress and the Schanz screw in the femur, placed through a small split in the vastus lateralis just distal to the greater trochanter.

When the posterior wall is very comminuted, it is not possible to restore all the small articular fragments with individual lag screws. In this situation, one can use spring hook plates (two-, three-, or four-hole one-third tubular plates with their tips cut off through a hole and the newly created prongs bent downward to create small hooks) (7). These plates are affixed in a loaded fashion underneath the posterior-wall buttress plate more medially, but with the spring-loaded lateral hooks providing a buttressing effect to the comminuted posterior wall.

Fractures involving the posterior column generally result in medial displacement and internal rotation of the posterior column as viewed from a posterior aspect. After debriding the fracture and removing all the comminuted fracture fragments and/or organizing hematoma, posterior column fracture reduction is accomplished by correcting the rotation with a Schanz screw in the ischium and the use of a pelvic reduction clamp in the greater sciatic notch to correct the medial displacement (Fig. 7). Once this has been accomplished, buttress plating is achieved from the sciatic buttress or greater sciatic notch down to the ischium. If combined with a posterior-wall fracture, the posterior column reduction should be addressed first followed by double plating, one plate for the column and one for the wall, as necessary. The adequacy of the posterior column reduction is assessed by digital palpation of the reduction relative to the quadrilateral plate through the greater and lesser sciatic notches.

Transversely oriented fractures with major displacement posteriorly or with involvement of the posterior wall are also accessed through a Kocher-Langenbeck approach. In these

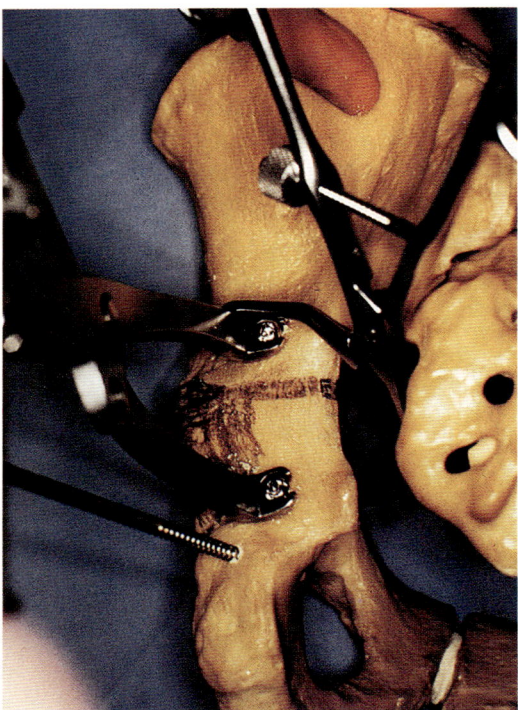

Figure 7. "Saw bones" pelvis in the prone position. Note the Schanz screw in the ischium, the Farabeuf clamp affixed to 4.5-mm screws proximal and distal to the transverse plus posterior wall fracture, and the pelvic reduction clamp in the greater sciatic notch.

fracture types, it is necessary to reduce not only the posterior column, but also the anterior displacement and malrotation. This is easier with a non-**T**-type transverse fracture pattern, where control of the inferior fragment posteriorly will also control anteriorly. This is obviously not the case in the **T**-type fracture, where control of the posterior column has no effect on the anterior column except possibly by ligamentotaxis through nondisrupted joint capsule. As in other fracture types, the columns are reduced first, and only then is the wall fracture, if present, reduced. This sequence of reduction allows visualization of the articular surface during and after reduction of the columns, which enables the surgeon to assess the accuracy of reduction of the articular surface and assure extra-articular hardware placement.

Pelvic reduction clamps are especially useful with displaced transverse fracture types. A 4.5-millimeter screw is inserted proximal and distal to the transverse fracture, from the posterior column (Fig. 7). By applying the pelvic reduction clamps, one can use these for distraction and debridement of the fracture line all the way to the anterior column and subsequently for manipulation and temporary reduction of the transverse fracture component. To control rotation, it is also necessary to place a Schanz screw into the ischium. Once it appears that there is reduction of the posterior aspect of the acetabulum, finger palpation in the quadrilateral plate through the greater sciatic notch all the way to the iliopectineal line is essential to assess the adequacy of the anterior reduction. If the anterior column is still malrotated or displaced, this can then be further corrected with the Schanz screw in the ischium or with a pusher or pelvic reduction clamp in the greater sciatic notch.

A 3.5-millimeter reconstruction plate is then placed along the medial border of the posterior column from the sciatic buttress to the ischium, using 3.5 cortical screws. A lag screw is then inserted across the obliquity of the transverse fracture line into the anterior column, paralleling the quadrilateral plate. This needs to be proximal to the thin part of the medial wall of the acetabulum and parallel to the quadrilateral plate. Finger palpation along the quadrilateral plate aids in assuring correct position for the screw. This should be checked fluoroscopically on the operating table, specifically looking at the obturator oblique view to assess its position in the anterior column and at the iliac oblique view to assure its extraarticular placement.

For a **T**-type fracture, indirect reduction of the anterior column is attempted through a Kocher-Langenbeck approach after an anatomical reduction of the posterior column. It is important to assure initially that none of the screws crosses into the anterior column. One can then place a small bone hook down the quadrilateral plate to pull the displaced portion of the anterior column into the acute angle, now reconstructed between the intact proximal anterior column and the stabilized posterior column. By inserting lag screws along the quadrilateral plate and using the bone hook and/or a pusher in the quadrilateral plate to control rotation of the anterior column, this can be reduced and stabilized to the posterior column.

Care must be taken to avoid intraarticular or intrapelvic placement of the lag screws. Again, the reduction and hardware placement need to be assessed very carefully, utilizing intraoperative fluoroscopy, including both the iliac and obturator oblique views. In addition, the adequacy of reduction is also assessed by finger palpation of the quadrilateral plate through the greater and lesser sciatic notches. With a finger placed along the quadrilateral surface, the hip joint is taken through a range of motion to check for crepitation in order to rule out intraarticular hardware insertion.

Following completion of the operative procedure, the wound is closed in a meticulous fashion. The tendons of the piriformis and obturator internus muscles are reattached at the greater trochanter along with the remainder of the short external rotators. The tendon of the gluteus maximus muscle is reattached at its insertion along the femur. Two suction drains are placed over the external rotators followed by closure of the iliotibial band and the fascia overlying the gluteus maximus muscle. A subcutaneus suction drain is inserted and the skin meticulously closed.

ILIOINGUINAL APPROACH

The ilioinguinal approach offers direct visualization of the iliac wing, the anterior sacroiliac joint, the entire anterior column, and the pubic symphysis (Fig. 8). The patient is placed in the supine position on a fluoroscopic table; he is supported on a bean bag and protected at all bony prominences. The incision begins at the midpoint of the iliac crest, follows the crest to the anterior superior iliac spine, and continues parallel to the inguinal ligament, ending 2 cm above the pubic symphysis (Fig. 9).

The proximal aspect of the approach is exposed first by releasing the lateral insertion of the external oblique muscle in the avascular plane between the insertion of the abdominal musculature and the origin of the tensor fascia lata and abductor muscles (Fig. 10). A subperiosteal dissection is carried out elevating the abdominal musculature along with the iliacus muscle to expose the internal iliac fossa (Fig. 11). A nutrient artery may be encountered along the iliac fossa during the dissection, requiring hemostasis. The iliac fossa is packed with a sponge and attention now directed to the inguinal dissection.

The external oblique aponeurosis is the most superficial layer encountered under the subcutaneous tissue and is incised 5 mm from its insertion on the inguinal ligament from the anterior superior iliac spine to the external inguinal ring (Figs. 10, 11). The inguinal canal terminates at the external inguinal ring where it transmits the spermatic cord in the male and the round ligament in the female. The ilioinguinal nerve should also be identified (Fig. 11). An inadequate closure of the floor of the inguinal canal can lead to a direct hernia. A sound closure of the insertion of the transversalis abdominis muscle and the internal oblique muscle to the inguinal ligament is necessary. The contents of the inguinal

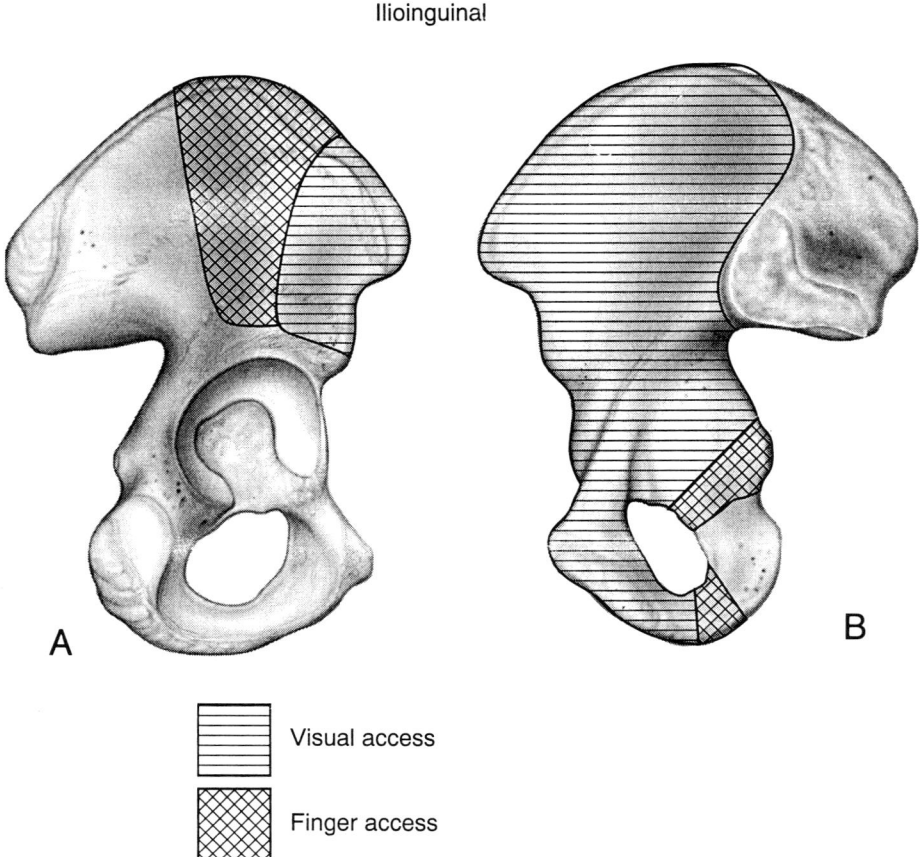

Figure 8. Access to the pelvis via the ilioinguinal approach, right side. (A) The lateral (outer) bony pelvis and (B) the medial (inner) bony pelvis.

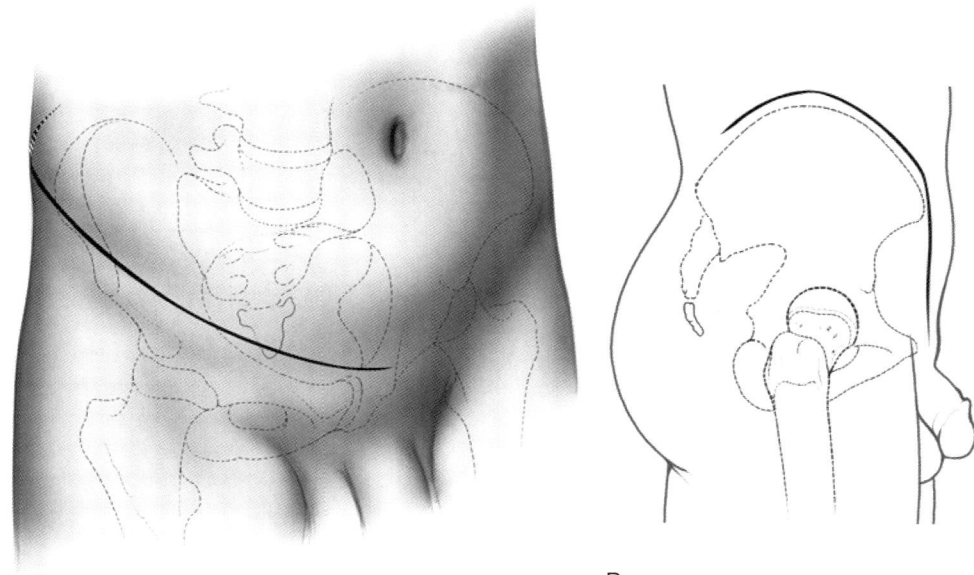

Figure 9. The ilioinguinal incision, right side. (A) Obturator oblique view. (B) Lateral view.

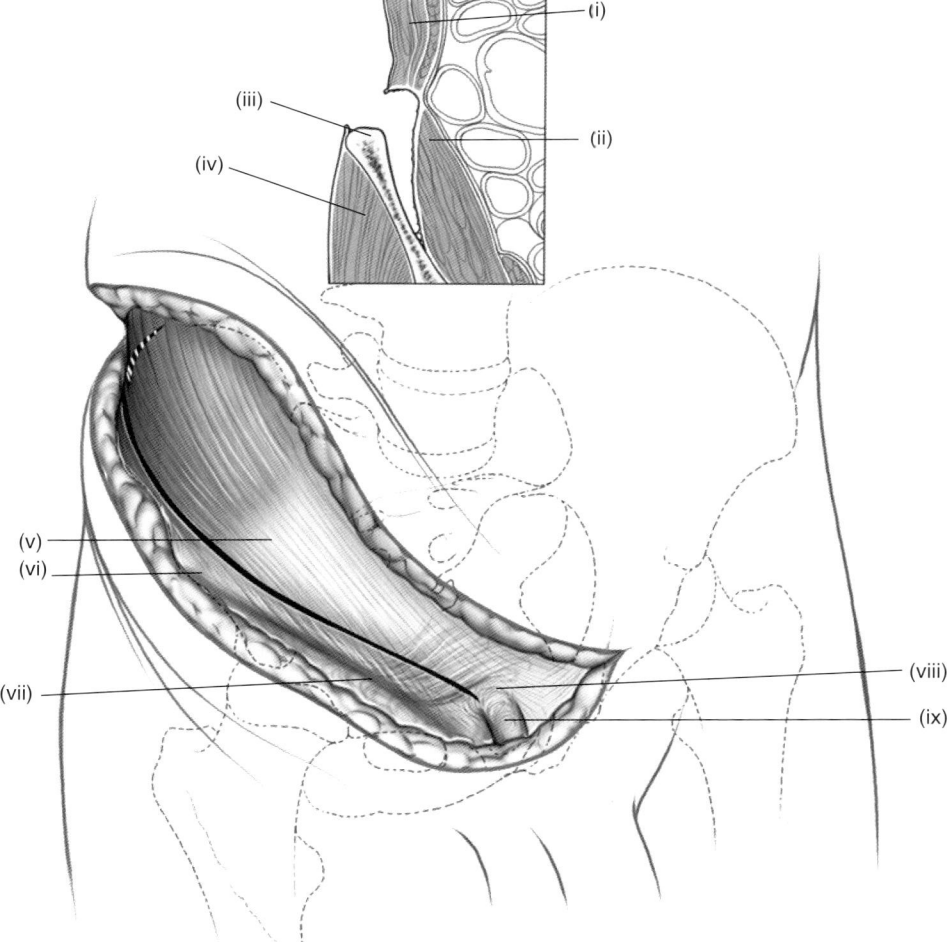

Figure 10. Exposure of iliac crest and external oblique muscle, right side. (i) Abdominal muscles freed from crest; (ii) Iliacus; (iii) Iliac crest; (iv) Gluteus medius; (v) External oblique; (vi) Anterior superior iliac spine; (vii) Inguinal ligament; (viii) Superficial inguinal ring; (ix) Spermatic cord.

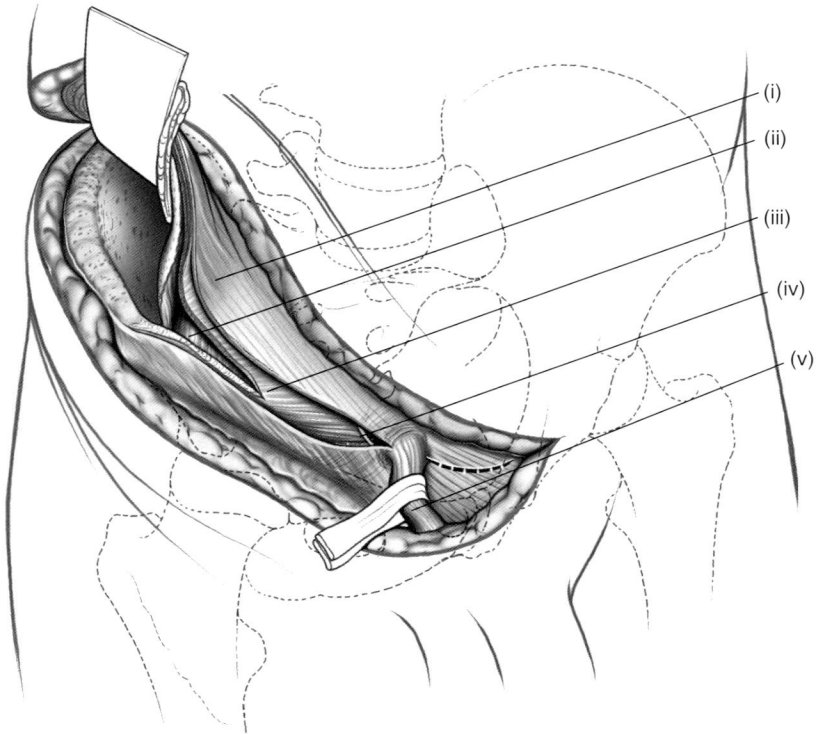

Figure 11. The inguinal exposure, right side: (i) External oblique, (ii) Iliopsoas, (iii) Conjoint tendon: internal oblique and transversalis fascia, (iv) Ilioinguinal nerve, (v) Spermatic cord.

canal (spermatic cord/round ligament and ilioinguinal nerve) are at risk during exposure of the external inguinal ring and should be carefully isolated and retracted with a Penrose drain (Fig. 11).

Lateral to the iliopectineal fascia, the conjoint tendon (internal oblique and transversalis abdominis muscles) is incised from the inguinal ligament with a 2-mm cuff (Fig. 12A). The lateral femoral cutaneous nerve is at risk immediately underneath the conjoint tendon just medial to the anterior superior iliac spine. The lateral femoral cutaneous nerve is at risk when mobilizing the transversalis abdominis and internal oblique muscles off the inguinal ligament just medial to the anterior superior iliac spine. The nerve can also be stretched during retraction. Patients should be warned preoperatively to expect this complication. Medial to the vessels, the conjoint tendon is then incised and the ipsilateral rectus abdominis muscle released from the pubic tubercle to the pubic symphysis (Figs. 12, 13). Associated anterior pelvic ring injuries may require fixation across the pubic symphysis necessitating a partial release of the contralateral rectus abdominis muscle. With anterior pelvic ring injuries, the rectus abdominis muscle may be avulsed off the pubic tubercle and rami, in which case the bladder is at increased risk of iatrogenic injury during the exposure. Release of the rectus abdominis insertion from the pubic rami and symphysis allows access to the space of Retzius (Fig. 12C).

We prefer to leave the conjoint tendon intact over the femoral artery, vein, and lymphatics to avoid any unnecessary dissection (Fig. 12A) and to protect them from undue retraction. Laterally the iliopsoas muscle and the femoral nerve are bluntly separated off the iliopectineal fascia and mobilized with a one-inch Penrose drain (not shown). The femoral vasculature and lymphatics are next carefully dissected off the pectineal fascia medially (Fig. 12), maintaining these structures as a unit with the overlying conjoint tendon

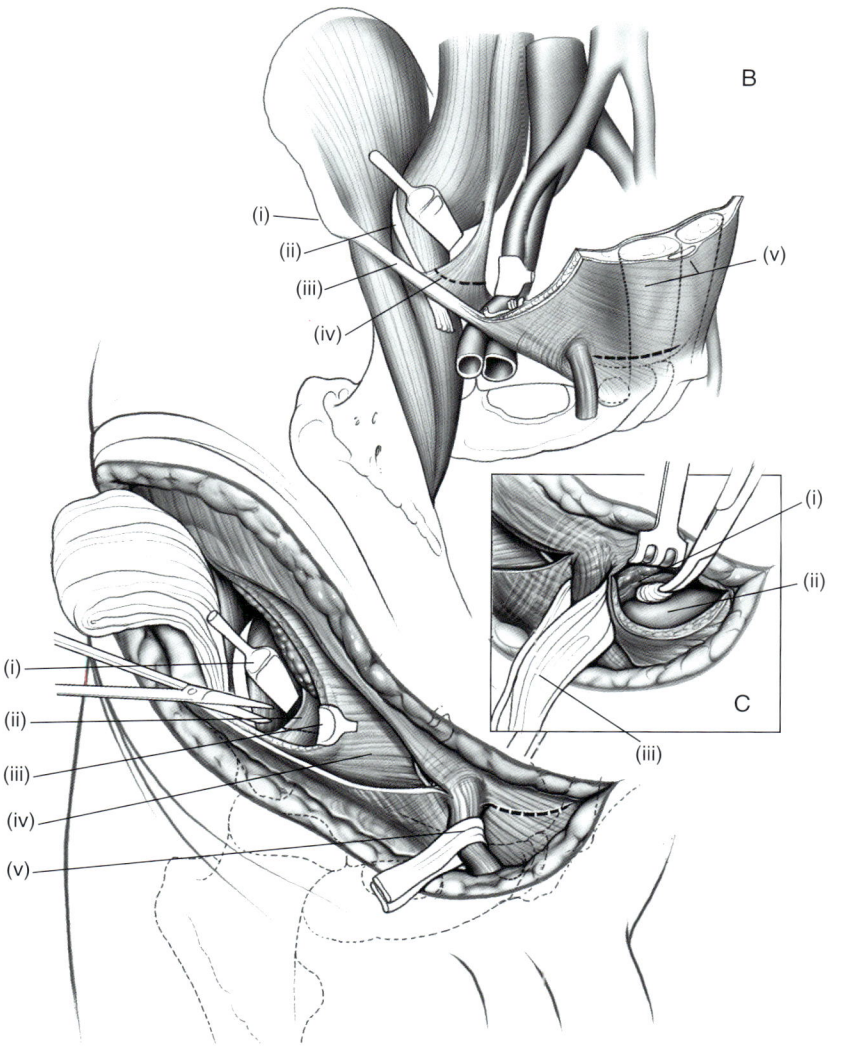

Figure 12. (A) Incision of iliopectineal fascia: (i) Retraction laterally of the iliopsoas, femoral nerve, and lateral femoral cutaneous nerve; (ii) Incision of the iliopectineal fascia off the iliopectineal eminence; (iii) Medial retraction of the femoral vessels; (iv) Conjoint tendon overlying external iliac vessels; (v) Penrose drain around spermatic cord. (B) Medial incision of rectus sheath: (i) Anterior superior iliac spine, (ii) Femoral nerve, (iii) Inguinal ligament, (iv) Iliopectineal fascia, (v) Rectus. (C) Exposure of superior pubis and symphysis: (i) Bladder and space of Retzius, (ii) Symphysis pubis, (iii) Penrose drain around spermatic cord.

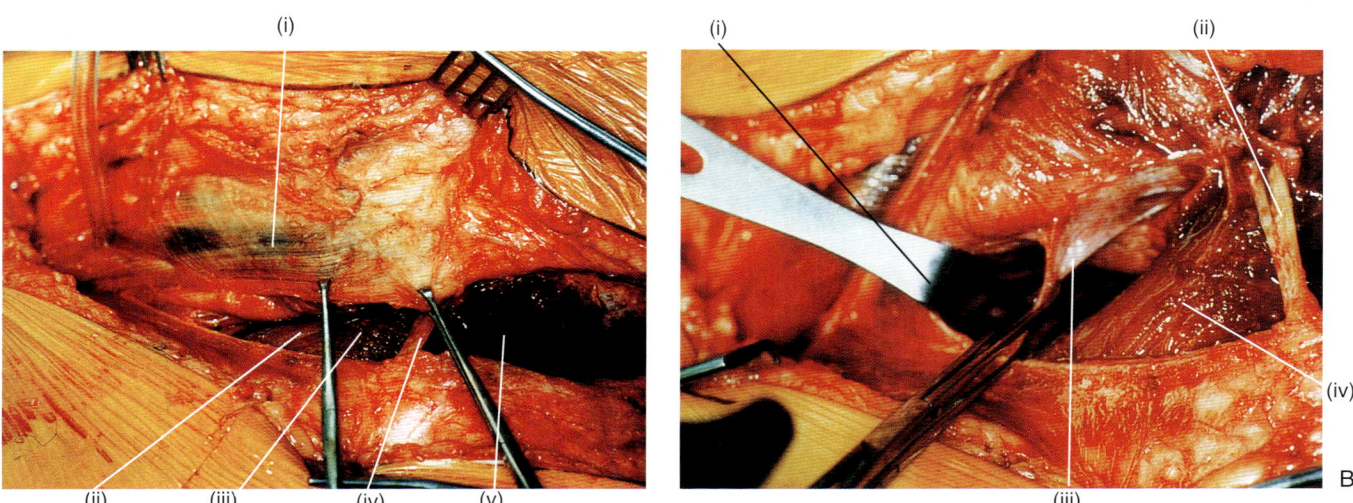

Figure 13. (A) Release of external oblique and conjoint tendons, left side. (i) External oblique and conjoint tendons; (ii) Femoral nerve; (iii) Iliopsoas muscle; (iv) Lateral femoral cutaneous nerve; (v) Iliacus muscle mobilized off inner table of the pelvic wing. (B) Excision of the iliopectineal fascia, left side. (i) Femoral vessels retracted and protected my blunt right angle retractor; (ii) Lateral femoral cutaneous nerve (iii) Iliopectineal fascia; (iv) Psoas muscle and femoral nerve.

(Figs. 13, 14). The femoral nerve is at risk during mobilization and excessive retraction of the iliopsoas muscle (Figs. 12A, B). Hip flexion will aid in relaxation of the iliopsoas muscle, minimizing the need for any undue retraction. Once the iliopectineal fascia is isolated (Figs. 12A, B), it is then excised off the pelvis brim from the pectineal eminence to just anterior to the sacroiliac joint. The iliopectineal fascia separates the true and false pelvis. Its excision allows access to the quadrilateral surface. A retropubic communication between the external iliac artery and the obturator or deep epigastric arteries called the corona mortis can be encountered during mobilization of the femoral vessels and should be ligated if identified. A broad Penrose drain is then passed around the femoral vessels, lymphatics, and the overlying conjoint tendon (Fig. 14).

The femoral vessels are at risk during mobilization of the vascular compartment off the iliopectineal fascia. They must be isolated with a wide ribbon Penrose drain and protected throughout the procedure (Figs. 14 to 16). Leaving the conjoint tendon intact over their surface protects them from undue dissection and retraction. It is important to search for the corona mortis, a variable retropubic anastomosis, which should be ligated if identified. The obturator artery is also at risk during exposure of the quadrilateral surface and must be protected with carefully placed retractors.

Access to the acetabulum through the ilioinguinal approach is now complete. Medial retraction of the iliopsoas muscle and femoral nerve allows access to the internal iliac fossa and anterior sacroiliac joint, the lateral window of the ilioinguinal approach (Fig. 14). The middle window is visualized by lateral retraction of the iliopsoas muscle and the femoral nerve and medial retraction of the femoral vasculature, allowing access to the pelvic brim, the quadrilateral surface, and the posterior column (Fig. 15). The medial window is exposed through lateral retraction of the femoral vasculature and lymphatics and allows ac-

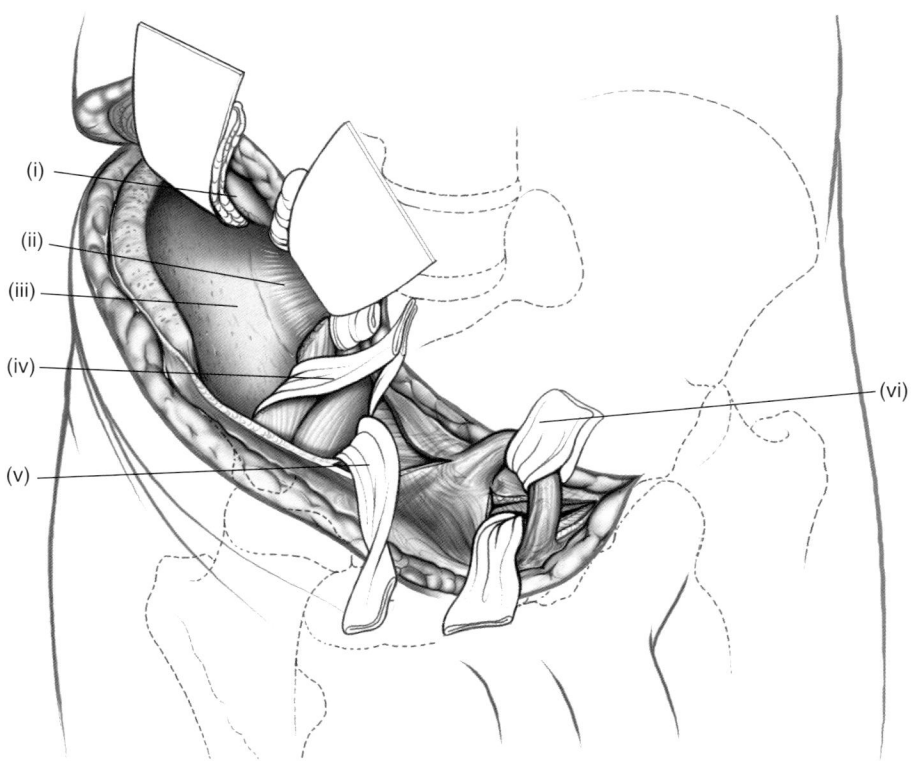

Figure 14. Lateral window of ilioinguinal, right side: (i) Iliopsoas muscle; (ii) Sacro-iliac joint; (iii) Internal iliac fossa; (iv) Penrose drain around ilopsoas, femoral nerve, and lateral femoral cutaneous nerve; (v) Penrose drain around femoral vessels; (vi) Penrose drain around spermatic cord.

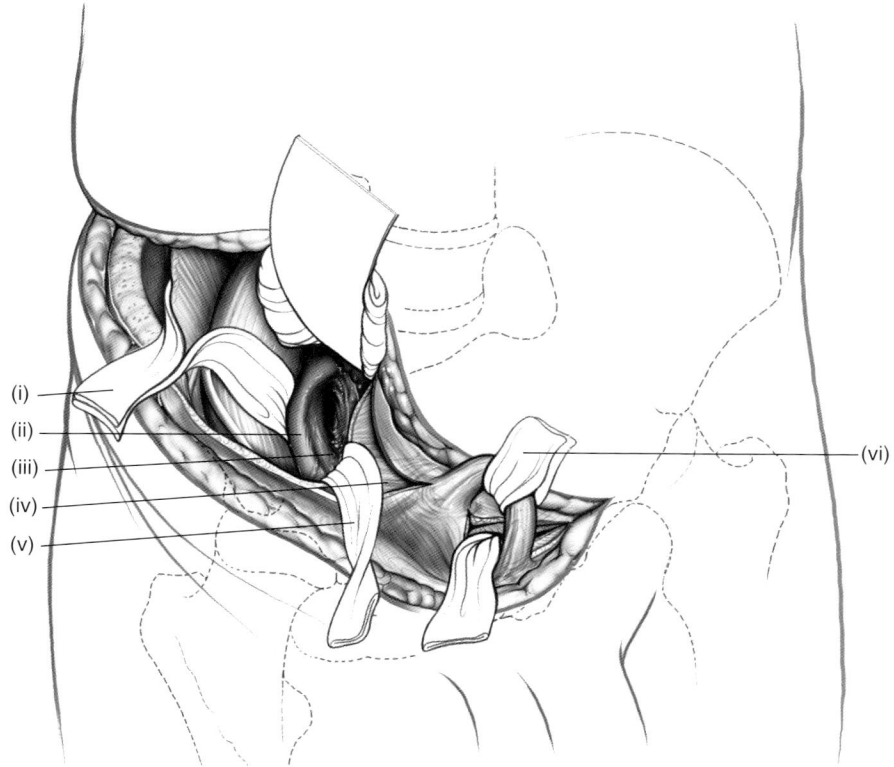

Figure 15. Middle window of ilioinguinal, right side: (i) Penrose drain around iliopsoas, femoral nerve, and lateral femoral cutaneous nerve; (ii) Pelvic brim; (iii) Iliopectineal fascia released down to iliopectineal eminence; (iv) Femoral vessels protected by their overlying internal iliac muscle; (v) Penrose drain around femoral vessels; (vi) Penrose drain around spermatic cord.

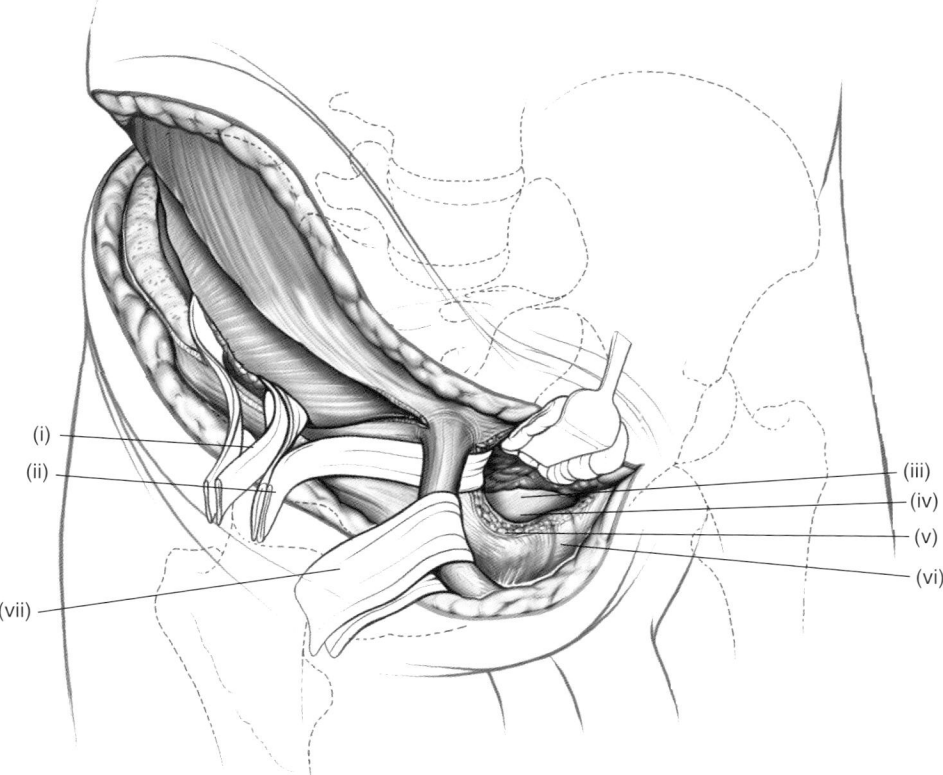

Figure 16. Medial window of ilioinguinal, right side: (i) Penrose drain around iliopsoas, femoral nerve, and lateral femoral cutaneous nerve; (ii) Penrose drain around femoral vessels; (iii) Bladder and Space of Retzius; (iv) Pubis; (v) Pubic tubercle; (vi) Symphysis pubis; (vii) Penrose drain around spermatic cord.

cess to the superior ramus and pubic symphysis (Fig. 16). The contents of the inguinal canal can be mobilized either medially or laterally as needed. The obturator vessels and nerves can be visualized through either the middle or medial window and require protection during exposure and reduction of the fracture. A limited subperiosteal exposure of the outer surface of the anterior iliac wing is occasionally needed for applying pelvic reduction clamps to control the posterior column.

Reduction of the acetabular fracture should be performed in a stepwise fashion according to the preoperative plan. Unlike most other articular fractures, acetabular fracture reduction proceeds from the periphery towards the joint in a sequential fashion. Because peripheral malalignment can result in major articular incongruence, reduction of each fracture segment must be performed painstakingly and exactly. This portion of the procedure can be aided by hip flexion in order to relax structures crossing anterior to the hip joint. A Schanz screw inserted through the lateral aspect of the femur into the femoral head followed by distal traction can also be extremely helpful as it can facilitate fracture reduction through ligamentotaxis. This is especially useful in cases where the femoral head has protruded through the quadrilateral surface. An accurate reduction of all the fracture fragments is imperative since the articular surface is not directly visualized through the ilioinguinal approach.

Anterior column and/or wall fractures are directly visualized through the ilioinguinal approach. Prior to attempted reduction, all the fracture lines are carefully irrigated and debrided with removal of fracture hematoma or small comminuted fragments. The hip joint is also irrigated, and loose fragments are removed through the displaced portion of the articular fracture. Starting at the iliac crest, the fracture is sequentially reduced. The iliac crest portion of the fracture can be reduced with pointed reduction clamps or specially designed pelvic reduction clamps. A gliding hole for lag-screw fixation can be created prior to fracture reduction in order to assure optimal lag-screw position in the thin cortical cap of the iliac crest. The iliac crest can then be stabilized either with the lag screw or with 3.5-mm reconstruction plates. The anterior column is then reduced to the intact iliac wing and temporarily stabilized with a Kirshner wire (and/or a 3.5-mm lag screw) into the sciatic buttress through the first window of the ilioinguinal approach.

Then, through the middle window, any anterior-wall fracture is reduced. Finally, any superior pubic rami and displaced pubic column fractures are reduced through the medial window. A 3.5-mm reconstruction plate can then be molded along the iliac fossa, across

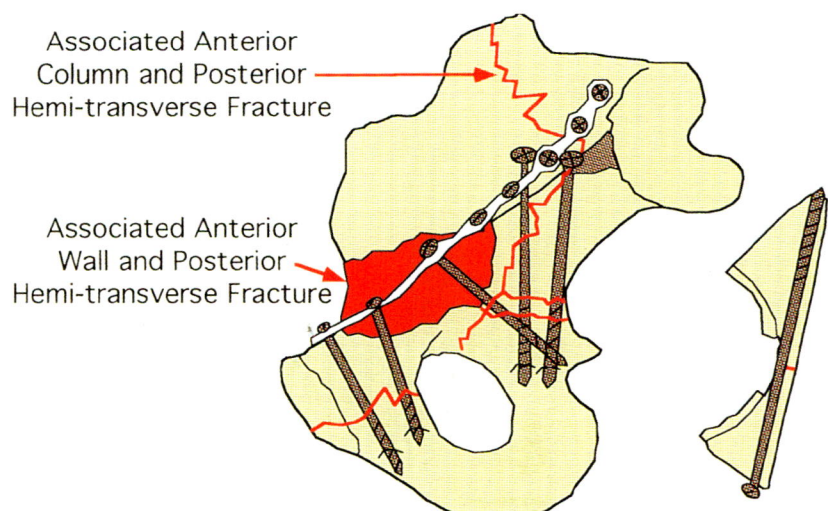

Figure 17. Example of contoured pelvic reconstruction plate, anterior screw placement, posterior screw placement, and posterior column lag-screw placement from an ilioinguinal approach, right side.

the iliopectineal eminence to the pubic tubercle and pubic column (Fig. 17). This should not cross the symphysis pubis, unless there are associated fractures in the pubic column anteriorly, or if there is involvement of the symphysis pubis with an associated pelvic injury. It is essential that the 3.5-mm reconstruction plate be perfectly molded, otherwise fixation of the plate to the pelvis can lead to a malreduction of the acetabular fracture.

The carefully molded 3.5-mm reconstruction plate is next stabilized to the internal iliac fossa, superior to the acetabulum, with 3.5-mm cortical screws and medially to the pubic tubercle and column (Fig. 17). It is then possible, along the pelvic brim, to insert 3.5-mm lag screws in the area of the sciatic buttress and quadrilateral plate, proximal to the acetabulum, providing stable fixation of the anterior column to the iliac wing and posterior column (Fig. 18). These need to parallel the quadrilateral plate. Fracture reduction is assessed by finger palpation of the quadrilateral plate. Fluoroscopy is necessary, including both the obturator oblique and iliac oblique views, to assess the adequacy of the reduction and confirm extraarticular position of the hardware.

Both-column acetabular fractures are also ideally approached and stabilized through the ilioinguinal approach. This requires an indirect reduction of the posterior column and hence cannot be performed if the fracture is more than two to three weeks old. In addition, significant involvement of the posterior wall, comminuted fractures of the posterior column, involvement of the sacroiliac joint, and the presence of lateral dome involvement preclude this approach and require an extensile exposure. Initially, the anterior column is reduced and stabilized with a 3.5-mm reconstruction plate as previously described (Fig. 17). This must be performed perfectly from the iliac crest to the symphysis pubis in order to provide an anatomic template for subsequent reduction of the posterior column to the reduced anterior column. If the anterior column fracture is not complete through the iliac crest, it may have to be completed in order to accomplish this reduction adequately. In addition, the anterior column segment of a both-column fracture, is shortened and externally rotated. To reduce the anterior column to the intact iliac wing (the "spur" sign), one needs to apply longitudinal traction using a Schanz screw in the femoral head, with the hip flexed.

Following anatomic reduction and stabilization of the anterior column, the rotated and medially displaced posterior column can next be reduced to the restored anterior column. This often requires lateral and anterior traction of the hip via the Schanz screw in the femoral head and specially designed pelvic reduction clamps with one tine placed on the outer surface of the ilium and the other tine, through the lateral or middle window of the il-

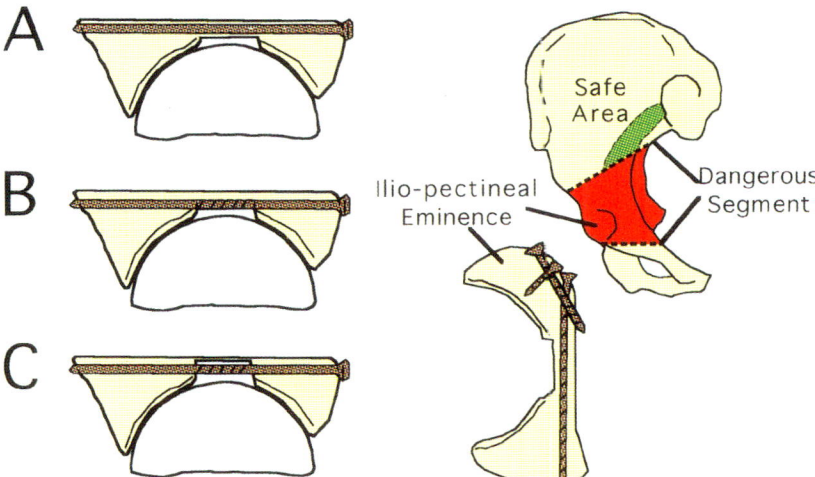

Figure 18. Safe and danger zones for anterior to posterior screw placement, right side (From: Letournel, E., Judet, R.: *Fractures of the acetabulum*. 2nd ed., In R. A. Elson (editor). Berlin, Heidelberg, New York, Springer-Verlag, 1993). A, B, and C all represent safe screws parallel to the quadrilateral plate, yet variable relative to the cotyloid fossa.

ioinguinal exposure, placed on the quadrilateral plate and/or posterior column (Fig. 19). In addition, a small bone hook placed down the quadrilateral plate and hooked around the ischial spine to pull the posterior column up to the anterior column may also be required. Following this reduction, 3.5-mm lag screws are inserted through the 3.5-mm reconstruction plate, from the pelvic brim superior to the acetabulum into the posterior column paralleling the quadrilateral surface (Fig. 17). These screws are directed from proximal to distal, aiming for the ischial spine.

Care must be taken to avoid intraarticular placement of these lag screws, which are often up to 110 mm long. This requires a careful appreciation of the location of the acetabulum relative to the fixed pelvic landmarks, i.e., inferior to the anterior inferior iliac spine and under the iliopectineal eminence. The adequacy of the reduction of the posterior column to the anterior column can be determined by palpation of the quadrilateral surface and the use of intraoperative fluoroscopy. The fluoroscopic views should include an AP pelvis, obturator and iliac oblique views; and a view parallel to the quadrilateral surface, aiming down the lag screw. Motion of the hip with a finger on the quadrilateral surface can also be utilized to assure the absence of any crepitation in the joint.

After completion of fracture reduction and fixation, drains are inserted into the space of Retzius, over the quadrilateral surface, and along the internal iliac fossa. The rectus abdominis muscle is reattached to the pubis. The floor of the inguinal canal is repaired by su-

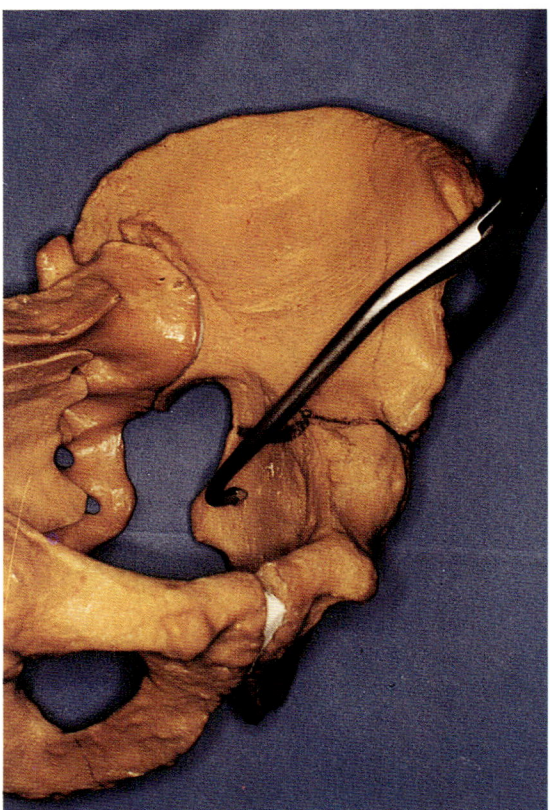
A

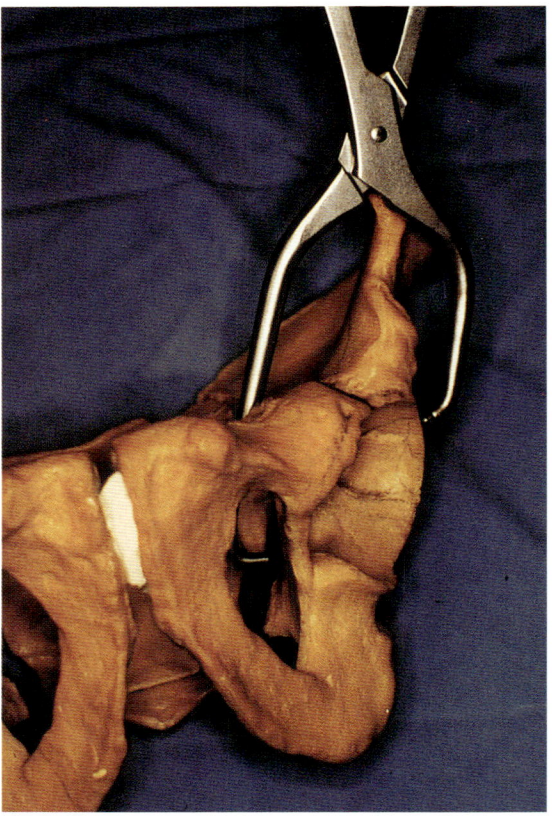
B

Figure 19. "Saw bones" left hemipelvis: using an offset large pelvic clamp (Synthes, Paoli, PA) to obtain reduction. The longer arm of the clamp is placed along the quadrilateral plate and the shorter arm inserted through an interval between the anterior inferior and anterior superior iliac spines to lie on the outer table of the iliac wing. (A) Iliac oblique view. (B) Obturator oblique view.

turing the conjoint tendons of the transversalis abdominis and the internal oblique muscles to the inguinal ligament with nonabsorbable sutures. The roof the inguinal canal is restored by repair of the external oblique aponeurosis and external inguinal ring allowing passage of the spermatic cord in the male and the round ligament in the female. The external oblique muscle is then reattached to the inguinal ligament and the iliac crest using nonabsorbable sutures. A superficial suction drain is inserted and the skin closed.

EXTENDED ILIOFEMORAL APPROACH

The extended iliofemoral is an anatomic approach that follows an internervous plane, reflecting anteriorly the femoral nerve-enervated muscles and posteriorly the muscles enervated by the superior and inferior gluteal nerves. The posterior flap is mobilized as a unit without damaging its neurovascular bundles (Fig. 20).

There are three main stages to the dissection: elevation of all the gluteal muscles with the tensor fascia lata, division of the external rotators of the hip, and an extended capsulotomy along the lip of the acetabulum. The end result is complete exposure of the outer aspect of the ilium and the whole posterior column to the upper part of the ischial tuberosity. Furthermore, the approach may be extended to allow a limited exposure of the internal iliac

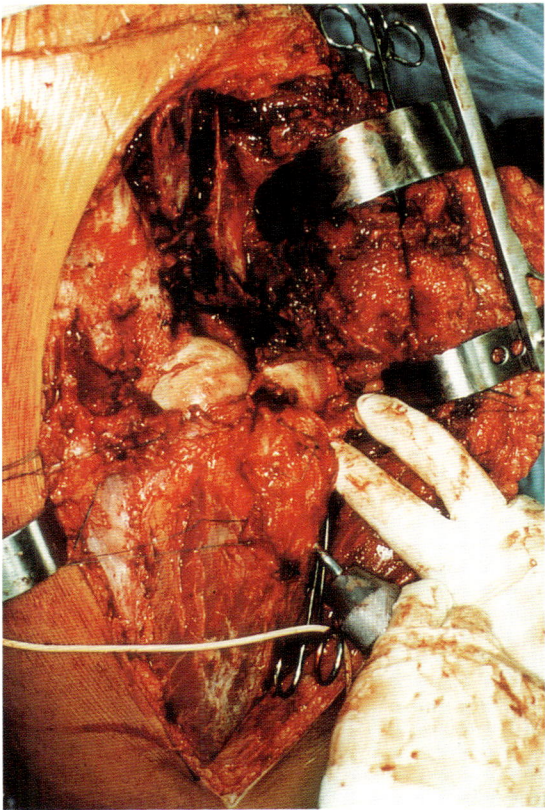

Figure 20. The extended iliofemoral approach for exposure of a comminuted left both-column acetabular fracture. The femoral head can be seen and there is a Schanz pin in greater trochanter, parallel with femoral neck.

Extended Iliofemoral

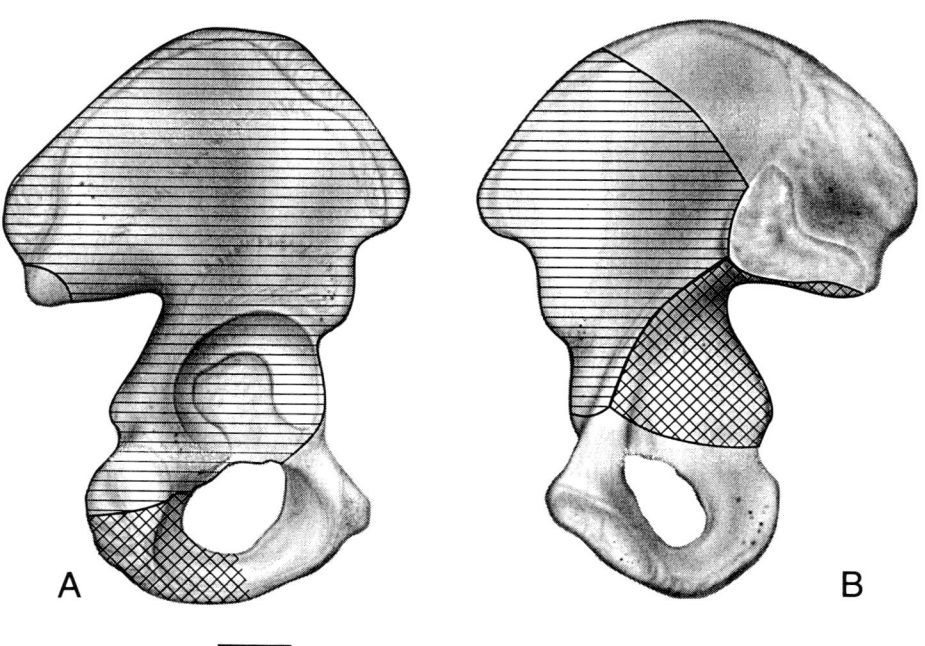

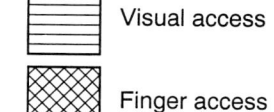
Visual access
Finger access

Figure 21. Access to the right pelvis via the extended iliofemoral approach. (A) The lateral (outer) bony pelvis, (B) the medial (inner) bony pelvis.

Figure 22. Skin incision. (A) The inverted-J skin incision, right side. (B) Anterolateral view: the inverted-J skin incision with distal extension for the extended iliofemoral.

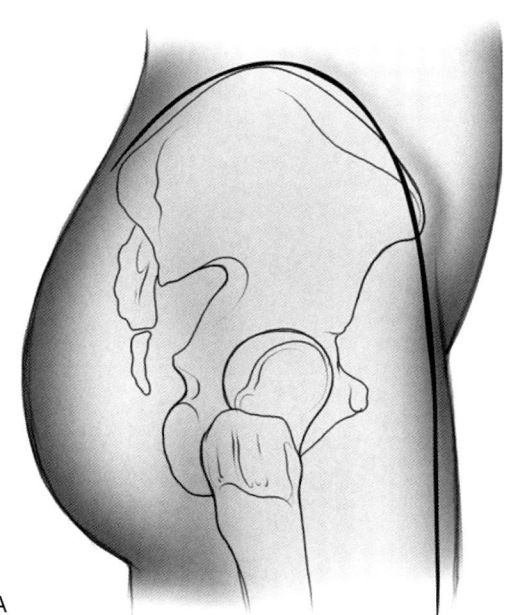
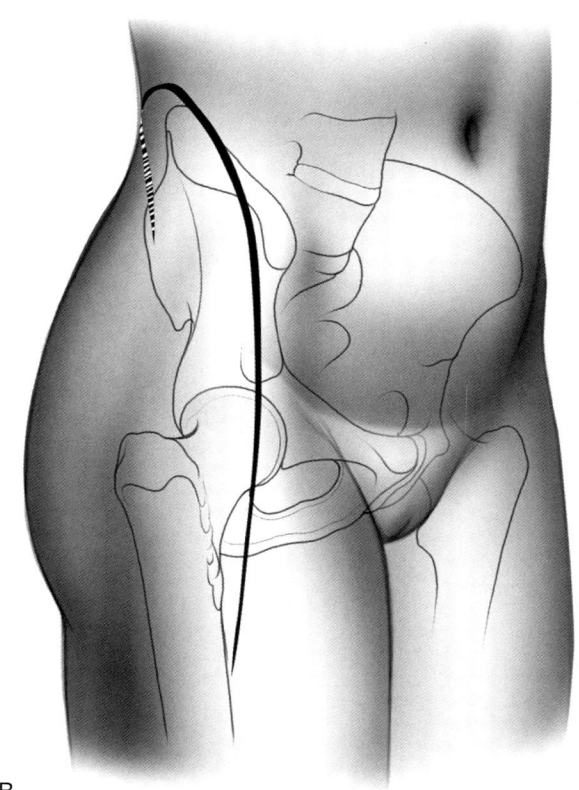

fossa and the anterior column to the level of the iliopectineal eminence. Thus, simultaneous extensile exposure of both columns is possible, which permits direct visualization of the reduction and fixation of the anterior and posterior columns (Fig. 21).

The approach is indicated for complex fracture patterns where exposure of both the anterior and posterior columns are needed. The patient is supported on a bean bag and placed in the lateral decubitus position on a radiolucent operating table. The hip is kept extended and the knee flexed throughout the procedure to minimize sciatic nerve injury.

The incision is in the form of an inverted J (Fig. 22A). It begins at the posterior-superior iliac spine and follows the iliac crest towards the anterior-superior iliac spine extending to the antero-lateral aspect of the thigh (Fig. 22B). The exposure begins in a stepwise fashion by first sharply releasing the tensor fascia lata muscle and the gluteus medius subperiosteally from the outer aspect of the iliac crest. The distal limb of the incision is carried over the fascia of the tensor fascia lata muscle (Fig. 23).

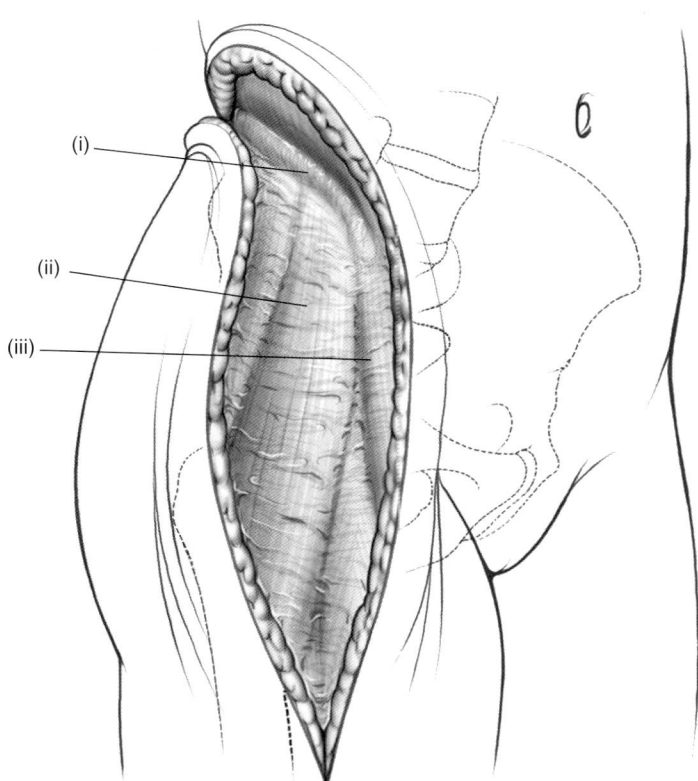

Figure 23. Exposure of right iliac crest and anterior distal limb. (i) Avascular "white line"; (ii) Fasia covering Tensor fascia lata muscle; (iii) Fascia covering sartorius muscle.

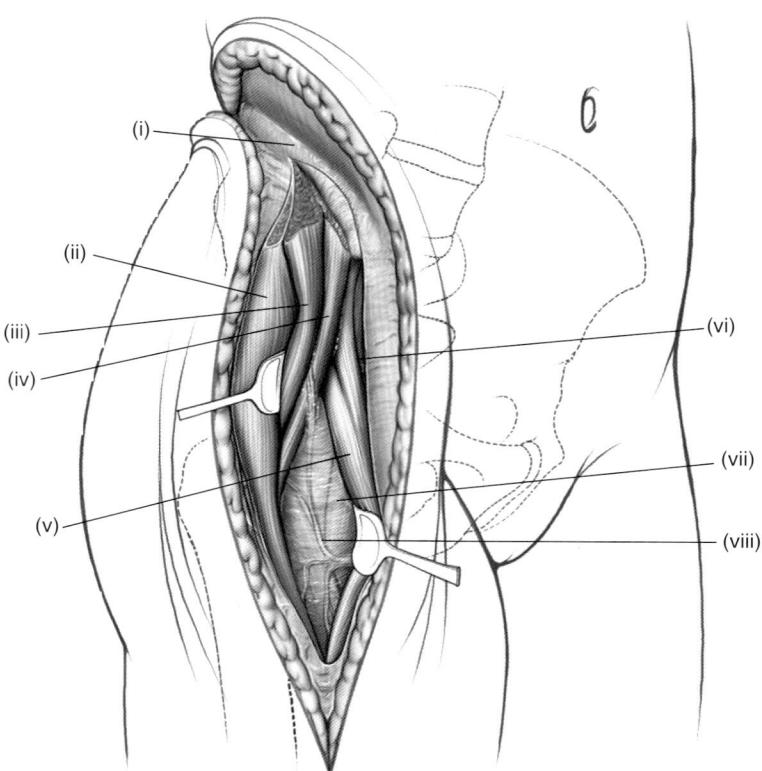

Figure 24. Subfascial reflection of tensor fascia lata and abductor muscle origins from right iliac crest. (i) Avascular "white line"; (ii) Tensor fascia lata muscle; (iii) Gluteus medius muscle; (iv) Gluteus minimus muscle; (v) Rectus femoris muscle; (vi) Sartorius muscle; (vii) "No name" fascia covering vastus lateralis; (viii) Ascending branch of the lateral femoral circumflex artery.

Having incised the fascia overlying the tensor fascia lata muscle, the muscle belly is reflected off the fascia and retracted laterally to expose the fascia overlying the rectus femoris (Fig. 24). The exposure stays lateral to the branches of the lateral femoral cutaneous nerve and therefore places them at minimal risk. The fascial layer overlying the rectus femoris muscle is divided longitudinally, the reflected head and direct heads of the rectus muscle are retracted medially exposing the fascia overlying the vastus lateralis muscle (Fig. 24). The ascending branches of the lateral femoral circumflex vessels are isolated and ligated beneath the fascia of the vastus lateralis muscle (Fig. 25).

The musculature along the external surface of the iliac wing is released up to the greater sciatic notch (Fig. 25). Superior gluteal neurovascular bundle injury can result from severe displacement of the sciatic notch due to a high transverse fracture with marked medial rotation or to an iatrogenic insult during surgery. The neurovascular bundle is at greatest risk during exposure of the greater sciatic notch and must be protected from undue traction or damage by retractors. The superior gluteal neurovascular bundle is at risk as it exits the greater sciatic notch (Fig. 26). Next, the gluteus minimus tendon is identified over the greater trochanter, tagged, and transected, leaving a small cuff for repair (Fig. 26). The gluteus minimus muscle also has attachments to the superior aspect of the hip capsule that need to be released. The gluteus medius tendon is tagged and transected, again leaving a small cuff for repair (Fig. 26). It is important to sequentially and carefully transect and label these structures for subsequent reattachment. The tensor fascia lata and gluteal muscles are held in continuity as a flap and reflected posteriorly to expose the external rotators (Fig. 26).

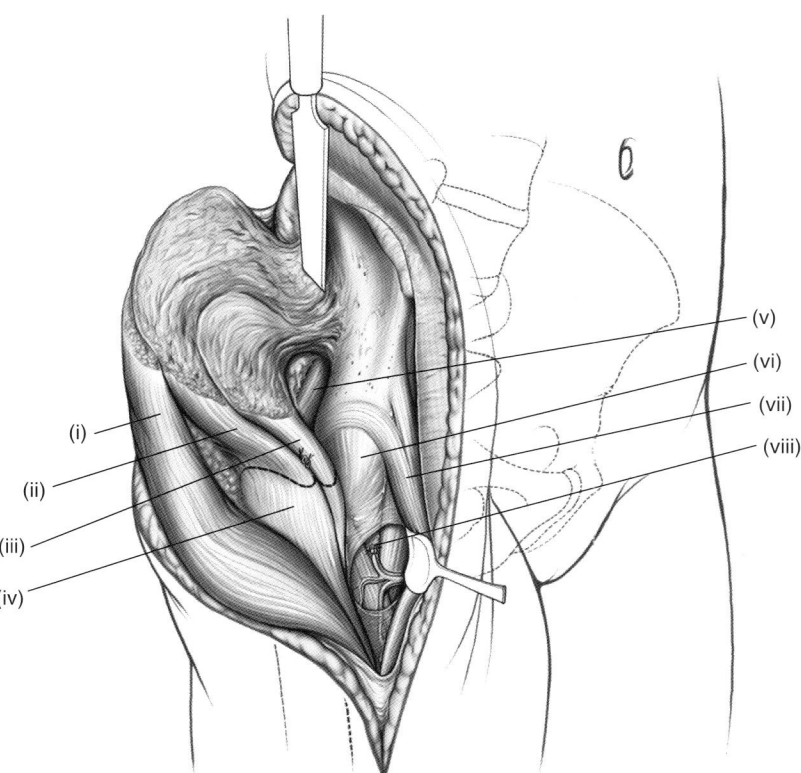

Figure 25. Proximally, the abductor and tensor fascia lata muscles have been stripped subperiosteally from the outer table of the right ileum. Distally, the ascending branch of the lateral circumflex artery has been ligated. The abductor insertions have been marked for release. (i) Tensor fascia lata muscle; (ii) Gluteus medius muscle; (iii) Gluteus minimus muscle; (iv) Greater trochanter; (v) Piriformis muscle; (vi) Hip joint capsule; (vii) Two heads of the rectus muscle; (viii) Ligated ascending branch of the lateral femoral circumflex artery.

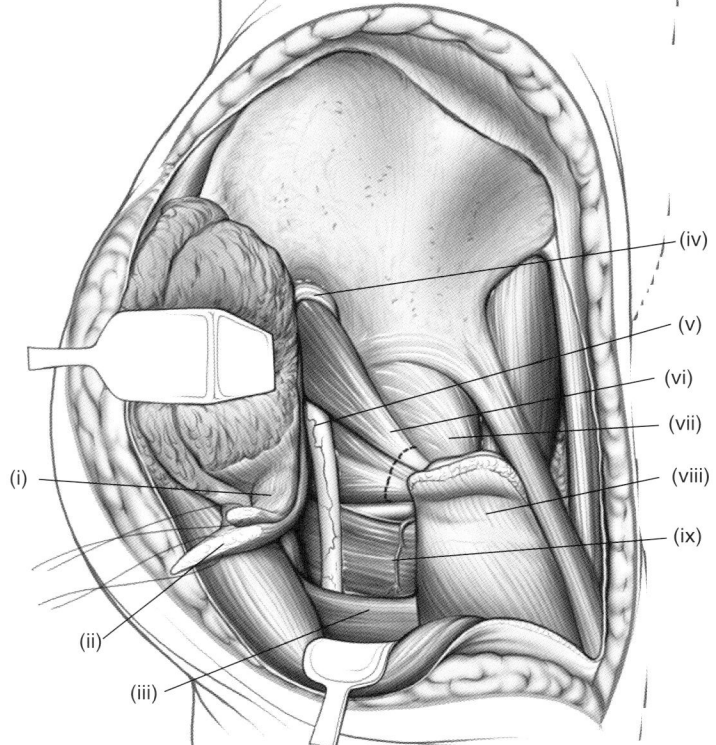

Figure 26. The abductors of the right hip have been tagged and their insertions into the greater trochanter released, allowing their muscle pedicle to be retracted to expose the sciatic nerve. The external rotators have also been marked for release. (i) Gluteus minimus tendon; (ii) Gluteus medius tendon; (iii) Gluteus maximus tendon: (iv) Superior gluteal neurovascular bundle; (v) Sciatic nerve; (vi) Piriformis and conjoint tendons; (vii) Hip joint capsule; (viii) Greater trochanter; (ix) Medial femoral circumflex artery overlying quadratus femoris.

The tendons of the piriformis muscle, obturator internus muscle, and the inferior and superior gemellus muscles are tagged and transected (Figs. 26, 27) similar to the Kocher-Langenbeck approach (Figs. 4, 5). Next, the tendinous femoral insertion of the gluteus maximus muscle is identified and transected with a cuff for repair (Fig. 27). The piriformis muscle is followed towards the greater sciatic notch and the obturator internus muscle to the lesser sciatic notch where retractors can be inserted allowing complete exposure to the posterior column of the acetabulum (Fig. 27). The sciatic nerve is at risk during exposure of the posterior column and needs to be identified along the belly of the quadratus femoris muscle as in the Kocher-Langenbeck approach, then protected behind the conjoint tendon (Fig. 27). Traction along the nerve should be avoided by maintaining the hip extended and the knee flexed at all times.

Further access to the acetabulum is available through an osteotomy of the superior and inferior iliac spines to release the sartorius and direct head of the rectus, respectively (Figs. 27, 28). The blood supply to the dome of the acetabulum is at risk during dissection at the anterior inferior iliac spine (27). The lateral femoral cutaneous nerve is at risk during exposure along the anterior superior iliac spine. It can also sustain a traction injury during mobilization of the soft tissues. Patients should be warned preoperatively to expect this complication. Visualization of the acetabular articular surface can be performed with a marginal capsulotomy leaving a cuff of tissue for repair followed by distraction of the hip joint with either a Schanz screw placed into the femoral head or with a femoral distractor (Fig. 29). The internal iliac fossa is further exposed by sharply releasing the external oblique muscle from the iliac crest (Fig. 28). The limits of the extended iliofemoral approach have been reached, and reduction of the fracture fragments can now be completed according to the preoperative

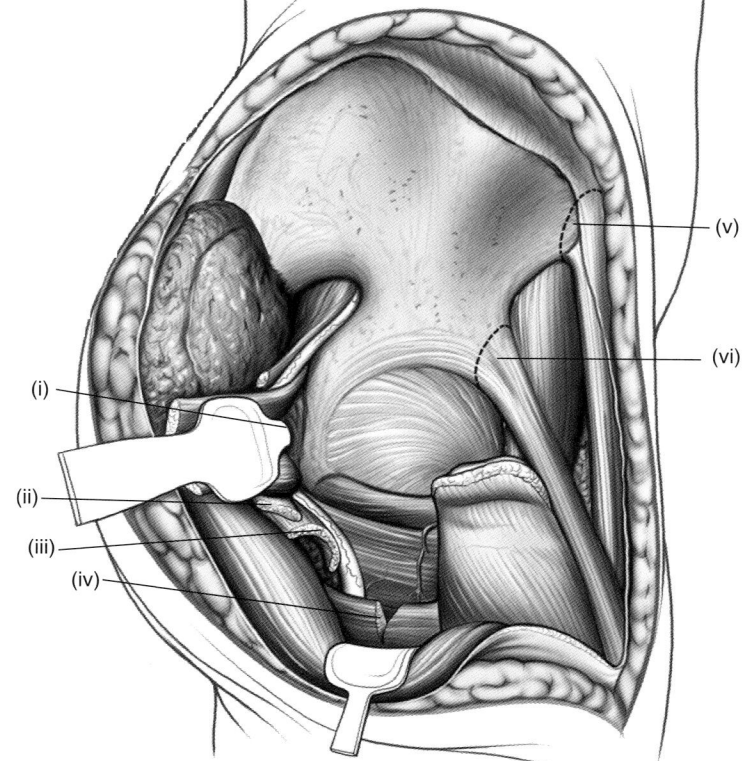

Figure 27. Retraction of right hip external rotator muscles and release of gluteus maximus insertion distally. Medially, the anterior superior and inferior iliac spines have been marked for either release or osteotomy. (i) Blunt Hohmann in lesser sciatic notch. The conjoint tendons have been positioned between the retractor and the sciatic nerve; (ii) Gluteus minimus tendon; (iii) Gluteus medius tendon; (iv) Partial release of gluteus maximus tendon; (v) Anterior-superior iliac spine and sartorius muscle origin; (vi) Anterior-inferior iliac spine and direct head of rectus femoris muscle.

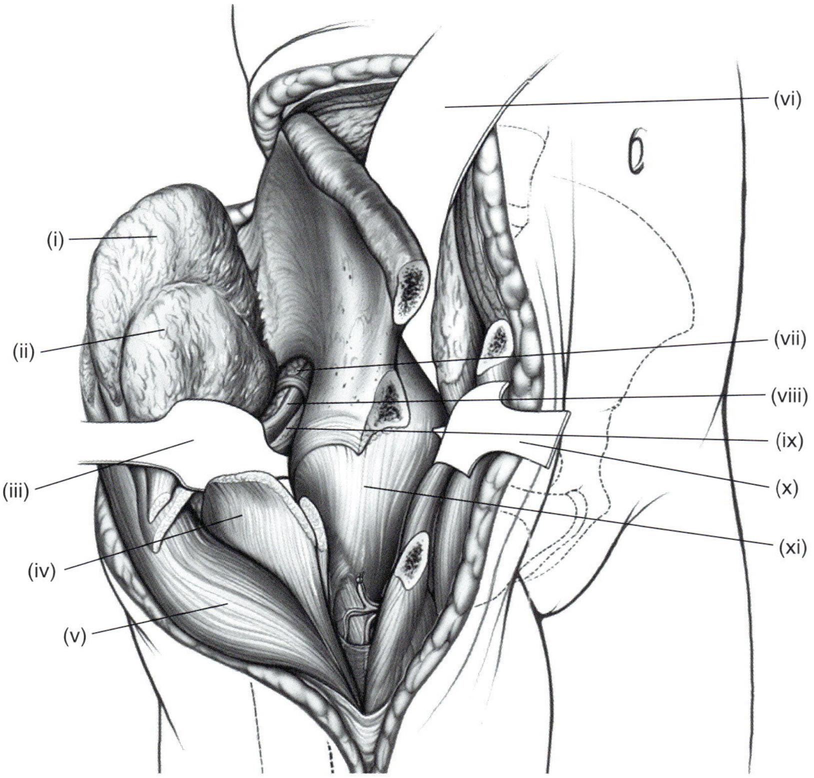

Figure 28. Complete exposure of right acetabulum. (i) Gluteus medius muscle; (ii) Gluteus minimus muscle; (iii) Blunt Hohmann in lesser sciatic notch; (iv) Greater trochanter; (v) Tensor fascia lata muscle; (vi) Malleable retractor under the iliacus muscle; (vii) Superior gluteal neurovascular bundle; (viii) Piriformis muscle; (ix) Sciatic nerve; (x) Spiked Hohmann retractor over the anterior capsule of the hip; (xi) Hip joint capsule.

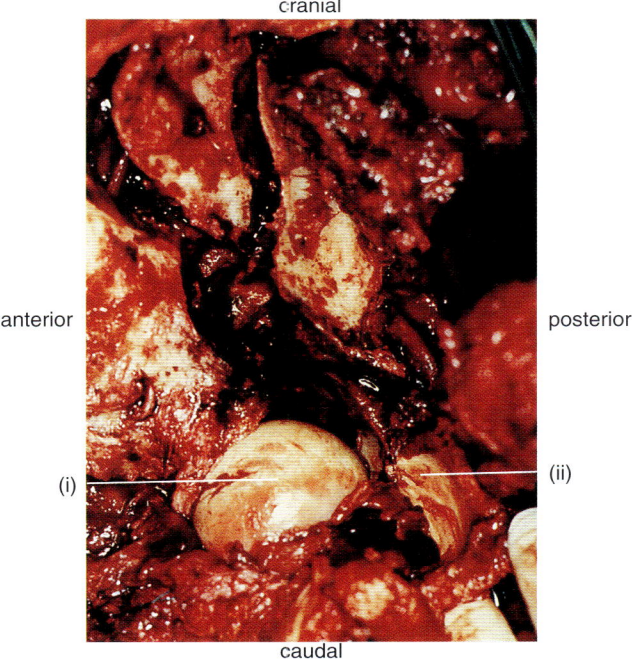

Figure 29. Close-up of acetabular joint exposure of patient. (i) Femoral head; (ii) Loose articular fragment.

plan. Medial exposure of the anterior column is limited by the iliopsoas muscle and the iliopectineal eminence. Therefore, further medial dissection without an ilioinguinal incision would place the femoral neurovascular structures at great risk (Fig. 28). It is important to keep the soft-tissue flaps moist with wet sponges throughout the procedure.

High, or transtectal, transverse, or **T** fractures, especially those with dome involvement, are often best reduced and stabilized through an extensile approach. This allows excellent access to the whole iliac wing, posterior column, and superior anterior column, hence providing direct visualization of the reduction and fixation of the acetabulum. Generally, for the transverse or **T**-type fractures, the pelvic reduction clamp with 4.5-mm screws, both proximal and distal to the posterior column fracture, allows distraction, debridement of the fracture surfaces. Additional control of rotation can be provided by a Schanz screw placed into the ischium as a "joy-stick." The adequacy of reduction of the posterior column can be assessed by direct visualization of the articular surface and also with digital palpation through the greater and lesser sciatic notches. As already discussed in the section on the ilioinguinal approach, reconstruction of the fracture generally proceeds centripetally from the periphery, i.e., from the top of the iliac wing towards to acetabulum (Fig. 30). Prior to definitive reduction, a gliding hole can be inserted into the proximal aspect of the posterior column from superior to inferior, assuring the correct position of the gliding hole in the middle of the posterior column. Following reduction, it is then possible to insert a 4.5-mm or 3.5-mm cortical lag screw down the posterior column. Additional stabilization is accomplished with a 3.5-mm reconstruction plate molded to the posterior column. With direct visualization of the acetabular articular surface, the anterior column can then be reduced. In a transverse fracture, there is a rotational malalignment of the columns, but in the **T**-type fracture pattern, the columns can be both separated and malrotated. Our approach to these complex fractures patterns involves lag-screw fixation of the two columns. Again, the gliding hole can be inserted from the lateral aspect of the iliac wing into the anterior col-

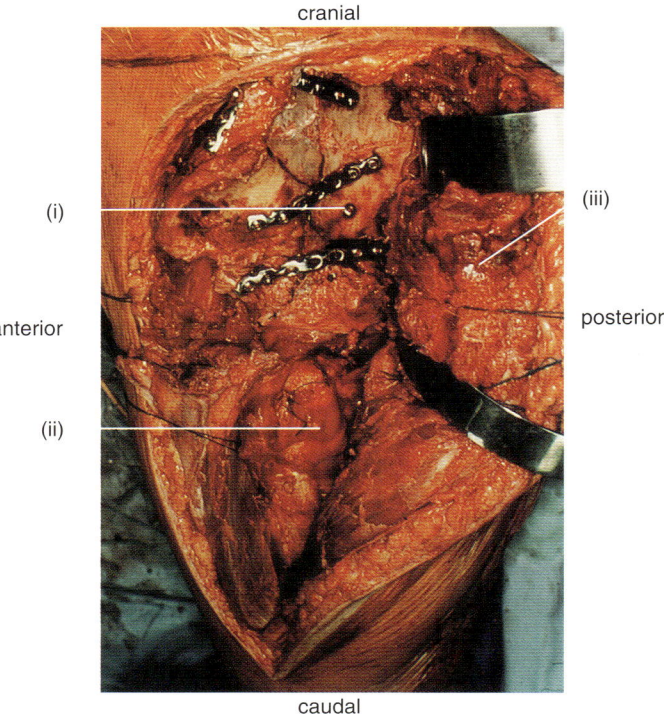

Figure 30. Reconstruction of comminuted left both-column acetabular fractures. Reconstruction proceeds centripetally from the periphery. (i) Anterior to posterior column lag screw; (ii) Greater trochanter; (iii) Abductor muscles and tensor fascia lata.

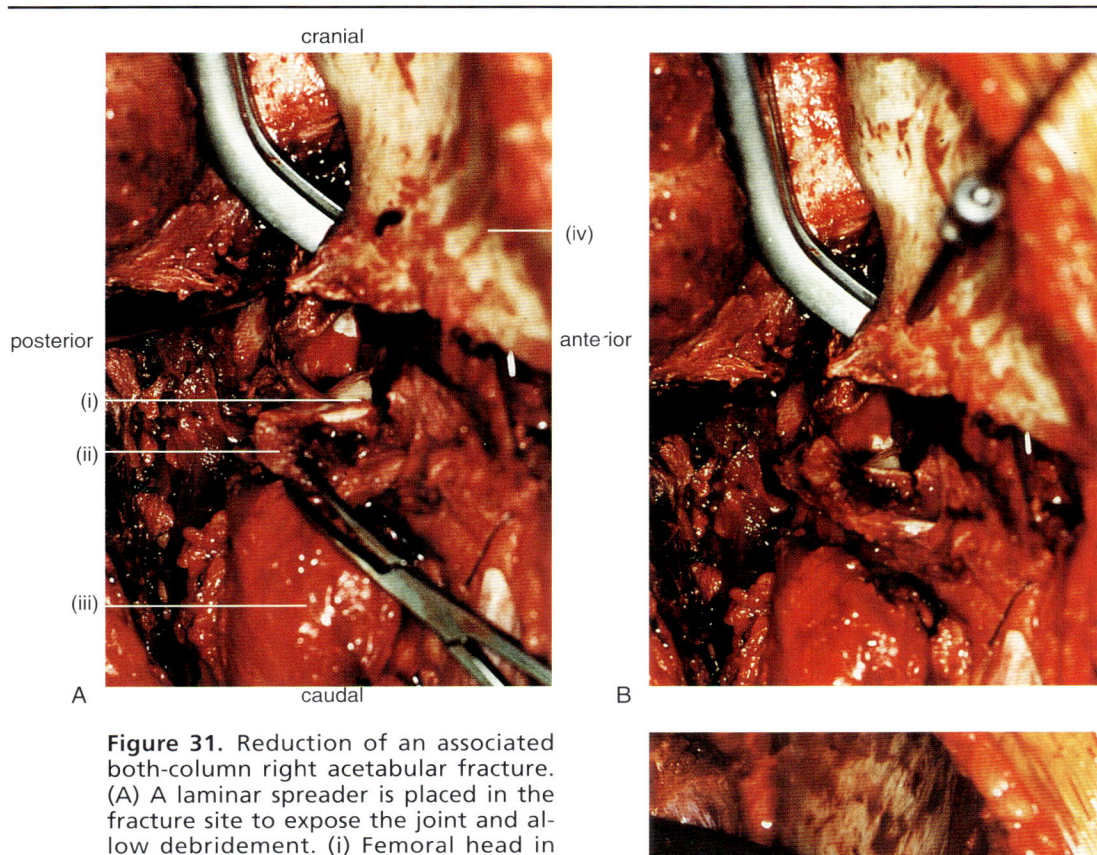
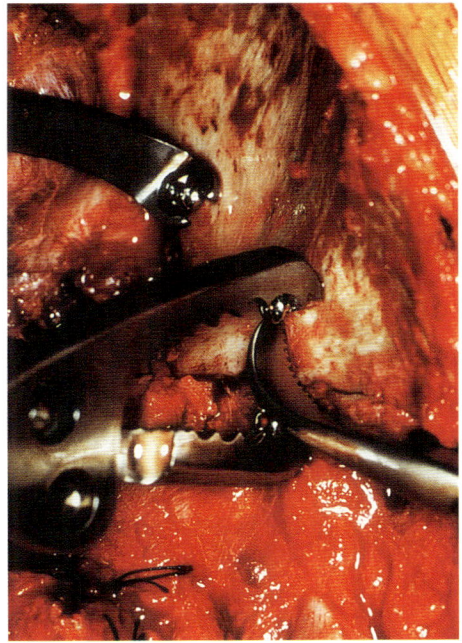

Figure 31. Reduction of an associated both-column right acetabular fracture. (A) A laminar spreader is placed in the fracture site to expose the joint and allow debridement. (i) Femoral head in joint; (ii) Superolateral dome fragment with capsular attachments; (iii) Greater trochanter; (iv) Intact iliac wing. (B) The gliding hole is predrilled for the anterior to posterior column screw. (C) A Farabeuf clamp affixed to screws is used to reduce the anterior column to the superolateral fragment, and a pelvic reduction clamp affixed to screws is used to reduce the anterior to the posterior column (posterior column portion not shown).

umn, superior and medial to the articular surface. Generally, this requires the insertion of a lag screw three finger breadths proximal to the superior aspect of the articular surface and one finger breadth posterior to the gluteal ridge on the outer aspect of the iliac crest. The lag screw is then angled from posterior-superior to anterior-inferior directly down the superior pubic ramus to secure both columns of the acetabulum. This can be accomplished with a 4.5 mm cortical screw in larger individuals or a 3.5 mm screw in smaller individuals. Care must be taken to assure that this screw remains extraarticular and does not penetrate the superior aspect of the anterior pelvis in proximity to the iliopectineal eminence, where the femoral vasculature is in close adherence. The use of intraoperative fluoroscopy for the insertion of this screw is mandatory. Lag screws can also be inserted anteriorly, into the intact ilium and superior posterior column (Fig. 31A).

For those associated both-column acetabular fractures, with a comminuted posterior column, posterior-wall involvement, lateral-dome involvement, or extension into the greater sciatic notch, an extensile approach is the approach of choice to assure an anatomical reduction of the acetabulum (Figs. 29 to 31). This mandates an anatomical reduction of all the fractures in the iliac wing, working from the periphery towards the acetabulum, as with the ilioinguinal approach. Once the iliac wing is stabilized with lag screws and/or by 3.5-mm laterally applied reconstruction plates, the posterior column is reduced to the iliac wing with direct visualization of the acetabular articular surface. The posterior column lag screw and 3.5-mm reconstruction plate fixation is accomplished as for **T**-or transverse-type fractures. The anterior column is then reduced to the intact posterior column. This can be accomplished with anterior to posterior 4.5-mm lag screws inserted from the antero-superior spine into the sciatic buttress, and/or anterior column lag screws from the lateral aspect of the iliac wing, as described previously. The adequacy of the reduction has to be assessed, both by direct visualization of the acetabulum, with finger palpation of the greater and lesser sciatic notches and quadrilateral plate, and, if necessary, in the internal iliac fossa. The use of fluoroscopy is essential to assure the adequacy of reduction and the position of the fixation.

An extensile approach is always necessary when open reduction and internal fixation of an acetabular fracture, which involves both the anterior and posterior columns, is performed 21 or more days after injury. Because of this delay in operative fixation, these cases are among the most difficult the surgeon can face. This is due to the need to meticulously take down varying amounts of organizing fracture hematoma and/or early callus in order to obtain an anatomical reduction of all the fracture lines in the iliac crest and acetabulum. Even with meticulous reduction and surgical stabilization, the results of late reconstruction of acetabular fractures are excellent or good in less than half of the cases (6).

After completion of the operative repair, drains are placed along the external surface of the iliac wing, along the posterior column, the internal iliac fossa, and the vastus lateralis muscle. The hip capsule is repaired, followed by reattachment of the tendinous femoral insertion of the gluteus maximus and the short external rotators. The tendons of the gluteus minimus and gluteus medius muscles are also sutured to their respective attachment sites on the greater trochanter. Reattachment of the origin of the gluteal muscles and the tensor fascia lata muscle to the iliac crest can be facilitated by hip abduction. The origins of the sartorius and direct head of the rectus femoris muscles are reattached at their osteotomy sites using lag screws through drill holes if such a medial exposure had been required. This is followed by reattachment of the external oblique muscle along the iliac crest. Subcutaneous drains are inserted prior to skin closure.

POSTOPERATIVE MANAGEMENT

Postoperatively, patients are maintained on intravenous cefazolin for 48 to 72 hours. Our postoperative anticoagulation regimen includes six weeks of Warfarin in conjunction with compression boots. Heterotopic ossification prophylaxis is important after posterior and extensile approaches, preferably with Indomethacin 25 mg orally three times each day for six weeks. Drains are not discontinued until output has tapered to 10 to 20 ml per eight-hour shift.

Patients are mobilized early during the postoperative period. They are allowed to dangle and sit on a chair within the first 24 to 48 hours following surgery. After removal of drains, they are started on a toe-touch to 20 lbs weight-bearing protocol with crutches for six to eight weeks. Over the ensuing (third) month there is gradual progression to full weight bearing. We do not use continuous passive motion during the postoperative period, since we have not had difficulty regaining hip motion in this patient population. Abductor strengthening along with gait training is initiated by the physical therapist during the postoperative period. Acetabular fractures with a concomitant neurologic injury can pose a difficult rehabilitation problem due to lack of motor activity or to neurogenic pain and frequently require treatment in conjunction with a pain management service.

We routinely obtain postoperative roentgenograms (anteroposterior pelvis and 45-degree oblique "Judet" views) and a CT scan to assess critically the fracture reduction and position of hardware.

Long-term clinical outcomes correlate closely with the type of reduction achieved during surgery. Letournel and Judet (5), in a review of 350 acetabular fractures with a 2- to 21-year followup, reported that an anatomic reduction was achieved in 74% of their patients, of whom 90% had a good clinical outcome. Of the 26% with an imperfectly reduced acetabulum, 55% had a good clinical outcome if the femoral head was situated under the dome, and only 11% if there was residual subluxation of the femoral head.

Even 10 years later, when reevaluating these patients, Letournel (25) continued to note rather gratifying results. In his review of 569 acetabular fractures treated within three weeks of injury, he achieved an anatomic reduction (a maximum of 1 mm of displacement on any of three views) in 74% of cases, with 82% of these patients having very good clinical outcomes at a followup of as much as 33 years. Of the 26% with an imperfectly reduced acetabulum, very good results were obtained in 54% of cases if the femoral head was centered under the dome, but in only 23% of cases where there was any residual subluxation of the femoral head.

Management of Complications

Complications following the operative treatment of acetabular fractures fall into early and late groups. The acute complications include iatrogenic sciatic-nerve injury, vascular injury, deep vein thrombosis, pulmonary embolism, infection, loss of reduction, and death. The late group includes heterotopic ossification, chondrolysis, avascular necrosis, and traumatic arthritis. De novo iatrogenic sciatic-nerve injury or worsening of a preexisting deficit is a significant problem. Patients at increased risk include those with preoperative sciatic nerve compromise and those with fracture patterns that involve the posterior wall or column (10,11). However, with the use of intraoperative sciatic-nerve monitoring using somatosensory evoked potentials, the incidence of iatrogenic sciatic-nerve injury has been reduced to 2% (10,11). This risk is further lessened by the addition of intraoperative monitoring of motor pathways (8).

Vascular injury, most commonly to the superior gluteal artery or the corona mortis, can occur during either the exposure or fracture reduction (6,10). In this situation, control of bleeding is crucial. Initially, packing of the area may provide hemostasis. Failing this, ligation of the bleeding vessel must be performed. Should a bleeding superior gluteal vessel retract into the pelvis in the midst of a posterior approach, then an osteotomy of the sciatic notch can be performed to identify and control the bleeding vessel. It is important to avoid the indiscriminate placement of suture ligations or clamps, due to the proximity of the superior gluteal nerve. Damage to this structure can result in significant loss of function.

A devastating complication following fixation of acetabular fractures is deep infection, with an incidence as high as 9% but probably nearer 4% to 5% (6,12,20). To minimize the incidence of postoperative infection, we advocate the use of prophylactic antibiotics, the use of multiple suction drains in all recesses to prevent hematoma formation, surgical evacuation of hematomas, and if present, debridement of the Morel-Lavalle lesion over the greater trochanter (6,16).

Another troublesome occurrence is loss of reduction during the early postoperative period. This is especially true in elderly patients with osteopenic bone where it is important to buttress the fractures adequately (9). Intraarticular hardware penetration has also been reported and can lead to rapid chondrolysis. We confirm hardware position using intraoperative Judet views and clinically by placing the hip through a range of motion with a finger placed along the quadrilateral surface to feel for any grating. We also obtain postoperative CT scans to confirm fracture reduction and hardware position.

The most common complication following the operative fixation of acetabular fractures is heterotopic ossification with an incidence ranging from 18% to 90% (6,12,22). While it causes functional limitation in only 5% to 10% of cases (20,25), heterotopic bone formation is particularly common and severe with the extended iliofemoral approach due to stripping of the external surface of the iliac wing (6,12,22). The ilioinguinal approach has the lowest incidence of heterotopic ossification (6,12).

We routinely prophylax all patients with Indomethacin if they undergo a Kocher-Langenbeck or an extensile approach. Indomethacin has been shown to decrease the incidence of heterotopic ossification in patients with acetabular fractures (6). We do not routinely prophylax patients who undergo fixation through an ilioinguinal approach, unless a limited subperiosteal exposure of the outer cortex of the ilium was performed for insertion of pelvic reduction clamps. Patients in whom Indomethacin is contraindicated can be treated with low-dose radiation therapy given in a single dose or multiple fractions (6,22,24).

The incidence of avascular necrosis following operative treatment of acetabular fractures has been reported to range from 3% to 9% (6,7,12), with the majority of cases identified between 3 and 18 months following surgery (6). Additionally, Letournel (6) has noted an increased incidence of avascular necrosis of the femoral head in cases presenting after three weeks and those associated with a posterior fracture/dislocation. In all probability, the fate of the femoral head is determined at the time of the injury. However, avascular necrosis must be differentiated from malreduction or screw impingement as a cause of femoral head disintegration.

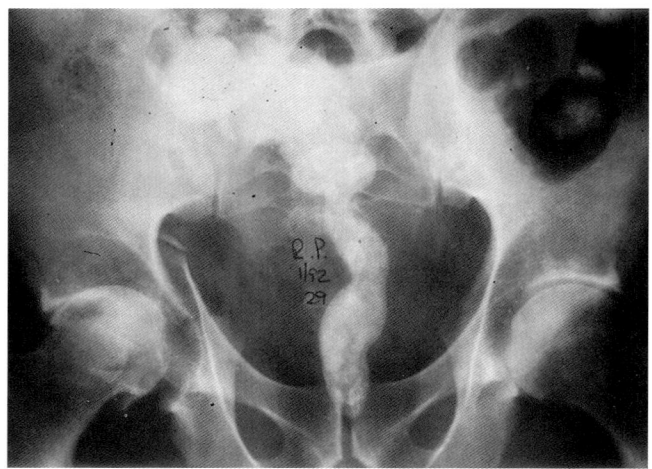
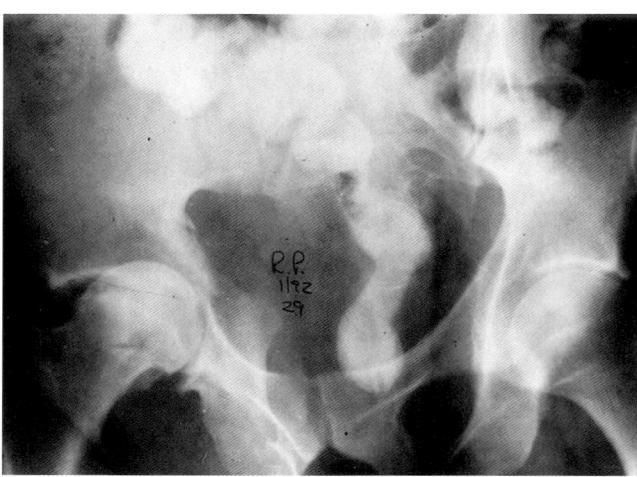

Figure 32. Preoperative radiographs of patient with comminuted transverse plus posterior wall right acetabular fracture. (A) AP pelvis. (B) Iliac oblique view. (C) Obturator oblique view.

5 ACETABULAR FRACTURES: SURGICAL APPROACHES AND TECHNIQUE

ILLUSTRATIVE CASE FOR TECHNIQUE

Kocher-Langenbeck Approach

This 29-year-old male presented with a right comminuted transverse plus posterior wall acetabular fracture, with associated partial greater trochanter avulsion (Fig. 32). Multiple intraarticular fragments and significant marginal posterior wall impaction were seen with CT scanning. A femoral distractor was used to allow removal of posterior wall fragments from the hip joint, the fracture was reduced, and stabilization was carried out with a 3.5-mm reconstruction plate and lag screws.

At one-year followup, healing and good maintenance of the reduction were noted, although slight hip-joint narrowing was observed (Fig. 33).

Extended Ilioinguinal Approach

This patient presented with an associated both-column fracture of the right acetabulum with dome comminution (Fig. 34A to C). The anterior column was initially reduced and

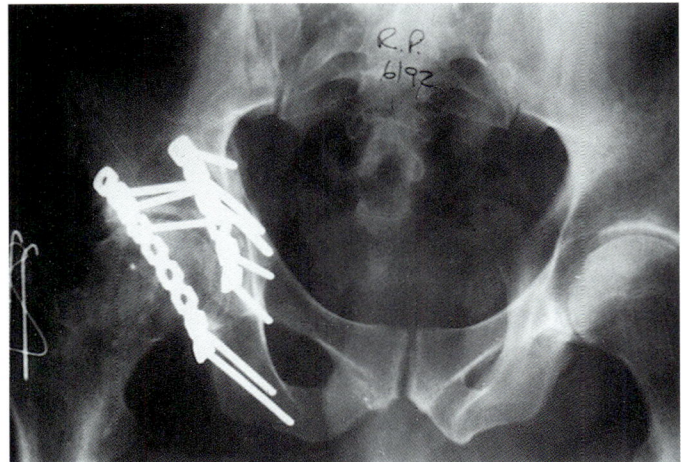
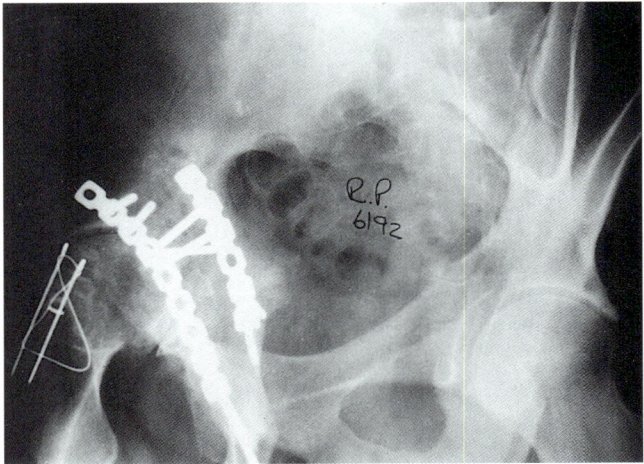
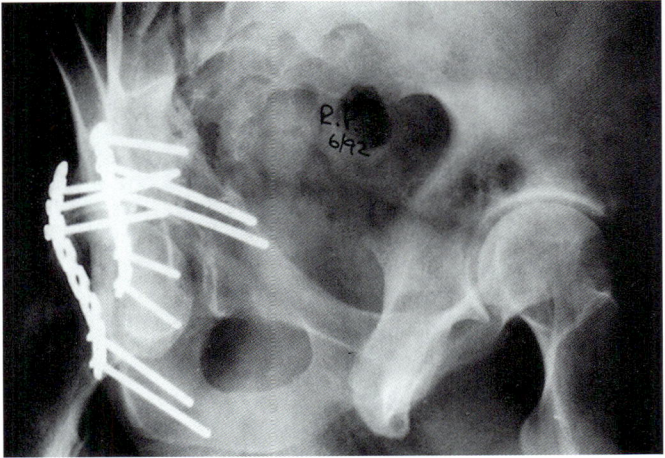

Figure 33. Radiographs showing one year followup of the patient in Fig. 31. (A) AP pelvis. (B) Iliac oblique view. (C) Obturator oblique view.

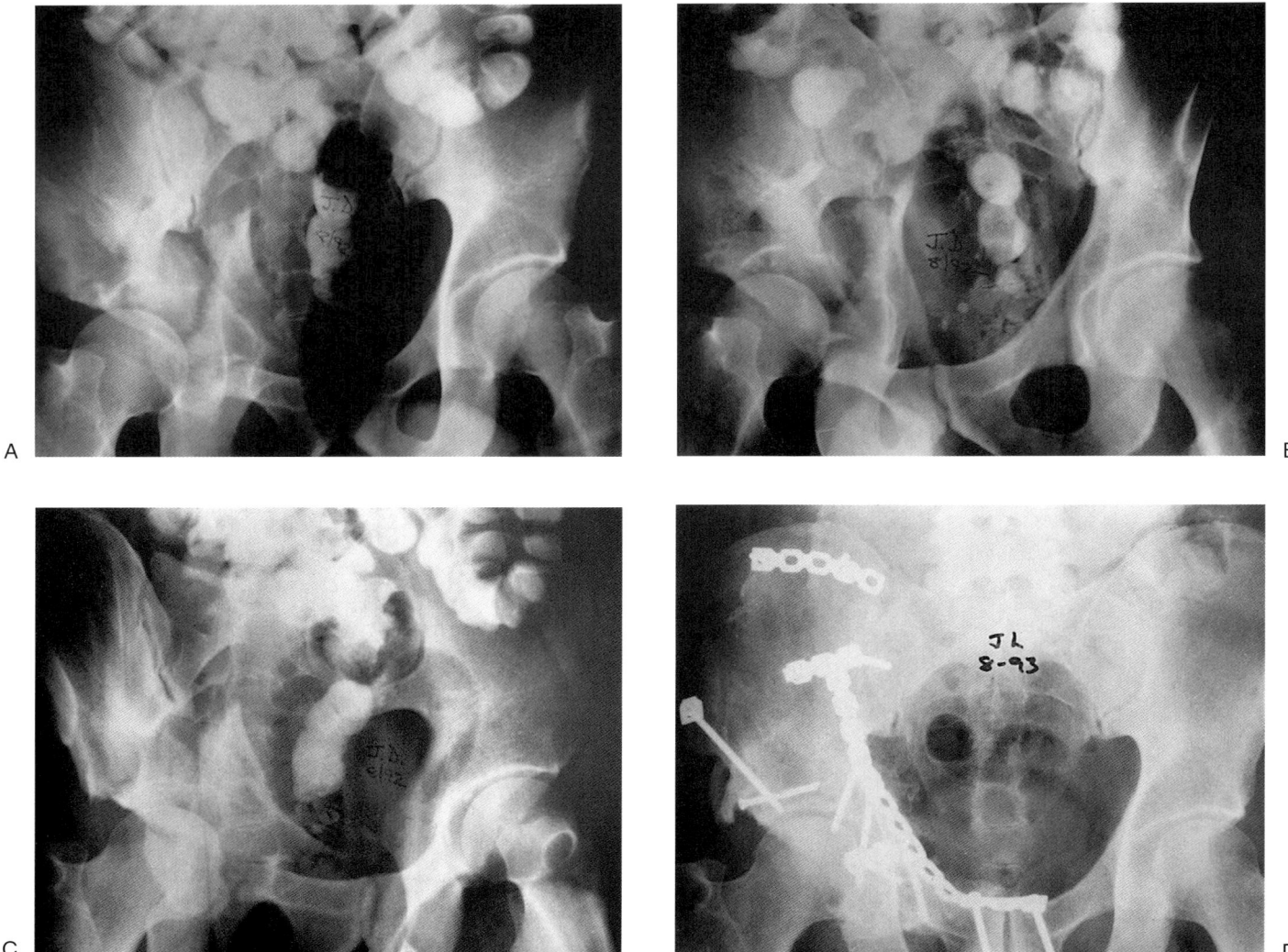

Figure 34. Radiographs of a patient treated for a comminuted associated both column fracture. (A) AP pelvis. (B) Iliac oblique view. (C) Obturator oblique view. (D) AP pelvis at one-year followup.

stabilized with a 3.5-mm reconstruction plate, and the posterior column with anterior to posterior lag screws. A percutaneous cannulated lag screw was placed through the abductor muscles into the dome fragment. Figure 34D shows the results one year postoperatively.

Extended Iliofemoral Approach

This 18-year-old female with an associated both-column right acetabular fracture was treated via an extended iliofemoral approach due to significant dome and superolateral acetabular involvement (Fig. 35). The fracture was reduced with direct visualization and stabilized with multiple plates and lag screws.

At one-year followup, a congruent reduction with healing, and maintenance of the joint space were noted (Fig. 36).

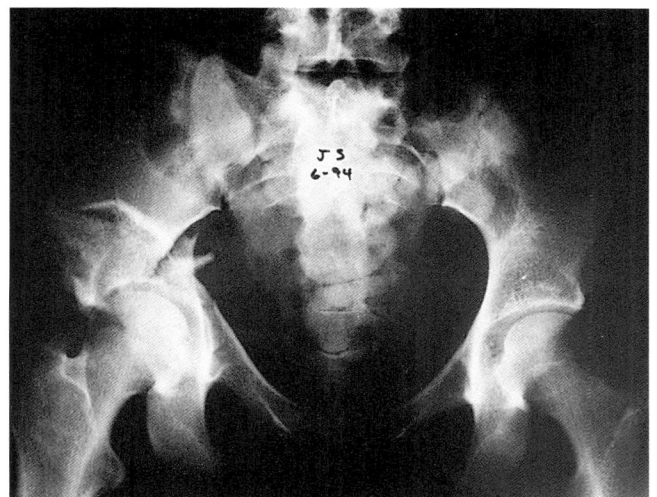
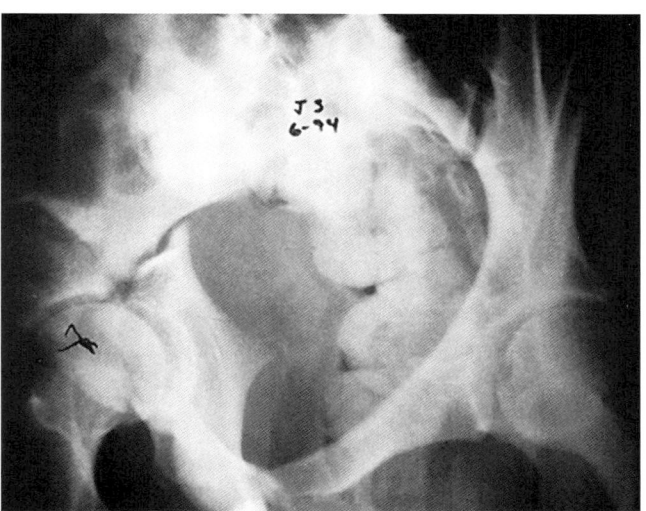
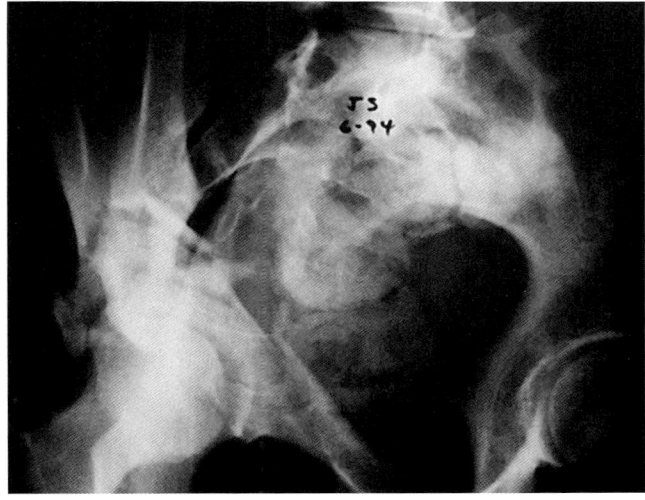

Figure 35. Radiographs of 18-year-old female treated for an associated both-column right acetabular fracture. Note the significant dome and superolateral acetabular fracture involvement. (A) AP pelvis. (B) Iliac oblique view. (C) Obturator oblique view.

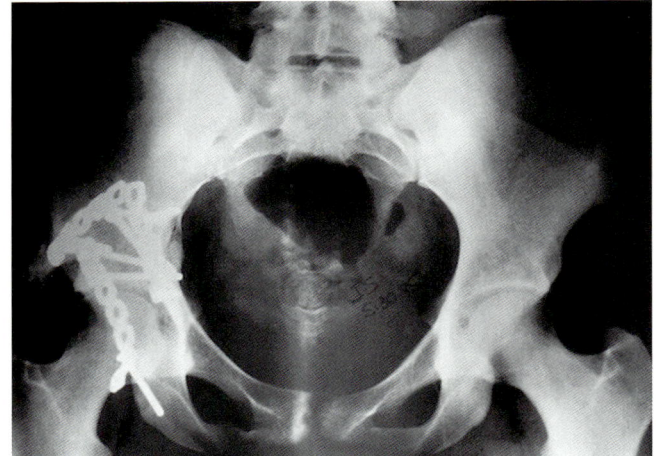
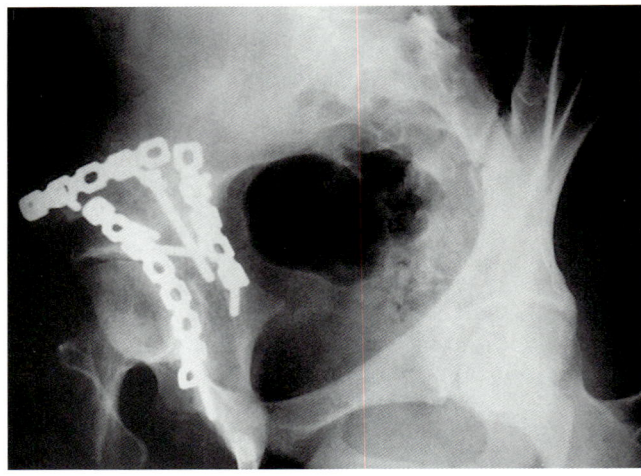
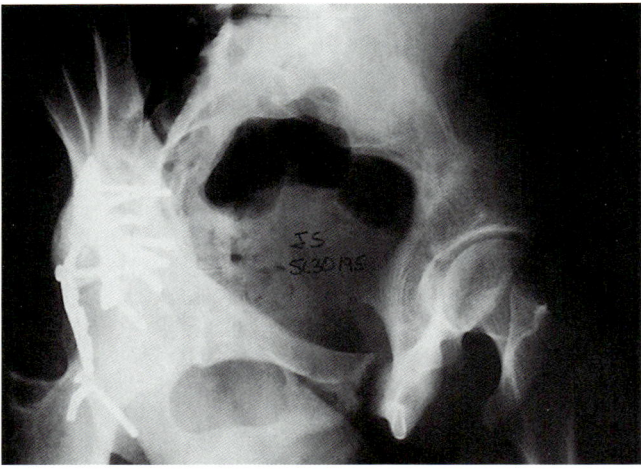

Figure 36. Radiographs showing one-year followup of patient shown in Fig. 34. (A) AP pelvis. (B) Iliac oblique view. (C) Obturator oblique view.

RECOMMENDED READING

1. Judet, R., Judet, J., and Letournel, E. Fractures of the acetabulum: Classification and surgical approaches for open reduction. Preliminary report. *J. Bone Joint Surg.*, 46(A):1615–1646.
2. Judet, R., and Lagrange, J. La voie postero-externe de Gibson Presse Med 66: 263–264, 1958.
3. Letournel, E. Acetabulum fractures: Classification and management. *Clin. Orthop.*, 151: 81–106, 1980.
4. Letournel, E. Surgical treatment of acetabular fractures. In: *The hip: Proceedings of the fifteenth open scientific meeting of The Hip Society*, pp. 157–180. St. Louis, C. V. Mosby Company, 1987.
5. Letournel, E., and Judet, R. *Fractures of the acetabulum.* Berlin, Springer-Verlag, 1981.
6. Letournel, E., and Judet, R. *Fractures of the acetabulum.* Berlin, Springer-Verlag, 1993.
7. Matta, J. M., Anderson, L. M., Epstein, H. C., and Hendricks, P. Fractures of the acetabulum: A retrospective analysis. *Clin. Orthop.*, 205: 241–250, 1986.
8. Helfet, D. L., Anand, N., Malkani, A. L., Heise, C. W., Quinn, T. J., Green, D. S. T., and Burga, S. Intraoperative monitoring of motor pathways during operative fixation of acute acetabular fractures. *J. Orthop. Trauma*, 11: 2–6, 1997.
9. Helfet, D. L., Borrelli, J. D., JR., Dipasquale, T. G., and Sanders, R. W. Stabilization of acetabular fractures in elderly patients. *JBJS*, 74(A): 753–765, 1992.
10. Helfet, D. L., Hissa, E. A., Sergay, S., and Mast, J. W. Somatosensory evoked potential monitoring in the surgical management of acute acetabular fractures. *J. Orthop. Trauma*, 5: 161–166, 1991.
11. Helfet, D. L., and Schmeling, G. J. Somatosensory evoked potential monitoring in the surgical treatment of acute, displaced acetabular fractures: Results of a prospective study. *Clin. Orthop.*, 301: 213–229, 1994.
12. Matta, J. M. Fractures of the acetabulum: Accuracy of reduction and clinical results. *JBJS*, 78(A): 632–1645, 1996.

13. Matta, J. M., Mehne, D. K., and Roffi, R. Fractures of the acetabulum: Early results of a prospective study. *Clin. Orthop.*, 205: 241–250, 1986.
14. Pennal, G. F., Davidson, J., Garside, H., and Plewes, J. Results of treatment of acetabular fractures. *Clin. Orthop.*, 151: 115–123, 1980.
15. Vrahas, M., Gordon, R. G., Mears, D. C., Krieger, D., and Sclabassi, R. J. Intraoperative somatosensory evoked potential monitoring of pelvic and acetabular fractures. *J. Orthop. Trauma*, 6(1): 50–58, 1992.
16. Hak, D. J., Olson, S. A., and Matta, J. M. Management of the Morel-Lavalle lesion. Presented at the third annual International Consensus on Surgery of the Pelvis and Acetabulum. Pittsburgh, October 5–11, 1996.
17. Stickney, J. L., and Helfet, D. L. Deep vein thrombosis prevention in orthopaedic trauma patients (abstract). *J. Orthop. Trauma*, 5(2): 227, 1991.
18. Montgomery, K. D., Potter, H. G., and Helfet, D. L. Magnetic resonance venography to evaluate the deep venous system of the pelvis in patients who have an acetabular fracture. *JBJS*, 77(A): 1639–1649, 1995.
19. Mayo, K. A. Surgical approaches to the acetabulum. *Tech. Orthop.* 4: 24–35, 1990.
20. Matta, J. M. and Merritt, P. O. Displaced acetabular fractures. *Clin. Orthop.*, 230: 83–97, 1988.
21. Johnson, E. E., Matta, J. M., Mast, J. W., and Letournel, E. Delayed reconstruction of acetabular fractures 21–120 days following injury. *Clin. Orthop.*, 305: 20–30, 1994
22. Bosse, M. J., Poka, A., Reinert, C. M., Ellwanger, F., Slawson, R., and McDevitt, E. R. Heterotopic ossification as a complication of acetabular fracture: Prophylaxis with low-dose irradiation. *JBJS*, 70(A): 1231–1237, 1988.
23. Leenen, L. P. H., Van Der Werken, C., Schoots, F. J., and Goris, R. J. A. Internal fixation of open unstable pelvic fractures. *J. Trauma*, 35: 220–225, 1993.
24. Skura, D. S., and Buchsbaum, S. Prophylactic low-dose postoperative irradiation for the prevention of heterotopic ossification in acetabular fractures. *Orthop. Trans.*, 16: 221, 1992 (abstract).
25. Mears, D. C., and Gordon, R. G. Internal fixation of acetabular fractures. *Techniques Orthop.*, 4(4): 36–51, 1990.
26. Brumback, R. J., Holt, E. S., McBride, M. S., Poka, A., Bathon, G. H., and Burgess, A. R. Acetabular depression fracture accompanying posterior fracture dislocation of the hip. *J. Orthop. Trauma*, 4(1): 42–48, 1990.
27. Chapman, M.W.: Effect of surgical approaches on the blood supply to the acetabulum. Presented at the First Annual International Consensus on Surgery of the Pelvis and Acetabulum. Pittsburgh, October 11–15th, 1992.
28. Geerts, W. H., Code, K. I., Jay, R. M., Chen, E., and Szalai, J. P. A prospective study of venous thromboembolism after major trauma. *N. Engl. J. Med.*, 332: 1448–1449, 1995.

Surgical Management of Intertrochanteric Fractures

James F. Kellam

INDICATIONS/CONTRAINDICATIONS

Restoration of function is the major indication for operative intervention of an intertrochanteric fracture. Function must be appropriately assessed with each individual patient. In a patient who does not walk, it may be quite suitable to treat the fracture nonoperatively (8). However, in a very active individual, surgery is indicated to allow the patient to maximize his/her function.

Contraindications to surgical intervention for intertrochanteric fractures include medical conditions that make the patient unsuitable for anesthetic intervention. A patient with a completely undisplaced and stable fracture who can use crutches and remain non-weight bearing may be treated nonoperatively. Last, if the function has not been changed because of the fracture, surgical intervention is inappropriate.

PREOPERATIVE PLANNING

The surgeon must be familiar with the anatomy of the proximal femur. The intertrochanteric region is composed of four segments. The proximal segment consists of the head and the neck and its capsular attachments causing it to align in a neutral or internally rotated position. The distal segment is the femoral shaft, which shortens and externally rotates. The other two segments represent variable-sized fragments of the greater and the

---

J. F. Kellam, M.D.: Department of Orthopedic Surgery, Carolinas Health Care System: Carolinas Medical Center, Charlotte, North Carolina 28232.

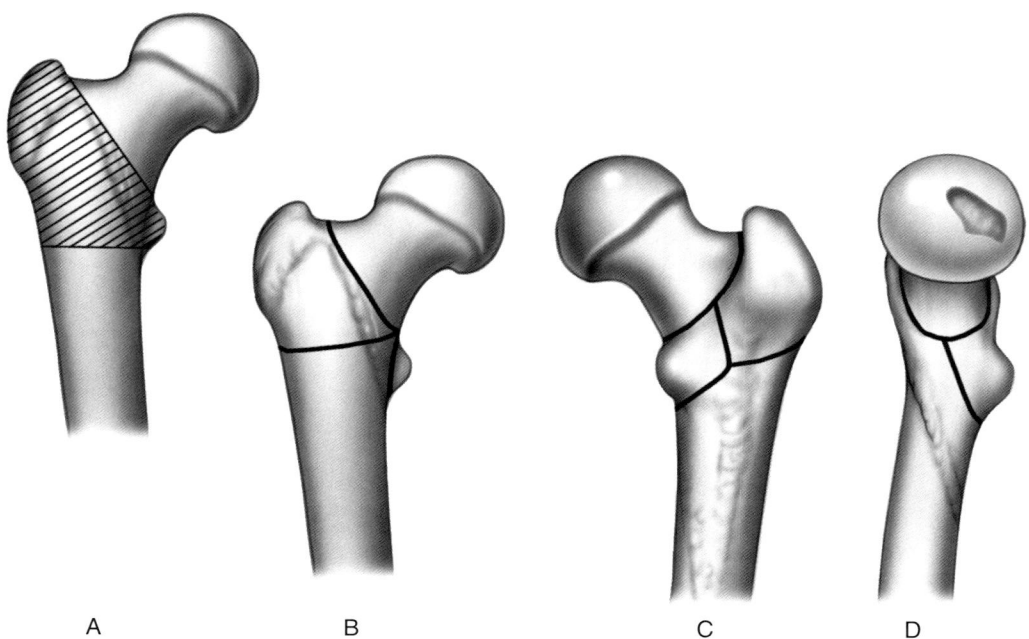

Figure 1. The proximal segment of the femur is defined by a line that transverses through the lower edge of the lesser trochanter. The trochanteric area can be defined as an area from the intertrochanteric line above to the distal limit of the proximal segment. This area can be divided into four segments: (A) neck and head, (B) distal shaft, (C) posterior medial fragment with lesser trochanter, and (D) greater trochanteric or intertrochanteric area.

lesser trochanter. The lesser trochanteric region, or posterior medial fragment, is responsible for the stability of the reduction (Fig. 1).

There have been numerous classifications of intertrochanteric fractures, aimed at determining which fractures represent potential problems for reduction or postreduction stability. To understand a classification and its implication for fracture care, one must appreciate the principle of fracture splintage. This is the equivalent to an intramedullary nail in a diaphyseal femoral fracture. Consequently, all the guidelines that apply to unlocked nailing are applicable. The major aim is to maximize the bony stability and minimize the stresses across the fracture site and the implant. Obviously, if two fracture surfaces are completely intact and concentrically reduced, the fracture will be stable with the implant in place. The assessment of the prereduction x-rays must determine how close the fracture pattern is to the matching of the two concentric fracture surfaces. The amount of comminution about the fracture surfaces will determine the final stability. This is usually represented by the size of the posterior medial fracture segment. The larger this fracture fragment becomes, the greater the instability at the fracture line. At present there are no data to determine how large this fragment has to be for instability to occur. Less than 50% loss of contact between the fracture fragments will allow a stable reduction and greater than 50% loss is probably unstable. If the posterior segment can be reduced and stabilized, then the fracture-implant stability will greatly increase (Fig. 2).

The other important distinction in assessing intertrochanteric fractures is to determine which is the primary fracture line. A certain group of fractures will have subtrochanteric extension, which will affect implant choice. In general, the most displaced fracture component is usually the primary fracture. Consequently, fractures can be looked upon as a major intertrochanteric fracture with subtrochanteric extension or as a subtrochanteric fracture with intertrochanteric extension.

Operative treatment requires an anatomical reduction and stabilization by splintage with a compression sliding hip screw. The preoperative x-rays include an anteroposterior view

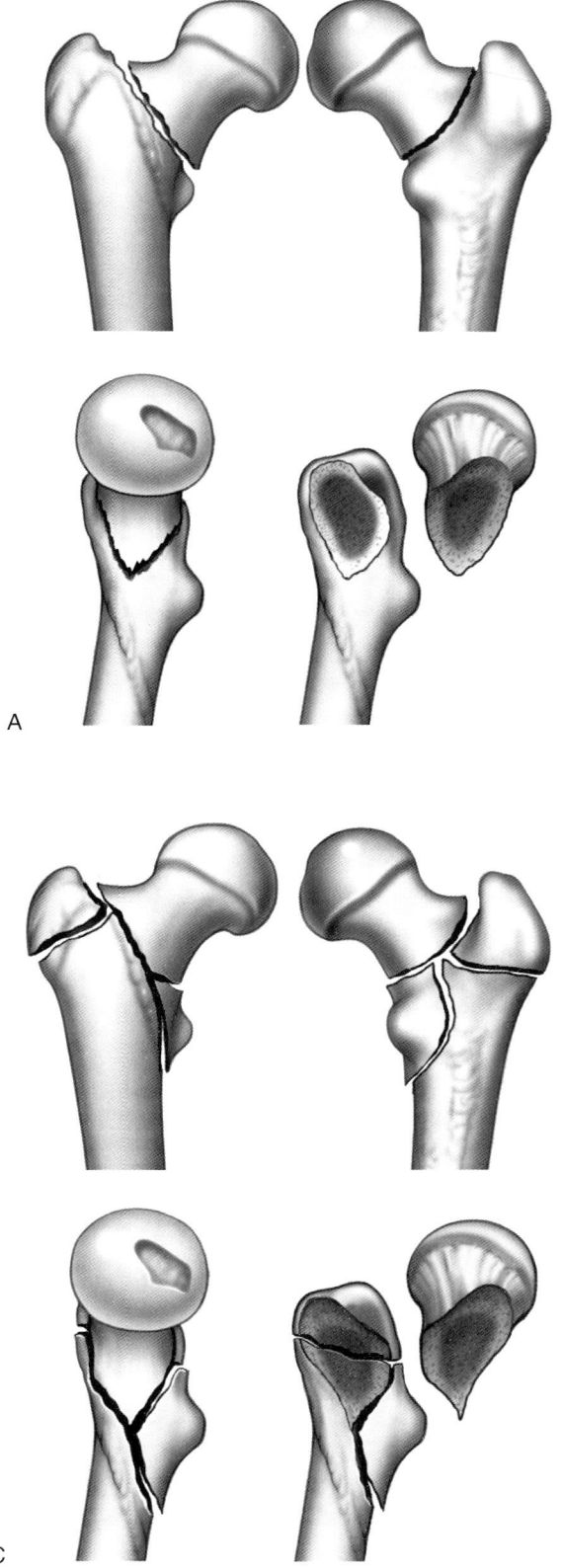
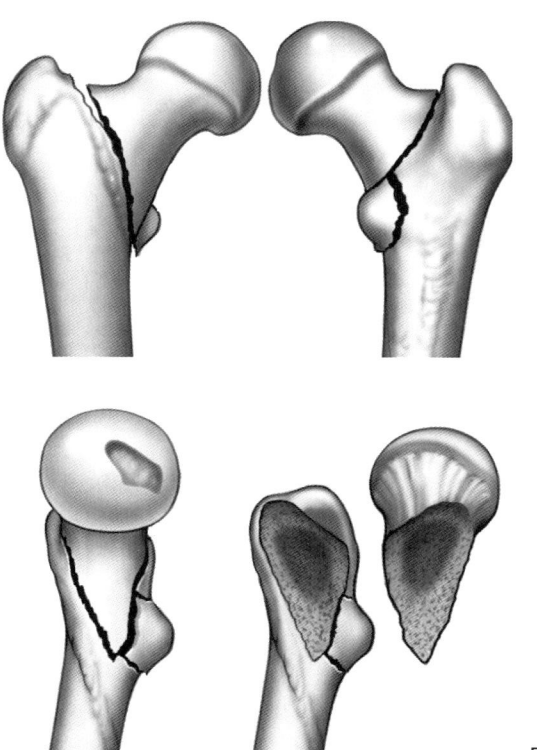

Figure 2. This group of figures demonstrates a visual representation of the concept of stability in the intertrochanteric region. It is essentially the position of two large surfaces of cancellous bone. Instability occurs as one or other of the sides of this construct is lost. (A) This represents a stable two-part intertrochanteric fracture. One can appreciate that this is stable, as there is no bone lost on either the distal fragment or proximal fragment, and on reduction two large surfaces of bone will be in contact. (B) This represents a stable construct; however, a small piece of the lesser trochanter has been removed through the fracture. Again one can appreciate the large contact bone representing a stable situation as the fracture surfaces impact. (C) This represents an unstable situation where over 50% of the fracture surface has been lost due to a fracture posterior medial fracture fragment. Again, at this point one can now see how instability would occur as the fracture tends to impact with minimal contact between the two major fracture fragments.

of the pelvis with the opposite uninjured hip visualized, an anteroposterior view, and a lateral view, preferably cross table, of the involved hip. From the uninjured hip, the plate angle is determined by the angle of the intersection of the line from the center of the head, center of the neck to the outer aspect of the lateral femoral cortex, and the line along the lateral femoral cortex. The length of the screw is determined by measuring the line from the center of the head to lateral cortex so that the screw tip is 10 mm from the subchondral plate, and the distal end is at the lateral femoral cortex. A plate with at least three holes distal to the fracture is necessary.

SURGERY

Anesthesia

Anesthesia will usually be determined by the patient's medical condition and other associated injuries. In the majority of elderly patients, the use of regional techniques such as spinal or epidural is recommended. When other associated injuries are present or the patient is unable to cooperate, a general endotracheal anesthetic may be indicated. Certainly, whatever technique is used, adequate muscle relaxation must be obtained during the procedure to facilitate reduction.

Patient Positioning

For fracture reduction of the hip, a reduction aid such as a fracture table is necessary. The surgeon must be familiar with the table and its mechanisms of reduction as well as assuring that the C-arm is compatible with the table so that excellent images in the anterior-posterior and lateral plane can be obtained. This compatibility should be reviewed each time

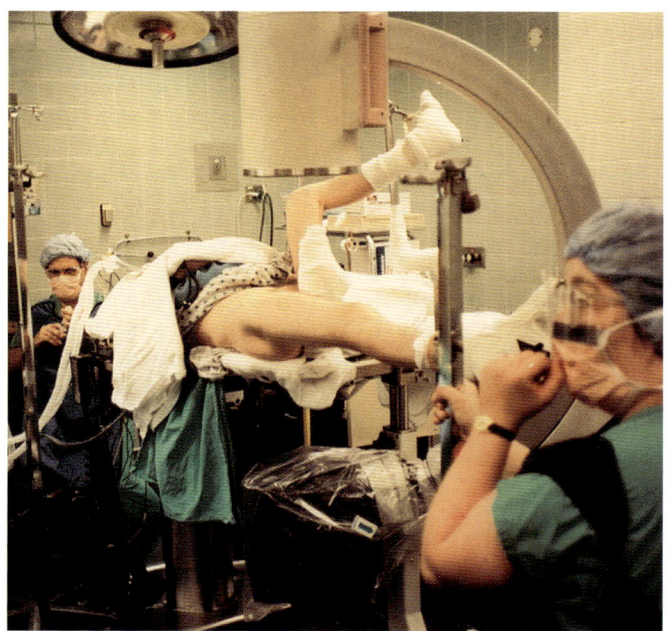
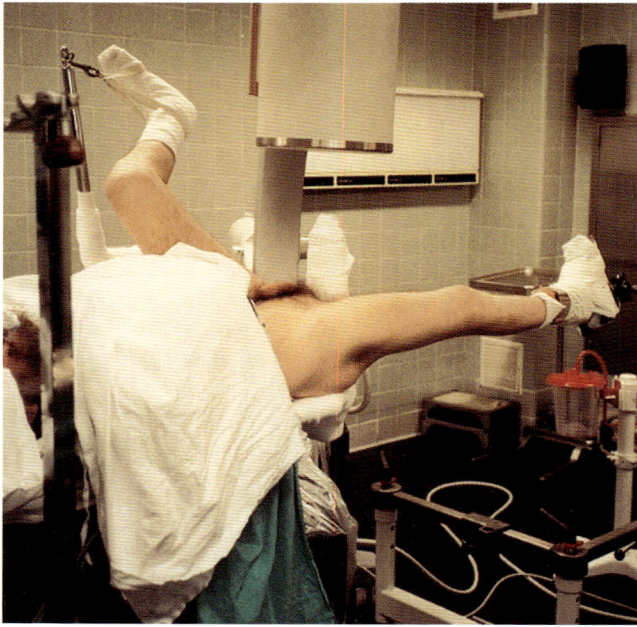

Figure 3 A, B. This figure shows the appropriate operative positioning for reduction and fixation of an intertrochanteric fracture. The patient is supine and in this picture the uninjured leg is placed in a well-leg holder which is abducted and flexed to 90° at the hip. This allows excellent access for the C-arm in between the legs for a good anterior-posterior view and lateral view of the hip.

the patient is positioned on the table. It is not acceptable to have the patient prepared and draped and then attempt to find the appropriate positions to visualize the fracture. Although an anatomical reduction can usually be achieved on a fracture table in the majority of elderly patients, the younger patient with a high-energy fracture with large fracture fragments may be better treated by an open technique on a radiolucent table. The patient in this situation would be placed in the supine position with a small roll under his buttock (Fig. 3). The advantage of doing this on a regular table is the freedom associated with the leg so that the reduction of the posterior medial fracture fragment is facilitated due to reduction of the tension across the hip secondary to the fracture table. Experience with the different techniques is most important.

Reduction Techniques

The patient is placed on the fracture table with the injured leg in boot traction. The well leg is placed in the well-leg holder, which will allow better access for a C-arm lateral than with the leg abducted and in extension at the hip (Figs. 3, 4). The reduction is then undertaken. This is an indirect reduction technique that is dependent upon the soft-tissue attachments about the hip region. As the leg is originally shortened, the first reduction maneuver is longitudinal traction in the externally rotated position. This will allow the distal fracture fragment to be pulled down until the appropriate length has been reestablished. Guides to appropriate length are usually the reestablishment of the medial arch of the calcar in the intertrochanteric region, and the tip of the trochanter should be level with the center of head

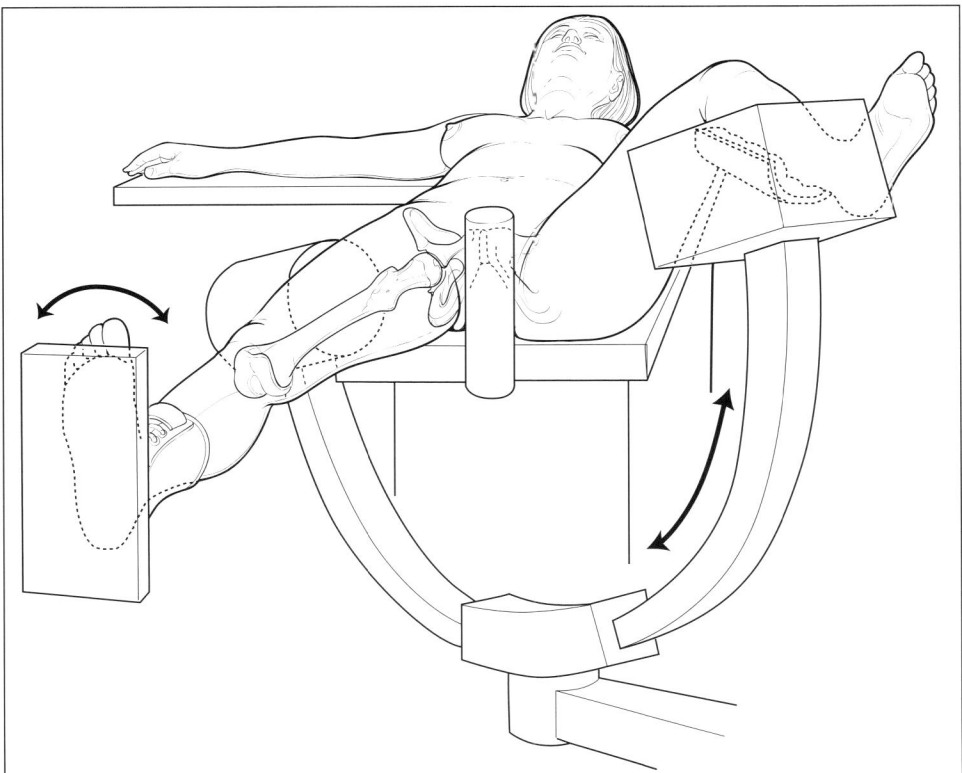

Figure 4. An alternate position for reduction and fixation is in the supine position with the well leg in abduction and extension through the hip. This means that the legs must be separated and the C-arm must be between them. This again will allow adequate anterior-posterior view but will hinder a true lateral of the proximal femur if this is required.

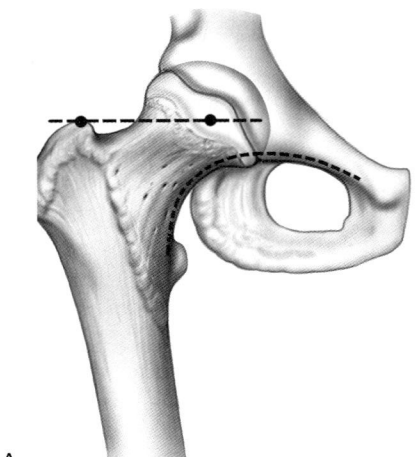

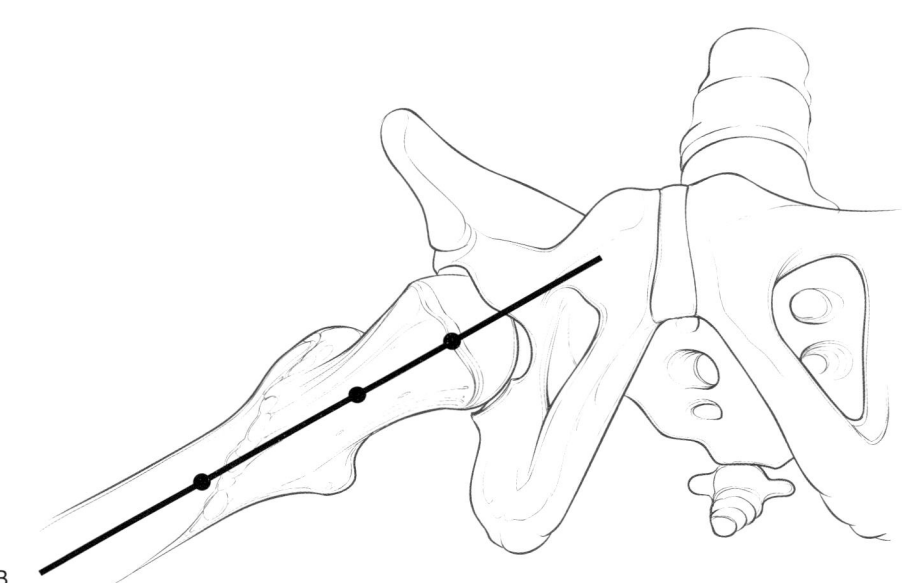

Figure 5. This figure represents the guides to an adequate reduction of an intertrochanteric fracture. (A) This figure shows on the anterior:posterior view how the medial calcar cortex region of the proximal femur is realigned so that the proximal fracture is reduced from the varus and the contour of Shenton's line is reconstructed. Note also that the tip of trochanter is centered into the center of the head. (B) This figure represents the lateral view. Note how a center point on the femoral shaft, femoral neck, and center of the femoral head are all lined up. Note that there is no apex anterior or posterior angulation. This represents an acceptable reduction on the lateral.

(Fig. 5). The reduction should be done under image intensification control so that the surgeon can get a feel of what is happening. At times, live images should be done if there is any question as to the method of reduction.

Once length has been obtained, the leg is rotationally corrected. As all fractures are displaced in external rotation, the first maneuver will be internal rotation. Normally, internal rotation to the neutral position, that is, the patella pointing upwards, will be undertaken. Beware of using the foot as a method of determining rotation as this will tend to be misleading because of the play of the ligaments at the ankle. At this point, if length is correct and rotation is neutral or slightly internally rotated, then a good reduction on the anterior-posterior view should be obtained. The C-arm should then be placed into the lateral position and the reduction confirmed. It may require some fine tuning of rotation to correct the lateral view. It must be remembered that length and rotation can be corrected in the anterior-posterior view, but rotation is the mechanism by which the reduction is improved in the lateral view.

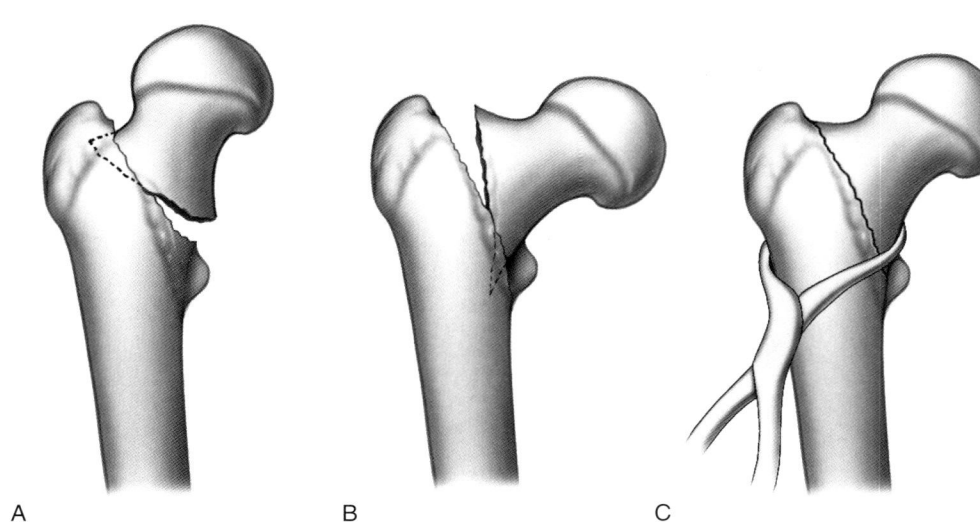

Figure 6. Impacted two-part shear fracture. This represents how the impacted shear fracture can hinder reduction with impaction either proximally or distally at the fracture line. (A, B) Normally an open reduction is required and this can then be held in position by a pointed reduction clamp extending from the inferior portion of the head neck fragment around onto the intact greater trochanter, or lateral femoral cortex. (C) This normally provides provisional stabilization for the fixation of the fracture.

Irreducible Situations

The Shear-type Fracture. The shear-type fracture resulting from high-energy causes a two-part fracture occurring along the intertrochanteric line. Normally this fracture can be reduced easily and will have excellent bone-on-bone contact. Occasionally, there will be impaction of the proximal fracture fragment into the upper aspect of the greater trochanteric region, or the inferior neck spike will be driven into the medullary canal in the region of the lesser trochanter. Because of either of these two problems, the fracture will be irreducible and disimpaction with traction or rotation will be unsuccessful. Open reduction of the fracture site is required, followed by provisional fixation using a pointed reduction clamp that spans the fracture, having one point on the inferior aspect of the neck or calcar region and one on the outer aspect of the femoral shaft or trochanteric region (Fig. 6).

Posterior Shaft Displacement. In many intertrochanteric fractures unstable due to the loss of a large posterior medial fracture fragment, the femoral shaft has a tendency to sag posteriorly secondary to gravity. The majority of these fractures can be reduced in the anterior-posterior plan to give length and appropriate rotation. On the lateral, the shaft tends to drift down, and it is very difficult to get the appropriate reduction. On the lateral view there should be colinearity between the shaft, the neck, and the center of the head. Any angulation posteriorly or anteriorly will lead to a malreduction and potential instability postoperatively. In order to overcome this posterior sag, it is usually necessary to lift the shaft up either manually or with an instrument. This is then confirmed on the lateral and AP C-arm views. The fracture is provisionally fixed using a 3.2-mm Steinmann pin or K-wire. This pin usually runs from the greater trochanteric region or superior trochanteric region into the superior aspect of the head. Be careful not to place this pin into an area where the compression screw will be going. The second stabilization wire will be the guide wire (Fig. 7 A, B).

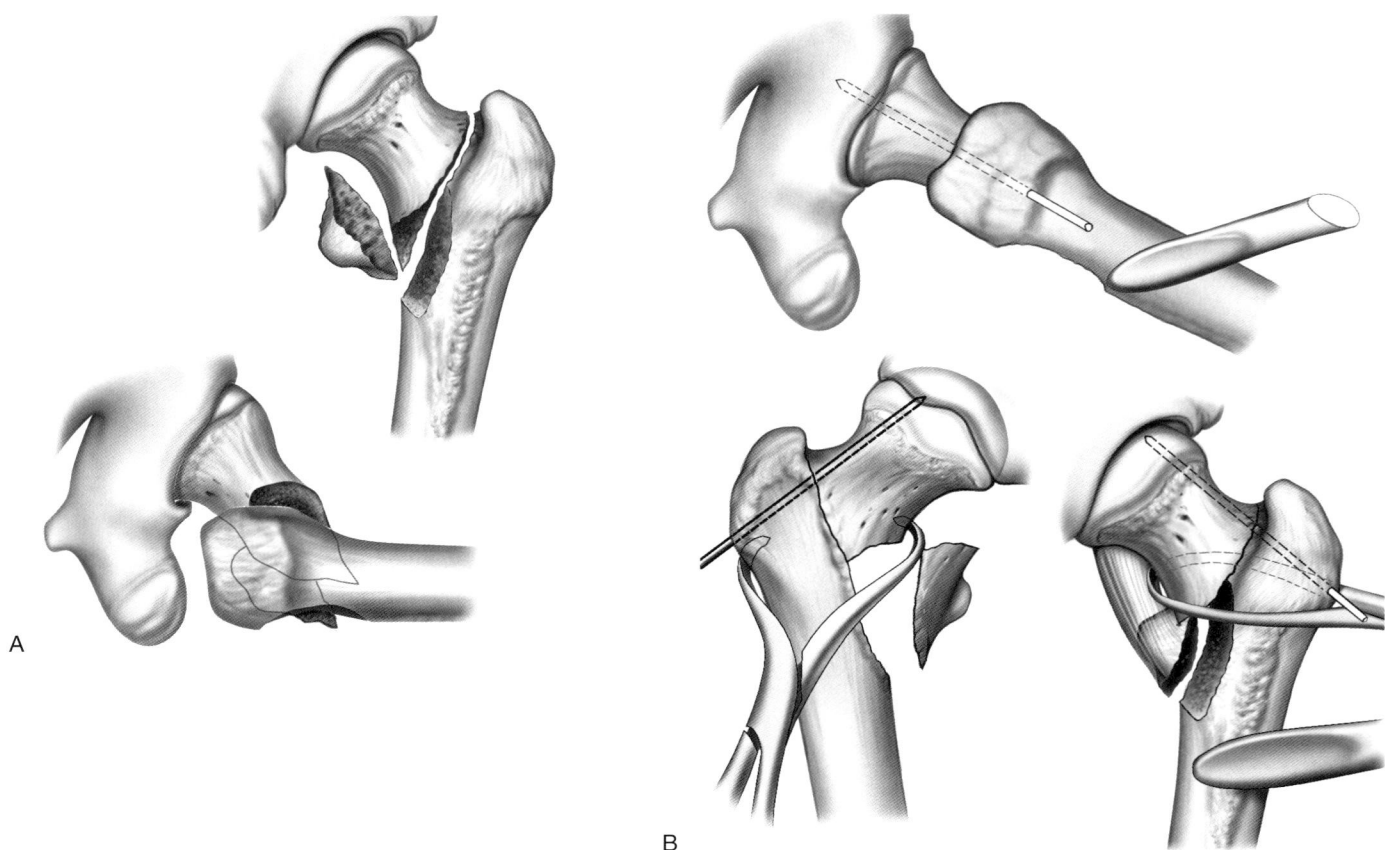

Figure 7. This figure demonstrates the problem of posterior shaft displacement. (A) The usual picture that is obtained at the time of reduction. On the anterior-posterior view a reasonable reduction can be obtained; however, on the lateral view there is discontinuity between the distal fracture fragment and the proximal and normally there is a posterior sag of the femur. (B) Demonstrates how an instrument can be placed under the distal femoral shaft segment and lifted up and a Steinmann pin or large K-wire used for provisional fixation by placing them through the greater trochanter and high into the head and neck. This may be supplemented by a pointed reduction clamp, which may reduce posterior medial fracture or the inferior neck region.

The posterior medial fracture fragment, secondary to the pull of the iliopsoas, displaces into a flexed position and is accentuated by the hip's being placed in extension. Although this fragment can normally be reduced from the posterior, dissection over the anterior aspect of the shaft may be required to identify the fracture fragment. A sharp hook can be used to pull the fragment into its normal position and to allow a K-wire to be placed from the shaft into the fragment for stabilization. This is performed following provisional fixation of the two major fracture fragments, or after the compression hip screw has been applied. Osteoporotic bone is best held in place with cerclage wires (Fig. 8 A, B); in normal bone a lag-screw technique can be used (Fig. 9).

Occasionally, certain fracture patterns will leave the greater trochanteric fracture fragment attached to the head–neck component. Because the external rotators are attached to the proximal fragment, external rotation and flexion displacement occur. Consequently, attempts to reduce this with internal rotation usually will not be successful. The fracture will best reduce in external rotation. If this does not provide adequate reduction, then limited open reduction is performed.

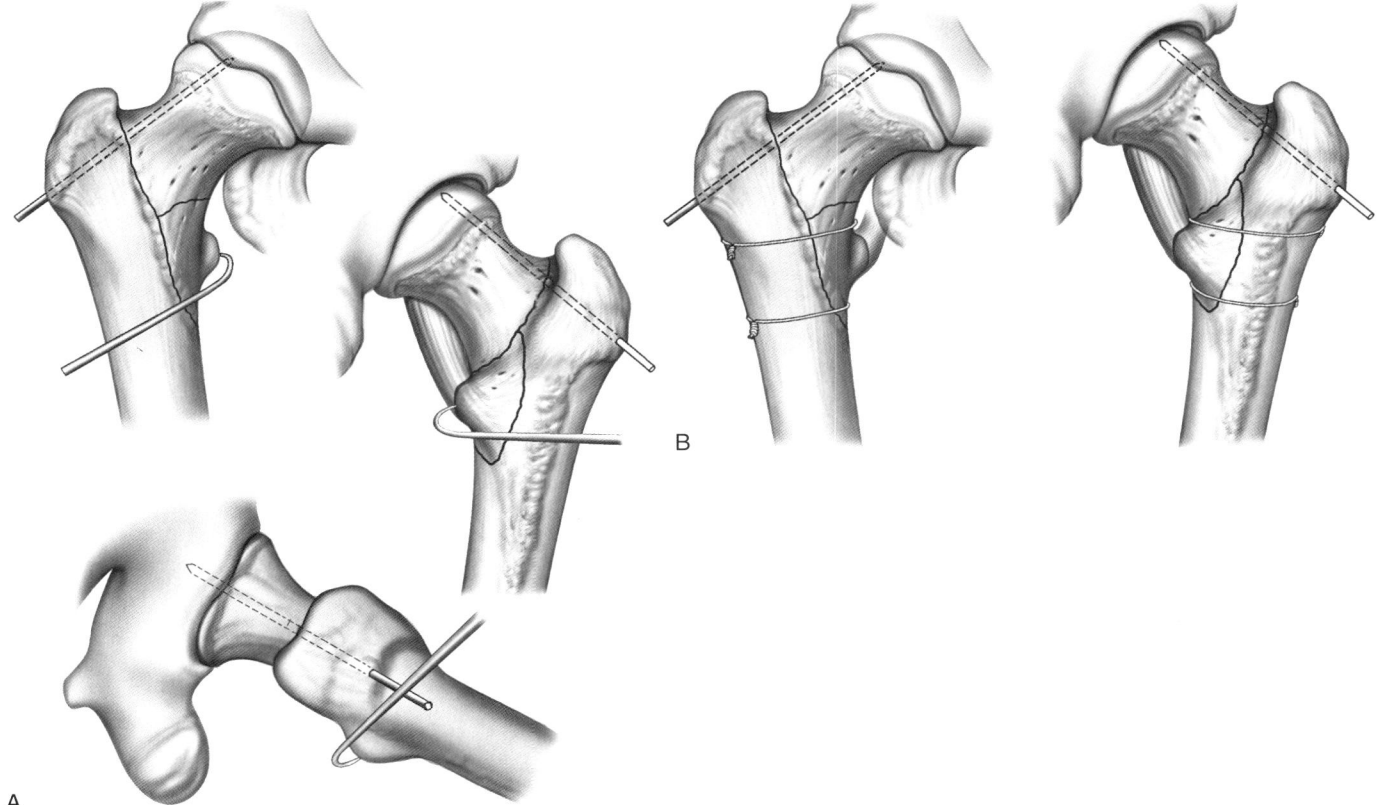

Figure 8. (A) The problem of the unreduced posterior medial fracture fragment is represented. This figure shows the mechanism of reduction of a large posterior medial fracture fragment. Either a sharp hook or pointed instrument can be passed over the anterior aspect of the shaft or through the posterior aspect and the fracture fragment hooked on and pulled down. (B) With the fracture fragment held in place a K-wire or Steinmann pin maybe placed into it to hold provisional fixation. Using wire passers and avoiding medial disruption of the soft tissue, two cerclage wires can be passed around this fracture fragment. One wire should be used to attempt to grab the fragment low at its apex to lock it into place, and the second wire should be passed either through or just above the tendon to hold the fragment in superiorly. These can be tied over the plate, or under the plate, or around the bone, as the situation allows.

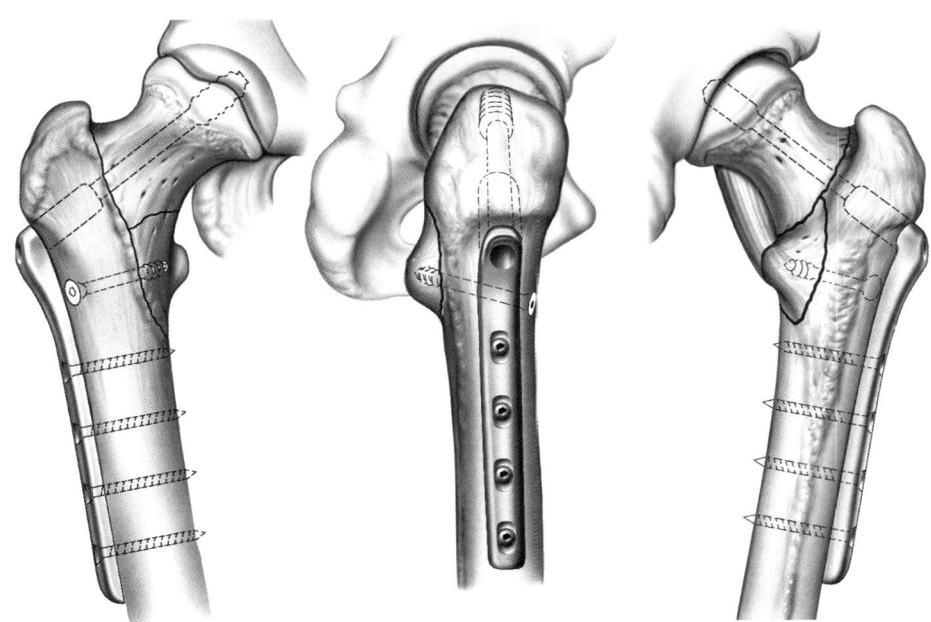

Figure 9. In bone of good quality, fixation of the posterior medial fracture fragment can be done with lag screws. This will provide interfragmentary compression. However, it is difficult to get the lag screw in through the plate and into the fracture fragment. Normally, this must be done separately and come from the anterior-lateral corner of the shaft into the posterior medial fracture fragment.

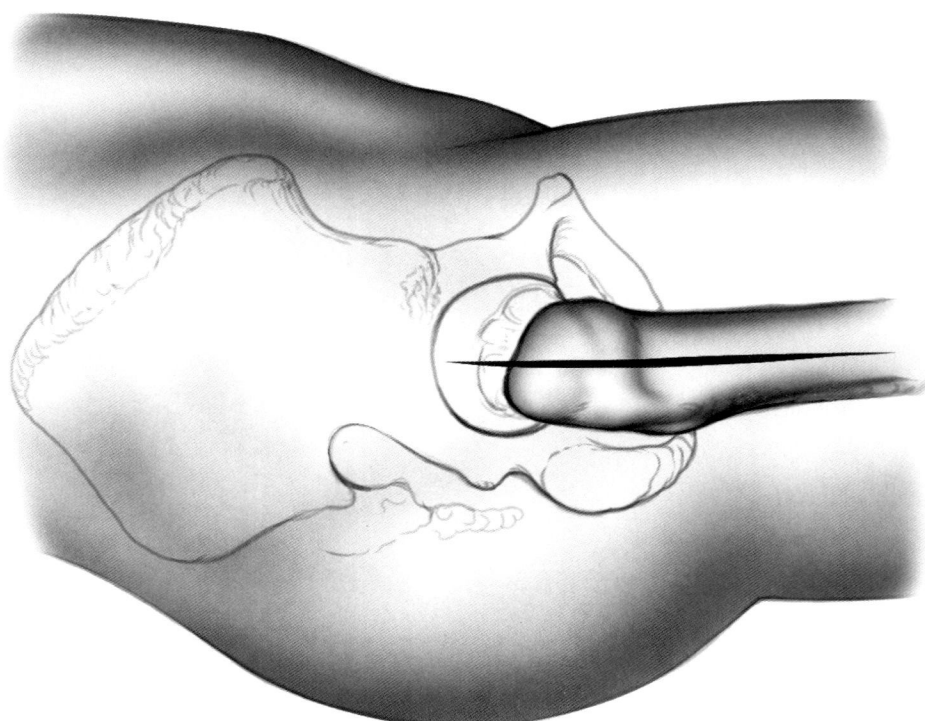

Figure 10. After the patient is placed on the fracture table and the reduction obtained, an incision is made distally 10 to 14 cm starting at the tip of the trochanter.

Exposure

The incision is a straight lateral approach to the proximal femur (Fig. 10). It commences at the tip of the greater trochanter and extends down the shaft approximately 10 to 14 cm. Remember to make this incision over the posterior half of the shaft as this facilitates exposure to the posterior aspect of the femur. The dissection exposes the fascia, which is split longitudinally revealing the vastus lateralis (Fig. 11).

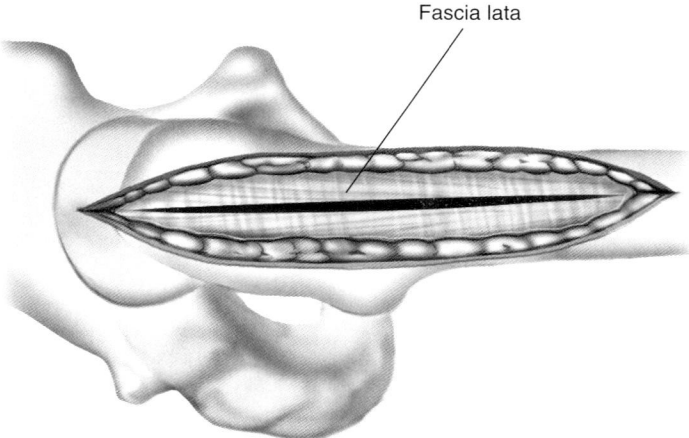

Figure 11. This incision is carried down to identify the deep fascia of the thigh.

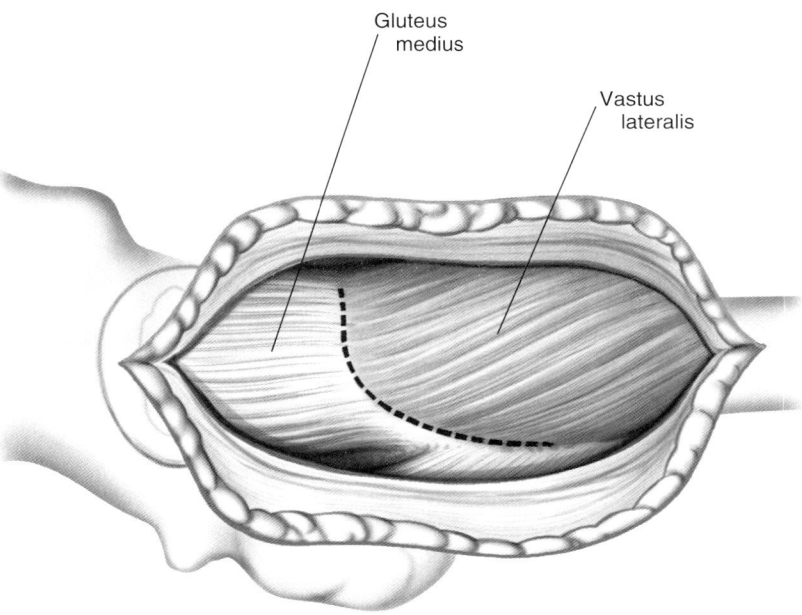

Figure 12. The fascia over the vastus lateralis is split in the direction of its fibers and retracted anteriorly and posteriorly. This reveals the vastus lateralis on the lateral aspect of the femur. This is best taken down by incising along the origin of the vastus lateralis and then along the posterior fascial covering of the muscle.

The origin of the vastus lateralis along the intertrochanteric ridge is freed by an incision performed parallel to the ridge and extending to the muscle's posterior attachment (Fig. 12). The facia overlying the vastus lateralis is split along the length of the incision. The insertion of the muscle from the femur is elevated by blunt dissection using a sharp periosteal elevator working into the acute angle of the muscle fibers. This technique, if done carefully, allows identification of the perforating vessels so that they may be ligated. The vastus lateralis is then reflected anteriorly to expose the whole lateral cortex of the femur (Fig. 13). The advantage of this approach is that it can be easily converted to a Watson-Jones approach to the anterior aspect of the hip if it is needed.

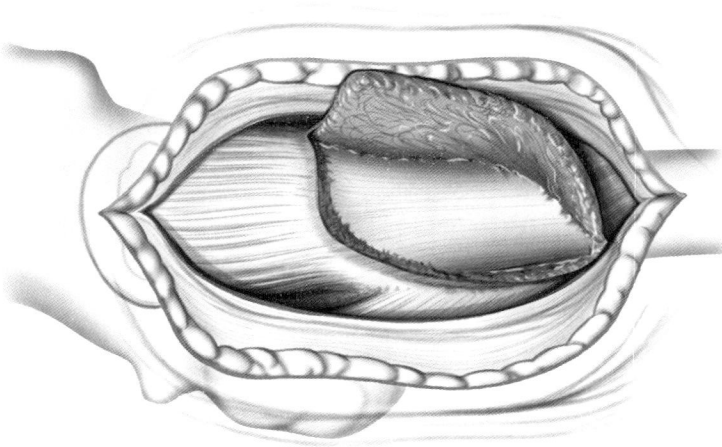

Figure 13. Using a sharp periosteal elevator working in the direction of the fibers, the muscle can be reflected anteriorly and any perforators ligated as they are discovered. This will reveal the lateral aspect of the femur and also the intertrochanteric area.

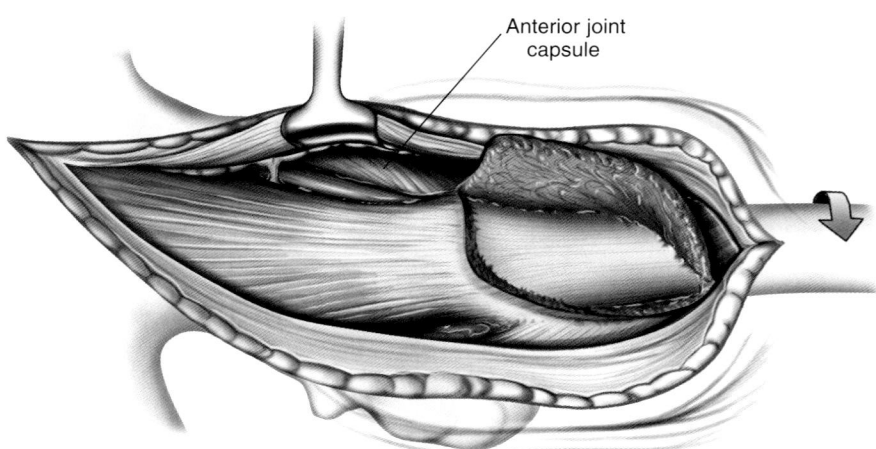

Figure 14. Extension of this incision to reveal the anterior aspect of the hip joint and the intertrochanteric fracture for open reduction can be accomplished by extending the incision proximally past the tip of the greater trochanter and identification of the interval between gluteus medius and tensor fascia lata. This interval is usually marked by fat, and under this the hip joint capsule will be seen. The dissection can then continue up onto the anterior wall of the acetabulum.

Fracture Stabilization

At this point, if an open reduction has to be performed, the fracture can be more fully exposed by moving anteriorly. The anterior capsule of the hip joint is approached and the intertrochanteric component of the fracture identified. If necessary, if the surgeon works posteriorly, the fracture can also be exposed (Fig. 14). With the fracture reduced and provisionally fixed, the insertion of the guide wire for the compression screw is undertaken (Fig. 15). The angle of the plate should have been determined from the preoperative plan. By use of this predetermined angle and the appropriate guide, the guide wire will be inserted. The guide should be placed directly on the lateral femoral cortex so that it is not angulated and is in the midportion of the lateral femoral cortex. To facilitate guide-wire placement, a free guide wire is placed at the determined angle along the anterior neck and

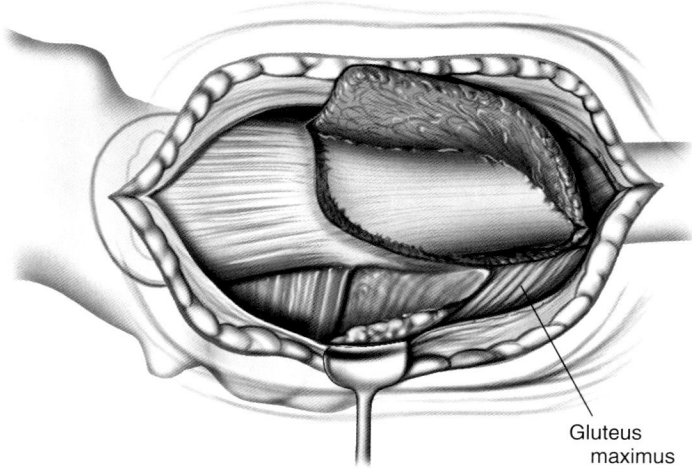

Figure 15. This figure represents the insertion of the gluteus maximus onto the femur. This is a broad-based strong structure that inserts on the posterior lateral aspect of the femur. It is directly opposite the lesser trochanter. This is usually an excellent landmark to determine the area to start the guide wire for compression-screw insertion.

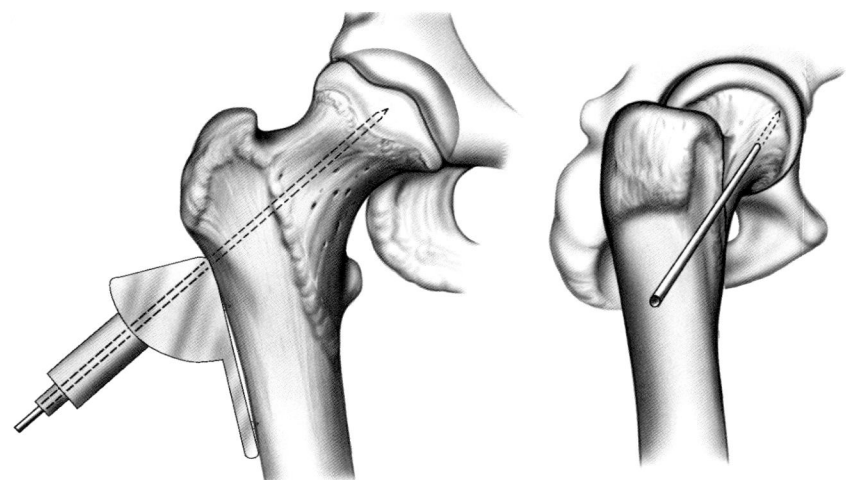

Figure 16. It is important that the angle of the plate be predetermined by templating. With this predetermined angle, then, the appropriate guide from the systems can be used to place a temporary guide wire up the anterior aspect of the neck. If this guide wire is placed into the center of the head and parallel to the neck and then tapped into the femoral head, it will serve as a temporary guide to the placement of the final guide wire. This technique is particularly helpful in minimizing operative time as well as assuring perfect placement of the screw.

impaled into the femoral head. Where the radiographic images of guide wire and lateral femoral cortex cross, the second guide wire is inserted through the bone (Fig. 16). This free wire will also allow determination of the anteversion. Anteversion can be confirmed by the angle of the C-arm in the lateral, which lines up the shaft, neck, and center of the head in a straight line. With these two guides, then, anteversion and placement of the guidewire is facilitated (Fig. 17).

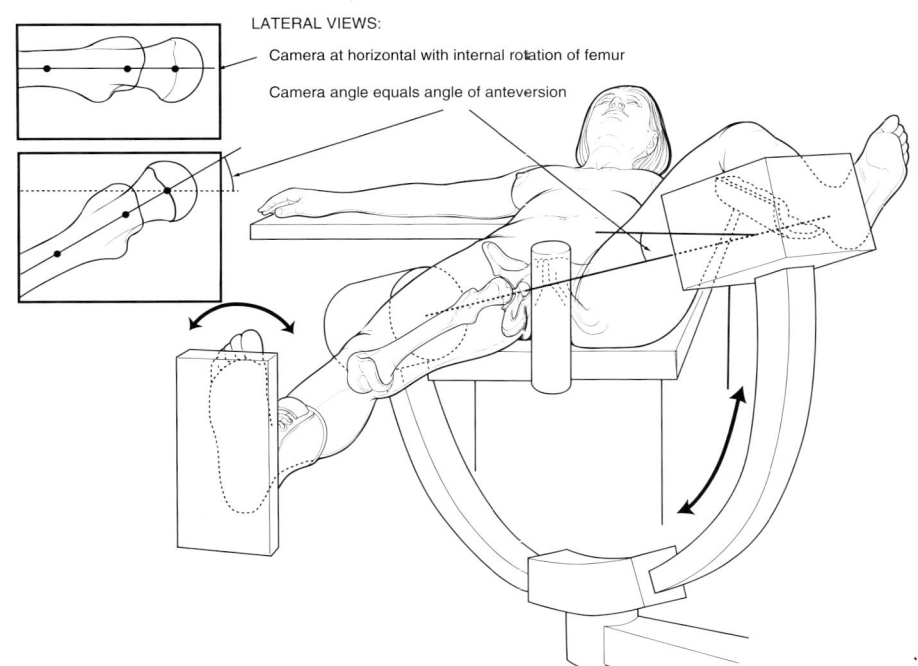

Figure 17. Another method of determining anteversion is the angle on the lateral view of which the C-arm obtains a true lateral view of the proximal femur. This true lateral view occurs when the shaft, neck, and head are perfectly lined up. The angle of rotation of the C-arm will determine where this occurs. Obviously the more external rotation of the leg with reduction, the more the C-arm will be tilted into external rotation. If the leg is internally rotated so that the patella is pointing upwards or about 20 degrees internally rotated, then the anteversion is removed, and when one places the guide wire in, it is directly parallel to the floor.

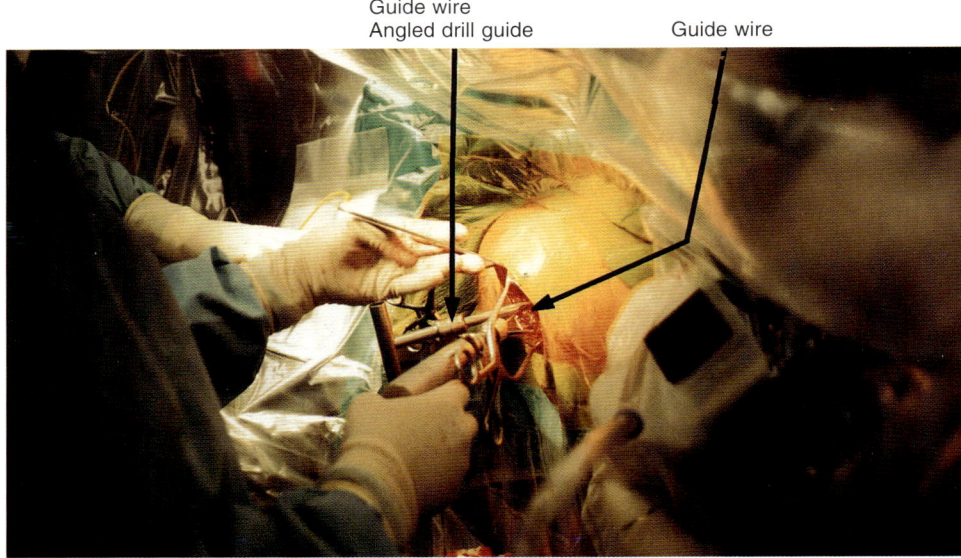

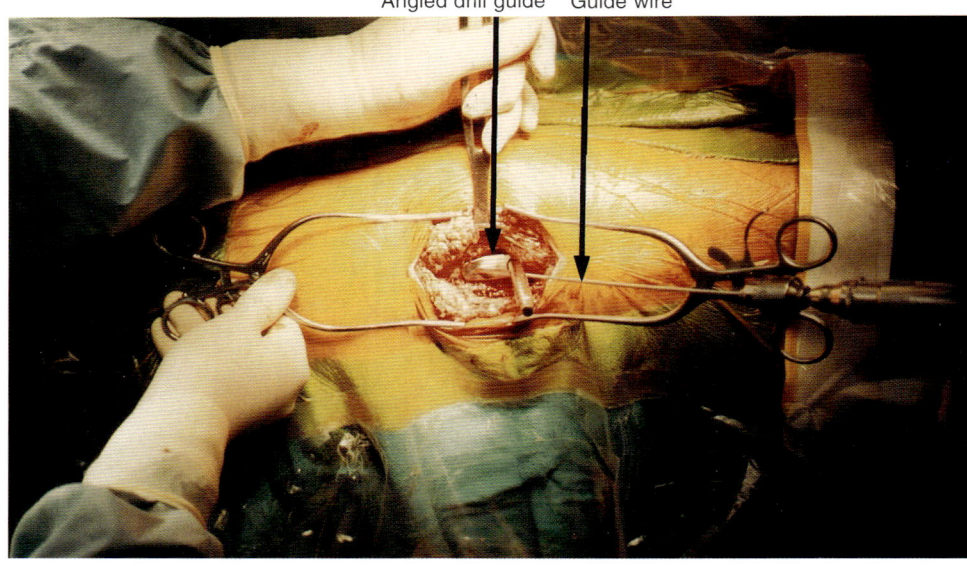

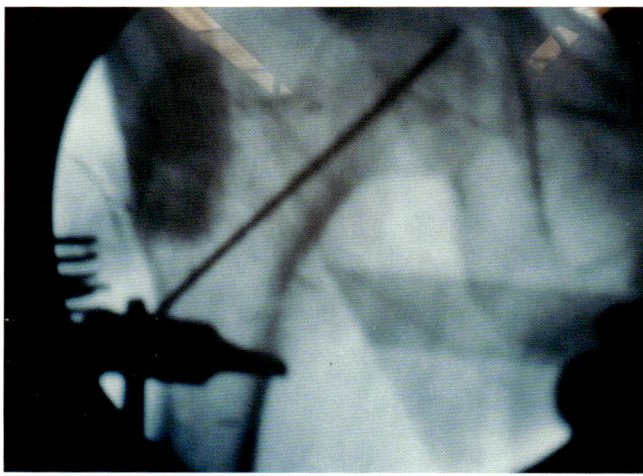
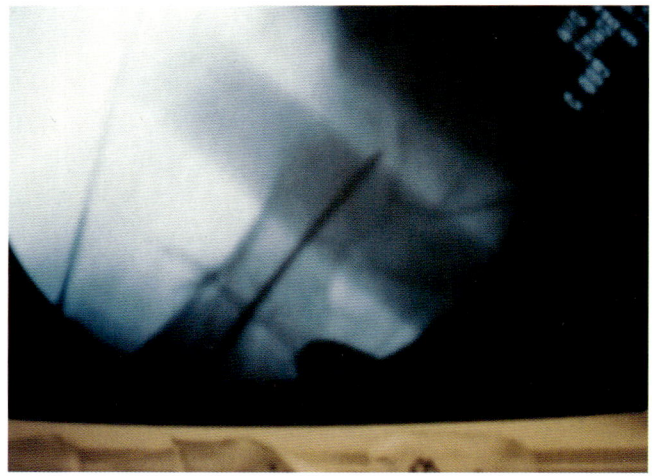

Figure 18. The correct insertion of the guide wire (arrows) is imperative with compression hip screw fixation to achieve an excellent result. This should be done using the appropriate guide wires and guides. (A, B) The guidewire guide is placed against the lateral femoral cortex. It is important that this be directly against bone and in the midportion of the shaft. Anteversion is determined as previously shown. (C, D) show excellent position of the guide wire. Note that this is in the center of the head in both views, and touches the subchondral plate, as well.

The position of the guide wire must be in the center of the head in both anterior-posterior and lateral views (Fig. 18 A, B, C, D). The threaded tip of the guide wire must touch the subchondral bone plate to assure the stable placement of the guide wire. If any error in placement is to occur, the only acceptable place for the guide wire to be is in the posterior inferior quadrant of the head. However, this should be avoided for fear of perforating the head itself if one is too close to the subchondral plate. The guide wire must not be placed across the articular surfaces of the hip joint into the acetabulum, as it may penetrate the inside of the pelvis or be amputated and then must be removed from the hip.

The Compression Screw Insertion

With the guide wire in place, most systems will allow the surgeon to measure the length of the screw. It is important to understand the system being used, for some of the them take into account the amount of guide wire protruding and some give a direct reading. What is important is that the threaded 10 mm of the guide wire is not overdrilled so as to prevent the guide wire from automatically coming out. Consequently, when measuring the screw, one should be guaranteed that the last centimeter of bone is left untouched.

With the appropriate measurement, the amount that must be drilled and reamed to allow compression screw insertion is set (Fig. 19). The reamer, which in most systems is a triple reamer, is then attached to a drill and is placed over the guide wire. During this procedure it is imperative that one be sure that the guide wire is straight, or amputation of the wire will occur. As well, the cannulation in the triple reamer must be checked to make sure that it is clean and will not stick or bind to the guidewire. Several images of the triple reamer being inserted are mandatory to make sure that it is in the proper track and is not advancing the guide wire. The reamer must then be fully inserted so that the lateral femoral cortex is opened and reamed to accept the plate. Once the reamer is in place, a lateral view should be checked. The reamer is then removed (Fig. 20).

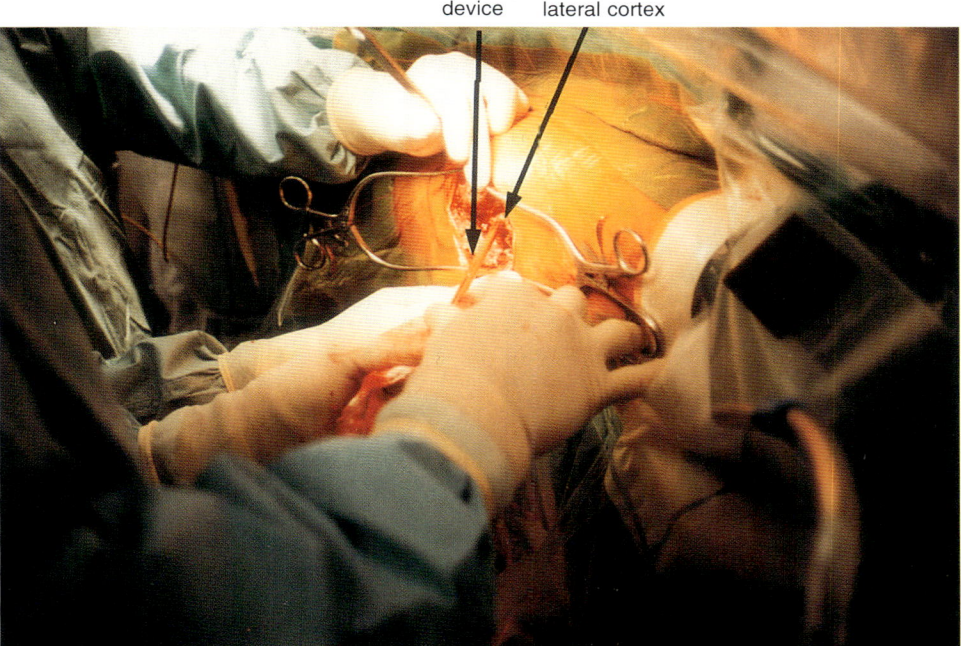

Figure 19. Using the appropriate measuring device the length of the guide wire is then determined. This will determine the length of the compression screw.

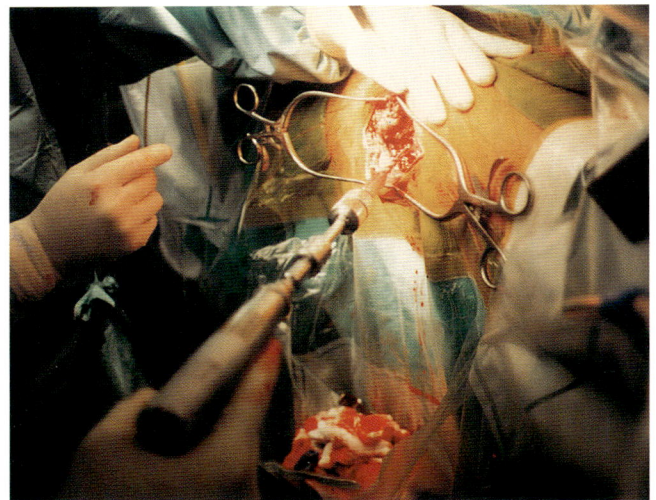
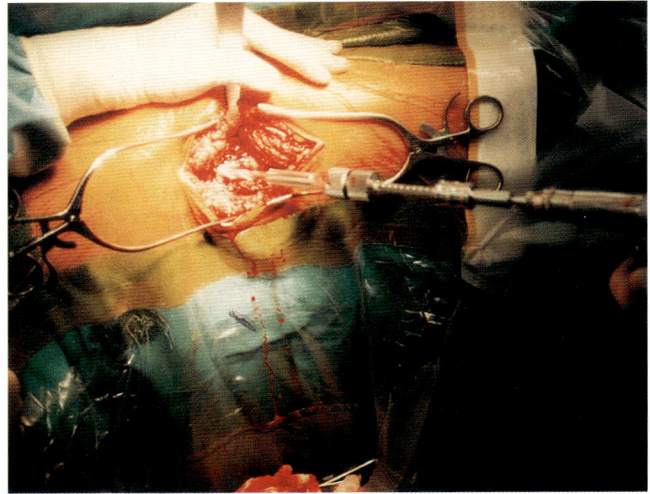
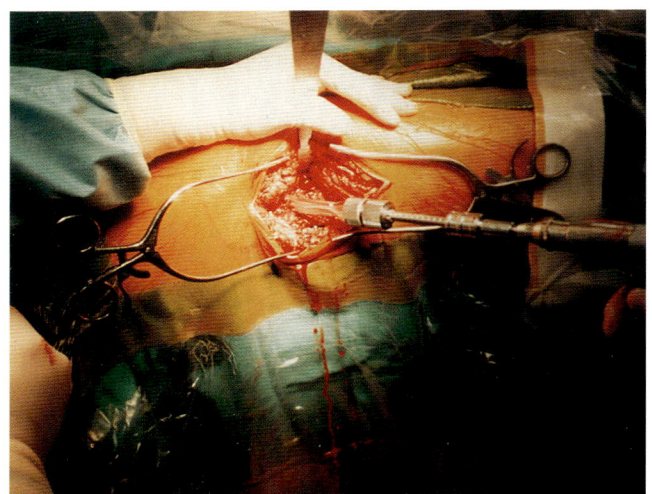
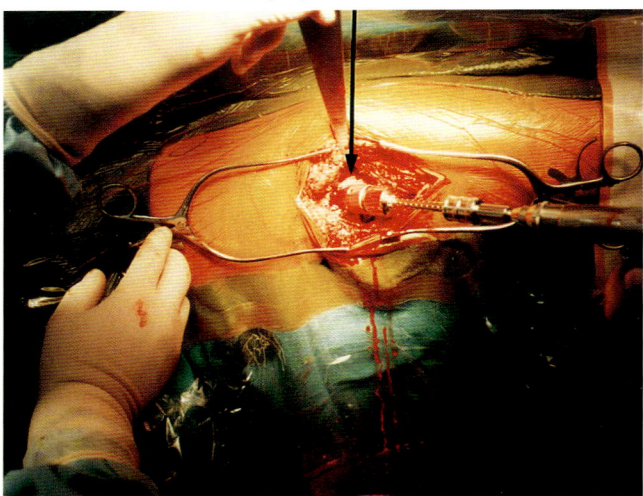

Triple reamer inserted up to bone to prepare channel for plate barrel

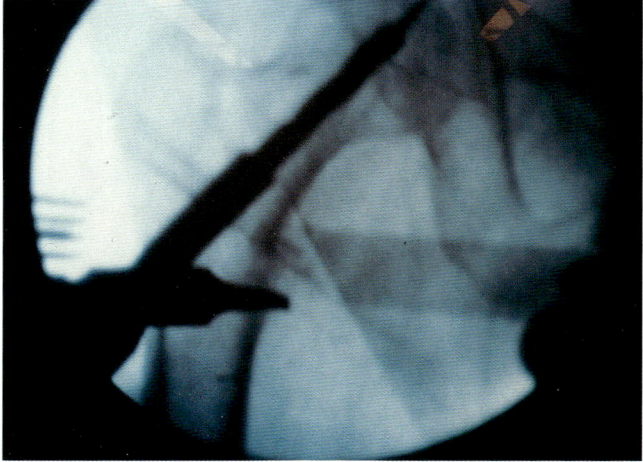

Figure 20. (A, B) The reaming to set the channel in the neck and head for the compression screw is then performed with a triple reaming device. This must be set to the exact length of the screw length. Care should be taken not to overdrill the threaded portion of the guide wire. (C, D) The reamer should be inserted as far as it will be allowed, and the surgeon must be absolutely certain that the flare portion of the last part of the reamer is allowed to contact the lateral cortex to open up the hole at this area to allow the plate to seat easily. (E) shows a visualization on the C-arm of the reamer. This is important to do several times throughout the procedure to guarantee that the guide wire has not been advanced and that the reamer is going in the appropriate channel.

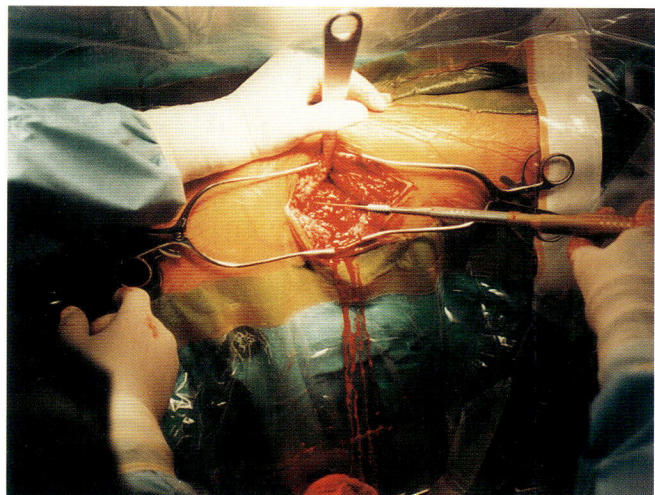
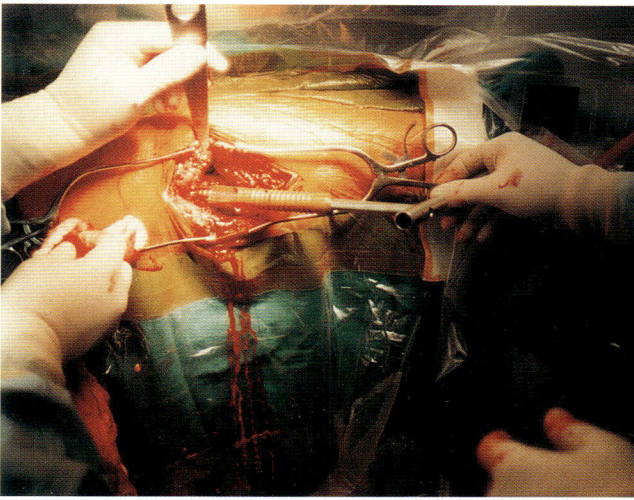
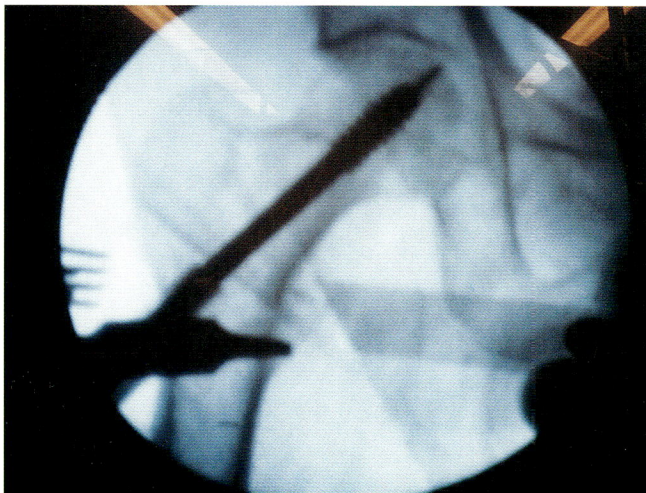

Figure 21 A, B, C. By means of the appropriate insertion handles and guides, the compression screw can then be seated over the guidewire. C-arm visualization must be undertaken to make sure that the screw is of the appropriate length and seats within 10 mm of the subchondral bone.

At this point the femoral head and neck may be tapped. Since the screw is going into the center of the head where the bone is the best, it is probably advisable in the majority of patients to tap the thread. Unless there is severe osteoporosis, most patients have suitable bone for screw purchase, and at times the insertion of an untapped screw may create a malreduction due to rotation as the blunt threads cut through the bone. This may lead to a malposition and loss of reduction at the time of screw insertion. Once the tract has been tapped, the appropriate length of screw is inserted. It must be remembered that if there is a gap, or the fracture is going to impact, then the screw will protrude through the barrel. This may cause discomfort for the patient, so one should make an estimate of the amount of impaction that will occur and shorten the screw the appropriate amount. However, one must make sure that at least half the barrel is filled by the screw. This will prevent the screw from cantilevering and galling to the plate barrel, thus preventing the sliding component of the system from working. The screw will then be inserted, and, depending upon the system, the handle of the screw insertion device should be aligned along the length of the femur (Fig. 21 A, B, C). All systems have a device that allows the plate to be inserted onto the screw.

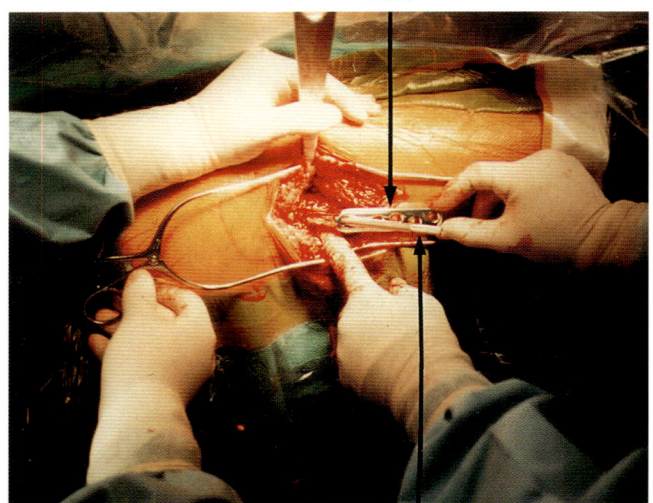 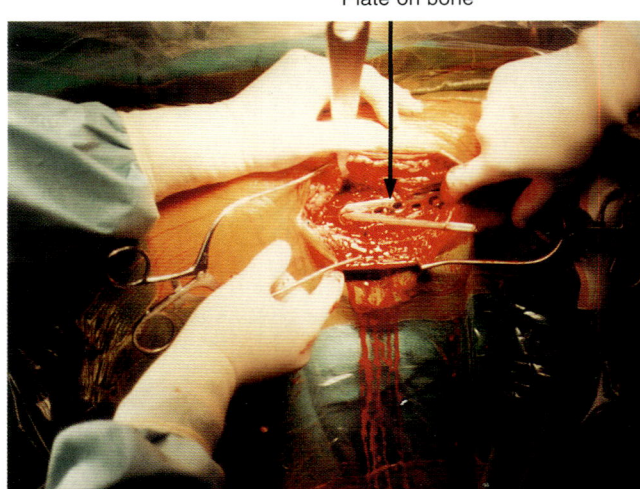

Figure 22 A, B. Following this, the chosen four-hole plate is slid over the appropriate extension device and centered onto the screw. Fine adjustment can be made at this point so that the plate lies directly along the lateral cortex. The plate should sit down easily. There should be no need for a clamp to hold the plate onto the bone.

Plate Insertion

The plate is slid up the guide onto the screw. The plate should slide onto the screw with hand pressure except for perhaps the last 2 to 3 mm, where it may be gently impacted by a hammer. It should then lie flush with the femoral shaft (Fig. 22). If it does not move easily or does not lie flush with the shaft, then either the wrong angle has been chosen, or there is bone blocking the insertion of the plate. Reevaluation of the hole around the compression screw will remove any debris and allow the plate to seat. Remeasuring of the angle will identify that problem. If one attempts to clamp the wrong-angled plate to the shaft, propagation of the fracture into the greater trochanter or into the subtrochanteric region may occur. At this stage one must accept the angle that is present and change the plate to fit the bone better. The plate is then fixed to the shaft. If a clamp is necessary, one should use a Verbrugge clamp, which will protect the medial soft tissues (Fig. 23).

Additional or Supplemental Fixation

With the fracture stabilized, it is appropriate to attempt to reduce the large posterior medial fracture fragment. This is performed as mentioned previously. In elderly patients with osteoporotic bone, the use of two cerclage wires to hold the fragment in place is usually advisable. One can be placed below the lesser trochanter over the fragment, and one can be placed above the lesser trochanter. This will lock the fracture fragment in place and either it can be tightened over the plate, or the plate can be slightly loosened and the wire placed under the plate and tightened and then the plate can be reapplied.

In bone that is not osteoporotic, the fracture can be reduced and provisionally fixed either with one cerclage wire or with a pointed clamp or K-wire and then stabilized with an interfragmental screw, which will compress the fracture. Depending on the size of the fracture fragment, one or two screws may be necessary. As this fragment is posterior medial and the plate is on the lateral surface, it is very difficult to lag the posterior medial fracture fragment successfully through the plate. The screw is usually at an angle to the fracture and will normally catch a small portion of it. It is much better to have the fracture provisionally reduced and then lag outside the plate from the anterior lateral corner of the femoral cortex into the posterior medial portion of the fracture fragment. This will give an interfragmen-

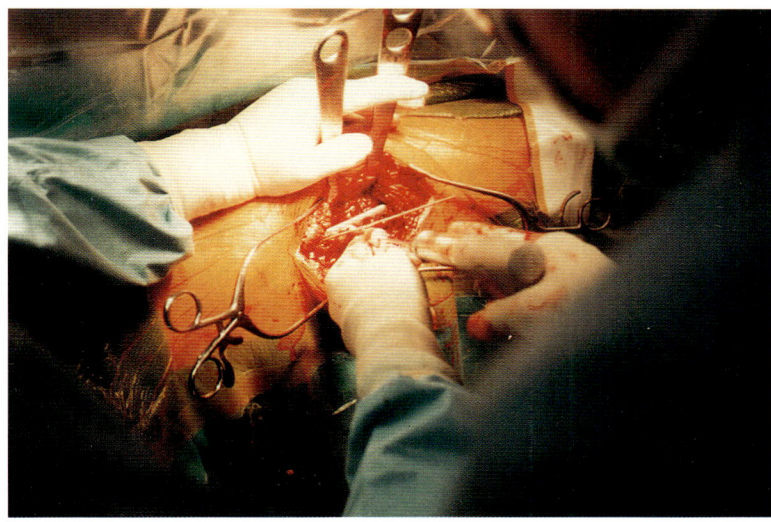

Figure 23. The plate is then affixed to the bone using the appropriate cortical screws.

tary screw that is at right angles to the fracture with much better compression. In rare incidences, the greater trochanter fracture fragment may be displaced. If this is the situation, the fracture should be reduced to reestablish the abductor mechanism. This can be done through a tension-band technique using 2-mm K-wires, which are placed through the tip of the trochanter in the substance of the gluteus medius insertion. These are impaled into the medial femoral cortical bone on either side of the compression screw. A 16-gauge wire, either one or two, is then passed around behind the tendon of the gluteus medius and the K-wires and then tied in a figure-eight fashion, either below the barrel of the plate or through a separate hole in the bone underneath the plate. Double tightening of this wire will maintain the reduction of the greater trochanteric fracture fragment. The K-wires are bent and hammered in so that they are impaled into the cancellous bone of the greater trochanter and lock the wire in place (Fig. 24).

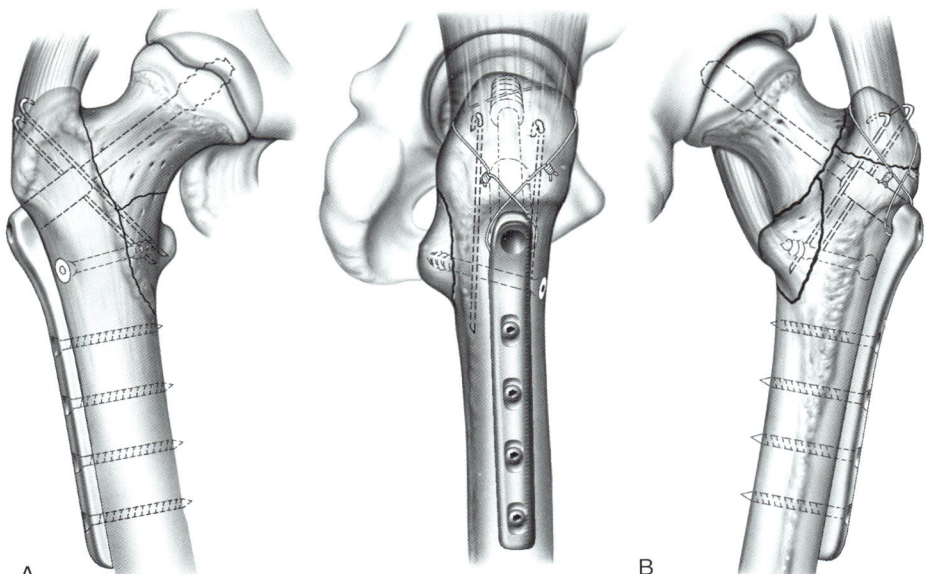

Figure 24. Occasionally, the greater trochanter is pulled off as a piece or may fracture during insertion of the plate. It may be necessary to reduce and fix this. (A) and (B) show that this can be done by means of a tension-band technique using two K-wires on either side of the barrel of the compression screw and a tension band wire through and around the barrel or bone to stabilize this fracture component effectively.

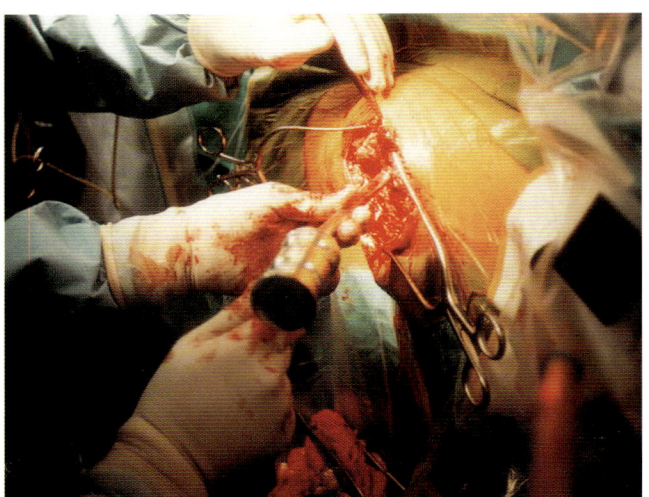

Figure 25. Interoperative stabilization by impaction of the fracture is imperative. This should be done under C-arm control and can occur either after traction has been released by impacting the fracture through taping a mallet onto an impactor over the greater trochanter, or plate, or by use of the interfragmental compression screw device through the plate. This should be visualized with the C-arm.

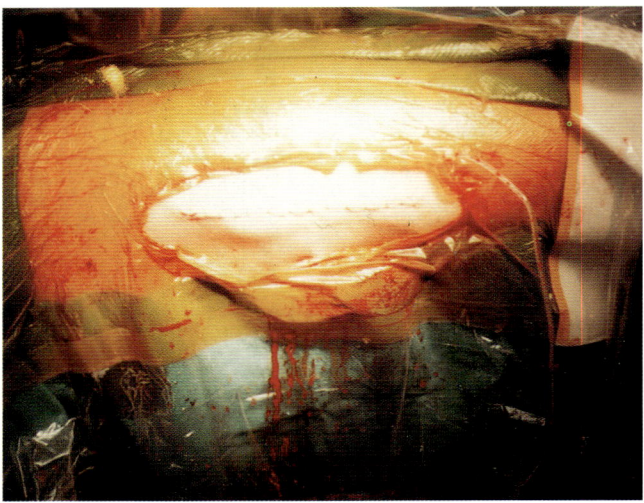

Figure 26. The wound is then closed in any manner of the surgeon's preference and a dressing applied.

Intraoperative Fracture Stabilization

At this point it is mandatory that the fracture be impacted. This provides the surgeon with control of the fracture impaction and enhancement of fixation stability. The surgeon releases the traction so that the knee has about 20 degrees of flexion, and with an impacting device curved to fit over the greater trochanter or to fit over the plate but not enter the barrel, impacts the fracture by gently hammering (Fig. 25). This allows the two main fracture components to collapse while visualized with the C-arm. The other technique is the use of the compression screw, which goes into the larger screw in the head. This is tightened against the barrel, and again the fracture fragments can be pulled together. Care must be taken throughout both procedures to watch that the screw in the femoral head is not loosened by hammering or pulled out due to the tightening of the intraoperative compression screw. The screw may be removed or left in place. If the original compression screw length has been such that over half of the barrel is filled, disengagement of the two components is highly unlikely. Therefore, the screw can be removed.

Closure

The wound is closed in layers with either running or interrupted sutures. Suction drains are left next to the bone and in the subcutaneous tissue, if it is indicated due to the injury or obesity. The skin is closed with staples. At this time the leg should be removed from the foot piece, and under the C-arm control the hip is put through range of motion in both the AP and lateral views to make sure that the fixation is stable and there has been no penetration of the screw into the hip joint (Fig. 26).

ALTERNATE TECHNIQUES

Intramedullary Hip Screw Concept

The implants are short intramedullary nails that are approximately 20 cm in length. They are constructed in a cloverleaf-type pattern with a proximal medial-to-lateral bow to allow for insertion through the tip of the greater trochanter. They have a larger proximal end that will allow the insertion of a compression hip screw into the head and neck component. Two screws placed distally will allow the system to be locked. The implant is inserted after reduction of the fracture and reaming of the canal (Fig. 27).

The patient position used is similar to that used for a conventional compression hip screw on the fracture table. There must be excellent access to the proximal femur, so that siting of the distal screws can be undertaken if it has to be done as a free-hand method. This will definitely necessitate the use of a well-leg holder. Fracture reduction is accomplished as previously described. One advantage of this system is that the placement of the guide wire into the distal fracture fragment in the unstable intertrochanteric fractures tends to help re-align this fracture, and the subsequent nail placement also tends to correct the posterior sag. Consequently, fractures can be reduced anatomically in the AP view, and the lateral can be corrected at the time of guide wire and nail insertion. However, it must be pointed out again that an anatomical reduction in both views is imperative.

The incision for this technique is about 5 to 8 cm long, starting at the tip of the trochanter and going proximal. This allows dissection down to the tip of the greater trochanter. The trochanter is opened using an awl. It must be opened at the tip, not going too far medially or laterally. The nail in the lateral view is started in the middle third of the greater trochanter. This position is confirmed with the C-arm. On a lateral view of the C-arm there should be equal amounts of the femoral head on both sides of the radiographic image of the awl. This will show that the starting point in the lateral is directly in the center of the neck. Once the starting point has been established, the guide wire is passed across the fracture site (Fig. 28).

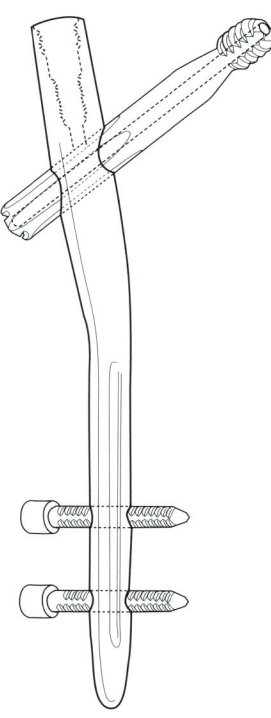

Figure 27. Intramedullary hip screw systems are composed of a short intramedullary nail with a medial lateral bend. This bend is variable between 6 and 10 degrees. The proximal end is expanded to allow the insertion of a solitary standard compression hip screw. Distal holes allow for distal locking. Some mechanism of fixation between the nail and the compression screw is provided to allow these to be a keyed system and prevent screw rotation in the head, but at the same time provide for sliding capabilities.

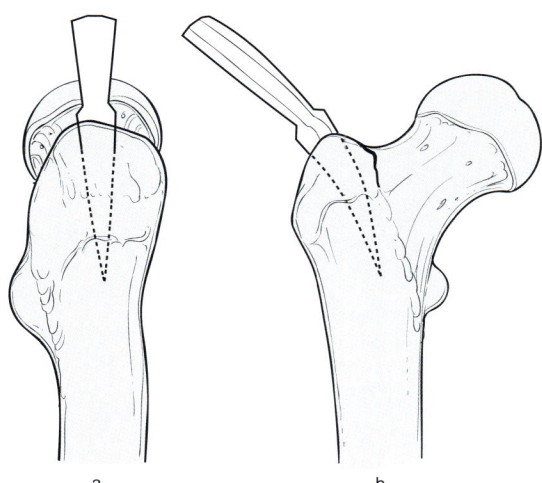

Figure 28 A,B. The starting position for the intra-medullary hip screw should be at the tip of the greater trochanter in the anterior posterior view. The awl should be inserted so that it takes up a place on the C-arm picture in the exact position where the proximal portion of the nail will sit. On the lateral the starting point is in the middle third of the greater trochanter. This will allow for the femoral head to be visualized on either side of the awl and will provide tract for the compression screw directly into the center of the head. This nail must not be inserted in the standard position for regular intramedullary nailing as this is to posterior.

The canal must be reamed for approximately 30 cm. This must be determined by C-arm control and measurement on the reaming device itself. There must be a minimum of 2 mm of overreaming as compared to the size of nail that is required. If the greater trochanteric region is unfractured, this area must be reamed to 17 mm to accept the proximal end of the nail. Greater trochanteric fracturing does not contraindicate the use of this nail because the soft tissues holding the fracture together have not been disrupted (Fig. 29).

Once the reaming has been finished, the appropriate templated nail is inserted. Preoperative planning can be carried out using templates to determine the size of the nail, which is usually a 130-degree angle, 12-mm diameter nail. The nail is pushed by hand into the canal so that the insertion handle sits down on the greater trochanter. This should place the compression screw hole at about the level of the inferior calcar. It normally looks as if it has gone too far; however, this is a radiological parallax problem, and the guide wire will be in the center of the head. With the nail in place and the appropriate angle guides attached, the compression screw can be inserted through the nail into the center of the head. This is done through a series of guides, taps, and reamers.

Technical concerns at this stage are that the guide wire and the reaming should be done by hand except in extremely hard bone. Entrapment of the reamer on the nail will occur because of slight nail rotation, and if power is being used, the risk of damaging the nail or the reamer or breaking the guide wire is present. Consequently, the reamer should be gently passed by hand across the nail and up into the head. The compression screw is then inserted so that it is within 1 cm of the subchondral bone and so that the outer aspect of the end of the screw is at the outer edge of lateral cortex of the femur. The screw cannot go inside the lateral femoral cortex, or sliding will not be achieved (Fig. 30 A, B). A device to lock the

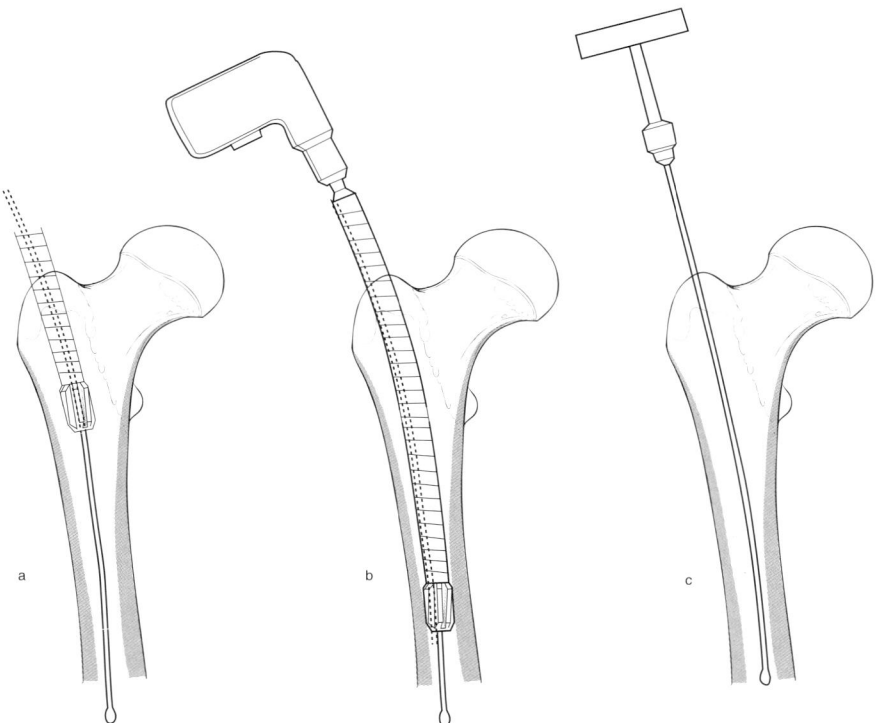

Figure 29 A,B,C. Following establishment of the entry portal, a guide wire should be passed down the femur to pass the isthmus into the distal portion, and the proximal 25 to 30 cm of the femur is reamed to a size 2 mm larger then the nail to be used. The proximal component of the area, particularly the intertrochanteric region, should be reamed to a size 17. If it appears that the nail will impinge in its wider portion in the trumpet area of entry into the isthmus, this area should also be reamed up to 17. This will prevent nail impingement as it is driven in.

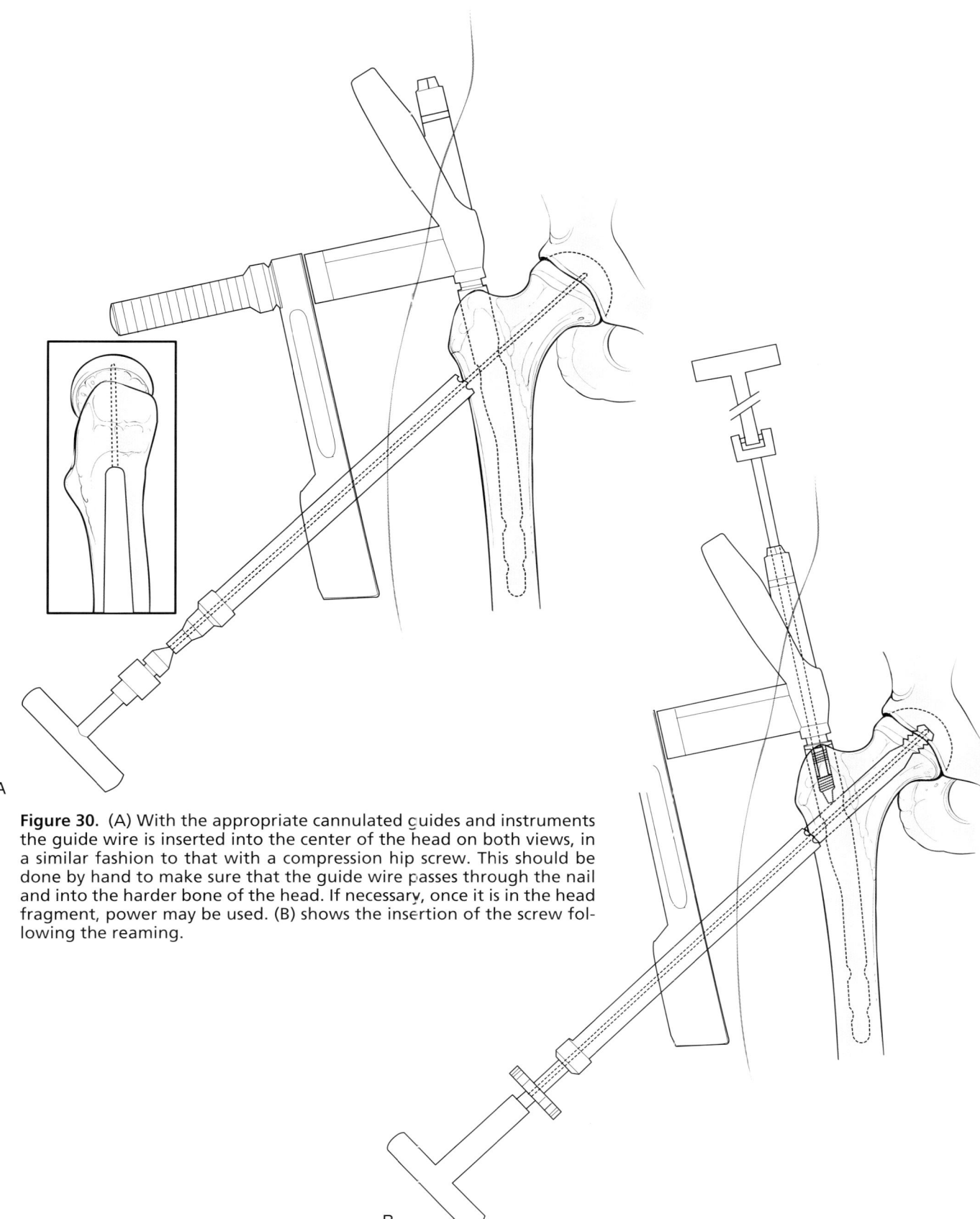

Figure 30. (A) With the appropriate cannulated guides and instruments the guide wire is inserted into the center of the head on both views, in a similar fashion to that with a compression hip screw. This should be done by hand to make sure that the guide wire passes through the nail and into the harder bone of the head. If necessary, once it is in the head fragment, power may be used. (B) shows the insertion of the screw following the reaming.

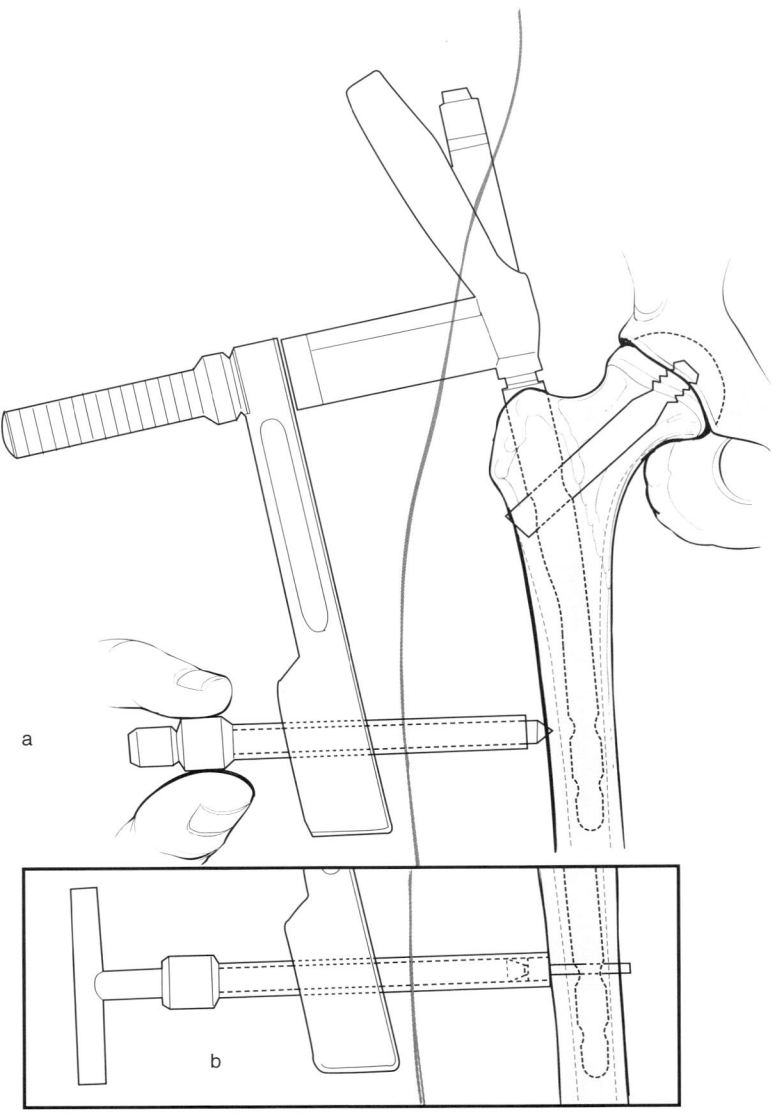

Figure 31 A, B. The distal locking of the nail. In the majority of fractures only one distal screw in the most proximal hole is required. If the fracture extends down to within several centimeters of the most proximal distal screw, two screws should be used. The locking should be done with the appropriate cannulated device and awl to perforate the cortex without hammering and with insertion of the drill and screw under C-arm control.

screw in place to prevent rotation is then inserted. Through an appropriate series of guides, the distal locking screws are inserted. When locking distally, a hammer must not be used to tap the awl to set the starting hole. This will cause microfractures down the femur and lead to potential postoperative femoral fracture (Fig. 31 A, B).

Warning

As this is an intramedullary device, there are several areas of concern that must be addressed. Because the nail is short and straight, patients who have significant anterior bow to their femurs or proximal femoral deformities may not be amenable to this procedure. If this is the elected procedure to be used, the smallest diameter nail will have to be inserted. Again it might require excessive reaming. This may force one to abandon this technique. It is also important to remember the lateral cortex of the greater trochanter cannot be reamed by allowing the starting point to drift posteriorly and lateral. This will allow the nail to fall from the back of the fracture, and then it will become very difficult to maintain the reduction and insert the compression screw into the head.

Open Reduction Internal Fixation

Occasionally it is necessary to do this as an open technique without a fracture table. In this situation the patient should be positioned on a radiolucent operating table and the C-arm brought in to get an AP view of the hip. A small roll should be placed under the buttock on the involved side. This will provide the ability to do a standard lateral approach to the femur as well as convert this to an anterior Watson Jones approach. In an open fashion, the fracture is reduced and then stabilized. With a C-arm and the radiolucent table, an anterior posterior view is very easy to obtain. If the fracture can be reduced and provisionally fixed with K-wires or interfragmental screws, then the appropriate frog lateral can be obtained as well. If the patient is rolled up to 40 degrees, a lateral view can be obtained by swinging the C-arm up under the table into its lateral position. If this is not possible, the lateral of the hip can be obtained by doing a frog-leg lateral of the proximal fracture fragment. If one places the guide wire up the femoral neck, one can obtain a frog lateral to determine the exact position of the guide wire. This usually means that the proximal fracture must be reduced. The compression hip screw can be put into position, the plate attached, and the distal fracture fragment then reduced to the plate. As well, this is a very viable technique for a 95-degree angle device such as a blade plate or dynamic compression screw (Fig. 32 A, B, C, D, E, F).

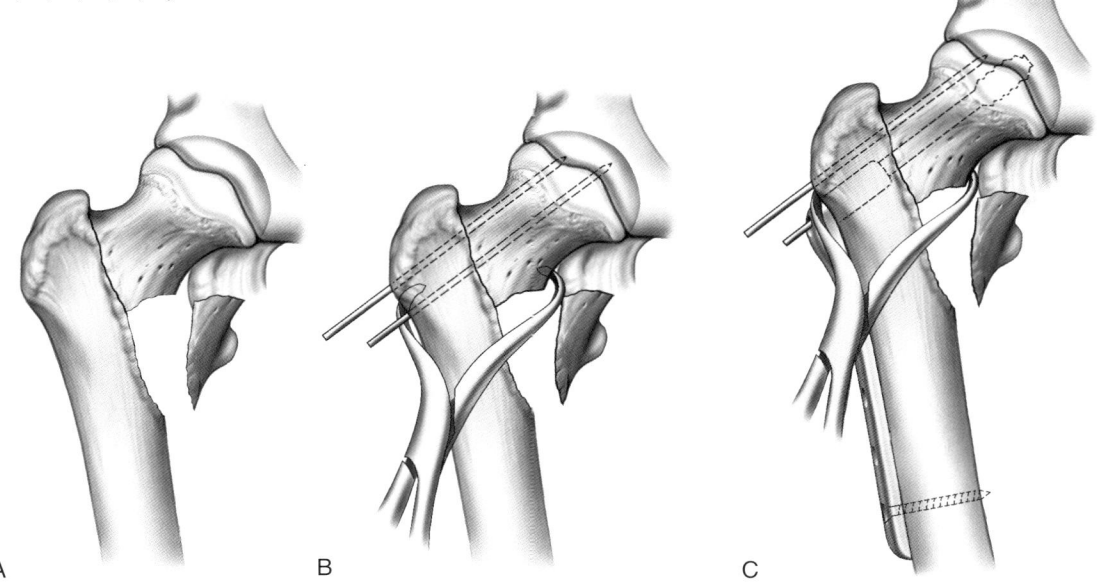

Figure 32. Open reduction and internal fixation of intertrochanteric fracture is performed through a standard lateral approach to the femur with the Watson Jones extension. Posterior dissection may be necessary to identify the posterior medial fracture fragment and to reduce it with an indirect soft tissue spearing technique. (A) This represents an unstable intertrochanteric fracture with a large posterior medial fracture fragment. (B) Following exposure in open reduction the proximal neck and head fragment is reduced to the major distal fracture fragment or trochanteric area. Provisional fixation is performed with K-wires. Appropriate anterior posterior view may be obtained with the C-arm and if the leg is then placed at 90 degrees of hip flexion and 20 degrees of abduction a lateral can be obtained. This will allow visualization of the position of the guide wire for compression screw insertion. (C) Following the insertion of the compression screw and plate which can then be affixed with one screw to the shaft. Using a sharp pointed instrument such as a dental hook or bone hook the posterior medial fracture fragment can then be reduced.

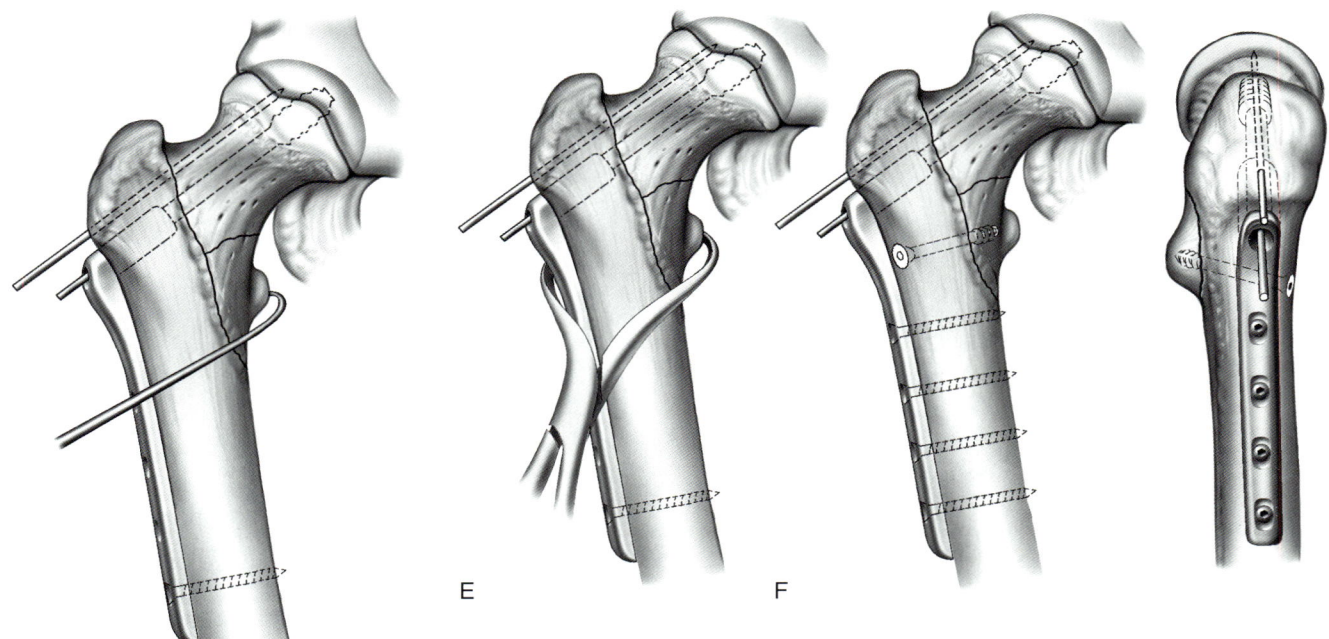

Figure 32. Continued (D, E) The posterior medial fracture fragment is then reduced using a sharp hook or dental pick and held in place by a pointed reduction clamp. With this in place then the appropriate interfragmental lag screw may be placed from anterior lateral femoral cortex into the posterior medial fracture fragment or cerclage wiring may be carried out. (F) On completion of this the plate is then finally affixed to the bone. Following this all the guide wires are removed and the incision maybe closed.

POSTOPERATIVE MANAGEMENT

The aim in all of these fractures is to achieve an anatomically stable reduction that is then stabilized by a splintage device. Because of the inability of the elderly patients to bear partial weight, the osteosynthesis must be strong enough to withstand weight bearing as tolerated in the immediate postoperative period. Within 24 hours the patient should be mobilized to a chair for several hours a day on an intermittent basis. Following this, the patient can then be mobilized to a walker, with weight bearing as tolerated on the involved leg. In any elderly fracture population group, a fracture hip program that addresses the psychosocial as well as the physical aspects of the patient must go hand in hand to improve rehabilitation of the patients. In the young individual, the use of partial weight bearing or non-weight bearing is quite acceptable because they can tolerate this. If there is good bone-on-bone contact, partial weight bearing with weight of leg can be commenced.

If the fracture fixation is stable, the patient will be seen in two weeks for suture removal, six weeks for radiographic control if weight bearing will be increased. A visit with radiographic control is performed at three months. Further followup occurs at six months and 12 months. Radiographic control will be determined by the patient's complaint and the status of fracture union. If the fixation is unstable, then radiographic control is mandatory at six weeks or earlier, depending upon patient symptomology. During this phase, physical therapy will be used to teach gait and the use of walking aids. It may be appropriate at the six-week period to institute muscle strengthening if fracture healing is progressing appropriately. This is most common in high-energy injuries where there is particular damage to the abductors of the hip.

Expected results are usually very good with a 95% union rate and in stable fractures with no significant leg-length or rotational abnormalities, if reduction is performed adequately. In an unstable fracture, shortening of up to 3 cm may occur, depending upon fracture instability, but healing will still be in the 95%-plus phase. Most elderly patients will take approximately one year to recover fully from this injury, but usually are off walking aids in about 3 to 4 months. They may continue to use a cane during this period for comfort and for confidence. Younger individuals usually are off all walking aids by 3 to 4 months and probably are returning to activity fairly quickly, unless there is significant soft-tissue damage from the injury.

COMPLICATIONS

Infection

It is uncommon with this approach to see major wound infections. However, it occasionally occurs, and rapid attention is necessary to treat this joint infection. Opening the wound, debridement, irrigation, and closure over drains or leaving it open after appropriate debridement must be undertaken.

Malunion

Because of the potential instability of the reduction, malunions will occur but are rarely significant. If the principles of an anatomical reduction and stable fixation with impaction at the time of surgery are obtained, these can usually be predicted and the patient can be consulted concerning this and be aware of any leg-length or rotational abnormality.

Nonunion

In intertrochanteric fractures nonunion is very rare, as these fractures are through cancellous, and bone healing is usually rapid. However, occasional nonunions will occur. The varus nonunions require a valgus osteotomy to reestablish dynamic compressive forces across a horizontal fracture line. If the nonunion is not in varus, simple compression will be enough with a bone graft.

Bone Failure

With inappropriate placement of the fixation and occasionally because of severe osteoporosis, the whole construct may collapse and fail. Consequently, close supervision in the first 4 to 6 weeks is relatively important. In situations where there is a concern, x-rays should be taken on a weekly basis for 3 to 4 weeks and then at six weeks. Early evidence of bone or implant failure can be identified and appropriate measures undertaken. Limitation of weight bearing, bed rest, traction, or revision may be necessary. If the fixation fails and the head is then destroyed by the screw cutting out, calcar replacement total joint may be necessary in the elderly. In the younger individual this must be undertaken by a different technique of internal fixation. With the appropriate techniques, good bone union is expected, and hip joint arthroplasty is not acceptable in this group unless the head is completely destroyed.

ILLUSTRATIVE CASE FOR TECHNIQUE

J. L. is a 69-year-old female. While playing golf she tripped and fell. Because of discomfort and pain in her hip region, she was unable to continue playing and was taken to the

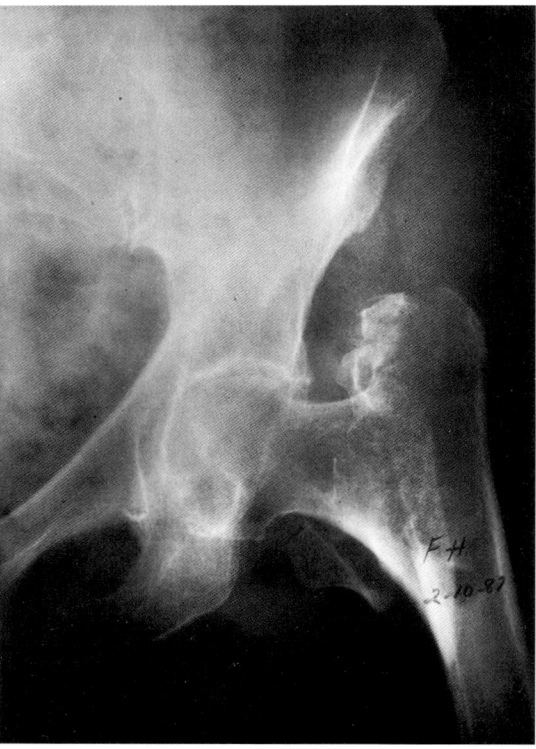

Figure 33. This figure represents the antero-posterior radiograph of an intertrochanteric fracture. It shows significant shortening and varus as well as external rotation with the greater trochanter in profile. The lesser trochanter is displaced.

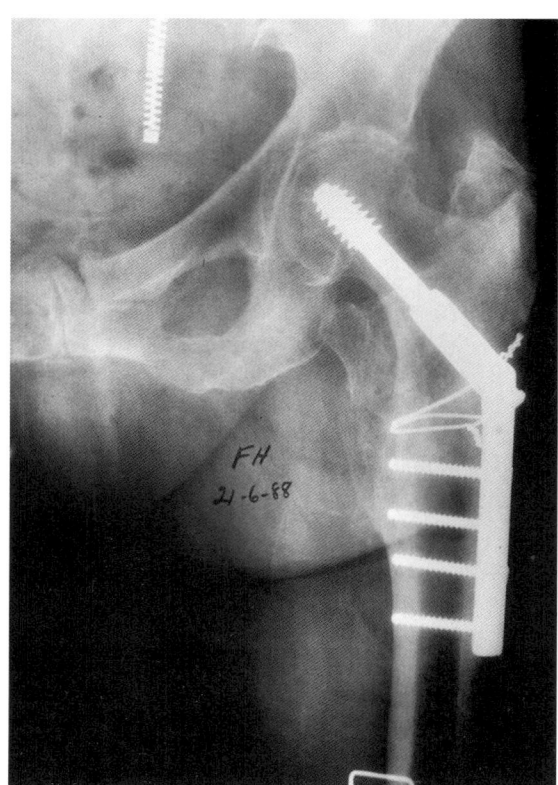

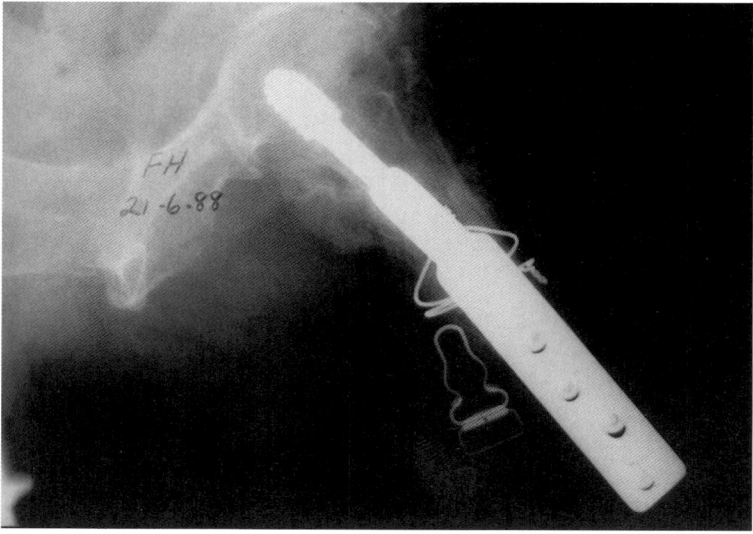

Figure 34 A, B. This represents the healed x-ray at a 6 month period. Note that the reduction has been obtained and cerclage wires applied to hold the calcar tip in place. These have created a stable reduction and there has been minimal collapse.

local hospital. Radiographs of her hip (Fig. 33) revealed an intertrochanteric fracture. This fracture was considered an unstable variety. She was otherwise healthy, and after appropriate examination to rule out any other potential life-threatening conditions, she was taken to the operating room. A closed reduction was obtained and the fracture was stabilized with a compression hip screw. Cerclage wires were applied around the tip of the calcar to hold it in place to increase the stability of the fixation.

Postoperative course was uneventful and at six months, radiograph (Fig. 34) showed union. There has been minimal collapse. At this stage she has abandoned the use of a cane and has returned to full functional activities.

RECOMMENDED READING

1. Bridle, S., Patel, A., Bircher, M., and Calvert, P.: Fixation of intertrochanteric fractures of the femur: A randomized prospective comparison of the gamma nail and the dynamic hip screw. *J. B. Joint S.*, 73(B): 330–334, 1991.
2. Chang, W. S., Zuckerman, J., Kumar, F., Frankel, V.: Biomechanical evaluation of anatomical reduction versus medial displacement osteotomy in unstable intertrochanteric fractures. *Clin. Orthop.*, 225: 141–146, 1987.
3. Clark, D. W., and Ribbans, W. J.: Treatment of unstable intertrochanteric fractures of the femur: A prospective trial comparing anatomical reduction and valgus osteotomy. *Injury*, 21: 84–88, 1990.
4. Davis, T., Sher, J., Horsman, A., Simpson, M., Porter, B., and Checketts, R.: Intertrochanteric femoral fractures: Mechanical failure after internal fixation. *J. Bone Joint Surg.*, 72(B): 26–31, 1990.
5. Foubister, G.: Outcome of proximal femoral fractures. *Sem. in Orthop.*, 5: 95–100, 1990.
6. Grosse, A., and Tagland, G.: *Gamma locking nail: Surgical Technique.* Howmedica, London. 1990.
7. Halder, S. C.: The gamma nail for peritrochanteric fractures. *J. Bone Joint Surg.*, 74(B):340–344, 1992.
8. Hornby, R., Grimley-Evans, J., and Varden, V. Operative or conservative treatment of the trochanteric fractures of the femur. *J. Bone Joint Surg.*, 71(B): 619–623, 1989.
9. Jensen, J. B.: Classification of trochanteric fractures. *Acta Orthop. Scand.*, 51: 803–810, 1980.
10. Jensen, J. B., Sonne-Holm, S., and Tondevold, E.: Unstable intertrochanteric fractures: A comparative analysis of four methods of internal fixation. *Acta Orthop. Scand.*, 51: 949–962, 1980.
11. Leung, K., So, W., Shen, W., and Hui, P., Gamma nails and dynamic hip screws for peritrochanteric fractures. *J. Bone Joint Surg.*, 74B: 345–351, 1992.
12. Meislin, R. J., Zuckerman, J., Kumar, F., and Frankel, V.: A biomechanical analysis of the sliding hip screw: The question of plate angle. *J. Orthop. Trauma*, 4:130–136, 1990.
13. Mohomend, N. Hearn, T., and Kellam, J: Biomechanical comparison of the gamma nail and the sliding hip screw. Proceedings sixth annual meeting of the Orthopedic Trauma Association, 1990: 57.
14. Rosenblum, S., Zuckerman, J., Kumar, F., and Fam, B.: A biomechanical evaluation of the gamma nail. *J. Bone J. Surg.*, 74(B): 352–357, 1992.
15. Walheim, J., Barrios, C., Stark, A., Brostrom, L., and Olsson, E.: Postoperative improvement of walking capacity on patients with trochanteric hip fractures.: *J. Orthop Trauma*, 4: 137–143, 1990.

7

Young Patients with Femoral Head Fractures

M. L. Chip Routt, Peter T. Simonian, and Sigvard T. Hansen

INDICATIONS/CONTRAINDICATIONS

Femoral head fractures are serious orthopaedic injuries that usually occur in association with hip dislocations after high-energy automobile or motorcycle accidents. The most common victims of these injuries are young adults (12), typically unrestrained occupants in the front seat of an automobile that is subjected to rapid deceleration. Eighty-two percent of hip dislocations are posteriorly directed with an 18% incidence of associated femoral head fracture (12). Anterior hip dislocations are far less common, yet 77% of anterior dislocations occur in association with femoral head fractures (5).

Femoral head fractures are grouped into two major categories. The most common type of injury is a shear (or cleavage) fracture associated with a posterior hip dislocation. The femoral head is fractured when the surface of the femoral head comes into contact with the acetabular rim at the moment of dislocation (Fig. 1A). Conversely, crushing fractures of the femoral head are associated with central acetabular fracture-dislocations. Impaction of the superolateral quadrant of the femoral head into the intact pelvic brim produces a depression or impression fracture of the articular cartilage in the cancellous bone of the femoral head (Fig. 1B). This type of injury is uncommon (2). Both types of femoral head fractures alter the spherical shape of the hip joint and create an anatomic predisposition to arthritis.

The goal of definitive treatment should be to restore normal hip anatomy by optimizing the contact area between the femoral head and the acetabulum. Normal anatomy cannot be restored unless the entire femoral head can be reconstructed. Accurate reduction of the femoral head fragments is vital to reduce the peak stresses on the articular cartilage, particularly after the weight-bearing surface has been disrupted. Most authors agree that femoral head fractures with more than 2.0-mm of displacement warrant operative intervention. Persistent widening of the hip joint space after closed reduction is caused by an

---

M. L. C. Routt, M.D. and P. T. Simonian, M.D.: Department of Orthopaedics, University of Washington Medical Center, Seattle, Washington 98195.

S. T. Hansen, M.D.: Department of Orthopaedics, Harborview Medical Center, Seattle, Washington 98104–2499.

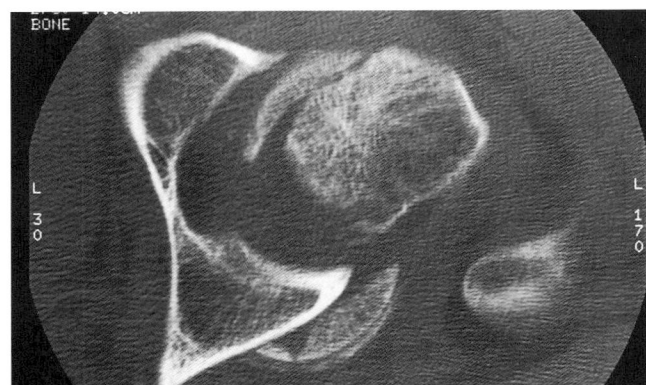
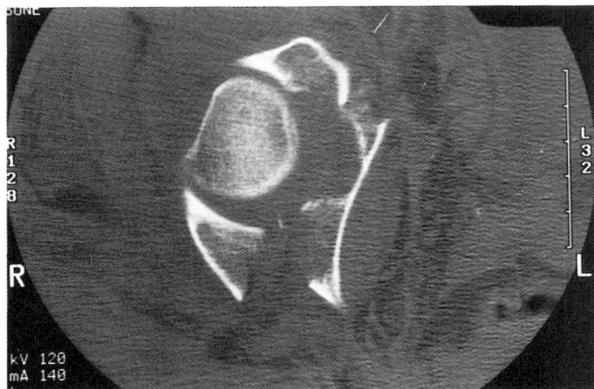

Figure 1. Femoral head fractures are grouped into two major categories: (A) the most common type of injury is a shear (or cleavage) fracture associated with a posterior hip dislocation. In this example, a cleaved portion of the femoral head is posterior to the acetabulum. (B) The more uncommon crushing fracture of the femoral head, which is associated with central acetabular fracture-dislocations. Impaction of the superolateral quadrant of the femoral head into the intact pelvic rim produces a depression or impression fracture of the articular cartilage and the cancellous bone of the femoral head.

obstruction such as a detached labrum or bony or chondral debris and is an absolute indication for arthrotomy (6). Roeder and DeLee (12) identified several situations in which operative intervention is indicated. These include inadequate closed reductions of the femoral head fracture or hip dislocations, significant fracture comminution, sciatic-nerve injury not present before closed reduction, femoral neck fracture, and involvement of the weight-bearing portion of the femoral head by a single large fragment (Fig. 2).

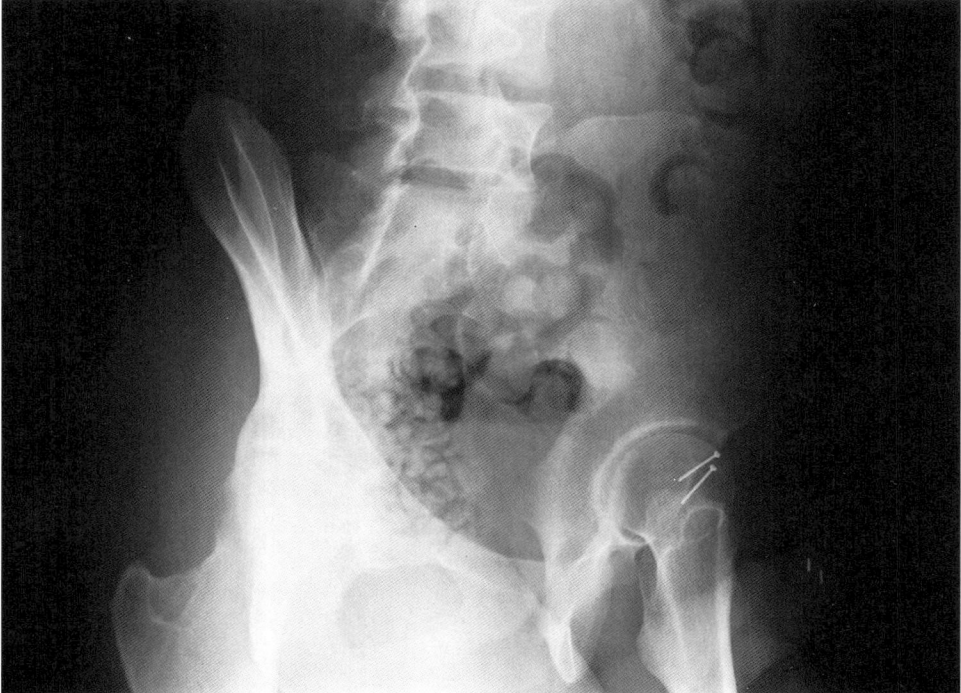

Figure 2. One of the indications for operative fixation of a femoral head fracture is involvement of the a single, large fragment of the weight-bearing portion. The large single fragment was fixed with two 1.5 mm screws.

Traction is recommended for stable and minimally displaced femoral head fractures. Elderly or inactive patients are also candidates for closed treatment. A traction device can be set up at home for patients who live in supportive home environments or those who are institutionalized.

Prosthetic Hip Replacement

Endoprosthetic replacement of the femoral head is reserved for elderly patients. Total hip replacement is indicated in the few individuals with underlying arthritis who sustain femoral head fractures.

PREOPERATIVE PLANNING

A team approach is recommended for optimal treatment of patients with these injuries. The history of injury is obtained from the patient or a paramedic who was present at the scene of the accident. The typical configuration of the lower-extremity deformity can be altered when the victim is removed from the scene of the accident. In the absence of an ipsilateral femoral neck fracture, reduction of a hip dislocation assumes the highest priority after ventilation and hemostasis. A careful prereduction neurological examination of the affected lower extremity should include an assessment of femoral and sciatic nerve functions. Atraumatic reduction maneuvers may be attempted after the patient is adequately relaxed. The patient's postreduction neurological function should be documented.

Associated Injuries

Nerve. Posterior hip dislocations can cause injury to the sciatic nerve by means of direct contusion, local hemorrhage, or traction due to displacement. Vigorous attempts at closed reduction can also cause nerve damage.

Femoral Neck. Associated traumatic femoral neck fractures can be occult or nondisplaced injuries. Good-quality admitting radiographs are critical for making an accurate diagnosis, and careful scrutiny of the prereduction radiographs usually reveals these fractures. Iatrogenic femoral neck fractures can result from forceful attempts at closed reduction. Closed reduction of a hip dislocation either with or without a femoral head fracture is contraindicated in the presence of a femoral neck fracture.

Posterior Wall Acetabular Fracture. A common injury triad consists of a femoral head fracture, a hip dislocation, and a posterior-wall acetabular fracture. High-energy forces producing these injuries can also cause comminution of the acetabular wall. A posterior acetabular-wall fracture rarely consists of a simple fragment but usually includes several osteochondral fragments. Impaction of cancellous osteochondral fragments into the posterior column may also be present (3). These findings influence management strategies.

Knee. Clinical findings that lead a discerning physician to suspect the presence of a femoral head fracture in a polytraumatized patient include patellar fracture, knee contusion, lacerations or ligamentous deficiency about the knee, and traumatic effusion.

Thoracic Aorta. This type of injury warrants maintaining a high index of suspicion for thoracic aorta injuries. Diagnosis is made from a high-quality chest radiograph and is further confirmed by arteriography. Prompt treatment is mandatory.

Femoral Shaft. The presence of an obvious femoral shaft fracture may obscure or prevent diagnosis of an ipsilateral femoral head fracture. Triage physicians frequently fail to obtain radiographs of the joints above and below a fracture. When a posterior hip dislocation occurs simultaneously with a femoral shaft fracture, the position of the proximal fragment of the femoral shaft fracture can alert the examiner to the presence of an associated femoral head injury. Proximal shaft fracture fragments associated with posterior hip dislocations are adducted, internally rotated, flexed, and shortened. Isolated femoral shaft fractures demonstrate a flexed, abducted, externally rotated proximal fragment deformity. These subtle clues are valuable for making an accurate diagnosis.

Imaging

Radiographs of the cervical spine, the pelvis, and the chest are taken during the initial resuscitation of all polytraumatized patients. A pelvic anteroposterior (AP) radiograph is examined to identify abnormalities and establish the need for more specific diagnostic studies. Femoral head fractures with associated posterior hip dislocations warrant AP, lateral and Judet oblique radiographic views of the hip and the proximal femur. Occult femoral neck fractures must be ruled out prior to closed reduction attempts. Postreduction, biplanar imaging of the hip is used to assess a concentric reduction.

Computerized axial tomography (CAT) scans of the pelvis, which also define the condition of the femoral head, are helpful in planning treatment. We recommend making 5-mm cuts through the pelvis, reserving 3-mm cuts for the femoral head and acetabular area. The CAT scans are useful for locating intraarticular loose bodies, classifying associated acetabular fractures, identifying occult posterior pelvic ring injuries, and planning the surgical exposure.

Moed and Maxey (10) recommended obtaining a CAT scan-directed Judet oblique radiographic view. The plain radiograph is obtained after a pelvic CAT scan reveals the presence of an oblique femoral head fracture. The patient is then oriented according to this degree of tilt similar to a Judet oblique radiograph. Radiographs taken with this direct tilt are the least expensive method of following the progress of these fractures, particularly when they are managed nonoperatively.

Injury Classifications

The usefulness of femoral head fracture classification schemes is variable because application of many schemes is often confusing, and treatment recommendations are inconsistent. As a result, clinical results following treatment of these injuries remain uniformly poor (9,13,15). There are numerous classification schemes for femoral head fractures and each scheme has some advantages. In 1954, Stewart and Milford (13) classified hip dislocations with femoral head and neck fractures as grade-IV injuries. Thompson and Epstein (15) classified posterior hip dislocations with associated femoral head fractures as type V. Brav (1) combined Thompson and Epstein's type-IV and -V injuries in his own classification, calling them type-III fracture dislocations. Pipkin (11) further subdivided Stewart and Milford's grade-IV fracture-dislocations into four types, according to the location of the femoral head fracture. Pipkin's classification (Fig. 3) includes:

Type I: Posterior hip dislocations with femoral head fractures caudad to the fovea capitis femoris

Type II: Posterior hip dislocations with femoral head fractures cephalad to the fovea capitis femoris

Type III: Type-I or -II dislocations with associated femoral neck fractures.

Type IV: Type-I or -II dislocations with associate acetabular rim fractures.

Although Pipkin's classification excludes anterior dislocations, it includes combination injuries and provides prognostic information.

Brumback (2) offered a detailed and comprehensive classification system which includes both anterior and posterior dislocations. He included combination injuries and severity grading in his system, as well as indentation fractures (Fig. 3):

Type 1 A posterior hip dislocation with femoral head fracture involving the inferomedial, non-weight bearing portion of the femoral head.

Type 1A With minimum or no fracture of the acetabular rim and stable hip joint after reduction.

Type 1B With significant acetabular fracture and hip joint stability.

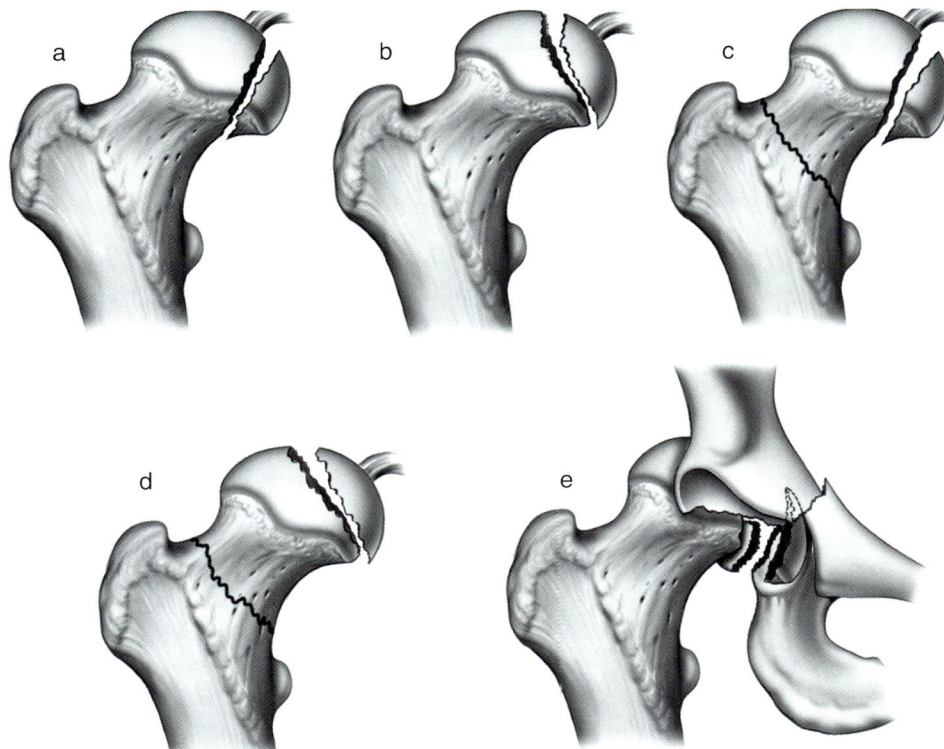

Figure 3. (A) Infrafoveal fracture; Pipkin I, Brumback 1A. (B) Suprafoveal fracture; Pipkin II, Brumback 2A. (C) Either A or B associated with a femoral neck fracture; Pipkin III, Brumback 3B. (D) Any femoral head configuration with an acetabular fracture; Pipkin IV, Brumback 1B, 2B.

Type 2 A posterior hip dislocation with femoral head fracture involving the superomedial, weight-bearing portion of the femoral head.
Type 2A With minimum or no fracture of the acetabular rim and stable hip joint after reduction.
Type 2B With significant acetabular fracture and hip joint instability.
Type 3 Dislocation of the hip (unspecified direction) with associated femoral neck fracture.
Type 3A Without fracture of the femoral head.
Type 3B With fracture of the femoral head.
Type 4 Anterior dislocation of the hip with fracture of the femoral head.
Type 4A Indentation type; depression of the superolateral weight-bearing surface of the femoral head.
Type 4B Transchondral type; osteocartilaginous shear fracture of the weight-bearing surface of the femoral head.
Type 5 Central fracture-dislocation of the hip with fracture of the femoral head.

SURGERY

Isolated Femoral Head Fractures

We recommend an anterior surgical approach for patients with femoral head fractures, without posterior acetabular involvement. The patient is positioned supine on a radiolucent operating table that is compatible with fluoroscopy. A soft lumbosacral support such as a small, folded blanket is placed under the patient to elevate the hip and allow wide access to

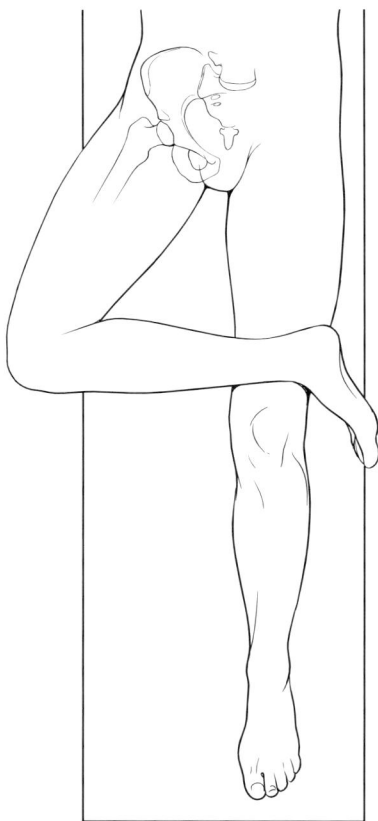

Figure 4. Draping of the leg free allows the "figure-of-four" position intraoperatively, which greatly enhances exposure.

the affected extremity and pelvic area. The fluoroscopy unit is positioned according to Moed's (10) recommendations for confirmation of proper positioning and facilitation of intraoperative imaging. The skin of the entire affected lower extremity and flank is prepared with antiseptic solution. Inclusion of the entire lower extremity within the surgical field is mandatory to allow unhampered manipulation of the hip joint intraoperatively (Fig. 4). The surgeon and the first assistant both wear headlamps. The patient is given an initial dose of a broad-spectrum intravenous cephalosporin, and the antibiotic is continued every 6 to 8 hours.

We use the Smith-Petersen anterior approach, which involves dissection between the femoral and gluteal innervated muscle groups (see Fig. 10). The skin incision, made parallel to the iliac crest, curves toward the lateral patella near the anterior-superior iliac spine (ASIS) (Fig. 5). If the skin around the ASIS is very thin, a more lateral skin incision is appropriate. The lateral femoral cutaneous nerve is protected during the exposure and retraction.

The interval between the sartorius and tensor fascia lata muscles is identified. The periosteal origin of the tensor fascia lata at the iliac crest is partially divided, and the gluteal and tensor fascia lata muscles are released subperiosteally from the lateral ilium as necessary. In certain patients these muscles can be retracted, rather than released. The tensor fascia lata muscle sheath is incised distally and the muscle fibers are retracted laterally, providing an approach to the ASIS from both arms of the incision (Fig. 6). Next, the deep or posteromedial fascia of the tensor envelope is incised to expose the rectus femoris muscle, which is retracted medially.

The next fascial layer separates the rectus femoris from the vastus lateralis. Dissection of this layer exposes the ascending branches of the lateral femoral circumflex artery. These often numerous vessels can be controlled entirely by ligature. Deep dissection is facilitated

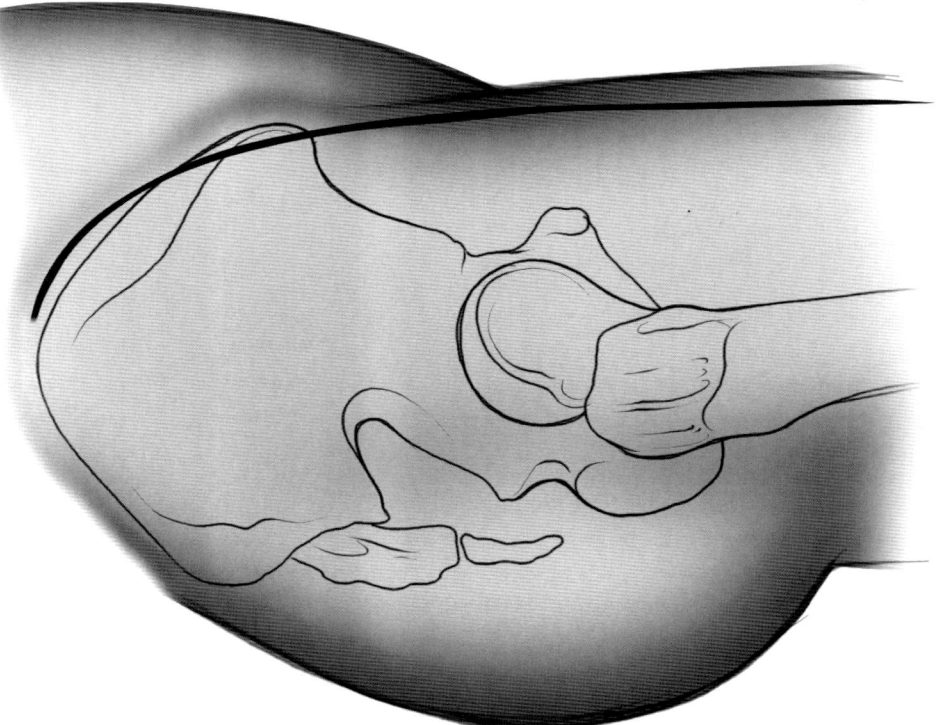

Figure 5. The skin incision is made parallel to the iliac-crest curves toward the lateral patella near the anterior-superior iliac spine. Redrawn by HT.

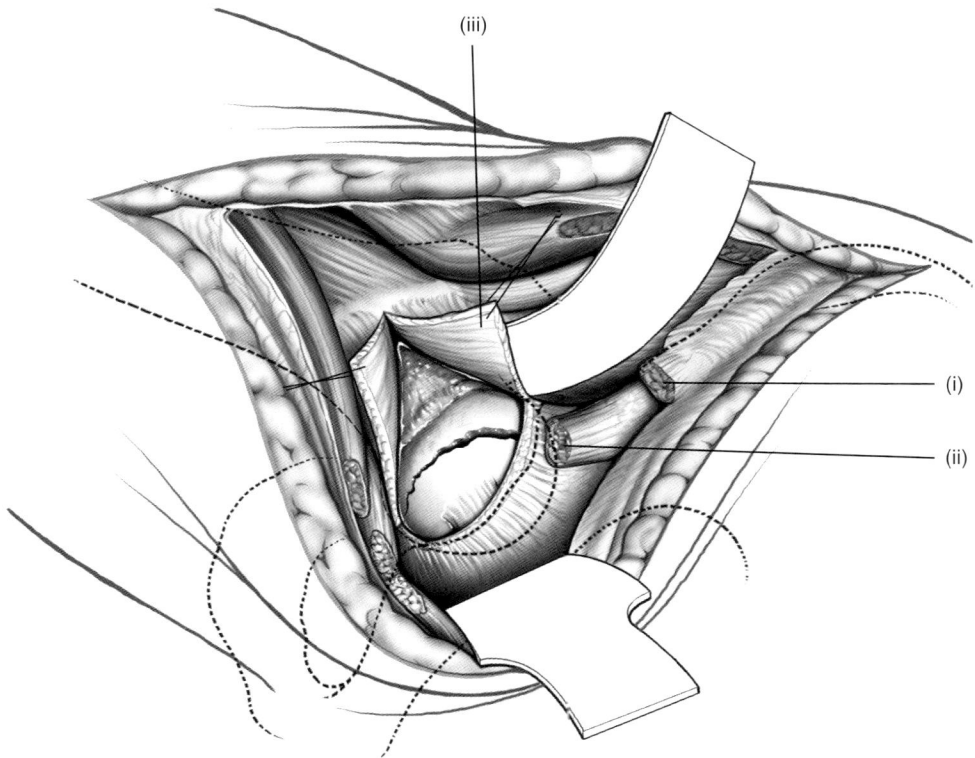

Figure 6. Deep exposure. The tensor fascia lata muscle sheath is incised distally and the muscle fibers are retracted laterally, providing an approach to the ASIS from both arms of the incision. Next, the deep or posteromedial fascia of the tensor envelope is incised to expose the rectus femoris muscle, which is retracted medially. An anterior **T**-type, **L**-shaped, or marginal capsulotomy is carried out to provide access to the joint. (i) Sartorius is not inside during the operation. (ii) Straight head and often the reflected head of the rectus femoris tendonis incised for exposure. (iii) Capsular edge is tagged with sutures.

by retraction of the gluteus minimus and medius muscles in addition to the tensor fascia lata muscle. When this approach is carried out, traumatic retraction and stripping of the abductor muscle should be limited to the amount necessary for visualization of the anterior hip joint and the femoral head.

The reflected head of the rectus femoris originates in the supraacetabular region and divides into capsular contributions. The reflected head is incised and retracted. An anterior **T**-type, **L**-shaped, or marginal capsulotomy is carried out to provide access to the joint (Fig. 6). The femoral head fracture is debrided of gathering hematoma. A Schanz screw is placed percutaneously at the level of the trochanteric line in order to distract the proximal femur distally and laterally and to improve joint visualization, irrigation, and debridement. Proper positioning of the proximal femur, usually into abduction and external rotation maximizes the exposure of the femoral head fracture. Narrow-diameter suction tips and headlamps are used to improve visualization, and dental hooks are used to manipulate the fracture fragments.

Small Kirschner wires are inserted away from the articular cartilage as provisional fixation to secure the reduction. The wires are placed away from the anticipated location of the surgical implants unless insertion of a cannulated screw is planned. Oblique fluoroscopic imaging is used to confirm adequate reduction at this point. The choice of fixation is variable and depends on the fracture pattern. In general, we use Herbert screws or countersunk

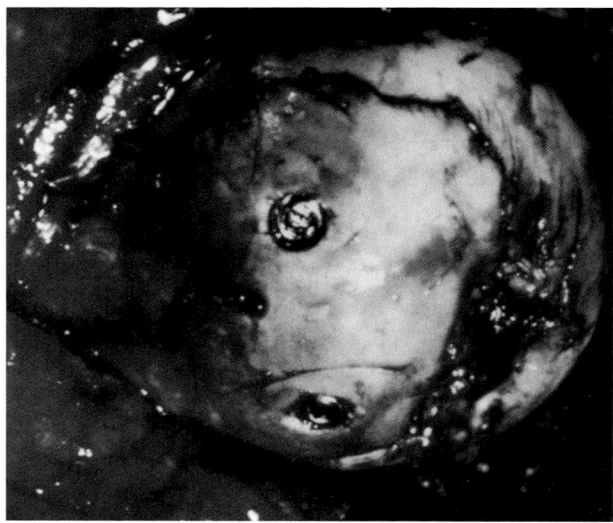

Figure 7. Reduction and fixation with two countersunk 3.5 mm cortical lag screws. Reprinted from *Orthopaedic Trauma Protocols*, (Hansen/Swiontkowski) p. 241, Fig. 3D.

3.5 mm or 2.7 mm lag screws. Miniature screws are also useful for small fragments. (Fig. 7). Some surgeons prefer to use 4.0-mm cannulated screws. Kirschner wires are not recommended for permanent fixation because they tend to migrate from their original position. Optimal placement of the screw has been achieved when the head of the screw can be located on the articular cartilage reflection. When cannulated screws are used, the provisional Kirschner wires serve two functions: they provide temporary fixation and guide strategic placement of the screw. Stability of the fixation is assessed under direct visualization during manipulation (rotation and compression) loading of the fracture fragment. The joint is thoroughly irrigated, and the capsule is anatomically aligned. The reflected head of the rectus femoris is often difficult to reapproximate perfectly. Both deep and subcutaneous suction canister drains are set in place, and the skin wounds (including the stab wound for the Schanz screw) are closed.

Concurrent Femoral Head and Neck Fractures

Patients with femoral neck and head fractures require special considerations. Closed reduction of a hip dislocation is contraindicated in these patients. The operative positioning is the same as that for an anterior approach, and reduction and fixation of the femoral head are carried out through the Watson-Jones approach with distal dissection, which exposes the proximal femur and femoral neck. The Watson-Jones approach is unpopular in general because the interval between the gluteal and tensor fascial lata muscles is not a true internervous plane and is difficult to identify. Nevertheless, the Watson-Jones anterolateral approach is preferred by some surgeons chiefly because ectopic bone formation is common after the Smith-Petersen approach. The skin incision is centered over the greater trochanter and extended distally in line with the femoral shaft. The proximal limb of the incision curves anteriorly and stops several millimeters short of the iliac crest. The vastus lateralis tubercle is identified through deep dissection. The interval between the gluteus medius and the tensor fascia lata is incised to allow anterior retraction of the tensor fascia lata and posterior retraction of the gluteus medius. A trochanteric osteotomy is not recommended. Dissection is continued along the femoral neck. The hip capsule is identified, and a T-type capsulotomy is carried out. Occasionally, the reflected head of the rectus muscle must be detached to allow full visualization of the femoral head fracture. The femoral neck fracture is reduced and stabilized temporarily with Kirschner wires or clamps. A proximal femoral Schanz screw is then used to carefully direct the open reduction of the hip joint. After the hip is reduced, the femoral neck fracture is anatomically reduced and definitively stabilized, by means of screw fixation with a lag technique. Placement of the lag screws is planned to prevent their interference with the femoral head fracture implants. The femoral head is then reduced and stabilized. Because manipulation of the proximal femur is necessary to visualize and reduce adequately the femoral head fracture, fixation of the femoral neck must be stable. Suction canister drains are inserted at wound closure.

Excision of Fracture Fragments

Excision of the fracture fragment(s) may be indicated in certain situations. Excision is usually reserved for femoral head fractures located caudad to the fovea centralis femoris (Pipkin type I) or fractures with significant comminution. This treatment option may also be beneficial in elderly patients who are not candidates for hip replacement for other reasons.

Concurrent Femoral Head and Posterior Acetabular Fractures

Displacement of the posterior wall, the posterior column, or associated posterior-wall and column acetabular fractures are indications for fixation through a Kocher-Langenbeck posterior approach. When a posterior approach is used because of posterior acetabular involvement and the fragment is difficult to visualize and reduce, the surgeon must resist the temptation to simply excise the fragment. Instead, an anterior exposure is added to facilitate fixation at the same operation. These exposures can be performed either simultaneously or sequentially.

POSTOPERATIVE MANAGEMENT

The patient is given indomethacin or postoperative low-dose irradiation (600 cGY), particularly when the abductor was stripped during the surgical exposure. Use of indomethacin is not recommended in polytraumatized or head-injured patients because it must be administered rectally, and the amount of absorption is unpredictable. For these patients we prefer to use irradiation targeted on the pericapsular abductor muscular origins.

Mobilization of the joint is started with continuous passive motion devices if motion is not contraindicated by other injuries. Hip flexion is limited to 60 degrees in patients with associated posterior acetabular injuries. After six postoperative weeks, hip flexion may be increased if radiographs show evidence of healing. Patient mobilization is dictated by the injury pattern. Weight bearing on the affected extremity is restricted to toe-touch, crutch-assisted gait. Hip strengthening exercises are carried out with physical therapy assistance. Activities are gradually increased toward a goal of independent gait at three postoperative months.

Routine AP, lateral, and Moed's CAT-directed oblique-plain radiographs are taken to follow the progress of fracture healing. Radiographs are obtained immediately postoperatively, at six postoperative weeks, and at three postoperative months. Hardware is usually left in place and not removed routinely.

Functional Outcome

Variations in classifications and inconsistent treatment regimens make functional results of most series difficult to compare. In addition to these difficulties, the followups of most series are erratic, and evaluations of the clinical results are not uniform (7,8,10,11). For example, Epstein, Wiss, and Cozen (8) stated that of the 46 patients in their series who had adequate followup, only 47% had a good result (8). Therefore, it remains inconclusive whether delayed reduction of a hip joint dislocation, poor reductions, femoral neck or acetabular involvement, nerve injury, or other factors are related to poor results in the management of femoral head fractures.

COMPLICATIONS

Avascular Necrosis

Since avascular necrosis is a potential complication of femoral head fractures, a discussion of anatomy must include vascular considerations. Trueta's femoral head vascular studies provide important information in this area (16). He identified three terminal arteries that supply blood to the femoral head:

1. The artery of the ligamentum teres from the obturator system
2. The lateral femoral circumflex terminal branch
3. The lateral epiphyseal artery, which is the terminal branch of the medial femoral circumflex artery

The lateral epiphyseal artery supplies blood to most of the weight-bearing area of the femoral head (Fig. 8). Trueta also carried out injection studies to demonstrate that blood supply going to the femoral head from the anterior hip capsule is negligible (16).

These anatomic considerations influence the management of femoral head fractures and posterior hip dislocations. Tension and occlusion injuries to the lateral epiphyseal artery mandate urgent reduction of the femoral head into the acetabulum. Connolly observed that posterior hip dislocations stretch the medial femoral circumflex vessel and that pressure from the edge of the disrupted posterior hip capsule or the acetabular labrum can occlude the lateral epiphyseal artery, jeopardizing the viability of the femoral head (4).

Blood supply to the displaced femoral head fragment is also disrupted by the injury. The ligamentum teres inserts onto the femoral head at the fovea centralis, and fracture fragments located inferior to the ligament are not tethered by soft tissues. The presence of fractures cephalad to the fovea suggests that the ligamentum teres might still be attached to the femoral head fracture fragment. Fractures occurring above the fovea are likely to disrupt the end arterioles of the lateral epiphyseal artery (14).

The incidence of avascular necrosis of the femoral head increases the longer the hip remains dislocated (8). The incidence of avascular necrosis of the femoral head is 13% for posterior hip dislocations and increases to 18% for posterior hip dislocations with associated femoral head fractures. The higher incidence is most likely attributable to high-energy injuries and severe soft-tissue disruption. Other factors contributing to avascular necrosis probably include delayed reduction, nonanatomical reduction of the fracture surfaces, and

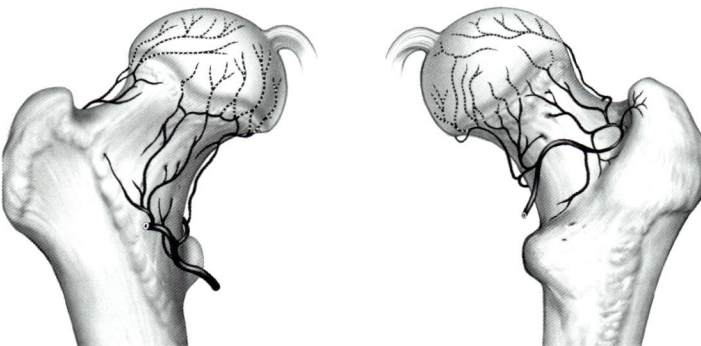

Figure 8. The lateral epiphyseal artery supplies blood to most of the weight-bearing area of the femoral head.

interposition of fragments or soft-tissue structures. Delayed reduction has also been associated with a higher incidence of ectopic bone formation (17).

Ectopic Bone

Heterotopic ossification formation is directly related to the amount of hip abductor retraction and stripping from the lateral ilium during the Smith-Petersen exposure. Low-dose targeted irradiation or indomethacin use has limited this to Brooker class I or less.

Malreduction

Comminution complicates the reduction of the femoral head fracture. The osteochondral and pure chondral fragments are often too small to stabilize. Fracture interdigitations cannot be used to improve reductions in such instances.

Implant

Small screws may be needed to secure many of these fractures. These screws are placed away from the articular cartilage whenever possible. Occasionally screws must be countersunk through the cartilage. Low-profile miniature screws or Herbert screws are advocated in these cases.

ILLUSTRATIVE CASE FOR TECHNIQUE

A 28-year-old female was injured in an automobile accident. She sustained pelvic ring fractures and a left femoral head fracture (Fig. 9A). She was treated operatively using a Smith-Petersen exposure. The femoral head fracture was comminuted and had several cartilage fragments with minimal remaining subchondral bone. Subluxation of the femoral head facilitated reduction and fixation. Small-diameter screws were used to stabilize the fragments. The miniature screws were countersunk beneath the articular cartilage. On her first postoperative day she received 800 cGys of irradiation targeted on the pericapsular hip

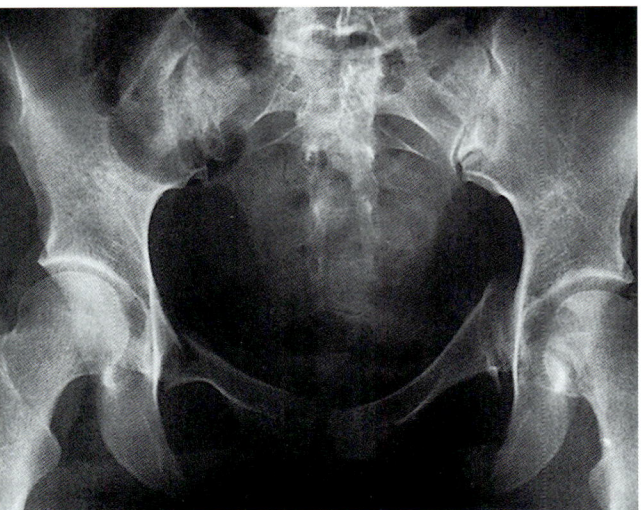 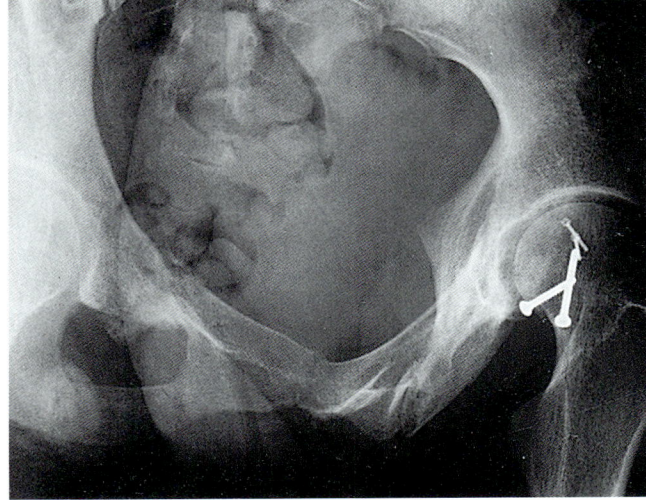

Figure 9. (A) A 28-year-old female was injured in an automobile accident. She sustained pelvic ring fractures and a left femoral head fracture. (B) Small-diameter screws were used to stabilize the fragments. The miniature screws were countersunk beneath the articular cartilage. (figure continues)

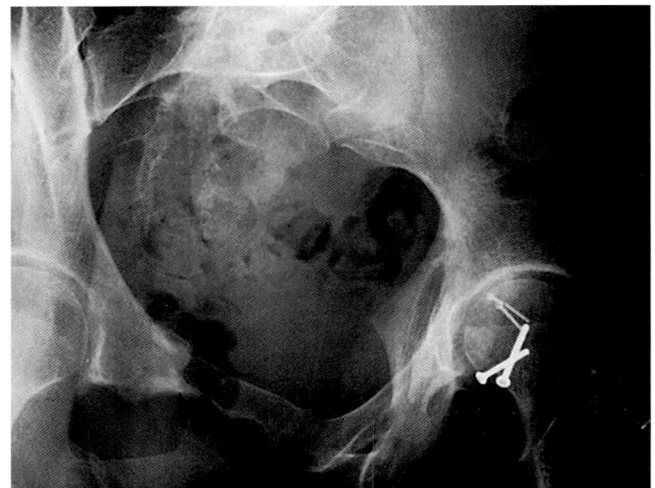
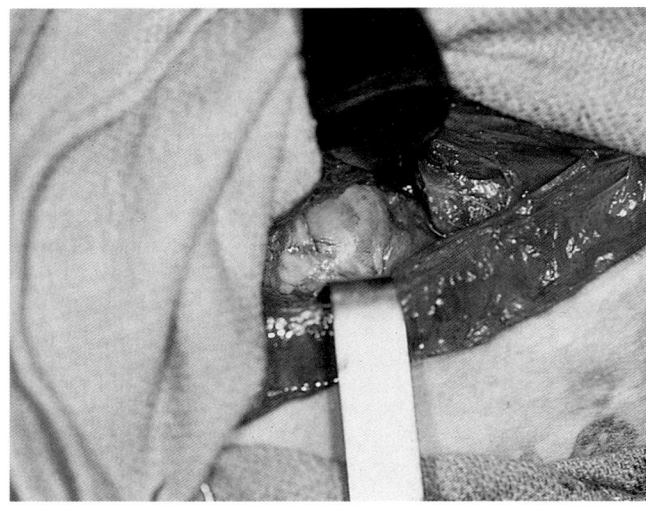

Figure 9. (continued) (C) She returned eight months after surgery complaining of left groin pain, and radiographs revealed a broken miniature screw. (D) At the time of broken screw removal, the femoral head fractures had healed and the cartilage surfaces were visibly smooth.

abductors. Because of the pelvic ring fractures, she was restricted to a chair for the first four weeks after surgery and then mobilized using crutches for an additional six weeks. She returned to work five months after injury to full duty. She returned eight months after surgery complaining of left groin pain. There were no constitutional symptoms. She used a single crutch to diminish her hip pain when walking. Her left hip was irritable to examination, with diminished active and passive motion. There was no swelling. Plain radiographs revealed a broken miniature screw. The screwhead and proximal portion were displaced into the fossa acetabuli. She underwent repeat joint exploration using the previous surgical wound and the broken screw fragment was removed without problems. The femoral head fractures had healed and the cartilage surfaces were visibly smooth. She returned to work six weeks later and remains asymptomatic.

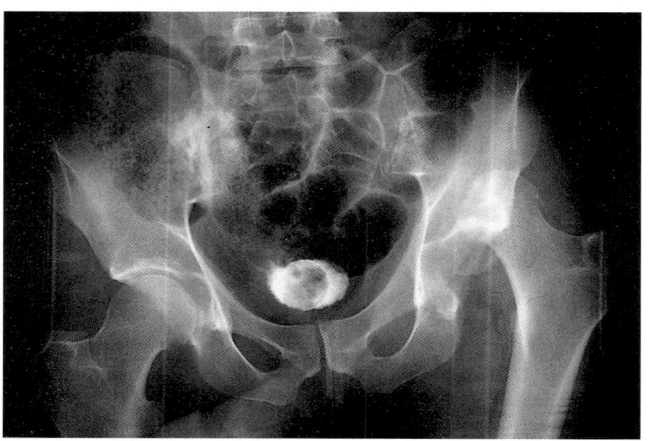
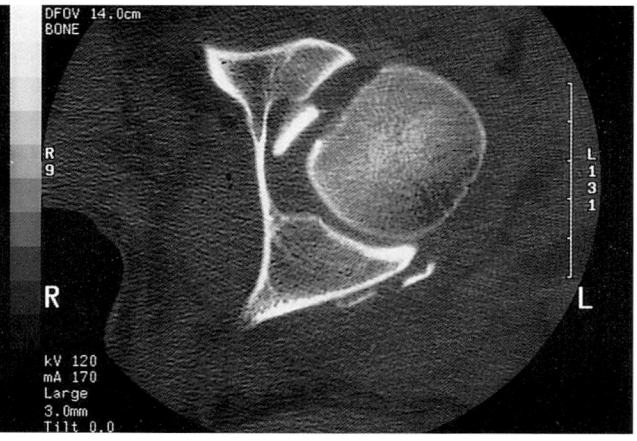

Figure 10. (A) This patient was injured in an automobile accident. An AP pelvis radiograph identified the femoral head fracture in association with a posterior hip dislocation and small posterior wall acetabular fracture (Pipkin type IV). A closed reduction was performed atraumatically and emergently using intravenous sedation. (B) A CT scan delineated the anterior femoral head fracture, intraarticular loose osteochondral fragments, and the small posterior wall acetabular avulsion fracture. The femoral head fracture fragment was displaced caudally onto the anterior femoral neck. (figure continues)

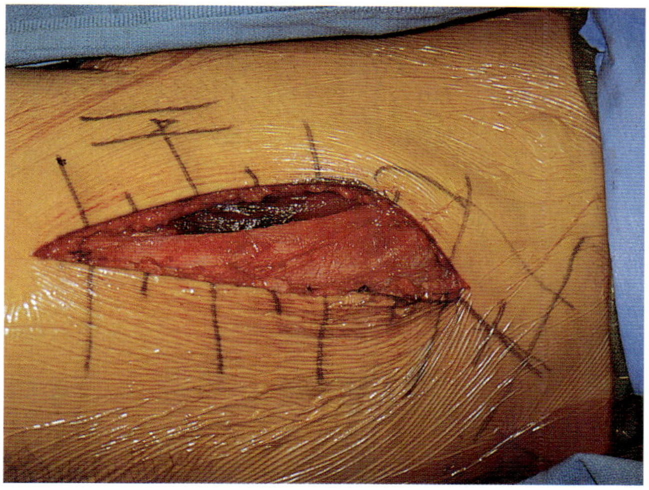

Figure 10. *(continued)* (C) This intraoperative photograph demonstrates the surgical exposure. The patient was in the supine position with his head to the reader's right and his feet to the left. The incision paralleled only the anterior portion of the iliac crest and then curved distally at the level of the ASIS. (D) The interval between the sartorius and tensor muscles was divided and retraction revealed the conjoined tendon of the rectus femoris deep within the wound. Subperiosteal elevation of the tensor muscle and hip abductors from the ilium was not necessary in this thin patient. (E) The conjoined tendon was incised and tagged for later repair. (F) The rectus femoris muscle was distally retracted. A "T-shaped" capsulotomy was carefully made to avoid femoral head direct injury. Capsular retraction improved visualization of the femoral head fracture fragment. (G) External rotation of the hip combined with distal longitudinal manual traction allowed the fracture fragment to be fully seen within the wound. *(figure continues)*

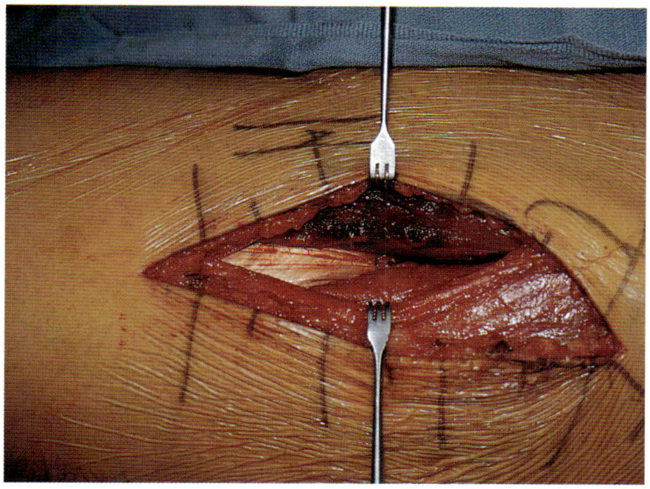

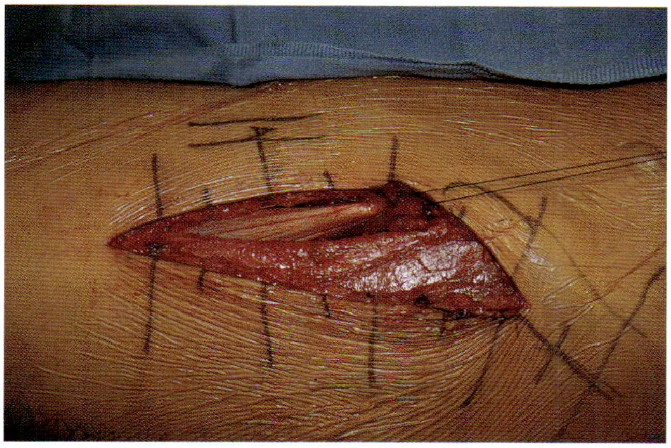

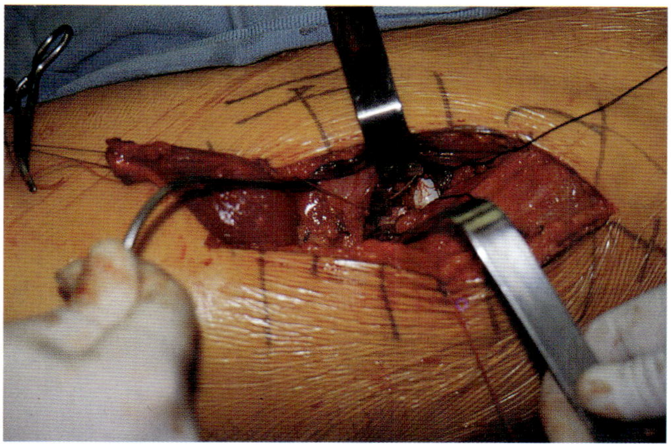

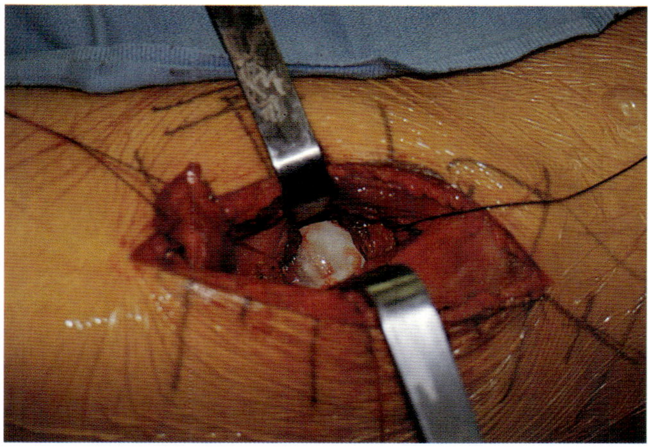

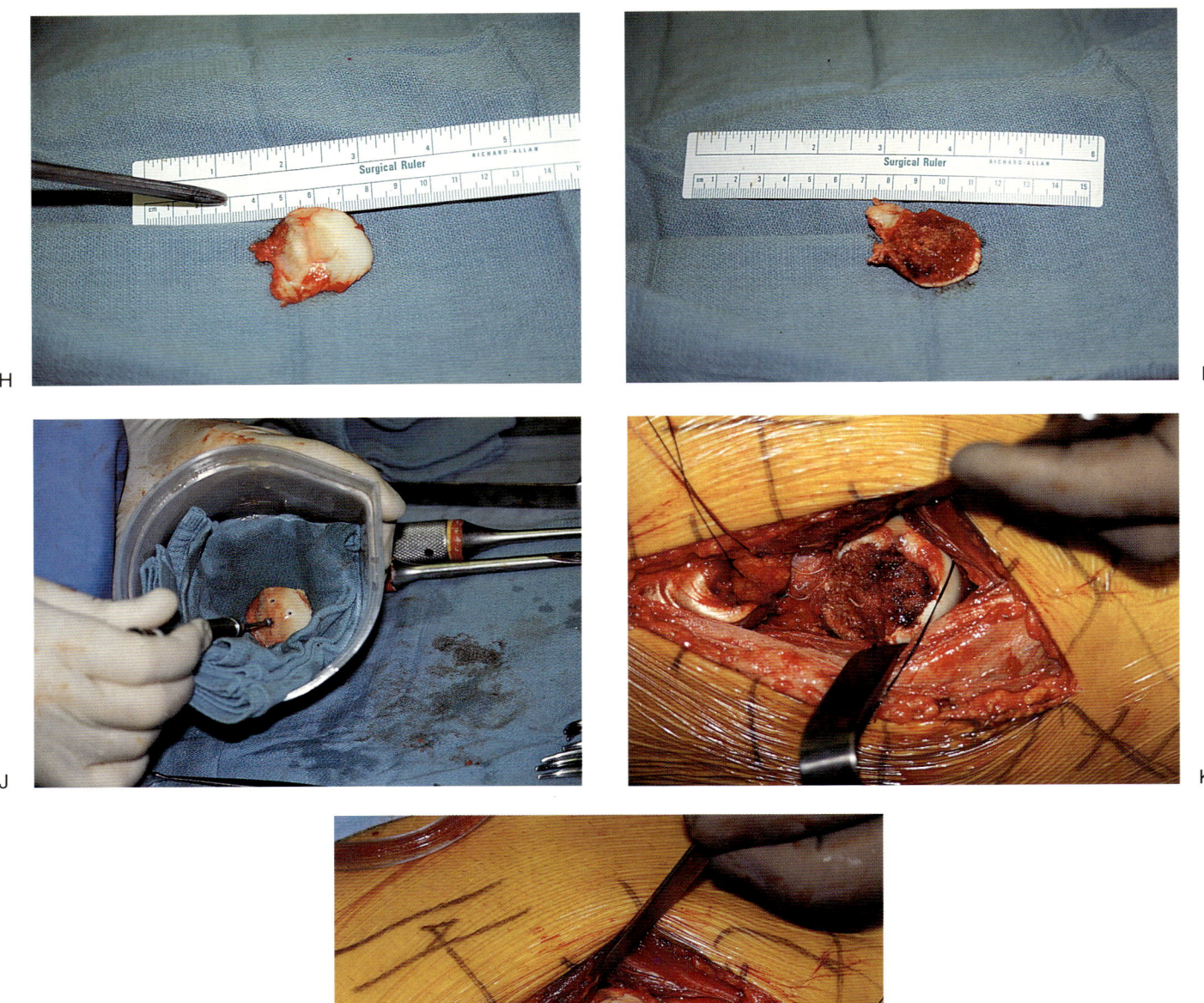

Figure 10. *(continued)* (H,I) The articular and cancellous surfaces of the fracture fragment are demonstrated. (J) The femoral head fracture fragment was prepared for fixation in a moistened towel within a container. The cancellous surface was cleansed of clot and organizing callus. Glide holes were strategically drilled in the fracture fragment and then countersunk. (K) Loose debris was removed from the hip joint. Pharmacological relaxation, manual distraction, and headlamp illumination were helpful to assure a thorough debridement. The proximal femur was next delivered into the wound using hip external rotation and abduction. The fracture site was cleansed and the fracture fragment reduced anatomically. Peripheral comminution did not complicate the reduction. (L) Small diameter lag screw fixation was used for this patient. The screws were countersunk to the level of the subchondral bone beneath the articular cartilage. The hip was then reduced and a smooth and stable full range of motion assured. The wound was irrigated and closed in layers over a drain. The rectus femoris tenotomy was repaired. Oral indomethacin caused gastrointestinal symptoms after one week and was discontinued. (figure continues)

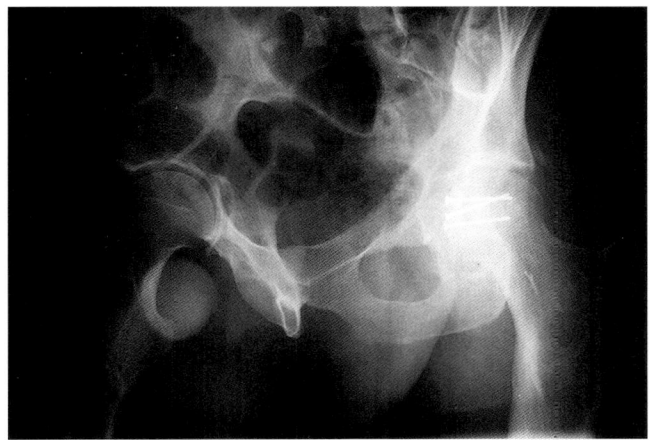 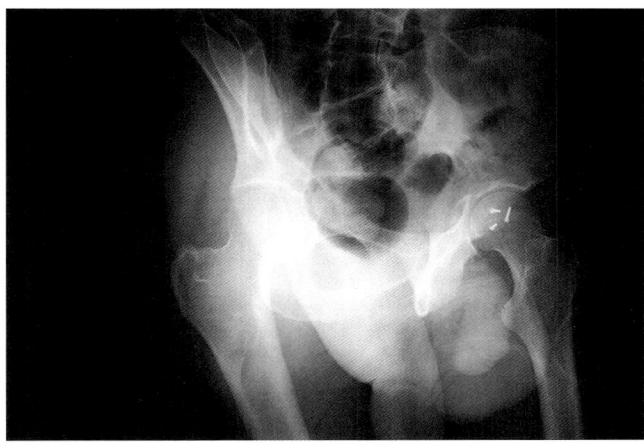

Figure 10. *(continued)* (M,N) Follow up Judet oblique radiographs confirmed healing and a spherical reduction.

RECOMMENDED READING

1. Brav, E. A.: Traumatic dislocation of the hip: Army experience and results over a twelve-year period. *J. Bone Joint Surg.* [Am], 44:1115, 1962.
2. Brumback, R. J., Kenzora, J. E., Levitt, L. E., Burgess, A. R., and Poka, A.: Fractures of the femoral head. In: *Proceedings of the 1986 Hip Society.* St. Louis, MO: CV Mosby, pp. 181–206, 1987.
3. Brumback, R. J., Holt, E. S., McBride, M. S., et al: Acetabular depression fracture accompanying posterior fracture-dislocation of the hip. *J. Orthop. Trauma,* 4:42, 1990.
4. Connolly, J. F.: Acetabular labrum entrapment associated with a femoral head fracture-dislocation. *J. Bone Joint Surg.,* 56A (8):1735, 1974.
5. DeLee, J. C., Evans, J. A., and Thomas, J.: Anterior dislocation of the hip and associated femoral head fractures. *J. Bone Joint Surg.* [Am], 62:960–964, 1980.
6. Epstein, H. C.: Traumatic dislocations of the hip. *Clin. Orthop.,* 92:116, 1973.
7. Epstein, H. C.: Posterior fracture dislocation of the hip: long term followup. *J. Bone Joint Surg.* [Am] 56:1103, 1974.
8. Epstein, H. C., Wiss, D. A., and Cozen, L.: Posterior fracture dislocation of the hip with fractures of the femoral head. *Clin. Orthop.,* 201:9–17, 1985.
9. Gross, A. E.: Reconstruction of the femur in revision arthroplasty of the hip. In: Galante, J. O., Rosenberg A. G., Callaghan, J. J. eds. *Total hip revision surgery.* New York: Raven Press, 1995.
10. Moed, B., and Maxey, J.: Evaluation of fractures of the femoral head using the CT-directed pelvic oblique radiograph. *J. Orthop. Trauma,* 7(2):189, 1993.
11. Pipkin, G.: Treatment of grade IV fracture dislocation of the hip. *J. Bone Joint Surg.* [Am], 39:1027–1041, 1957.
12. Roeder, L. F., and DeLee, J. C.: Femoral head fracture associated with posterior hip dislocations. *Clin. Orthop.,* 147:121–130, 1980.
13. Stewart, M. J., and Milford, L. W.: Fracture dislocation of the hip: An end result study. *J. Bone Joint Surg.* [Am], 36:315, 1954.
14. Swiontkowski, M. F., Thorpe, M., Seiler, J. G., and Hansen, S. T.: Operative management of displaced femoral head fractures: Case matched comparison of anterior versus posterior approaches for Pipkin I and Pipkin II fractures. *J. Orthop. Trauma,* 6(4):437–442, 1992.
15. Thompson, V. P., and Epstein, H. C.: Traumatic dislocation of the hip: A survey of 204 cases covering a period of 21 years. *J. Bone Joint Surg.* [Am], 33:746, 1951.
16. Trueta, J., Harrison, M. H. M.: The normal vascular anatomy of the femoral head in adult man. *J. Bone Joint Surg.* [Br], 35:442–461, 1953.
17. Watson-Jones, R.: *Fractures and joint injuries.* 5th ed. Churchill Livingstone, New York, 1976.

PART III

Alternatives to Total Hip Arthroplasty

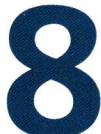

Reconstructive Osteotomies of the Pelvis for the Correction of Acetabular Dysplasia

Michael B. Millis

INDICATIONS/CONTRAINDICATIONS

Developmental dysplasia of the hip still represents the most common single etiology of osteoarthrosis of the hip (1,10). Arthroplasty offers a good solution for the painful arthritic hip in the older or inactive patient. Unfortunately, the dysplastic acetabulum, particularly if subluxation is present, will often deteriorate to painful, irreversible arthrosis as early as the end of the third decade of life, much too early for arthroplasty to be a satisfying choice. This poor natural history of uncorrected hip dysplasia is a strong argument for timely correction of the offending malalignment (6,7).

The predominant malalignment in residual hip dysplasia in the young adult patient is usually on the acetabular side. Unless ischemic necrosis from treatment in infancy has complicated the picture, excellent congruity and an excellent range of motion are often preserved at the time the patient first becomes symptomatic, (which can be as early as age 14 or 15, but may be as late as 25 or 30).

M. B. Millis, M.D.: Department of Orthopaedic Surgery, The Children's Hospital, Boston, Massachusetts 02115.

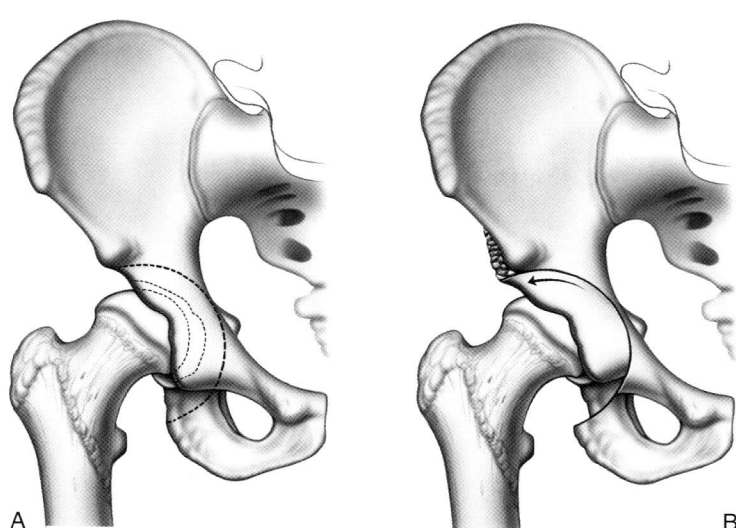

Figure 1 A, B. The spherical acetabular osteotomy employs spherical chisels to osteotomize the acetabulum at a distance of 15 to 20 mm from the articular surface. The blood supply to the isolated acetabular fragment comes from branches of the acetabular artery and from the intact hip joint capsule.

The two osteotomies to be discussed, the spherical acetabular osteotomy (SAO) (Fig. 1) (5,11,12,13) and the periacetabular osteotomy (PAO) (Fig. 2) (2), are powerful techniques for reorienting a dysplastic acetabulum that is functionally malaligned, yet has preserved a congruous relationship with the femoral head. It is assumed that the radiographic cartilage space is still reasonably wide, radiographic arthrosis is still slight or absent, and a good range of motion is preserved.

These osteotomies are therefore of reconstructive type (5,6,15), meaning that their primary indication is during the phase of hip disease before irreversible degenerative change has taken place. Specifically, these procedures are indicated in situations where the prognosis is poor without timely surgery, but can be greatly improved by the osteotomy. These procedures are not so clearly indicated for joints in which arthrosis is well established. Their best indication is in the relatively young patient, under age 30, in whom arthrosis is inevitable without the surgery. Wagner considers acetabular redirectional osteotomy relatively contraindicated in patients older than 25 to 30 years of age (17,18). Ganz et al. are operating on much older patients who otherwise have an indication for these procedures, but the long-term results in patients with this widened age indication are not yet known (2,16).

In general, spherical acetabular osteotomy or periacetabular osteotomy are indicated in mature patients with congruous acetabular dysplasia with lateral and anterior center-edge angles less than about +10 degrees. Patients with milder dysplasia can often be treated satisfactorily by simple innominate osteotomy.

Spherical acetabular osteotomy is contraindicated if the capsule must be opened, because the capsule carries a major portion of the blood supply to the osteotomized spherical acetabular fragment. Both osteotomies are contraindicated before closure of the triradiate cartilage because proximity of the osteotomies to this physis can cause premature closure.

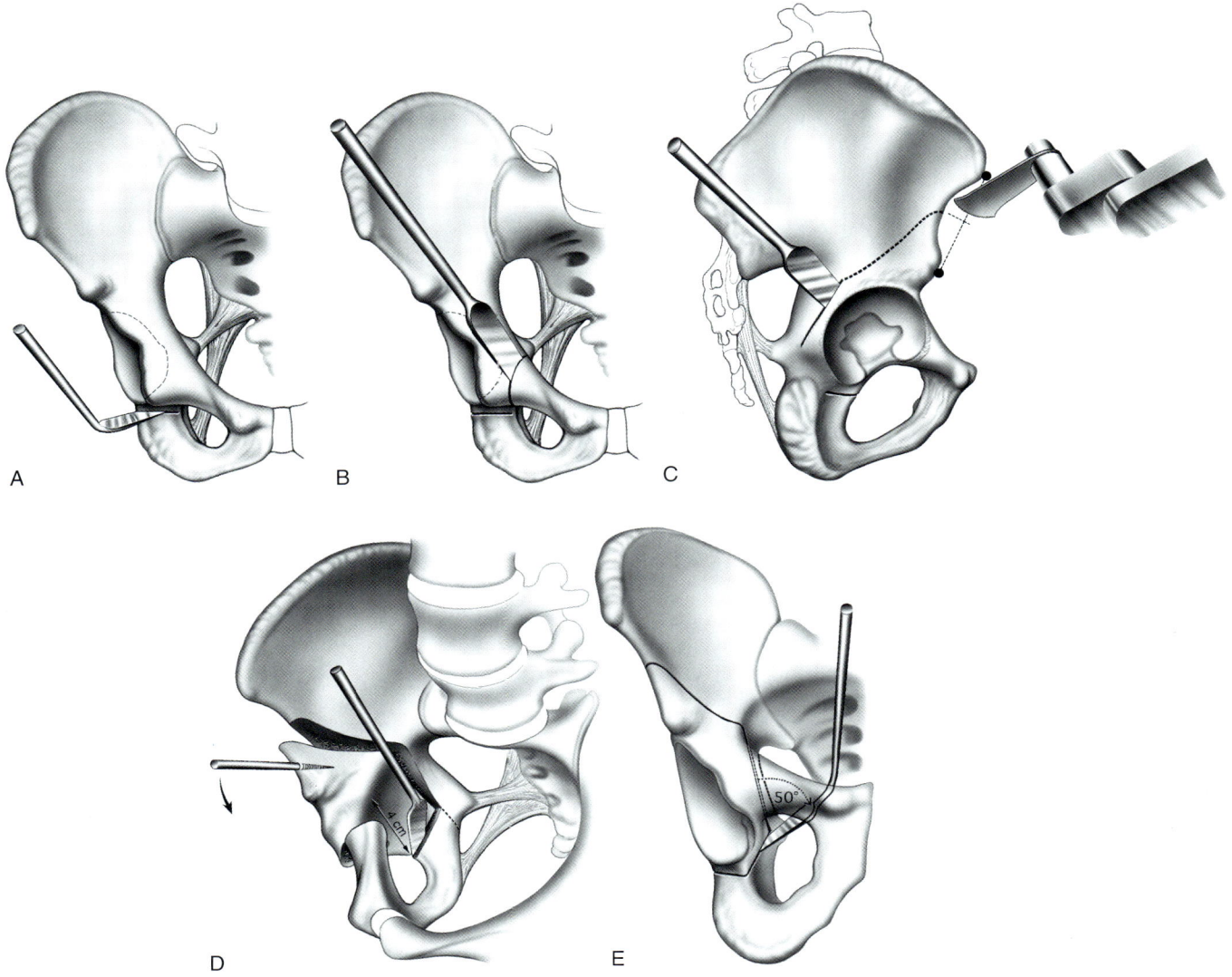

Figure 2 A, B, C, D, E. The Bernese periacetabular osteotomy was devised by Ganz et al. Reproduced with permission from Ganz, R. et al: A new periacetabular osteotomy for the treatment of hip dysplasias: Technique and preliminary results. *Clin. Orthop.* 232:26–36, 1988.

PREOPERATIVE PLANNING

Ian McNab's statement that "the incision is not as important as the decision" represents the first stage of preoperative planning, in which one must decide whether the patient, and his hip, qualify for this type of complex surgery, which is at least as much prophylactic as it is therapeutic. The patient must understand the philosophical basis as well as the mechanical basis for this surgery.

Assuming the patient is appropriate for acetabular redirection, with prearthrotic acetabular dysplasia, then a detailed analysis must take place before the surgery is performed. Specifically, one must first decide whether the patient is in the reconstructive category, meaning that the malalignment, and therefore the prognosis, can be normalized. One must evaluate the proximal femur and indeed the entire distal limb, to decide whether femoral realignment is indicated. While no amount of femoral realignment can compensate for an oblique acetabulum, leaving the proximal femur excessively anteverted or in valgus can compromise the result of an otherwise perfectly performed acetabular realigning procedure.

Evaluation of the dysplastic acetabulum itself should include the following plain radiographs: AP pelvis, AP hip in abduction, and faux profil view of each hip (Fig. 3). These studies allow one to characterize the amount of lateral and anterior deficiency on the acetabular side, and to confirm that no significant incongruity or hinge abduction is present. Remember that the lower limits of normal for the lateral center-edge angle of Wiberg is approximately 24 degrees in females and about 28 degrees in males, with the average center-edge angle being approximately 35 degrees. The anterior center-edge angle, as measured in the faux profil view, has a lower limit of normal of 20 degrees.

The plain radiographic views are usually supplemented in our institution by a three-dimensional CT scan, which can be used with appropriate software to simulate various amounts and directions of acetabular reorientation (3,8,9).

An important element in the analysis of the preoperative imaging studies is the determination of whether simple reorientation of the acetabulum is indicated or whether some degree of medialization is also required. At a relatively early stage, the dysplastic hip joint center may migrate laterally and anteriorly, with a resulting increase in unit load from the increased length of the body-weight lever arm.

Both the SAO and PAO allow virtually unlimited acetabular reorientation. The SAO can be modified through the use of a supplemental Chiari-like osteotomy cut to allow medialization (13). This medialization is accomplished only at the expense of some shortening, though. The PAO is easily modified to allow medialization, without modifying the procedure in any way other than sometimes requiring a supplemental small fragment reconstruction plate along the medial wall of the pelvis, in addition to the standard three screws (2).

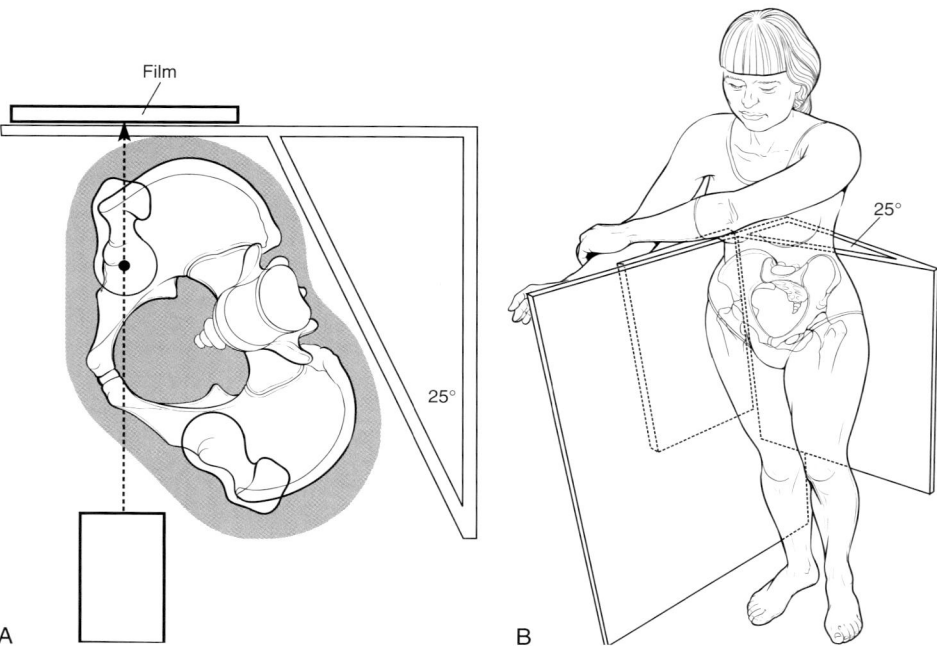

Figure 3 A, B. Diagram of the faux profil view of Lequesne and deSeze. A frame may be constructed to hold the patient in the desired standing position, with the pelvis rotated 25 degrees toward the beam from the straight lateral position. The patient stands with the right foot parallel to the plane of the film. The center of the cassette is behind the hip that is to be examined.

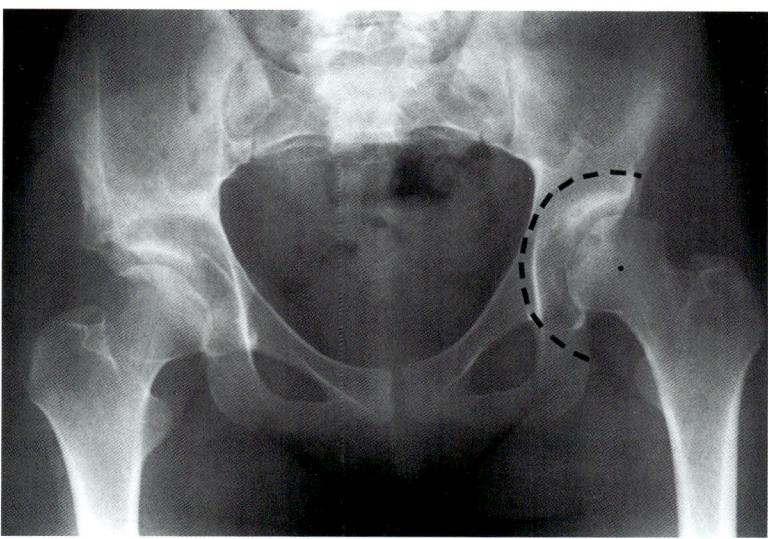

Figure 4. A surgical template similar to a Mose guide allowing for approximately 15% magnification on a standard AP pelvis film is used to outline a proposed spherical acetabular osteotomy of radius 40 mm, maintaining a distance of 15 to 20 mm between the proposed osteotomy line and the articular surface of the acetabulum. In the dysplastic acetabulum ideal for correction with spherical osteotomy, the articular surfaces of both femoral head and acetabulum are spherical, and the centers of rotation of both femoral head and acetabulum lie at the same point. The greater the deviations from ideality in these parameters, the greater the difficulties in both planning and technical execution of the osteotomy.

In general, we have employed spherical acetabular osteotomy in patients with dysplastic but spherical joints, who require acetabular reorientation without medialization. We have tended to employ the periacetabular osteotomy in patients whose joints are not so nearly spherical, whose arthrosis is more than minimal, or both, in whom some degree of medialization was felt to be indicated.

If SAO is chosen, the preoperative AP radiograph of the pelvis should be templated (Fig. 4). The spherical osteotomy is drawn, maintaining a distance of 15 to 20 mm from the joint surface. The radius of the ideal osteotomy is noted, as is the planned point of entry and angle of entry of the chisel on the lateral wall of the ilium. The available acetabular chisels (manufactured by Aesculap) have either a 40-mm or 50-mm radius of curvature, mandating a spherical osteotomy with these parameters (Fig. 5).

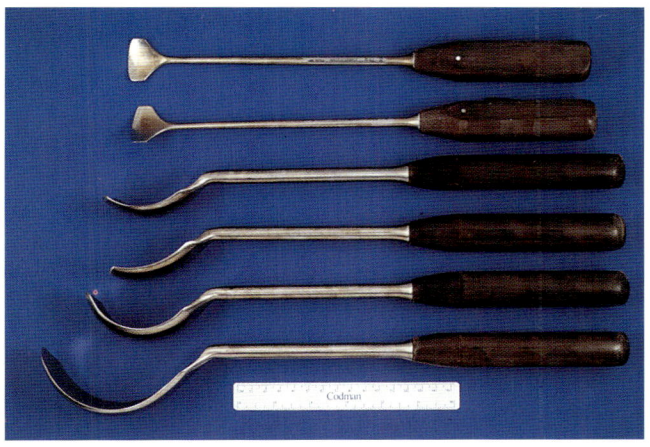

Figure 5. The spherical acetabular chisels employed in the Wagner modification of spherical osteotomy are manufactured by Aesculap and have either a 40-mm or 50-mm radius of curvature. Both a short and long blade are available in each radius of curvature. There is a special starting chisel corresponding to each radius of curvature.

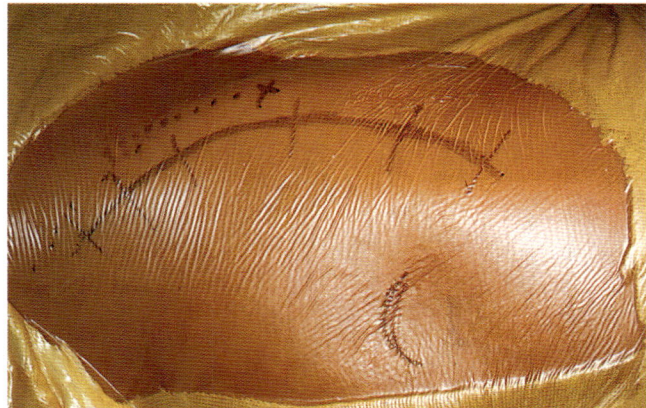

Figure 6. The skin incision for the anterior approach of Smith-Petersen (right hip) is convex anteriorly and located lateral to the iliac crest, with its central portion 2 to 3 mm lateral to the anterior superior spine. It is extensile and useful for either spherical acetabular osteotomy or periacetabular osteotomy.

SURGERY

Spherical Acetabular Osteotomy

The patient is positioned supine on a radiolucent table, elevated a few centimeters off the table by radiolucent padding. The operative extremity and flank are prepped and draped free. A plastic incisional Betadine-impregnated drape is employed.

Surgical Approach. The skin incision is semicircular, convex anteriorly, centered approximately 2 cm lateral to the anterior superior spine (Fig. 6). The deep approach is by the method of Smith-Petersen. The lateral femoral cutaneous nerve is carefully protected by entering the interval between sartorius and tensor within the fascial envelope of the tensor. This allows the tensor and the abductors to be reflected atraumatically off the lateral wall of the ilium posteriorly and proximally enough to allow a blunt Hohmann retractor to be placed in the sciatic notch as the leg is allowed to abduct slightly and extend to relax the sciatic nerve. This allows the outer wall of the pelvis to be exposed anterior to the sciatic notch and posterior to the capsule (Fig. 7).

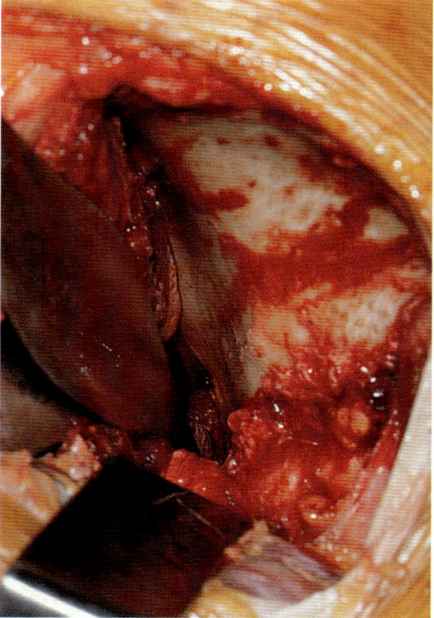

Figure 7. A careful atraumatic exposure of the lateral wall of the right ilium is achieved by gentle reflection of the abductors off the lateral aspect of the iliac crest, maintaining the leg in slight abduction and extension. Exposure of the posterior column of bone posterior to the hip joint capsule and anterior to the sciatic notch is both possible and desirable.

The medial portion of the exposure requires the hip to be flexed, as the sartorius and iliacus are reflected medially off the anterior portion of the medial wall of the ilium. The capsular iliacus is carefully dissected off the anterior capsule. The capsule should not be opened, since it carries the major blood supply to the osteotomized acetabulum. A subperiosteal dissection is carried out along the superior pubic ramus with a Cobb elevator, carefully protecting the iliopsoas and the femoral neurovascular structures with a blunt retractor. As the dissection is carried medially over to and beyond the iliopectineal eminence, a spiked Hohmann retractor is gently impacted into the superior pubic ramus. The placement of this retractor can be facilitated by making an initial hole medial to the iliopectineal eminence with a large, smooth Steinmann pin or a drill bit.

Using the spiked Hohmann as a retractor and keeping the hip flexed, the placement of a blunt Hohmann retractor into the supero-lateral corner of the obturator foramen is possible (Fig. 8). A second blunt Hohmann retractor is also placed more proximally, below the brim of the pelvis, to be placed within the sciatic notch medially.

With the lateral, posterior, and medial portions of the dissection thus accomplished, one can place the guide wire and carry out the osteotomy.

Next, a smooth Steinmann pin is drilled into the supraacetabular ilium approximately 20 mm above the joint line, as determined with the image intensifier (Fig. 9). The position of this Kirschner wire is adjusted as necessary, in accordance with the preoperative plan. Next, the Aesculap starting chisels are employed to mark the outline of the osteotomy on the outer surface of the ilium, beginning just above the anterior inferior spine and working posteriorly. The osteotomy should remain the same distance from the capsule at each point. Straight or curved osteotomes may be employed to deepen the outline of the osteotomy on the lateral iliac cortex.

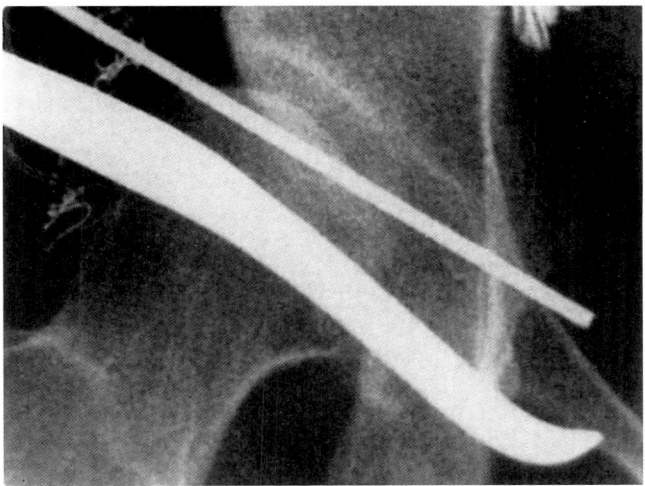

Figure 8. To confirm that the medial dissection is extensive enough, the extent of the subperiosteal exposure of the superior pubic ramus should be marked with a Kirschner wire and the image intensifier employed to confirm that the Kirschner wire lies medial to the radiographic tear drop. A blunt Hohmann retractor placed in the superolateral corner of the obturator foramen facilitates the medial exposure.

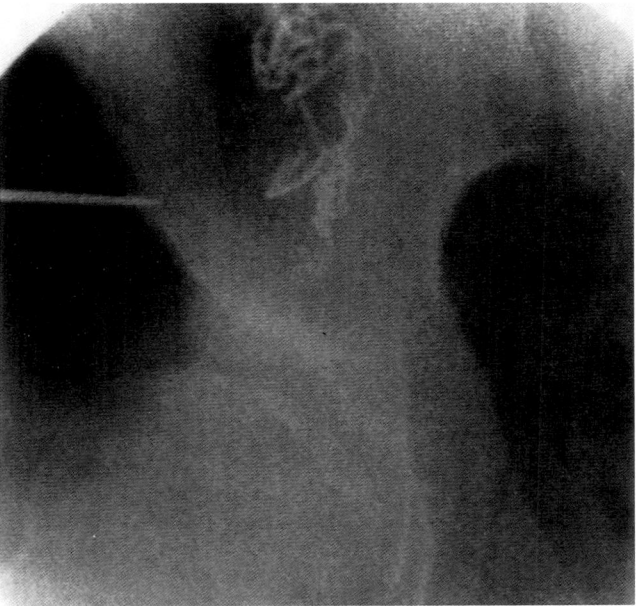

Figure 9. A guide wire is placed into the lateral iliac cortex approximately 20 mm directly proximal to the joint surface. The level and attitude of this guide wire should allow a perfect placement of the osteotomy outline on the lateral iliac cortex.

The appropriate-sized spherical acetabular chisel is then selected, and the acetabular osteotomy itself is begun. The one-third spherical gouge is employed first, with the cut beginning from lateral to medial, then from anterolateral to posteromedial, and from anterior to posterior. As the osteotomy is begun in each direction, the image intensifier is positioned so that the beam travels perpendicular to the direction of the cut, so that the attitude of the cut may be precisely controlled (Fig. 10 A, B).

In all but the most thick pelvis, it is necessary for the acetabular chisel to exit the medial wall of the ilium before reentering the pelvis just medial to the iliopectineal eminence as the chisel travels from lateral to medial. Careful protection of the psoas tendon and the femoral neurovascular structures is mandatory during this stage. Hip flexion and the use of the spiked Hohmann in the superior pubic ramus are important (Fig. 11 A, B).

The chisel blade must be visualized as it reenters the bone. It is prudent to notch the point at which the gouge will reenter the pelvis with a curved osteotome, as one becomes certain of the points at which the blade will reenter the pelvis.

If the attitude of the osteotomy has been appropriately controlled and small changes in direction of the chisel made as indicated, then the direction that the acetabular gouge takes after it reenters the pelvis will be appropriate. A distance of 15 to 20 mm is maintained between the spherical osteotomy and the joint surface.

It is usually necessary to replace the one-third spherical gouge with the hemispherical gouge (180 degrees curvature) to complete the last portion of the osteotomy far inferomedially. This portion of the osteotomy is not performed under direct vision, but the sound of the chisel as it is being impacted with the mallet gives one a good sense of when the last cortex is being encountered and cut.

Placing bone spreaders within the osteotomy cleft facilitates the completion of the last portions of the osteotomy.

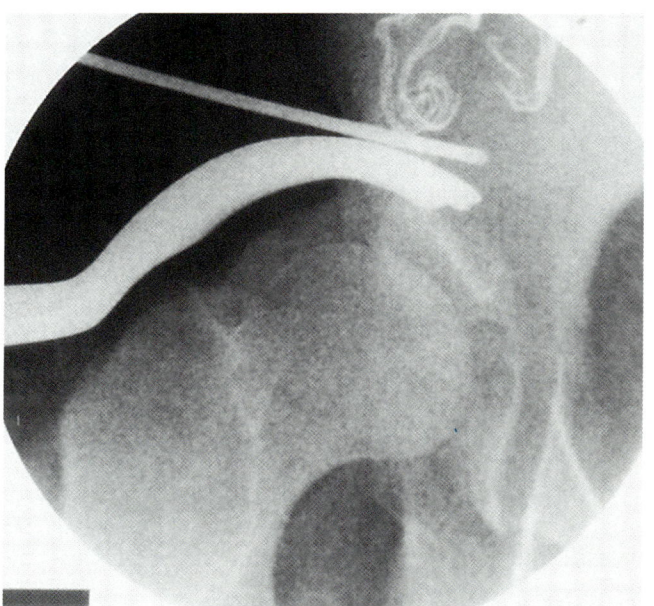
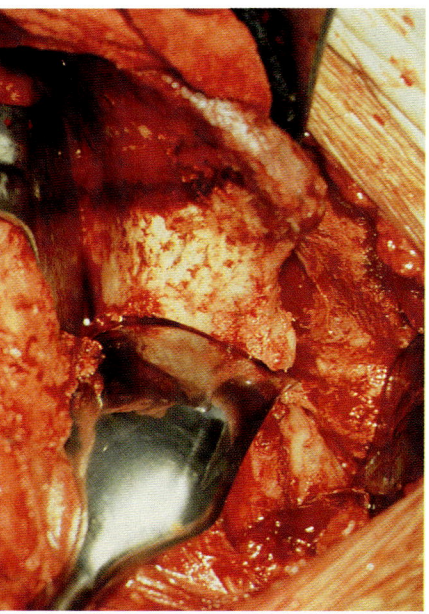

Figure 10. After the cortical osteotomy is made with the starting chisel, the appropriate spherical chisel is employed to deepen the cut for 1 to 2 cm. At this point, the image intensifier should be employed to confirm that the osteotomy lies at the appropriate level and is in the appropriate direction. (A) Radiographs showing initial portion of the osteotomy, beginning just below the guide wire. (B) Spherical chisel in situ, directed medially and slightly posteriorly.

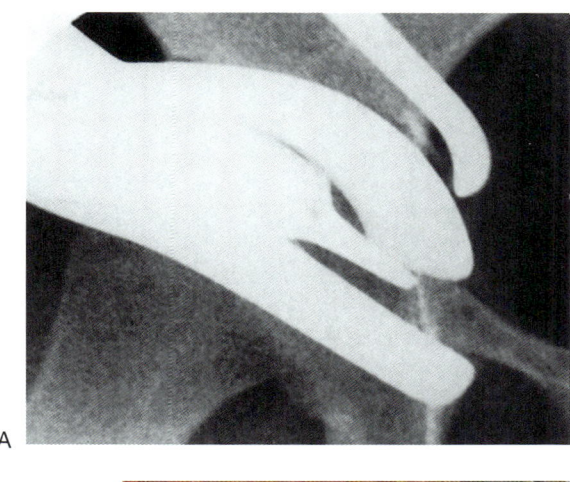
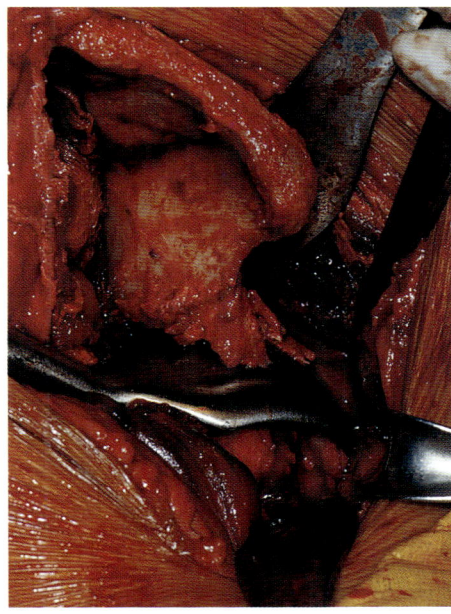

Figure 11. Reentry of spherical acetabular chisel into superior pubic ramus and medial ilium. (A) Radiograph illustrating appropriate direction of acetabular chisel toward tear drop. (B) Acetabular chisel *in situ* reentering superior pubic ramus more than 1 cm medial to iliopectineal eminence.

Displacement of the Osteotomy

The osteotomy is displaced by using bone spreaders within the osteotomy cleft and placing a rake or small Hibbs retractor on the anterolateral edge of the raw surface of the acetabular fragment. This is necessary to stretch the reflected capsular fibers that otherwise limit the amount of displacement. The fragment should, however, be relatively free to rotate at this point, and there should be no tendency to hinging. Any tendency for the fragment simply to hinge anterolaterally as it is pulled indicates that there is a small bridge of bone remaining uncut. If this is the case, the acetabular gouge should again be reinserted, carefully, into the osteotomy cleft and gentle tapping carried out with the mallet until the remaining bony bridge is divided.

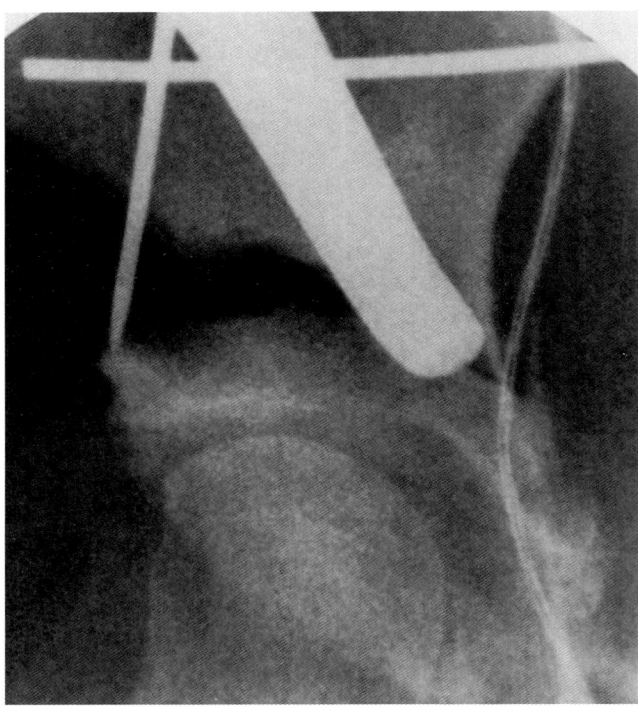

Figure 12. Provisional fixation of displaced acetabular osteotomy fragment transverse Kirschner wire above joint defines transverse plane of body.

A smooth Kirschner wire is then drilled from the iliac crest into the acetabular fragment for provisional fixation. A straight Kirschner wire is then placed across the front of the pelvis, held by a steri-strip to each anterior superior spine to give radiographic reference to the transverse plane of the pelvis. One can then use the image intensifier or a plain AP radiograph of the pelvis, to determine the coverage that has been achieved (Fig. 12). An oblique view can be also be taken with the image intensifier to simulate the faux profil view. The sourcil should lie transversely. The center-edge angle should be normal, greater than 25 degrees.

Fixation of the Osteotomy

After appropriate acetabular realignment has been confirmed, definitive fixation is carried out. The standard fixation is two modified, large-fragment, AO pronged semitubular plates with the prongs impacted into the free surface of the acetabular fragment, and two bicortical screws in each plate holding the implant to the outer wall of the ilium (Fig. 13A and B). These implants will provide satisfactory internal fixation once the abductor muscles have been reconstructed over the iliac crest and muscle tone returns to the patient. An additional oblique screw or Steinmann pin may be employed if needed. Any spaces in the osteotomy cleft are then packed with bone graft taken from the medial wall of the ilium.

Wound Closure. After copious irrigation of the wound, the iliacus and medial periosteum are reapproximated over the iliac crest to the abductor origin and lateral periosteum. Drill holes may be made through the iliac crest to supplement the abductor repair as required. Suction drains are placed, and the more superficial tissues are closed routinely. Bulky sterile dressings are applied, following which an Ace spica bandage is applied. The patient is transferred to bed and is placed on a small pillow to maintain slight flexion of the hip and knee and further lateral rolls are placed to prevent external rotation of the hip in the

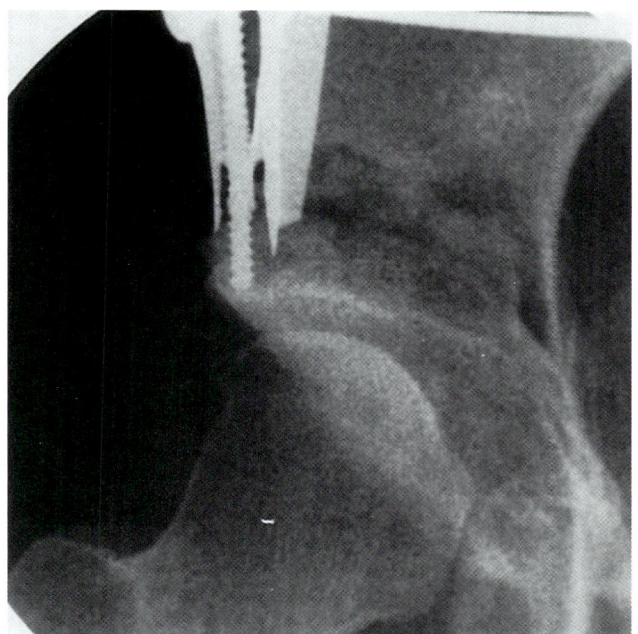 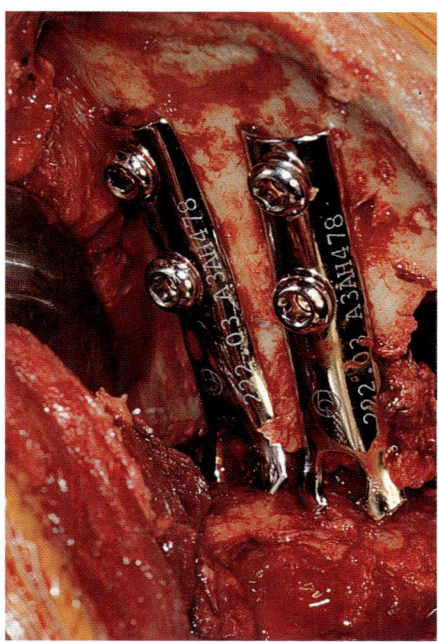

Figure 13. Definitive fixation of osteotomy with two pronged modified three-hole one-third tubular AO plates and screws. Sharp prongs impacted into cancellous surface of acetabular fragment. (A) Radiograph showing definitive fixation. Transverse wire above joint defines horizontal axis. (B) Definitive fixation.

early postoperative period. No longitudinal traction is applied, to minimize the risk of displacement of the osteotomy.

SURGERY TECHNIQUE

Periacetabular Osteotomy

The patient is positioned supine on a radiolucent table elevated a few centimeters off the table by radiolucent padding. The operative extremity and flank are prepped and draped free. A plastic incisional Betadine-impregnated drape is employed. The incision is identical to that in the basic anterior approach. As an alternative, the ilioinguinal approach may be employed (4,6,7).

Certain modifications may be employed in the anterior approach itself, specifically osteotomizing a small flake of bone off the anterior superior spine to carry the sartorius and anterior iliacus medially. A small flake of bone may also be reflected off the lateral portion of the anterior superior spine to reflect the tensor and anterior portion of the abductors laterally and posteriorly. These small osteotomies may facilitate postoperative healing and recovery of muscle function (see Addendum at the end of this chapter).

The medial portion of the exposure for the periacetabular osteotomy is almost identical to that carried out by Wagner for the spherical acetabular osteotomy, including exposure of the superior pubic ramus to and beyond the iliopectineal eminence, facilitated by placing a spiked Hohmann retractor into the superior pubic ramus. The medial and lateral walls of the ilium are cleared subperiosteally as in the usual anterior approach.

Anteriorly and distally, it is necessary to dissect into the interval between the psoas tendon and the capsule, distal to the rim of the pelvis. Placing a long-handled scissors into this gap allows one to palpate the ischium with the tip of the scissors at the level of the so-called

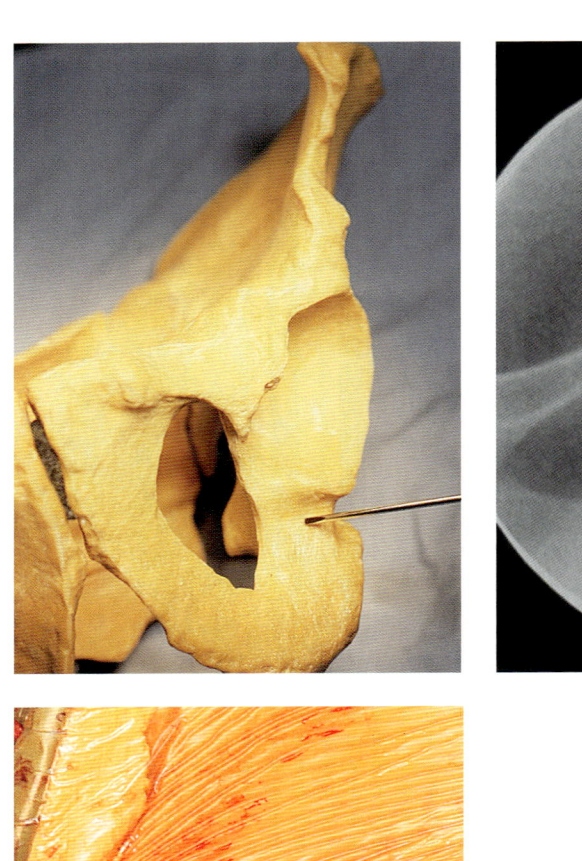
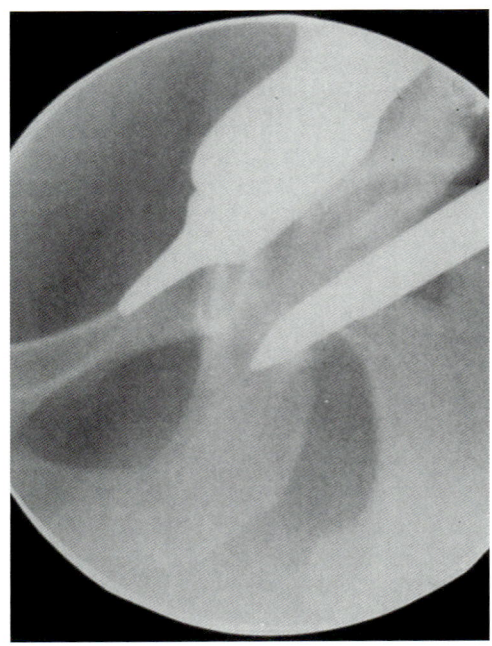
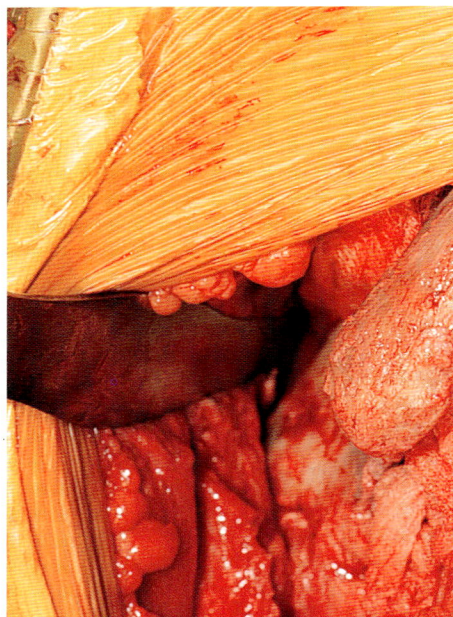

Figure 14. Medial dissection must enter interval between psoas tendon and medial capsule, extending down to the infracotyloid groove of the ischium directly below the hip joint capsule. (A) Level of infracotyloid groove demonstrated by tip of Kirschner wire on skeleton. (B) Tip of long-handled scissors lies on infracotyloid groove, as confirmed by image intensifier. (C) Scissors lying in interval between medial capsule and psoas tendon. Anterior superior spine is top center in photograph showing this anterior view of left hip. Handle of scissors is out of picture to left. Richardson retractor is just distal to scissors.

infracotyloid groove. One can use the edge of the scissors to feel the lateral edge of the obturator foramen medially. The image intensifier can be used to confirm the location of the tip of the scissors (Figs. 14 A to C). This point is well distal to the obturator nerve, which lies superiorly in the obturator foramen.

Sequence of the Osteotomies. The osteotomies are facilitated by the use of special osteotomes manufactured by Synthes, which are angled 30 degrees at a point four cm from the tip of the osteotome. The osteotomes come in two widths, 15 and 20 mm (Fig. 15).

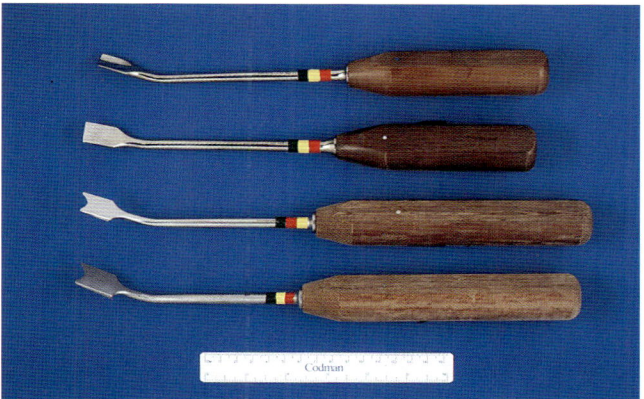

Figure 15. Special osteotomes useful for performing Bernese periacetabular osteotomy. The two lower osteotomes are angled 30 degrees at a point 4 cm from their tips. The notched heads are available in widths of 15 or 20 mm, (manufactured by Synthes). The two upper gauges have slightly different shaped heads and curved shafts (manufactured by Aesculap).

The first portion of the osteotomy is a scoring of the body of the ischium in an anterior to posterior direction, performed at the level of the infracotyloid groove. To perform this osteotomy, the osteotome is carefully inserted into the interval between the capsule laterally and the psoas tendon medially until the tip of the osteotome comes in contact with the infracotyloid groove just below the acetabulum and just lateral to the obturator foramen. The position of the osteotome tip is confirmed using the image intensifier (Fig. 16 A, B). Next, the osteotome is impacted to a depth of at least 15 to 20 mm in a posterior direction, to cut through both the medial and lateral walls of the ischium.

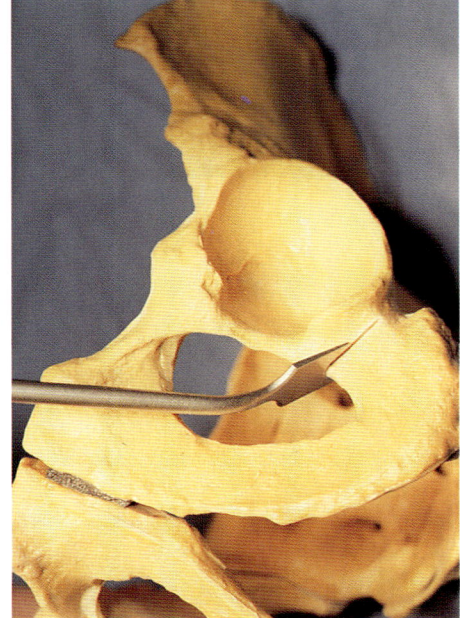
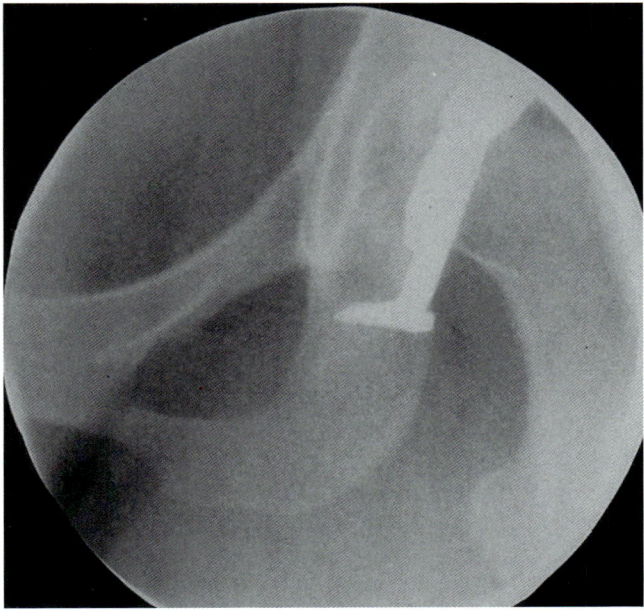

Figure 16. Osteotomy of infracotyloid groove. (A) Notched Synthes osteotome is placed at point on infracotyloid groove previously identified by tip of scissors. (B) Location and attitude of osteotome tip confirmed with image intensifier.

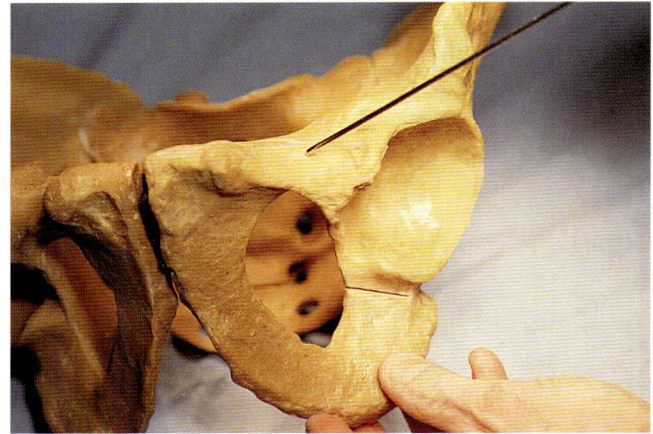
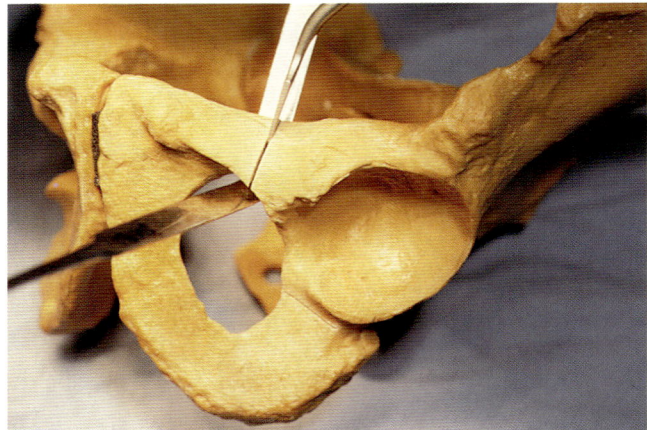
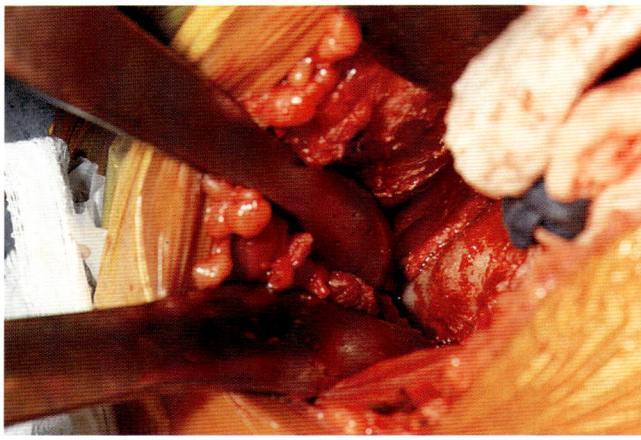
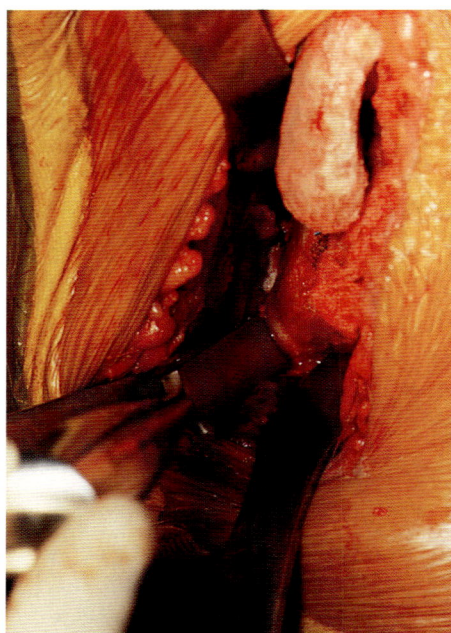

Figure 17. Osteotomy of superior pubic ramus. (A) Desired placement of superior pubic ramus osteotomy is depicted by tip of Kirschner wire lying at least 1 cm medial to iliopectineal eminence. This point lies medial to the radiographic tear drop and may be confirmed with the image intensifier. (B) Two Hohmann retractors are placed deep to superior pubic ramus to protect obturator nerve during osteotomy cut of superior pubic ramus. (C) Intraoperative photograph showing spiked Hohmann retractor impacted into left superior pubic ramus medial to superior pubic osteotomy with supplemental blunt Hohmann retractors meeting just under superior pubic ramus. (D) Osteotomy of superior pubic ramus with osteotome.

The second osteotomy is a complete cut through the superior pubic ramus (Figs. 17 A to D). This cut is made by flexing and adducting the hip and replacing the spiked Hohmann retractor into the superior pubic ramus at least 1 cm medial to the medialmost extent of the iliopectineal eminence. Two blunt Hohmann retractors are placed anteriorly and posteriorly just under the superior pubic ramus at the top of the obturator foramen to protect the obturator nerve. A straight, broad osteotome is positioned on the superior pubic ramus just lateral to the spiked Hohmann. The image intensifier confirms the location of the osteotome, before a complete osteotomy through the superior ramus is made. This osteotomy should be made at a point that is just medial to the teardrop, as seen in the AP projection on the image intensifier. The great tendency here is to make this cut too far lateral and to enter the joint medially. The cut *must* be made well medial to the iliopectineal eminence.

The third portion of the osteotomy is the supraacetabular portion, which is similar in direction to the anterior portion of the Salter innominate osteotomy, though more proximal (Fig. 18 A, B). The outline for this cut is made along the lateral cortex of the ilium, ap-

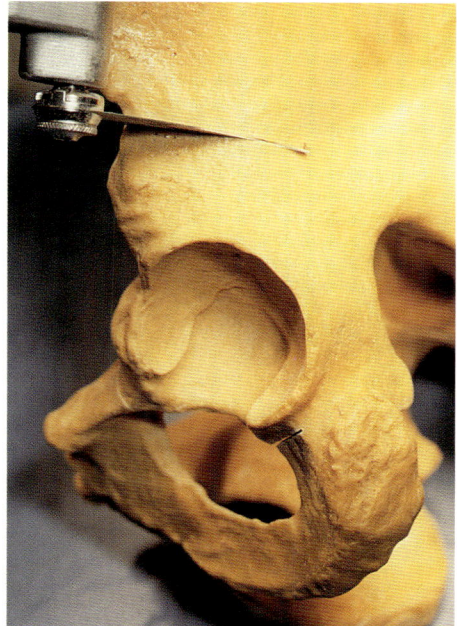 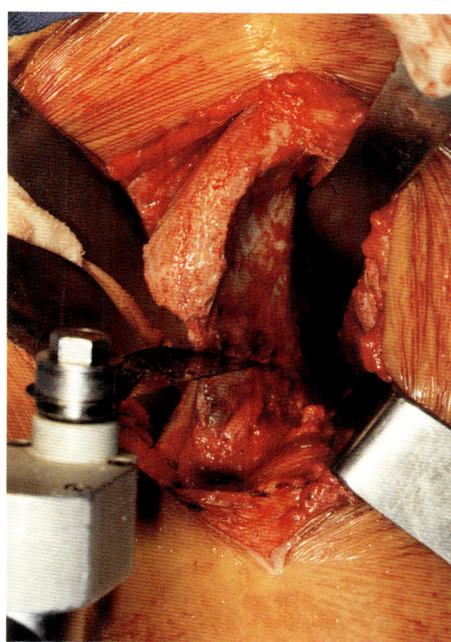

Figure 18. Osteotomy of ilium. (A) Oscillating saw cut begins halfway between anterior superior and anterior inferior spine, directed straight posteriorly, extending to a point just posterior to capsule. (B) Anterior view of left hip, showing oscillating saw making anterior-to-posterior iliac osteotomy.

proximately halfway between the anterior superior and anterior inferior spines, directed posteriorly toward a point just proximal to the most proximal extent of the sciatic notch. This cut is made to a depth approximately equal to that of a large saw blade on the oscillating AO saw. The soft tissues are carefully protected medially and laterally while this cut is made.

Next, a single Schanz screw is inserted from anterior to posterior, beginning anteriorly at a point just proximal to the anterior inferior spine but just distal to the anterior osteotomy (Fig. 19).

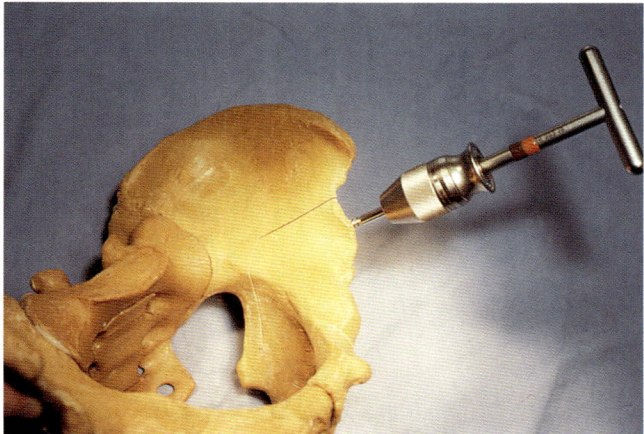

Figure 19. Placement of Schanz screw parallel to iliac osteotomy and just inferior to it.

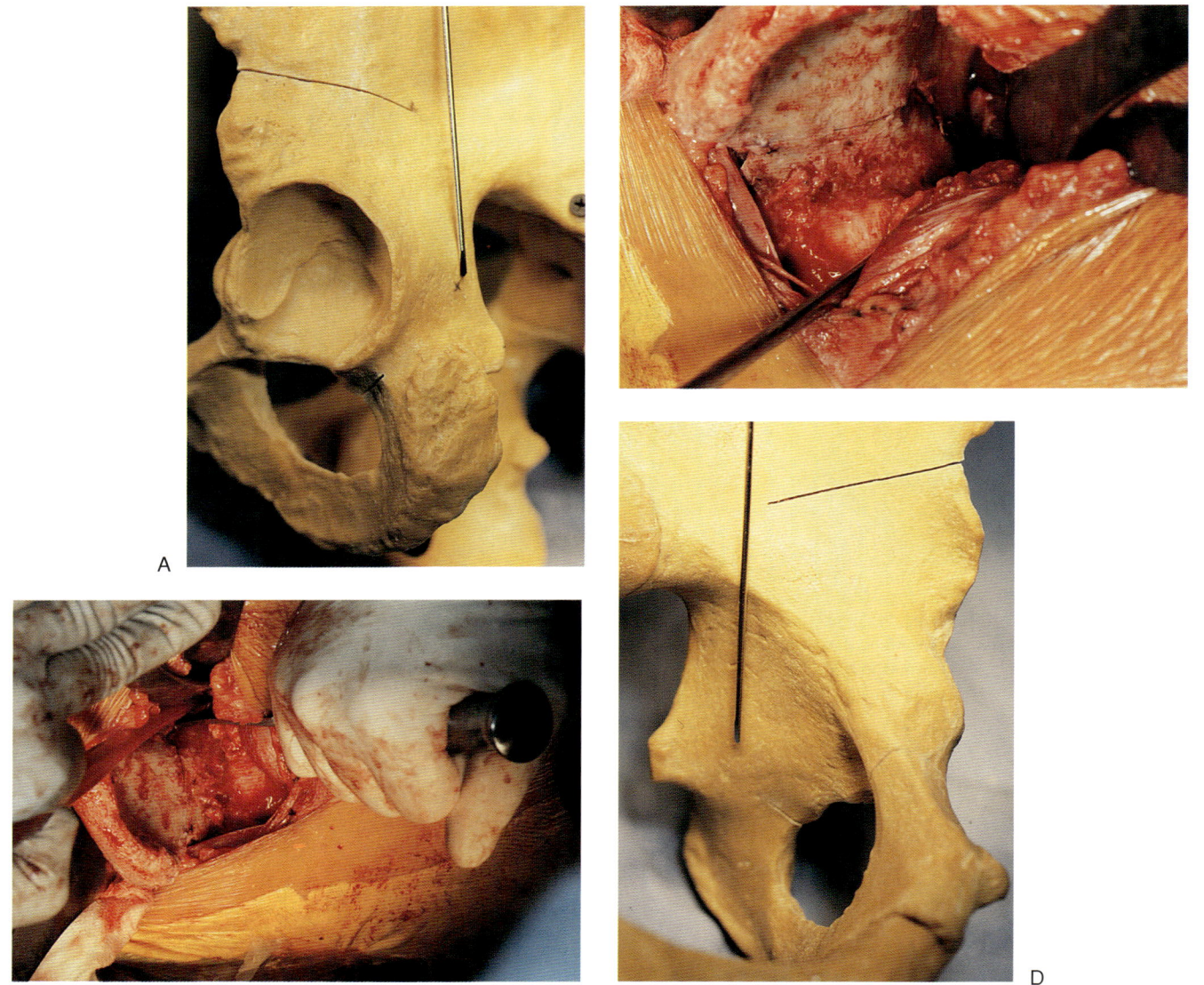

Figure 20. Posterior leg of osteotomy. (A) Smooth Kirschner wire illustrate direction of posterior leg of osteotomy, at an angle of approximately 110 degrees to first leg and parallel to the anterior edge of sciatic notch. The osteotomy lies along a line approximately halfway between the posterior capsule and the sciatic notch. (B) Curved osteotome beginning posterior leg of osteotomy along lateral iliac cortex. Anterior superior spine lies in top center of photograph. Patient's head is to the right of photograph. (C) The extent of the posterior leg of osteotomy may be seen on lateral cortex, directed parallel to anterior aspect of sciatic notch. (D) Smooth Kirschner wire illustrates direction and placement of medial aspect of posterior limb of osteotomy, extending over the pelvic rim to a point 4 cm below it. *(Figure continues on next page)*

The posterior leg of the osteotomy (Fig. 20) is made at an angle of 110 to 120 degrees with the anterior leg and is marked along both the medial and lateral walls of the ilium with an osteotome. This portion of the osteotomy parallels the anterior edge of the sciatic notch and lies half way between the sciatic notch and the posterior capsule. The initial 15 to 20 mm of this posterior leg are completed by deepening the osteotome cut from lateral to medial and from medial to lateral until they join.

8 RECONSTRUCTIVE OSTEOTOMIES OF THE PELVIS

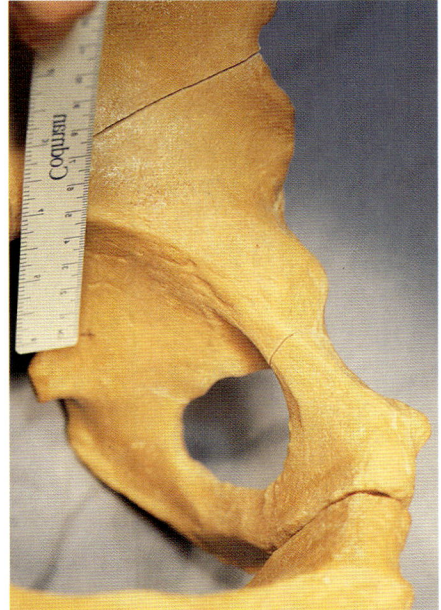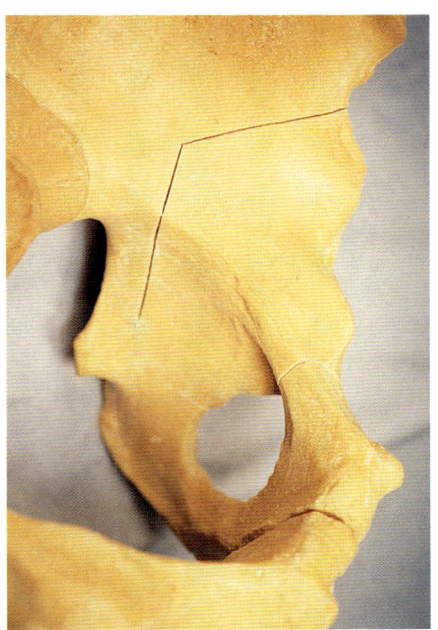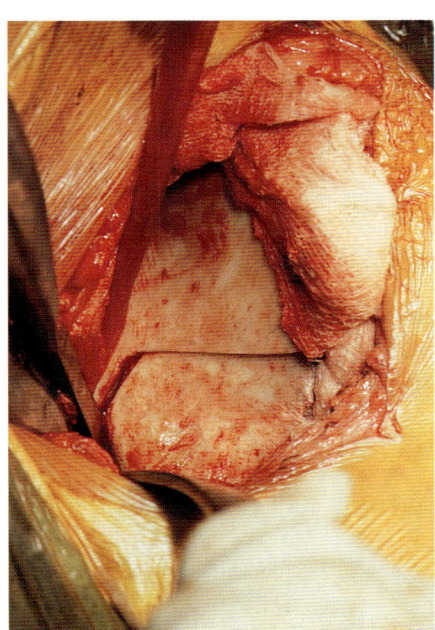

E,F G

Figure 20. *(continued).* (E) Distal extent of medial aspect of posterior leg of osteotomy should lie at least 4 cm below pelvic brim. (F) Completed posterior limb of osteotomy from medial aspect. (G) Intraoperative photo of posterior limb and posterior corner of osteotomy from medial aspect.

Next, bone spreaders are placed in the posterior portion of the anterior osteotomy from both lateral and medial (Fig. 21). At this point, it can be demonstrated that the periacetabular fragment is nearly free. This further freeing up occurs as the posterior leg of the osteotomy propagates down toward the ischial spine. (This is dotted line in Fig. 1C.)

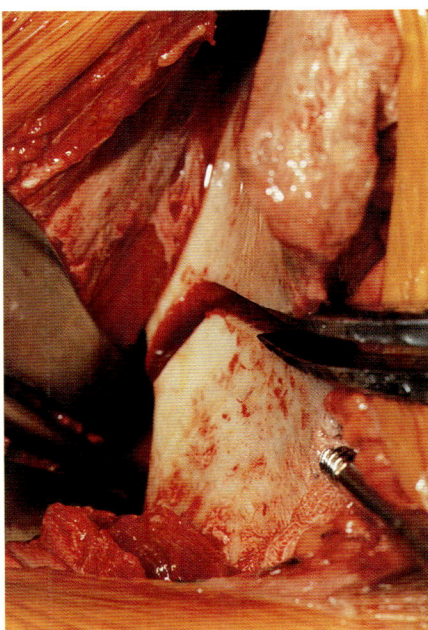

Figure 21. Initial distraction of posterior portion of osteotomy with bone spreader. Anterior superior iliac spine is at top right. Schanz screw entering anterior inferior iliac spine is at lower right.

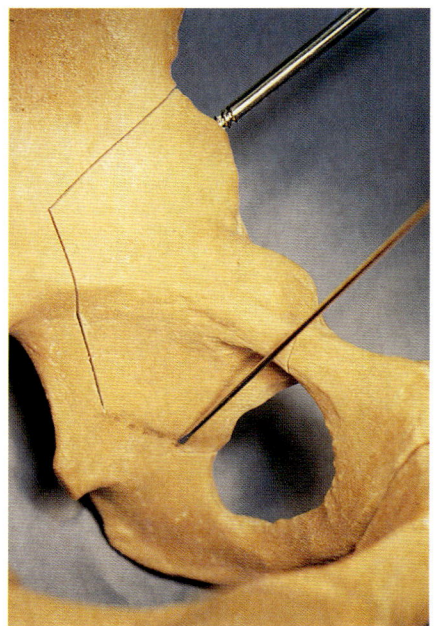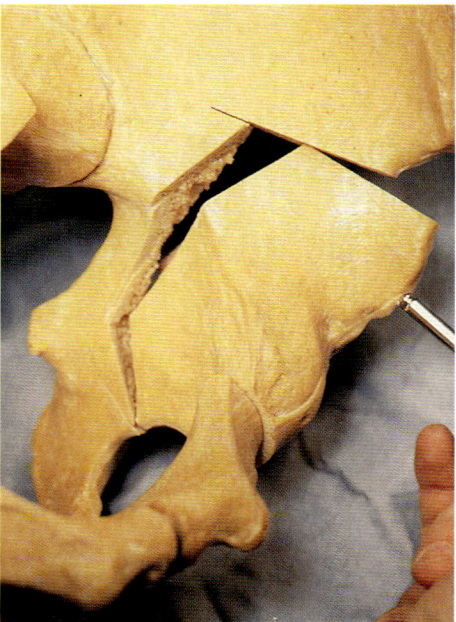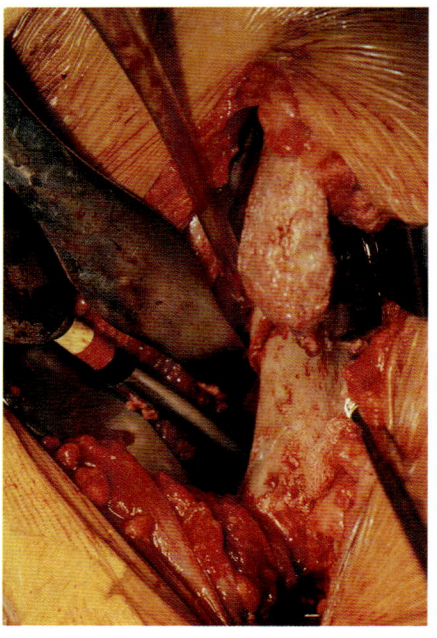

Figure 22. Delineation of medial osteotomy. (A) Tip of Kirschner wire marks level of medial osteotomy, four centimeters below brim of pelvis and parallel to it. (B) Medial osteotomy performed with angled osteotome, with tip of angle about 50 degrees to medial cortex. Cut begins posteriorly at end of posterior leg of osteotomy and advances anteriorly toward obturator foramen. (C) Intraoperative photo of medial osteotomy in progress.

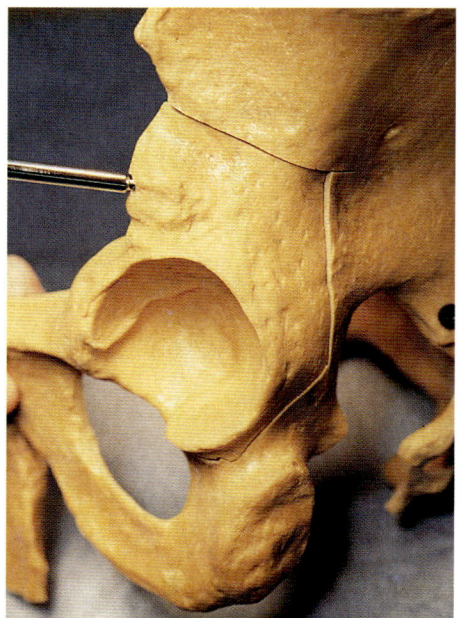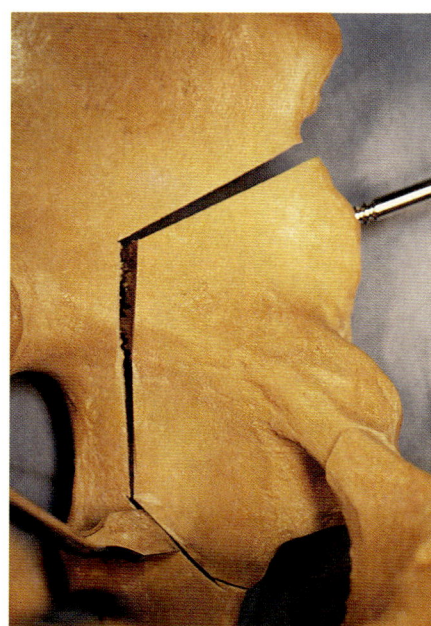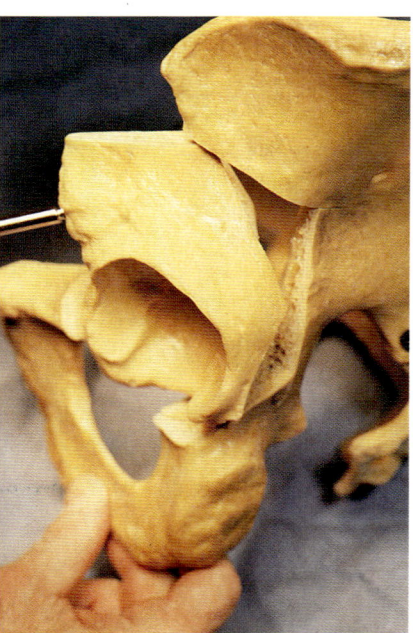

Figure 23. Completion of osteotomy. (A) Placement of anterior Schanz screw assists in completing osteotomy (lateral view). (B) Depressing Schanz screw in freeing up fragment (medial view). (C) Completion of osteotomy with anterior rotation (lateral view).

The last portion of the osteotomy is made with the angled chisel along the medial wall of the pelvis (Fig. 22 A, B, C). The hip is flexed and adducted, and blunt Hohmann retractors are placed deep medially, with one anteriorly placed into the medial lateral corner of the obturator foramen and the most posterior placed medially into the sciatic notch. The osteotome is applied 4 cm below the brim of the pelvis and oriented at 50 degrees to the quadrilateral plate of the pelvis. This last osteotomy is made beginning posteriorly at the deepest extent of the previously made posterior leg of the osteotomy and continuing anteriorly until the edge of the obturator foramen is reached. This osteotomy must be made at *least* 4 cm below the brim of the pelvis, and the angle of the chisel blade with the quadrilateral space must be no more than 50 degrees, or the hip joint may be entered.

As this last cut is completed, and the posterior bone spreaders are opened a bit, and the Schanz screw is levered in a distal direction, the previously incomplete osteotomy is completed, though certain soft-tissue attachments remain (Fig. 23 A, B, C).

Displacement of the Osteotomy

The anterior Schanz screw is used to reorient the acetabular fragment into any desired position. To assist in the displacement, a second, smaller Schanz screw may be inserted from lateral to medial into the posterior portion acetabular fragment behind the joint. A pelvic reduction clamp (Synthes) is also helpful in rotating the acetabulum. At this point, one can decide whether one wants simply to rotate the acetabulum in place over the femoral head, varying the amount of lateral rotation versus anterior rotation as desired; or one may medialize as desired, in which case, the axis of rotation of the osteotomy is at a point proximal to the osteotomy. As Ganz has pointed out, (Fig. 24) one should avoid having the axis of rotation of the osteotomy distal to the hip joint center, in which case one would be lateralizing the joint, which is biomechanically undesirable.

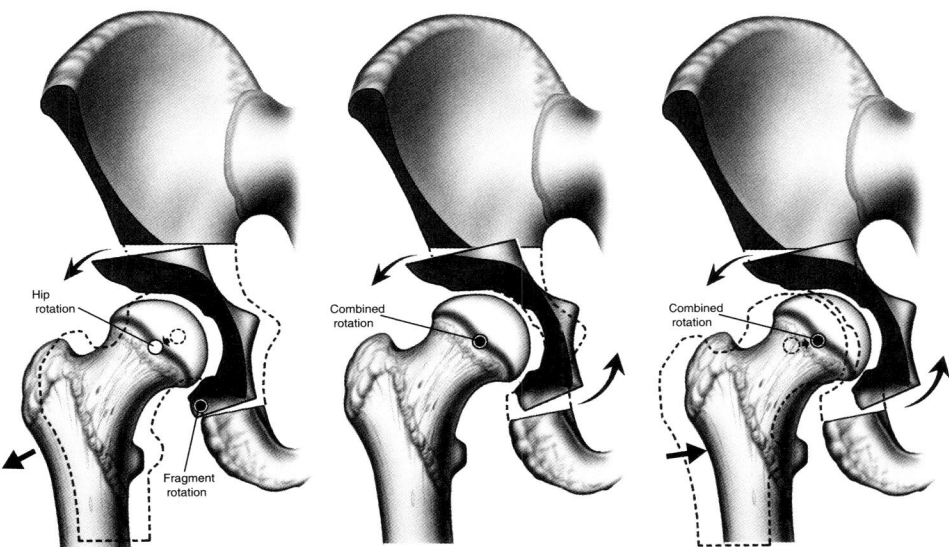

Figure 24. Diagram of right acetabular redirection. Effect of the location of the center of adduction-rotation on medial-lateral displacement of the acetabular fragment. Redrawn from a new periacetabular osteotomy for the treatment of hip dysplasia: Technique and preliminary results. *Clin. Orthop.*, 232:26–36, 1988). A distal center of rotation with a proximally easily visible correction results in biomechanically undesirable lateral displacement. If the fragment is rotated around the center of the head, there is neither medial nor lateral displacement. Proximal location of the center of rotation results in a medial displacement of the femoral head in a barely visible displacement of the supraacetabular osteotomy lines. The medial displacement may be beneficial and intentionally desirable intraoperatively.

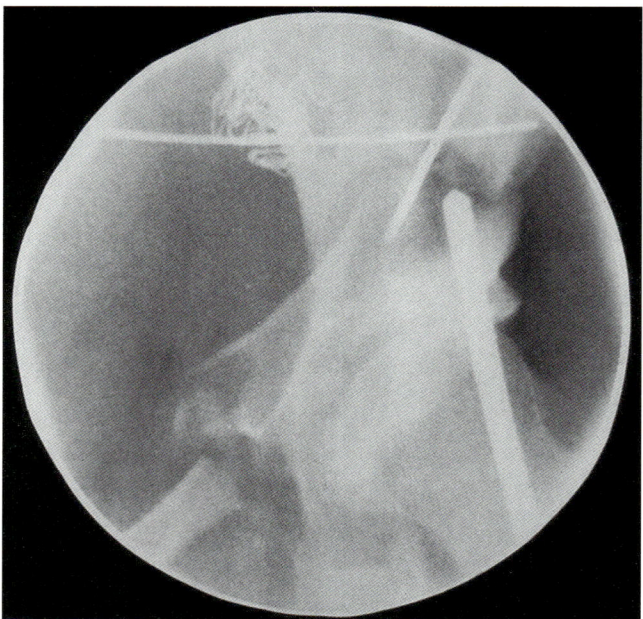

Figure 25. Image intensifier view of provisionally fixed osteotomy. Transverse Kirschner wire defines horizontal axis. A-P radiograph of pelvis offers even more security.

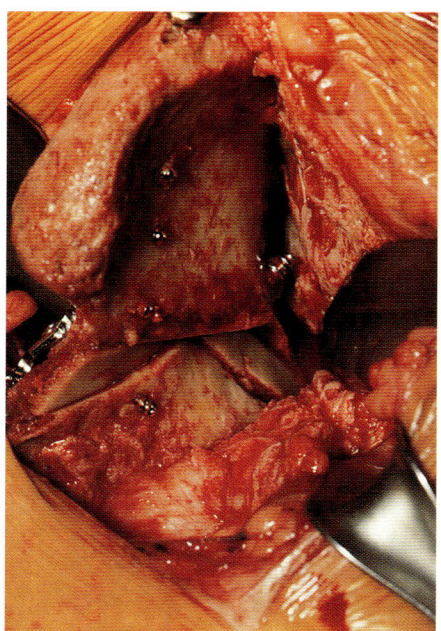
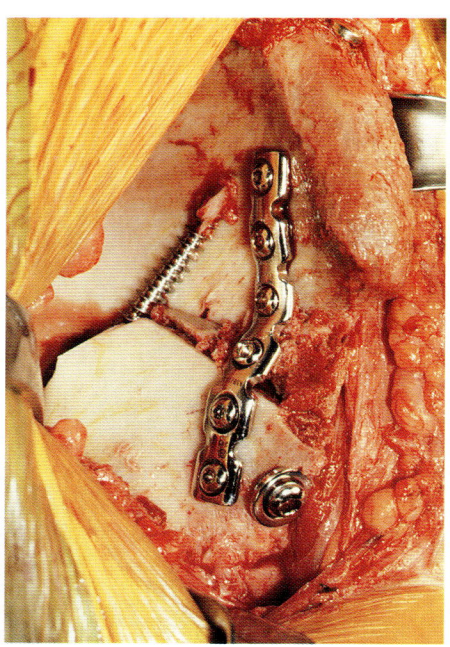

Figure 26. Definitive fixation. (A) Lateral view of left hip after final fixation. Interposition graft in anterior gap. Multiple cortical screws and reconstruction plate visible from antero-lateral aspect. (B) Medial aspect of osteotomy with definitive fixation. Well seen is anterior-to-posterior fully threaded cancellous screw entering acetabular fragment just above joint and below osteotomy line and passing into posterior column. Contoured small fragment reconstruction plate and screw shown on medial wall of ilium and acetabular fragment. Long iliac screw seen passing from posterior aspect of iliac crest into posterior column of distal fragment. Note medialization of the acetabular fragment.

Fixation of the Osteotomy

Next, provisionally fix the acetabular fragment with one or two Steinmann pins, and take an AP radiograph of the pelvis or carefully controlled C-arm view of the pelvis to confirm that the desired reorientation has been achieved (Fig. 25). An additional oblique view may be taken with the image intensifier to confirm that anterior coverage is as desired. The position of the fragment is adjusted as indicated. Next, the provisional fixation is replaced with definitive fixation. This usually consists of three cortical or cancellous screws. It is often desirable to place one long cortical or fully threaded cancellous screw from anterior to posterior, passing from the region of the anterior inferior spine in a posterior direction into the posterior column. One or two additional screws are placed from the iliac crest into the acetabular fragment, usually passing posterior to the joint. A reconstruction plate can be placed on the medial wall of the ilium and the medial wall of the acetabular fragment if needed (Fig. 26).

The anterior portion of the acetabular fragment is trimmed, if it is prominent. Bone graft is taken from the medial wall of the ilium to pack in any gaps in the osteotomy, particularly in the area of the superior pubic ramus, to reduce the chances of a delayed union or nonunion.

Wound Closure

The wound is irrigated copiously and closed in layers over suction drains (Fig. 27). Careful reconstruction of the abductors over the iliac crest is carried out. Small-fragment screws may be employed to reattach the bone fragments taken with the sartorius and tensor.

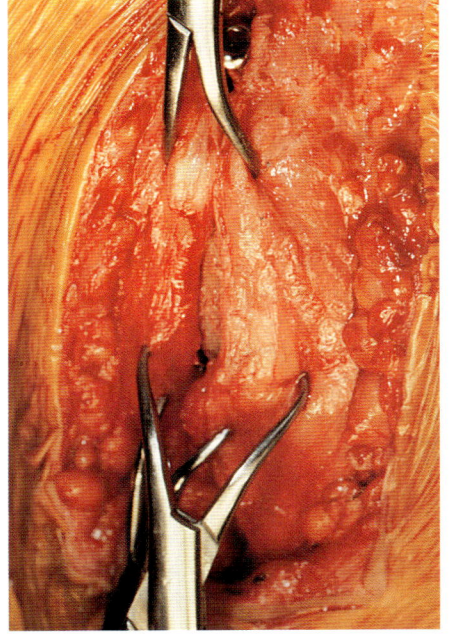
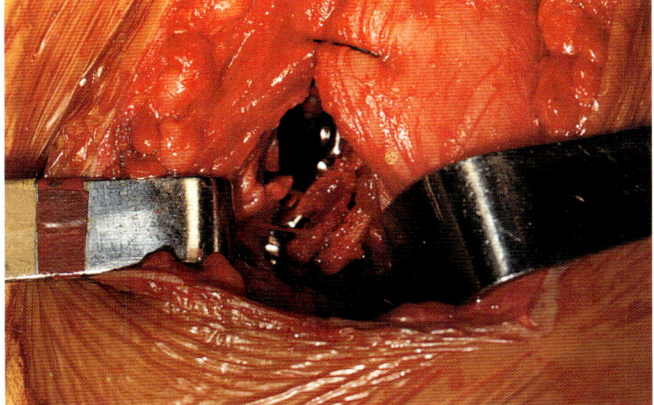

Figure 27. Careful closure is carried out in layers. (A) Careful reapproximation of abductors over iliac crest is carried out with multiple sutures, drill holes in iliac crest are used if needed. (B) Sartorius-tensor interval seen. This interval is usually drained.

POSTOPERATIVE MANAGEMENT

The patient is allowed to sit on the second postoperative day. A partial weight-bearing gait, which has been taught preoperatively, is begun thereafter. Fifteen to 20 pounds of weight is taken with two crutches for the first three postoperative months. A touch-down or non-weight-bearing gait is absolutely prohibited. After three months, according to radiographic healing and return of abductor strength, weight bearing is progressed to one crutch, then to a cane, and then to full weight bearing.

For those patients who have undergone periacetabular osteotomy, weight bearing may be advanced a bit more quickly due to the greater stability achieved by the more extensive internal fixation. Vigorous range of motion and resistive exercises are avoided for at least 6 to 8 weeks, after which weight bearing can be increased if radiographic healing is noted.

The postoperative physical therapy is simple, emphasizing function much more than formal strengthening or range of motion. Almost without exception, these patients preoperatively have good strength and an excellent range of motion. Resistive exercises are avoided for at least 3 months.

Spherical Acetabular Osteotomy

Achievement of the desired acetabular redirection has been nearly universal in our experience (5). Both undercorrection and overcorrection occurred primarily very early in our learning, both before adequate freeing up of the reflected capsular fibers was appreciated and before precision in intraoperative control of the acetabular fragment was achieved routinely. Some slight limitation of flexion and abduction is usually noted for the first 6 to 12 postoperative months. Since these patients tend to be constitutionally ligametously lax, they routinely have regained the sense of full flexion and abduction, except for two patients of our first four, who were overcorrected into extension.

Preoperatively, 83% of our patients had some pain. At last followup, average five years postoperative, only 15% had some pain, and there was only one whose pain was unimproved by the surgery. Average preoperative lateral center-edge angle was 9 degrees; average postoperative center-edge angle was 30 degrees.

Periacetabular Osteotomy

Periacetabular osteotomy is a much more recently developed technique, and, therefore, our experience is more limited, although the redirections achieved with it have been satisfying. The amount of acetabular redirection possible with this procedure is approximately equivalent to that which we have achieved with spherical acetabular osteotomy. Virtually all patients have had restoration of the sourcil to a horizontal alignment. Medialization of the joint center as much as 2 cm has been possible as well.

Reduction in pain and preoperative limp has been universal. Elimination of any preoperative limp and preoperative pain has been usual, though this has been dependent upon the amount of preoperative arthrosis (16). Patients with spherical heads and spherical but dysplastic acetabular can be expected to have long-lasting and probably permanent relief of symptoms and prevention of osteoarthrosis, assuming that perioperative complications have been avoided and restoration of acetabular alignment to normal has been achieved.

COMPLICATIONS

The potential complications, which must be actively avoided, are the same for both spherical acetabular osteotomy and periacetabular osteotomy.

1. Intraarticular osteotomy can result from either misdirecting an osteotomy cut into the hip joint or by an inadvertent fracture into the acetabulum occurring during performance of the osteotomy. This type of complication can be avoided by meticulous attention to maintaining a minimum distance between osteotomy line and the acetabular articular surface of at least 10 mm. In joints with early arthrosis, the periacetabular osteotomy technique may be preferable to the spherical osteotomy, because the oscillating saw is less likely to lead to uncontrolled fracture through a sclerotic acetabulum than is a cut made by the spherical gauges.
2. Vascular injury represents a second major potential complication. Vessels potentially at risk include the femoral vessels, the obturator vessels, and superior gluteal vessels. While there has been no recognized major vascular lesion in our series, damage to the femoral vessels has been reported anecdotally from other series in association with the ilioinguinal approach. Careful attention to keeping the hip flexed and adducted during the medial portions of the exposure, as well as attention to careful handling of the medial soft tissues, should minimize the risk of a major vascular complication.
3. Neurologic injury represents a third major category of complication. The femoral nerve is at some risk during the periacetabular osteotomy when one is approaching both the superior pubic ramus and the infracautaloid groove. Keeping the hip flexed and adducted and the knee extended, is helpful in reducing tension on the femoral nerve. In addition, completely releasing the origins of the rectus femoris from the anterior inferior spine will allow both the rectus and the femoral nerve to retract distally and medially, reducing the risk of neurapraxia.

   The obturator nerve is very close to the underside of the superior pubic ramus, and it must be carefully protected by elevators during the portions of both acetabular osteotomies that involve the superior pubic ramus.

   The sciatic nerve could theoretically be injured during each of the osteotomies if either gauge or chisel is malpositioned. Careful positioning of retractors to protect the sciatic nerve in the notch is important, as well as maintaining the hip extended during those portions of each osteotomy that are performed close to the sciatic notch.

   The lateral femoral cutaneous nerve is at risk of injury during every anterior approach to the hip. The incidence of postoperative dysesthesia from damaging this nerve can be reduced by carrying out the dissection into the sartorius-tensor interval from within the fascial envelope of the tensor.
4. Heterotopic ossification historically has been reported frequently with anterior approaches to the hip. In our series of cases, heterotopic ossification in the abductor muscles has been quite rare, and mild when it has occurred. Care in handling the abductors is important in minimizing heterotopic ossification. Of course, our more recent approaches, have emphasized leaving the abductors attached to the iliac crest, will likely reduce our already low incidence of heterotopic ossification even further.
5. Malalignment, or imprecise correction of the osteotomized acetabulum, represents the last major complication. With these powerful techniques of acetabular realignment, one can relatively easily overcorrect the dysplastic acetabulum as well as undercorrecting it. Careful image-intensifier control of the final position of the acetabulum in both the anteroposterior and faux profil projections is important before final fixation is achieved. Ganz has emphasized the advisability of obtaining an anteroposterior plain radiograph of the entire pelvis intraoperatively, before the final osteosynthesis is in place.

ILLUSTRATIVE CASE FOR TECHNIQUE

Spherical Acetabular Osteotomy

This female adolescent with no history of childhood hip disease had an onset of bilateral groin pain at the age of 14 (Figure 28 A). She underwent a right spherical acetabular os-

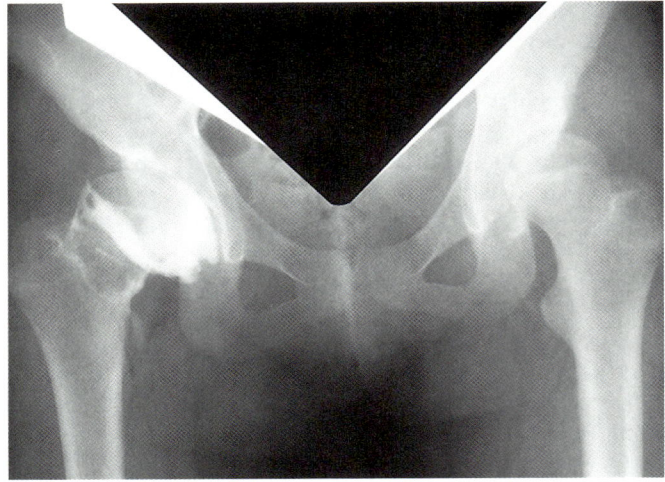
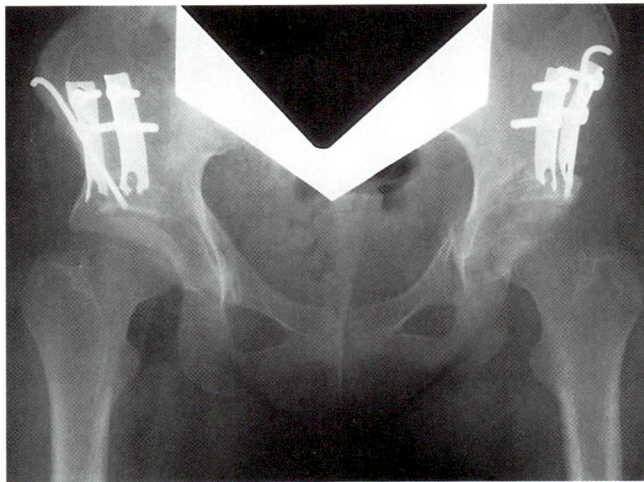
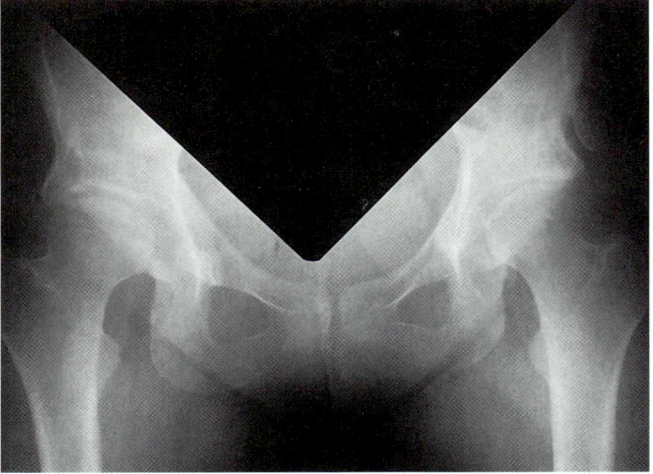

Figure 28. (A) Preoperative radiograph of 14-year-old female. (B) Early postoperative radiograph 7 months after right spherical osteotomy and 1 month after left spherical osteotomy. (C) Postoperative view 5 and 6 years after osteotomies.

teotomy at age 15 and a left spherical acetabular osteotomy at age 16 (Figure 28B). At followup five years after the left hip osteotomy and six years after the right hip osteotomy, she remains pain free with no limp or limitation of motion. She is fully active.

The cartilage space and bone structure remain normal (Figure 28C). Correction of the lateral center-edge angle was from approximately plus 5 degrees to more than 30 degrees bilaterally. Similar correction was noted on faux profil views (not shown here).

ILLUSTRATIVE CASE FOR TECHNIQUE

Periacetabular Osteotomy

A 20-year-old college student had no history of childhood hip disease but a four-year history of progressive bilateral thigh pain during activity (the left greater than right). Radiographic views showed anterior subluxation and anterior uncovering (Fig. 29 A, B).

The patient underwent a periacetabular osteotomy. Postoperative views showed good correction and anterior coverage (Fig. 29 C, D).

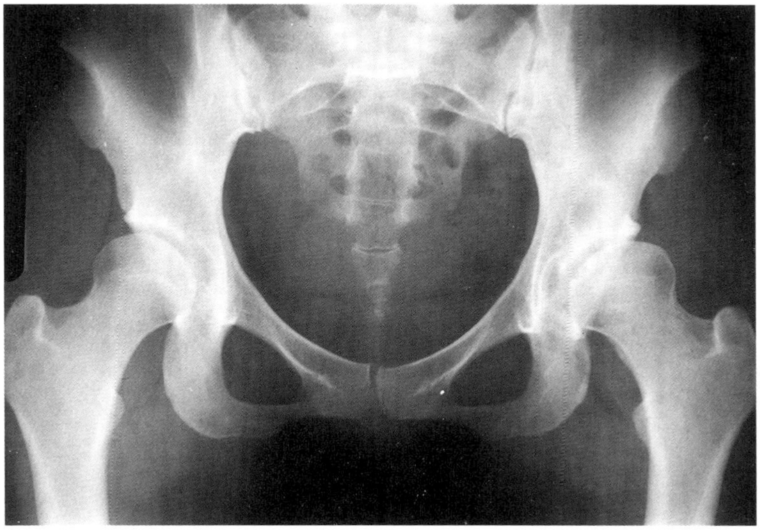

Figure 29. (A) Preoperative view shows large left supraacetabular cyst and early sclerosis. Preoperative lateral center-edge angle is 7 degrees. (B) Preoperative faux profil view shows anterior subluxation and anterior uncovering (anterior c-e angle less than zero degrees). (C) Postoperative correction of lateral center-edge angle to 31 degrees. Weight-bearing surface of acetabulum now horizontal. Medialization of left hip joint center of nearly one centimeter achieved. (D) Postoperative faux profil view shows good anterior coverage (anterior c-e angle is more than 20 degrees).

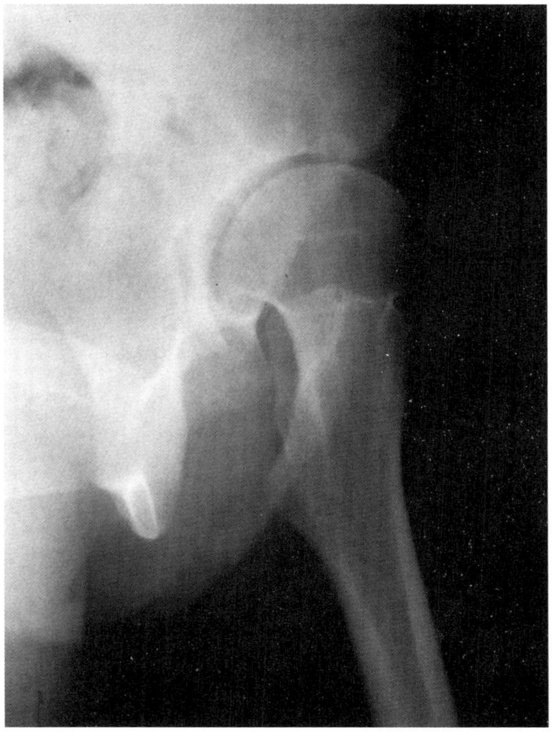

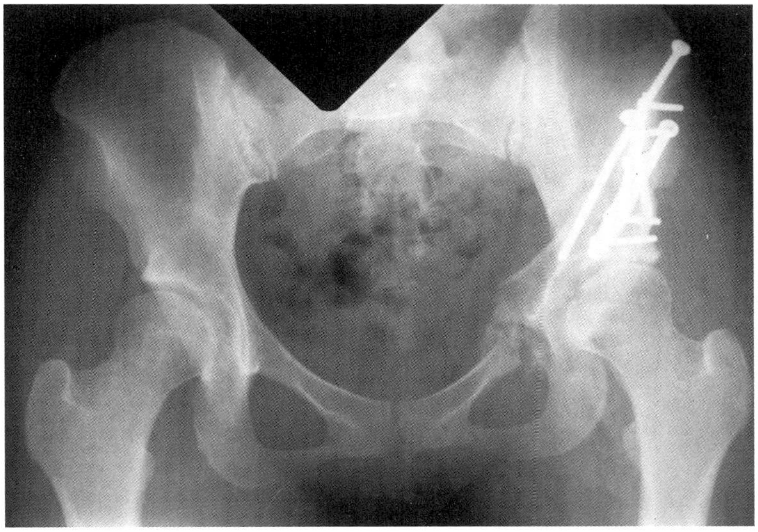

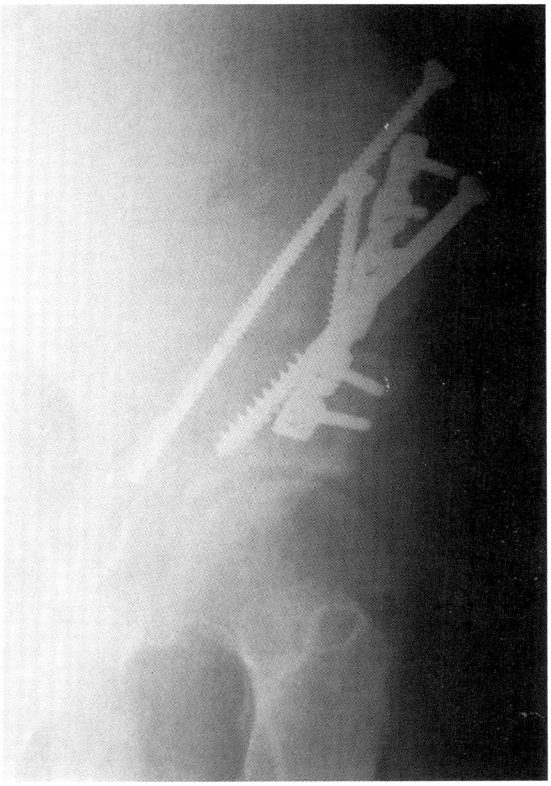

Addendum: Over the past 3 years, we have employed the so-called "direct anterior approach" in which the osteotomy of the anterior superior spine is carried out to carry the sartorius and iliacus medially, but absolutely no stripping is carried out of the abductors off the iliac crest. Only a very small window is made along the lateral ilium, without disturbing the abductor origin, in order to allow the saw cut of the supra-acetabular ilium to be made without injuring the abductor muscles. The direct anterior approach can be made either with or without an ilioinguinal dissection medial to the psoas muscle. While the direct anterior approach does greatly improve the postoperative recovery of abductor functioning following periacetabular osteotomy, there is less direct visualization of the relationship of the posterior osteotomy line to the acetabulum and therefore should be employed only after some experience has been gained through the more surgeon-friendly Smith-Petersen approach.

RECOMMENDED READING

1. Aronson, J.: Osteoarthritis of the young adult hip: etiology and treatment. *Instr. Course Lec.*, 55:119–125, 1986.
2. Ganz, R., Klaue, K., Vinh, T. S., and Mast, J.: A new periacetabular osteotomy for the treatment of hip dysplasias: technique and preliminary results. *Clin. Orthop.*, 232:26–36, 1988.
3. Klaue, K., Wallin, A., and Ganz, R.: CT evaluation of coverage and congruency of the hip prior to osteotomy. *Clin. Orthop.*, 232:15–25, 1988.
4. Macnicol, M., ed. *Color atlas and text of osteotomy of the hip.* Mosby-Wolfe, London, 1996.
5. Millis, M. B., Kaelin, A., Curtis, B., Schluntz, K., and Hey, L.: Spherical acetabular osteotomy for the treatment of acetabular dysplasia in adolescents and young adults. *J. Pediatr. Orthop.* Part B. 3:47–53, 1994.
6. Millis, M. B., Poss, R., and Murphy, S. B.: Osteotomies of the hip for the prevention and treatment of osteoarthritis. *J. Bone Joint Surg.* 77-A:426–437, 1995.
7. Millis, M. B., Poss, R., and Murphy, S. B.: Osteotomies of the hip in the prevention and treatment of osteoarthritis. *AAOS Instructional Course Lec.* 45:209–226, 1996. AAOS, Park Ridge.
8. Millis, M. B., and Murphy, S. B.: Use of computed tomographic reconstruction in planning osteotomies of the hip. *Clin. Orthop.* 274:154–159, 1992.
9. Murphy, S. B., Kijewski, P., Millis, M. B., and Harless, A.: Acetabular dysplasia in the adolescent and young adult. *Clin. Orthop.*, 261:214–223, 1991.
10. Murphy, S. B., Ganz, R., and Mueller, M. E.: The prognosis in untreated hip dysplasia: factors predicting outcome. *J. Bone Joint Surg.* 77-A:985–989, 1995.
11. Ninomiya, S., and Tagawa, H.: Rotational acetabular osteotomy for the dysplastic hip. *J. Bone Joint Surg.* 66A:430–439, 1984.
12. Ninomiya, S.: Rotational acetabular osteotomy for the severely dysplastic hip. *Clin. Orthop.*, 247:127–137, 1988.
13. Tonnis, D.: A modified technique of triple pelvic osteotomy. *J. Ped. Ortho.*, 1:241–249, 1981.
14. Tonnis, D.: Triple pelvic osteotomy, pp. 370–381, In: *Congenital dysplasia and dislocation of the hip.* Springer-Verlag, Heidelberg, 1984.
15. Tonnis, D.: Treatment of residual dysplasia after developmental dysplasia of the hip and prevention of early coxarthrosis. *J. Pediatr. Orthop.* Part B. 2:133–144, 1993.
16. Trousdale, R. T., Ekkernkamp, A., Ganz, R., and Wallrichs, S. L.: Periacetabular and intertrochanteric osteotomy for the treatment of osteoarthrosis in dysplastic hips. *J. Bone Joint Surg.* 77-A:73–85, 1995.
17. Wagner, H.: Experiences with spherical acetabular osteotomy for the correction of the dysplastic acetabulum. *Prog. Orthop. Surg.*, 131–146 Springer-Verlag, Heidelberg, 1978.
18. Wagner, H.: Spherical acetabular osteotomy for the correction of the dysplastic acetabulum: long-term results of 100 patients followed 14 to 25 years. Fourth Harvard Medical School Continuing Education course on Osteotomy of the Hip and Knee, Boston, MA, May, 1992.

9

The Intertrochanteric Osteotomy

Robert Poss and Alastair Younger

INDICATIONS/CONTRAINDICATIONS

Intertrochanteric osteotomy may be beneficial in treating developmental dysplasia, some posttraumatic disorders, and avascular necrosis. In young and active patients an osteotomy can allow patients to meet their functional needs without the pitfalls of total hip arthroplasty in the young age group. Our indications center in three areas affecting young adults causing symptomatic hip problems with a poor prognosis if left untreated.

Developmental Dysplasia of the Hip

Developmental dysplasia is associated with anatomical abnormalities of the acetabulum and proximal femur. Recently, the importance of acetabular redirection in the surgical treatment of this problem has been recognized. In many patients a simultaneous acetabular *and* proximal femoral osteotomy is required. In some patients with minimal acetabular deformity a proximal femoral osteotomy alone will suffice.

Patients with minimal arthritic involvement are helped most by acetabular and proximal femoral redirectional osteotomies. These patients experience progressive symptoms. At presentation they are fully functional and have a full range of motion. Radiographs will show a congruous hip joint with poor femoral head coverage. Adaptive bony or cartilaginous changes have not yet occurred. For these patients a timely intervention (reconstructive osteotomy) should result in a long term good outcome.

In patients with arthritic changes indicated by joint space narrowing and osteophytes, the indications for osteotomy, as opposed to arthroplasty, are less clear. Some patients may develop an ovoid or elliptical femoral head as a secondary change. These patients have significant symptoms compromising their function and have limited joint range of motion. The prognosis for a successful *salvage* osteotomy is less certain than that for a successful *reconstructive* osteotomy. The decision between osteotomy or total hip arthroplasty must

---

R. Poss, M.D. and A. Younger, M.B., CH.B., M.SC., F.R.C.S.C.: Department of Orthopedics, Brigham and Women's Hospital, Boston, Massachusetts 02115.

be made on a case-by-case basis, with both the patient and surgeon aware of the advantages and disadvantages of each procedure.

Posttraumatic Arthritis

Some traumatic conditions lead to an incongruous hip joint. If congruency can be restored, these patients will benefit from intertrochanteric osteotomy. Clinical and radiographic examination will allow the surgeon to identify patients in whom congruency can be achieved.

Osteonecrosis

Patients with stage III osteonecrosis can benefit from an intertrochanteric osteotomy. The osteotomy can remove the necrotic lesion from the weight-bearing surface or result in containment of a small central lesion. In our review, 80% of patients have enjoyed pain relief without progression of osteonecrosis at a minimum of five years follow-up.

Osteotomies for all three conditions are contraindicated in patients suffering from inflammatory arthritis. Older patients (over the age of 50) are better served by total hip arthroplasty, regardless of diagnosis. In general, patients with disease of the hip not of mechanical origin (i.e., degeneration secondary to focal overload of articular cartilage) are poor candidates for femoral osteotomy. Patients with avascular necrosis and extensive femoral head involvement are not candidates for an osteotomy, as no noninvolved segment can be rotated into the weight-bearing zone. Patients with earlier stages of avascular necrosis may be better served by observation as 80% will not progress. Careful follow-up will identify the 20% progressing, and the intertrochanteric osteotomy can be done at the appropriate stage.

PREOPERATIVE PLANNING

Success is completely dependent on accurate preoperative planning. In developmental dysplasia, the goal of surgery is to restore congruency and normal biomechanics. Preoperative anteroposterior (AP) and false profile views of the hip are essential. Fluoroscopic examination will determine whether congruency can be achieved. The examiner can determine whether a laterally placed femoral head will reduce with hip abduction. Hips with secondary arthritic changes may no longer have spherical femoral heads. These hips may become less congruous with abduction when they "hinge" on the superior acetabulum. These hips may become more congruent in adduction.

Patients suffering from osteonecrosis require AP and frog lateral views of the affected hip. A CT scan will allow the size and position of the affected segment to be localized and the redirectional osteotomy planned. The CT scan is therefore the procedure of choice for preoperative planning. An MRI scan is sensitive in the diagnosis of osteonecrosis, but the image is not clear enough to plan the procedure.

Candidates for osteotomy must have enough motion to accommodate the planned correction. For example, if a patient requires 30 degrees of abduction to make the joint congruous, then the patient should have at least 50 degrees of preoperative abduction to leave 20 degrees of abduction range after a varus osteotomy. Varus osteotomies result in loss of abduction and a gain of adduction. The extent of the varus correction should allow for 10 to 20 degrees of abduction after the osteotomy.

Angular corrections can be made to improve the functional arc of motion both in the sagittal and coronal plane. A flexion arc of at least 90-degree range is a prerequisite for an intertrochanteric osteotomy. A flexion contracture can be neutralized by an extension osteotomy in addition to abduction and adduction corrections in the coronal plane.

Intertrochanteric osteotomy does not result in a change in total range of motion, but arcs of motion can be changed to favor functional needs. The goal of osteotomy is therefore to change the patient's range of motion to within the functional arc of motion.

A suitable candidate for osteotomy therefore has an arthritic or prearthritic abnormality of the hip joint correctable by redirectional osteotomy with a sufficient range of motion. In addition, the patient should understand the alternatives, risks, and benefits of the procedure.

The surgical procedure is planned as the final stage of preoperative assessment. With the help of a tracing of the femur, the osteotomy can be customized to the patient's anatomy and needs. We favour impaction of the osteotomy, as this reduces the angulation at the level of the osteotomy and maintains preoperative leg lengths. The effect of the planned osteotomy on leg lengths can be determined using the femoral tracing. The type of plate fixation that best accomplishes the technical goals is chosen. By mapping out the surgery on paper beforehand, the surgeon reduces the real operation to a technical exercise that plays out a well-rehearsed script.

Patients are encouraged to predeposit autologous blood. The average loss during the procedure is 2 to 3 units. The need for heterologous blood is minimized. Preoperative antibiotics, usually a cephalosporin, are given preoperatively and for 24 hours postoperatively.

SURGICAL TECHNIQUE

To reduce the risk of infection, the procedure should be performed in an operating room designed for total hip arthroplasty. Our hospital is equipped with ultraviolet light to reduce the number of viable airborne organisms.

Patient Positioning

Utilizing a Watson-Jones anterolateral approach, we prefer to perform an intertrochanteric osteotomy with the patient supine. The patient is positioned on a five-foot-long radiolucent osteotomy table. The osteotomy table is an extension of a regular operating table; it allows the anesthetist access to the patient's airway. The lower extremity is positioned on the radiolucent table so that the whole pelvis and lower limb can be visualized using the image intensifier. A small pillow is placed under the buttock so that the skin hangs free. The ipsilateral arm is folded out of the way over the patient's chest to make room for the surgeon and two assistants on the operative side of the patient (Fig. 1). Figure

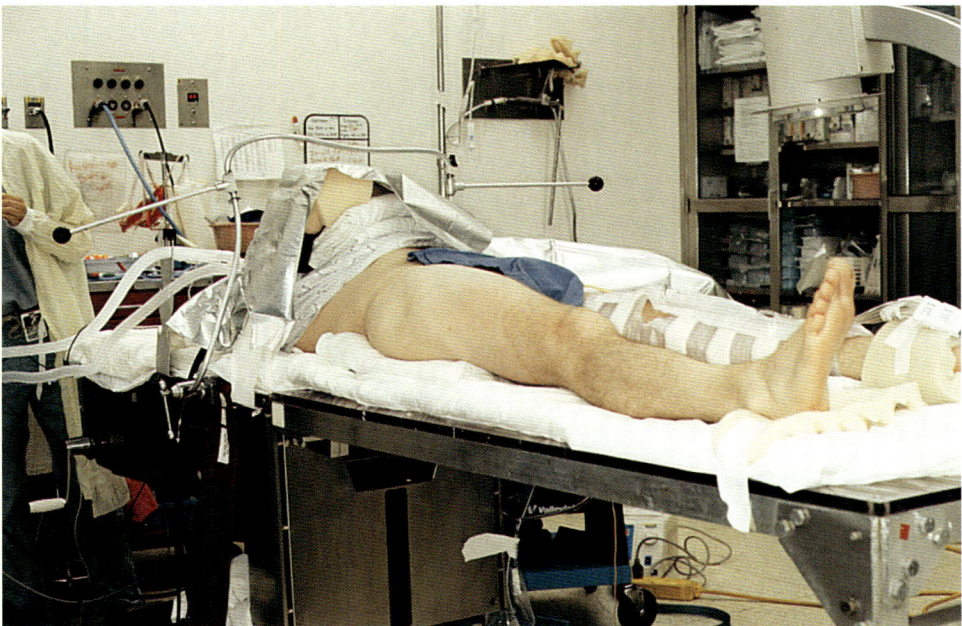

Figure 1. The patient is positioned with the ispilateral arm over the chest. No arm board is used on the operative side so that the wound can be accessed by two surgeons and the image intensifier.

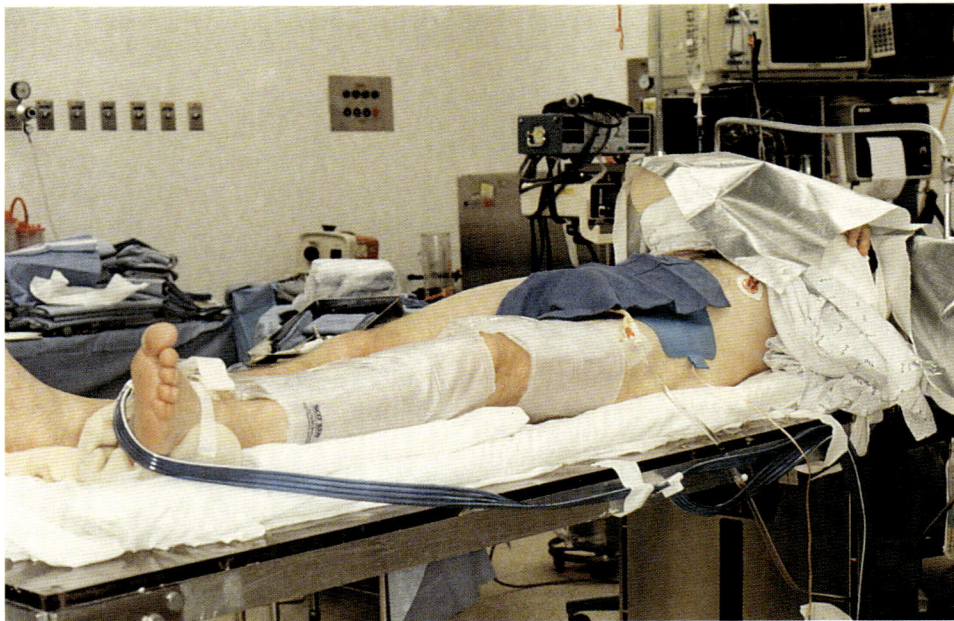

Figure 2. A view from the opposite side of the bed. An insulated warming blanket is used. Pneumatic compression stockings are used on the opposite leg during the case.

2 shows the position of the patient from the nonoperative side. A pneumatic compression stocking is used to prevent venous thrombosis. Bony prominences are well padded. An indwelling Foley catheter is placed to prevent bladder distention; it causes less urinary sepsis than intermittent catheterization. All patients are given epidural regional anesthesia supplemented by a light general anesthetic as necessary. An insulated blanket or warm air blanket is used to maintain body temperature.

Exposure

The extremity is free-draped exposing the pelvis and including the iliac crest (Fig. 3). If the hip joint is to be opened or a capsulotomy performed, then the full incision illustrated

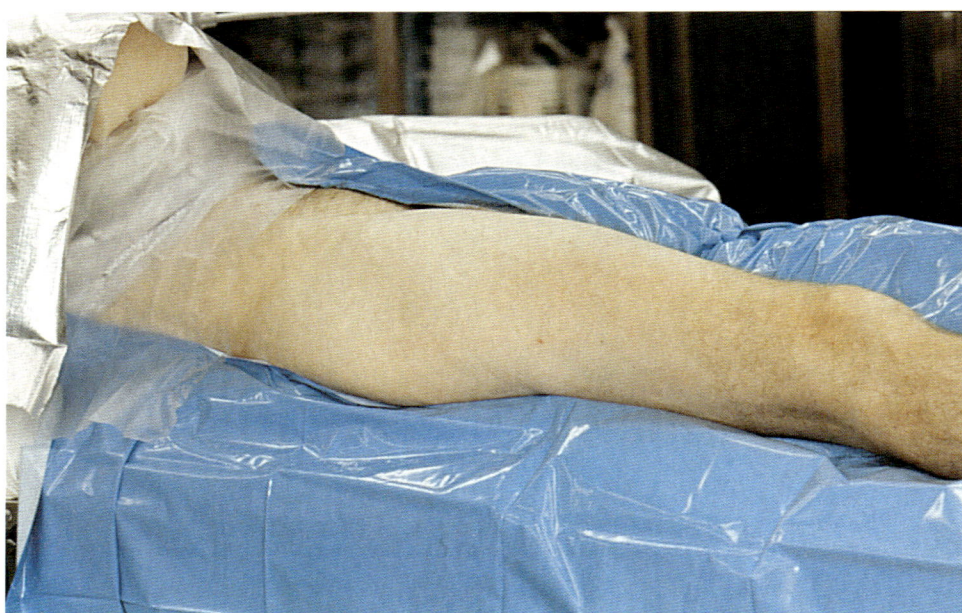

Figure 3. The pelvis is draped to above the level of the iliac crest. The leg is free draped.

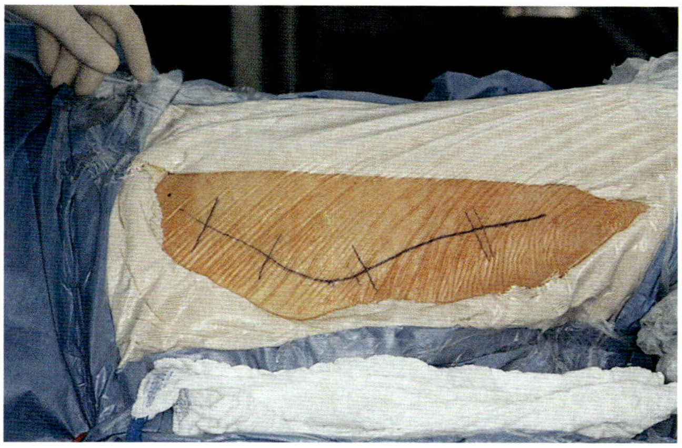

9 THE INTERTROCHANTERIC OSTEOTOMY

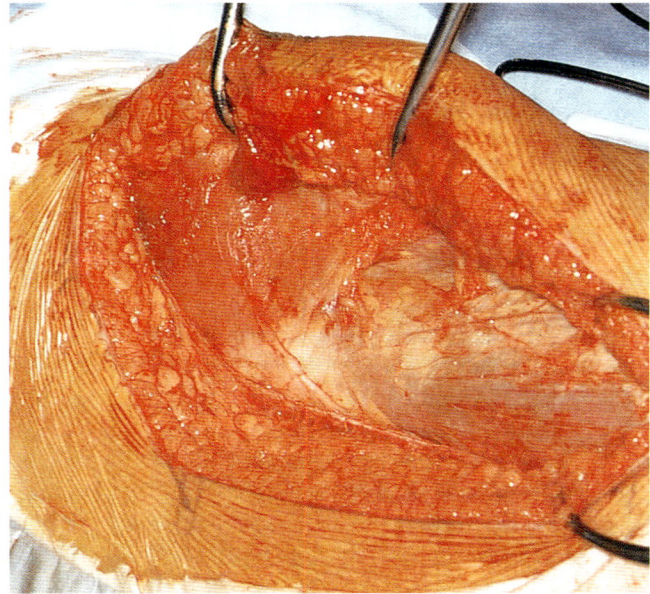

Figure 4. The full incision is illustrated extending 10 cm above and 15 cm below the greater trochanter.

is used. This incision extends 15 cm from the tip of the trochanter distally along the shaft of the femur. The proximal part of the incision extends from the greater trochanter 10 cm towards the anterior superior iliac spine (Fig. 4). The iliotibial band and the tensor fascia lata are incised in the line of the skin incision. The anterior flap is retracted using two bone hooks. The retraction will open the plane between the tensor fascia lata and anterior border of gluteus medius (Renato Bombelli, M.D., personal communication) (Fig. 5).

The anterior capsule is easily exposed by placing retractors along the medial and lateral borders of the femoral neck. In a flexion osteotomy a wide anterior capsulectomy must be performed to allow the proximal fragment to hyperextend (Fig. 6). If the capsulotomy is not performed, a flexion contracture of the limb will result, and the osteotomy will not bring the osteonecrotic segment off the weight-bearing portion of the joint. If the intertrochanteric and periacetabular osteotomy are performed in conjunction, the arthrotomy should be performed through the iliofemoral or ilioinguinal approach used for the acetabular procedure.

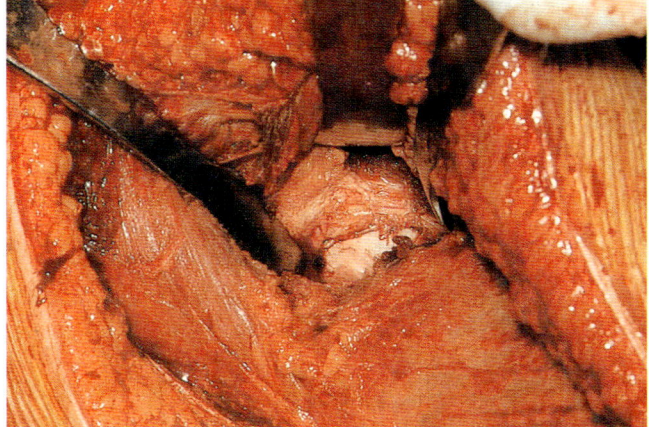

Figure 5. The anterior flap is retracted with two bone hooks. The plane between tensor fascia lata and gluteus medius opens up.

Figure 6. The anterior capsule is easily visualized. A capsulotomy can be performed if required.

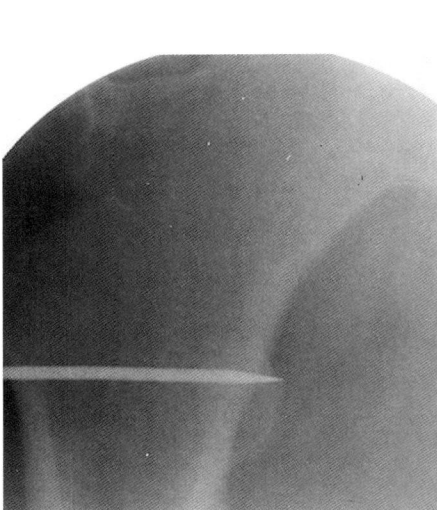

Figure 7. Radiographs show correct placement of the first Steinmann pin at the level of the osteotomy.

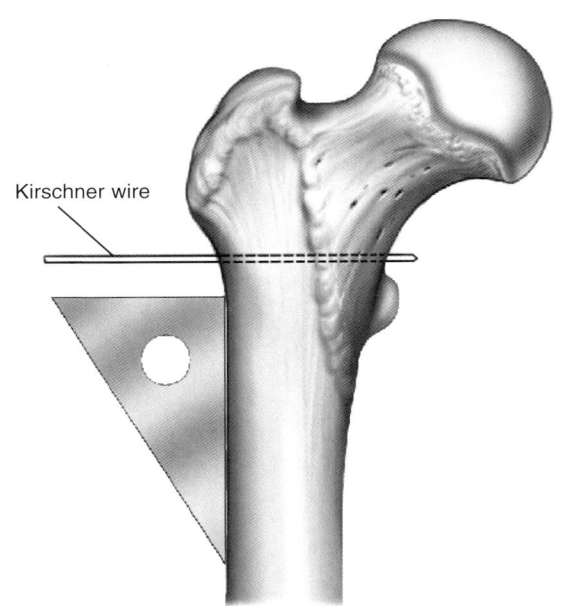

Figure 8. Perpendicular placement of the Steinmann pin at the osteotomy site is achieved using the 90 degree triangle as a guide.

Techniques

The procedure requires x-ray control by means of an image intensifier. A Steinmann pin is placed perpendicular to the long axis of the femur at the level of the proximal border of the lesser trochanter. It is vital that the osteotomy be performed at this level (Figs. 7 and 8). All other pin placements are indexed off this initial pin. A second Steinmann pin is placed starting at least 1.5 cm above the first pin on the lateral femoral cortex. This pin marks the position of the blade of the blade plate and is angled depending on the required correction (Fig. 9).

Blade plates of different angles are available from 90 to 130 degrees in 10-degree increments. The angle chosen should allow central placement of the blade in the femoral neck after the correct angular correction. The correct plate should match the one chosen by preoperative templating. The entry point is 1.5 cm above the osteotomy site to maintain a lateral cortical bridge that can buttress up against the plate and prevent cut-out of the blade and loss of fixation. An additional Steinmann pin is placed parallel to the anterior surface of the femoral neck in line with the desired direction of the seating chisel. The two proximal Steinmann pins allow correct orientation of the seating chisel in two planes (Fig. 10).

The femoral shaft is exposed by elevating the vastus lateralis muscle from the lateral intermuscular septum. The perforating vessels are identified and ligated. The origin of the vastus lateralis is lifted from the vastus tubercle and retracted anteriorly. The proximal shaft, the greater trochanter, and the femoral neck are now exposed. This allows placement of the blade plate (Fig. 11).

A channel is prepared for the seating chisel. The entry hole on the lateral femoral cortex is opened with a drill and rongeur. The entry hole should allow insertion of the chisel parallel to the cortices of the femoral neck. The greater trochanter usually lies posterior to the femoral neck, requiring an entry hole anterior to the middle of the greater trochanter. Increased femoral anteversion will require a more posterior entry hole on the lateral femoral cortex. Careful examination of the fluoroscopic lateral view will allow the correct starting point to be determined. The channel is angled into flexion or extension if a flexion or extension osteotomy is required. For the more common flexion osteotomy, the guide is ro-

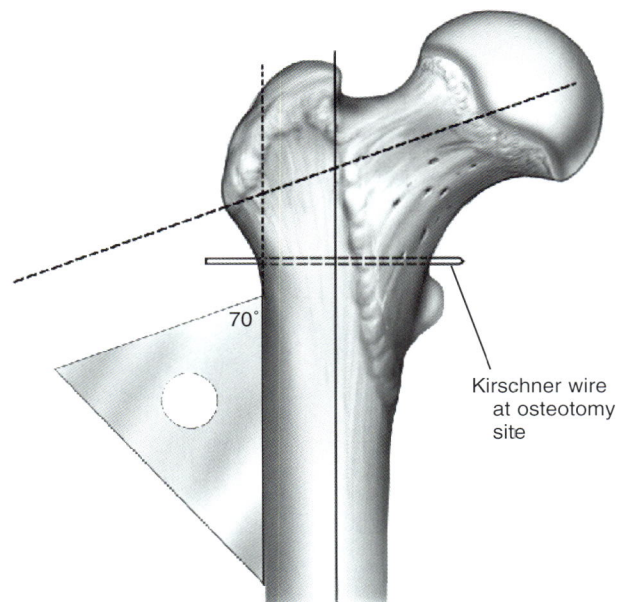
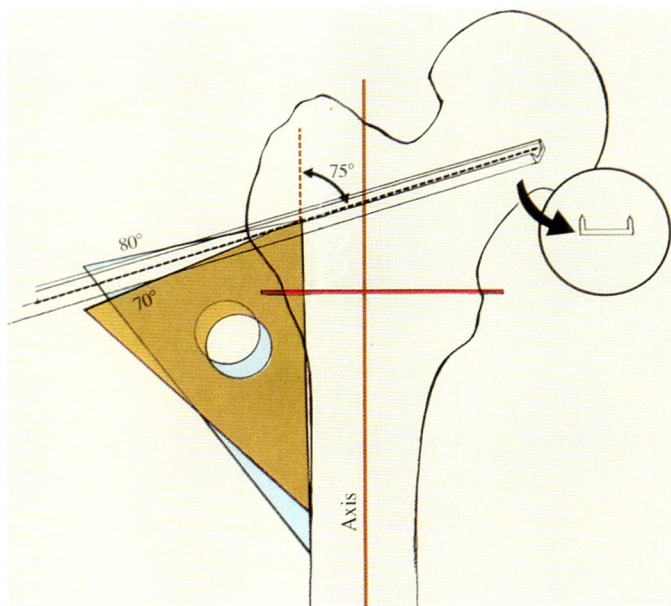

Figure 9. The osteotomy has to be performed at the proximal border of the lesser trochanter. The seating chisel should be placed 1.5 to 2 cm proximal to the osteotomy site on the lateral femoral cortex. These are two important technical considerations in performing the osteotomy.

Figure 10. A Steinmann pin acts as a guide for the seating chisel in both planes.

tated anterior to the long axis of the femur by the required amount. The entry hole must be larger than the cross-section of the blade so that it does not engage the lateral femoral cortex. The seating chisel is slowly advanced parallel to the proximal Steinmann pin under radiological control. The chisel should advance relatively easily. If it does not, the chisel's position should be checked on both views, as the chisel may be hitting the cortex of the neck. The chisel should be easily removable from the tract *before* the osteotomy is performed, as a tightly seated chisel will be hard to remove once the proximal fragment is free. After ensuring that the chisel can be removed from the tract, the osteotomy is performed. The osteotomy is performed parallel to the long axis in both planes along the wire seated

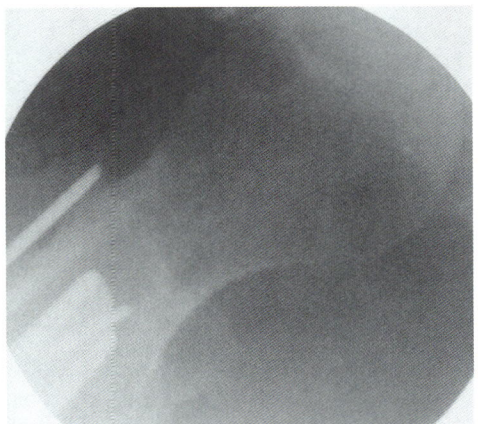

Figure 11. The proximal femoral shaft, the greater trochanter and the femoral neck are exposed allowing accurate placement of the blade plate.

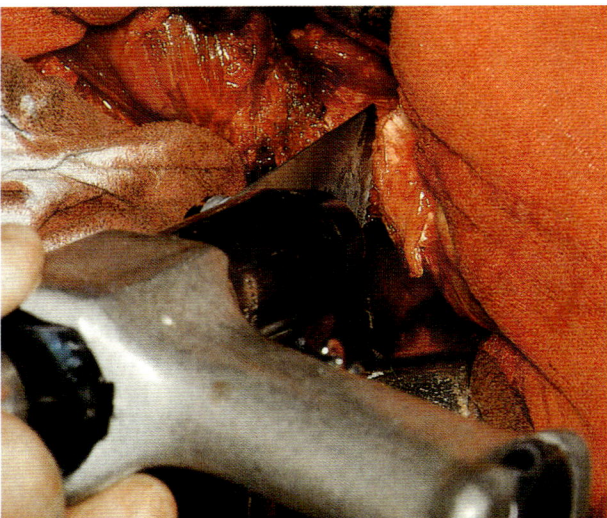

Figure 12. The osteotomy is perpendicular to the long axis of the femur in both planes.

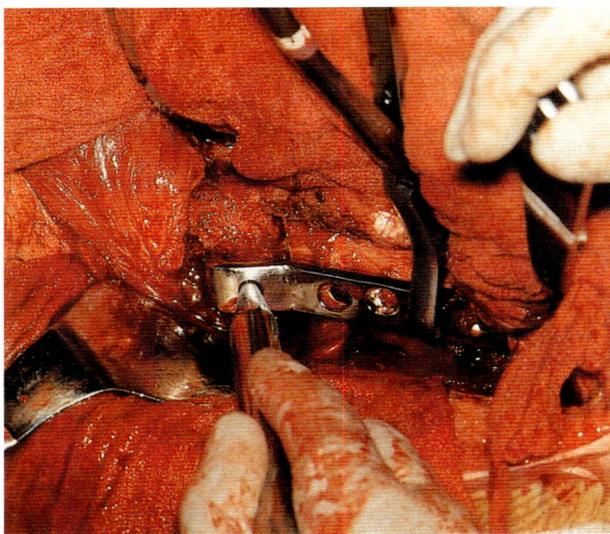

Figure 13. The seating chisel is left loose within its track before the osteotomy is performed. It is removed and the blade plate immediately placed by hand into its track.

into the proximal border of the lesser trochanter (Fig. 12). The osteotomy is performed at this level to leave enough bone proximally for fixation, while the osteotomy is still performed in cancellous bone to encourage prompt union.

After the osteotomy is completed, the two fragments are distracted to make sure that all of the medial soft tissue is disrupted. Two wide osteotomes are inserted into the osteotomy and levered apart. The seating chisel should not be used to distract the proximal fragment. When the fragments are free, the seating chisel is removed and the blade plate immediately inserted into the same tract (Fig. 13).

Recently, we have performed a direct impaction of the proximal and distal fragments. An impaction osteotomy does not change the length of the limb, unlike a wedge resection, and prevents the deformity associated with a wedge resection. For a flexion osteotomy, a direct impaction osteotomy will result in a straight femoral canal after remodeling, making a subsequent total hip arthroplasty easier to perform. A wedge resection causes greater deformity and can complicate a subsequent total hip arthroplasty. An indent is made on the medial cancellous bone on the distal fragment to allow impaction of the fragments for a varus osteotomy. The plate is brought parallel to the long axis of the femur. The proximal fragment is inserted just within the medial cortex, and the fragments are compressed. The external compression device is used to achieve compression (Fig. 14). A supplementary proximal screw should be used for valgus osteotomies using plates angled 100 degrees or more. Before fixation of the distal fragment, rotational alignment should be checked. This can be referenced to a mark along the axis of the femur made before the osteotomy is performed. In some cases derotation is performed: The amount required can be determined using the difference in internal and external rotation measured preoperatively, so that both arcs are equal postoperatively.

After reduction, screw fixation of the femur is performed with at least eight cortices being transfixed. An arthrotomy should be performed if the patient requires a flexion osteotomy to release the capsule and allow full extension of the hip. Degenerative changes in the joint requiring debridement will also require a joint arthrotomy. The capsule should be released off the acetabular side to prevent compromise of the femoral head blood supply. The labrum should not be damaged during the exposure. The capsule will require a longitudinal split, which should be performed over the anterior neck to avoid the major retinacular vessels.

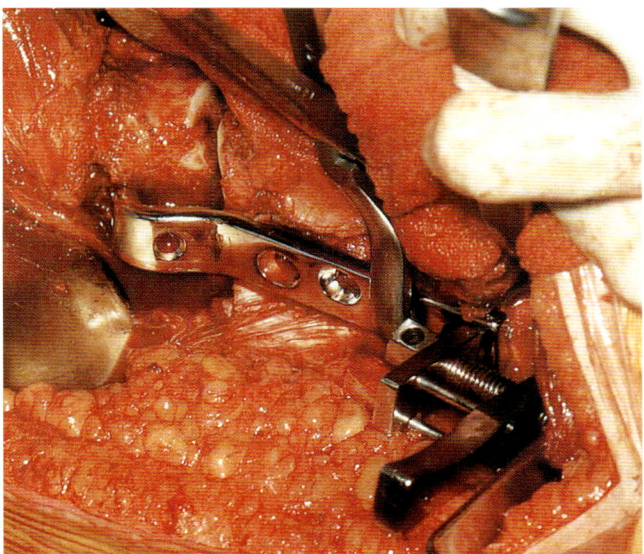

Figure 14. The osteotomy is reduced and held with bone holding forceps.

After completion of the arthrotomy the longitudinal split in the capsule is repaired. The origin of the vastus lateralis is reattached to a periosteal cuff left on the vastus ridge using interrupted absorbable sutures. The posterior border of the vastus lateralis is repaired to the intermuscular septum with a running absorbable suture. Drains are not used if the wound is dry. The fascia lata is repaired with interupted sutures. Our routine skin closure includes a closure of the deep fascia with interrupted absorbable sutures, followed by a subcutaneous and subcuticular closure. Steri strips are used on skin.

POSTOPERATIVE MANAGEMENT

The operated limb is placed in pillow suspension on transfer to the hospital bed in the operating room. This is continued for 24 to 48 hours depending on patient comfort. Rapid mobilization of the patient to partial weight-bearing using two crutches precedes discharge. Active assisted range of motion is encouraged. The weight-bearing status is reassessed at the six-week review. Clinical and radiographic examination will allow the progress to bony union to be assessed. With simple varus osteotomies, union is usually seen by six weeks. More complex osteotomies may take 12 weeks to heal. Weight bearing is gradually increased at 6 weeks to a single crutch and then to a cane, depending on patient comfort. Strengthening exercises are begun.

In our experience, patients reporting an almost immediate loss of rest pain tend to do well. If correct indications are chosen, early symptomatic relief is seen. Warfarin prophylaxis for deep vein thrombosis is continued for six postoperative weeks.

Patients with pre-existing degenerative disease may require an osteotomy to delay the progression of arthritis and provide interim symptomatic relief. These patients must understand the possibility of delayed total hip arthroplasty. If over five years' of improved function is achieved, then the procedure has been worthwhile.

COMPLICATIONS

Incorrect patient selection and technical errors are the two major errors in subtrochanteric femoral osteotomy.

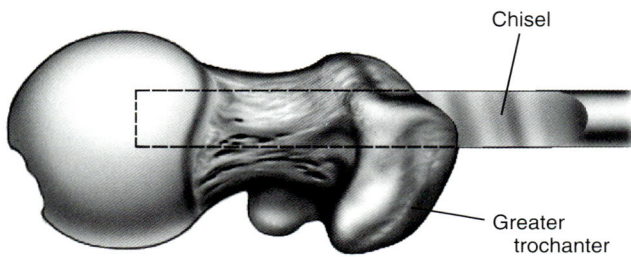

Figure 15. The blade is inserted parallel and just posterior to the anterior femoral neck. Because the greater trochanter is a posterior structure, the entry hole will lie anterior to the midline to avoid perforation of the posterior cortex, which can disrupt the blood supply to the femoral head.

Patients selected for the procedure should demonstrate clinical and radiographic signs of mechanical overload. The fluoroscopic examination must show improved congruency and mechanics with a maneuver compatible with an osteotomy. The patient must be fully educated as to the risks, benefits, and goals of the procedure. The alternative procedures should be explained, including the role of nonoperative management.

Technical errors are prevented by surgeon experience. Some of the pitfalls may be avoided by practicing the procedure on a cadaver.

Incorrect placement of the seating chisel is avoided by preoperative planning. A 1.5 to 2 cm bone bridge is left on the lateral femoral cortex on the proximal fragment. The lateral cortical entry hole for the chisel should be correctly placed with correct flexion or extension. The entry hole should allow the chisel to be centrally placed within and parallel to the femoral neck. Penetration of the posterior neck can cause damage to the ascending branch of the medial circumflex femoral artery, which supplies the retinacular vessels on the lateral and posterior femoral neck. If the surgeon is unsure, a guide wire placed along the proposed track will allow the position to be checked, as changing the position of the chisel is hard to achieve once a track has been made. Once the chisel is inserted, the anterior neck is used as a guide, while the path is checked in both fluoroscopic views (Fig. 15). The seating chisel should be removed and manually placed within its tract before the osteotomy is performed.

Malposition of the osteotomy can lead to delayed union or nonunion of the osteotomy site. More distal placement of the osteotomy leads to a greater chance of nonunion. External rotation deformity can occur if the rotational alignment is not checked and marked.

In our series of 140 osteotomies, observation of technical detail has resulted in union in 142 of 144 osteotomies. The two delayed unions were managed by changing the plate for a longer plate. No nerve palsies were seen in this series.

CASE ILLUSTRATION

A 40-year-old man who works at a sedentary job experienced the onset of right hip pain one year prior to consultation. The patient's symptoms became acute after heavy exercise over one weekend. He subsequently gave up sports, but his hip became progressively more painful. His history was negative for risk factors associated with osteonecrosis.

The patient's range of motion was almost normal with 135 degrees of flexion, a 10-degree flexion contracture, 50 degrees of abduction, 30 degrees of adduction, and 20 degrees of internal and external rotation in extension.

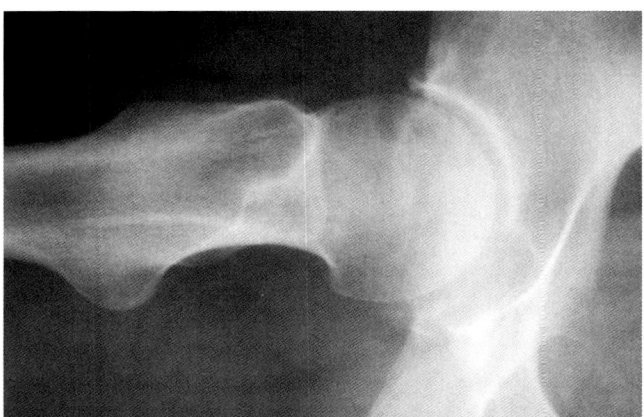

Figure 16. The cystic lesion seen on the lateral view.

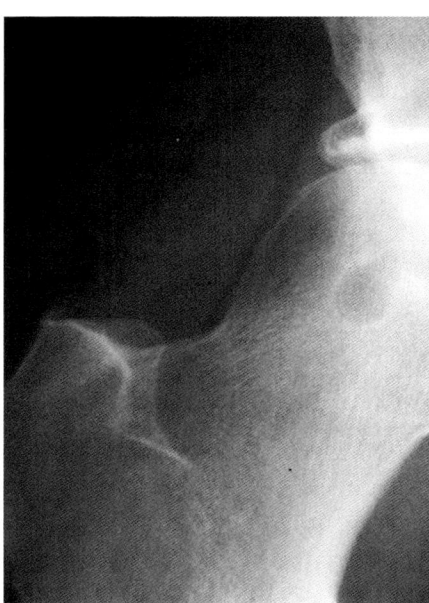

Figure 17. The cystic lesion seen on the anterior view.

The radiographs showed a cystic lesion visible on both views (Figs. 16 and 17). The MRI showed changes consistent with osteonecrosis (Fig. 18). A cystic lesion with a section of collapse was localized to the anterior femoral head (Fig. 19).

The patient was considered a good candidate for osteotomy as he was increasingly symptomatic and had an isolated osteonecrotic segment on the anterior femoral head which was removed from the weight-bearing surface by a flexion osteotomy.

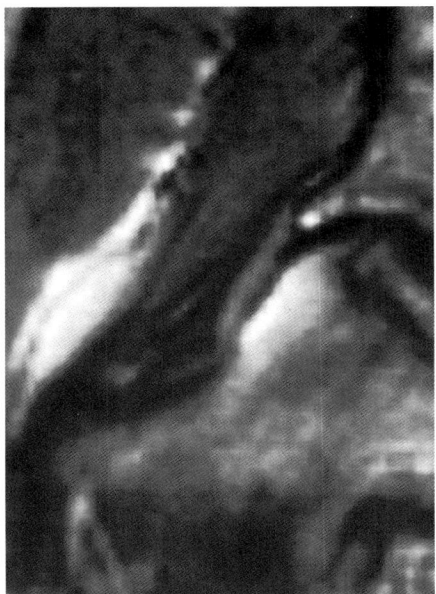

Figure 18. The magnetic resonance image shows changes consistent with avascular necrosis.

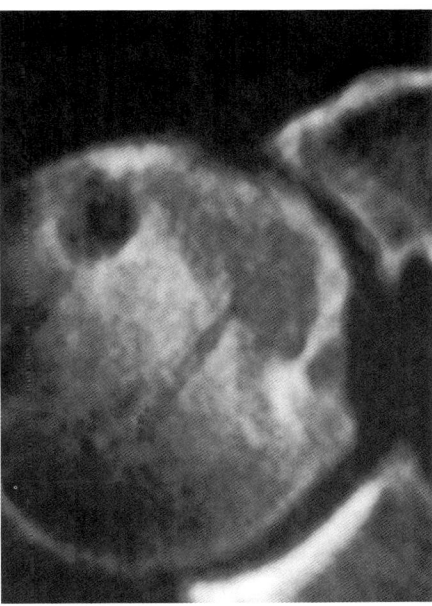

Figure 19. The CT scan identifies the area of subchondral collapse and confirms the position of the cystic lesion within the anterior portion of the femoral head.

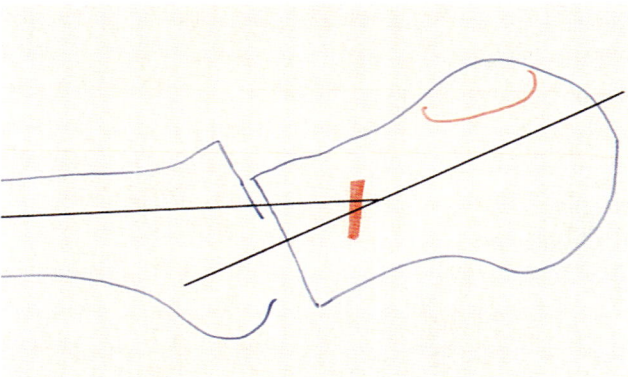

Figure 20. The seating chisel is introduced rotated into flexion (counterclockwise on the right) by 30° to the long axis of the femur. When the plate is aligned with the long axis of the femur 30° of hyperextension of the proximal fragment will have been achieved. This illustration shows the deformity created after a wedge excision. We would presently perform a direct impaction of the osteotomy.

The goal of surgery was to deliver 50% of the lesion away from the superior acetabulum. A 30-degree flexion osteotomy was planned (Fig. 20). By rotating the drill guide anteriorly by 30 degrees from the neutral position around the blade insertion site, the reduction was achieved once the plate was placed parallel to the femoral shaft. Thirty degrees of hyperextension of the femoral head occurred when the patient stood in the anatomic position, removing some of the osteonecrotic segment from the weight-bearing area.

At surgery a wire was first placed perpendicular to the long axis of the femur at the level of the proximal end of the lesser trochanter. The second wire marked the entry point of the seating chisel and was placed along the parallel to the anterior cortex of the neck at least 1.5 cm above the first wire at the lateral femoral cortex. In this case, it was parallel to the first wire in the AP plane as no varus or valgus correction was planned (Fig. 21). The seating chisel was placed parallel to this wire (Fig. 22). After the osteotomy had been performed, the blade plate was introduced by hand into the track of the chisel and the osteotomy was reduced (Fig. 23).

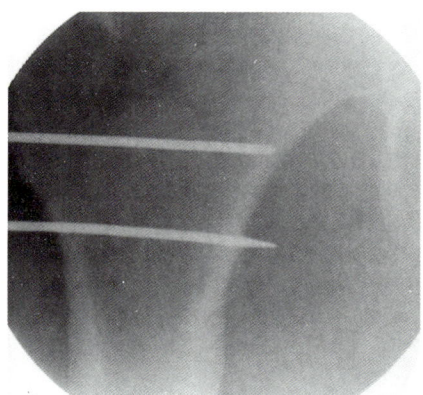

Figure 21. The two Steinmann pins are placed parallel to each other on the anteroposterior view.

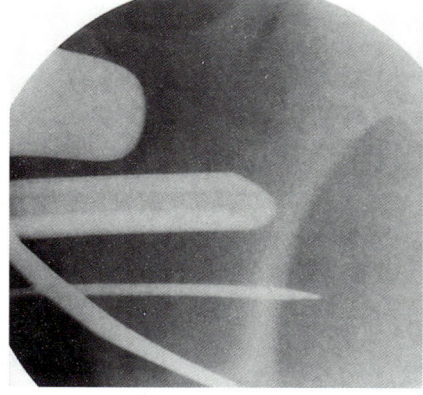

Figure 22. The seating chisel is placed parallel to the second wire in both planes.

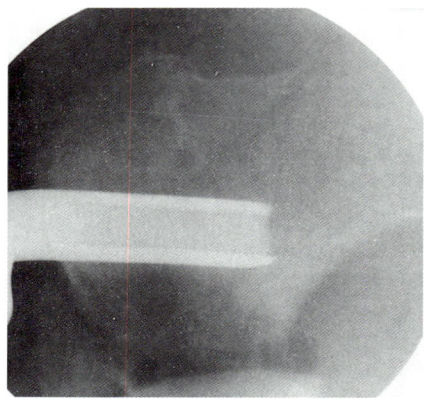

Figure 23. The blade plate is introduced into the seating chisel track. This shows the blade in profile before rotation of the proximal fragment.

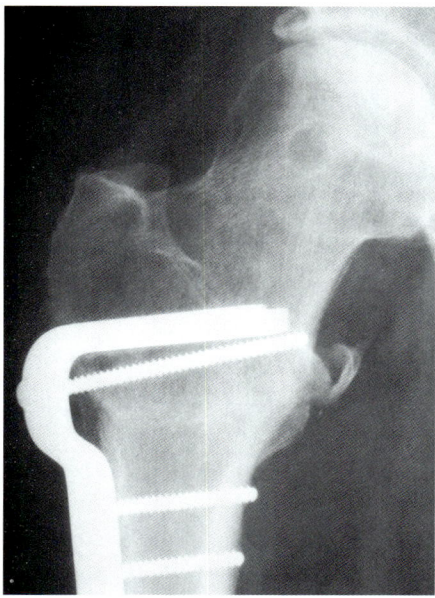

Figure 24. A postoperative lateral view shows a healed osteotomy.

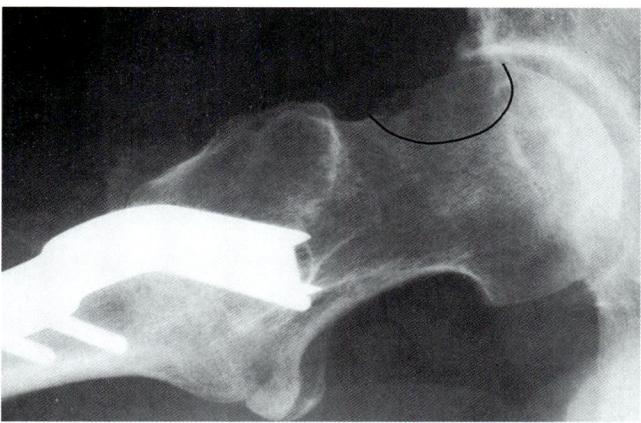

Figure 25. A postoperative anterior view confirms that the cystic lesion was delivered from the weight bearing sector of the acetabulum.

One year later the patient is almost pain free. He has a mild limp after exercise and is still finding some late improvement in his abductor strength. He has been able to return to walking 18 holes of golf. Radiographs show that the required correction was achieved (Figs. 24 and 25).

Clinical examination shows equal leg lengths and a pain-free range of motion. His flexion is now reduced to 95 degrees. He has full extension and 30 degrees of abduction and adduction. External rotation is 20 degrees and internal rotation now 5 degrees. The blade plate will be removed after eighteen months.

RECOMMENDED READING

1. Aronson, J.: Osteoarthritis of the young adult hip: Etiology and treatment. *Inst. Course Lec.*, 35:119–128. CV Mosby, St. Louis, 1986.
2. Bombelli, R.: Osteoarthritis of the hip. 2nd ed. Springer-Verlag, Berlin, 1983.
3. Ganz, R., Klaue, K., Vinh, T. S., and Mast, J. W.: A new periacetabular osteotomy for the treatment of hip dysplasias. Technique and preliminary results. *Clin. Orthop.*, 232:26–36, 1988.
4. Hadley, N. A., Brown, T. D., and Weinstein, S. L.: The effect of compact pressure elevations and aseptic necrosis on long-term outcome of congenital hip dislocation. *J. Orthop. Res.*, 8:504–513, 1990.
5. Harris, W. H., and Kirwan, E.: The results of osteotomy for early primary osteoarthritis of the hip. *J. Bone Surg.*, 46–B:477, 1964.
6. Harris, W. H.: Etiology of osteoarthritis of the hip. *Clin. Orthop.*, 213:20–33, 1986.
7. Langlais, F., Roure, J. L., and Maquet, P.: Valgus osteotomy in severe osteoarthritis of the hip. *J. Bone Joint Surg.*, 61–B(4):424–431, 1979.
8. Lequesne, M., and de Sèze, S.: Le faux profile du bassin: Nouvelle incidence radiographique par l'étude de la hanche. Son utilité dans les dysplasies et les différentes coxopathies. *Rev. Rhum. Mal. Osteartic.*, 28:643, 1961.
9. Mankin, H. J., Dorfman, H., Lippiello, L., and Zarins, A.: Biochemical and metabolic abnormalities in articular cartilage from osteoarthritic human hip. II. Correlation of morphology with biochemical and metabolic data. *J. Bone Joint Surg.*, 53A:523–537, 1971.
10. Miegel, R., and Harris, W. H.: Medical displacement intertrochanteric osteotomy in osteoarthritis of the hip. *J. Bone Joint Surg.*, 66–A:878–887, 1984.
11. Millis, M. B., Poss, R., and Murphy, S. B.: Osteotomies of the hip in the prevention and treatment of osteoarthritis. *American Academy of Orthopaedic Surgeons Instr. Course Lec.* 41:145–156, 1992. AAOS, Park Ridge.
12. Morscher, E. W.: Intertrochanteric osteotomy in osteoarthritis of the hip. In: *The Hip*. Proceedings of the Eighth Open Scientific Meeting of the Hip Society. CV Mosby, St. Louis, 1980.

13. Moskowitz, R. W., Howell, D. S., Goldberg, V. M., and Mankin, H. J.: *Osteoarthritis: Diagnosis and Medical/Surgical Management.* 2nd ed. WB Saunders, Philadelphia, 1992.
14. Pauwels, F.: *Biomechanics of the Normal and Diseased Hip.* Springer-Verlag, Berlin, 1976.
15. Poss, R.: The role of osteotomy in the treatment of osteoarthritis of the hip (Current Concepts Review). *J. Bone Joint Surg.*, 66-A: 144–152, 1984.
16. Radin, E. L., Ehrlich, M. G., Chernack, R., Abernethy, P., Paul, I. L., and Rose, R. M.: Effect of repetitive impulsive loading on the knee joints of rabbits. *Clin. Orthop.*, 131:288–293, 1978.
17. Schatzker, J.: *The Intertrochanteric Osteotomy.* Springer-Verlag, Berlin, 1984.
18. Schneider, R.: Results of intertrochanteric osteotomies in patients with coxarthrosis 12–15 years after surgery. In: *Joint Preserving Procedures of the Lower Extremities. Progress in Orthopedic Surgery* (Vol. 4) Weil, H. H., ed. Springer-Verlag, Berlin, 1980. pp. 39–43.
19. Stulberg, S., Harris, W., and MacEwen, G. D.: Unrecognized childhood hip disease. A major cause of idiopathic osteoarthritis of the hip. In *The Hip.* Proceedings of the third open scientific meeting of the Hip Society (Vol. 3). CV Mosby, St. Louis, 1975.
20. Tsahakis, P. J. Brick, G. W, Poss, R., Reilly, D. T., and Thornhill, T. S.: Proximal femoral osteotomy in the treatment of stage III osteonecrosis of the hip. Presented at the 60th Annual Meeting of the AAOS, February 20, 1993, San Francisco, CA.
21. Wagner, H.: Osteotomies for congenital hip dislocation. In: *The Hip.* CV Mosby, St. Louis, 1976. pp. 45–66.
22. Wagner, H.: Experiences with spherical acetabular osteotomy for the correction of the dysplastic acetabulum. *Progress in Orthopaedic Surgery*, 2:131, 1978.

10

Arthrodesis: The Vancouver Technique

Robert W. McGraw, Clive P. Duncan, and Christopher P. Beauchamp

INDICATIONS/CONTRAINDICATIONS

Arthrodesis is one of the alternatives to hip arthroplasty. Though infrequently advocated, it remains a valuable operative solution for treating a variety of conditions affecting the young hip. Regardless of apparent improvement in prosthetic design and arthroplasty technique, it should be considered with caution in the young in view of ongoing problems with loosening, breakage, disassembly, and rapid wear leading to osteolysis.

Arthrodesis of the hip is ideally indicated in the young, unskilled male manual laborer with monarticular hip disease. Contraindications to this operation are low back pain and ipsilateral knee disease.

The Vancouver technique for hip arthrodesis is simple and precise. Immediate mobilization and early protected weight bearing are permitted. Concentric reamers are used to achieve maximum coaptation, and a cobra plate is used to achieve rigid internal fixation. Medialization is achieved by reaming, thereby avoiding complex pelvic osteotomies. Trochanteric osteotomy with anatomic relocation preserves the abductors for possible future conversion to total joint arthroplasty. Supplementary immobilization such as hip spica is not necessary.

PREOPERATIVE PLANNING

Appropriate clinical and laboratory investigation should be carried out to ensure that the hip disease is monarticular and no significant pathology exists in the thoracolumbar spine or ipsilateral knee. It is important to measure leg lengths carefully and anticipate changes that will occur as a result of the permanent position of the hip joint.

R. W. McGraw, M.D., F.R.C.S.C and C. P. Beauchamp, M.D., F.R.C.S.C: Department of Orthopaedics, Vancouver Hospital and Health Science Centre, Vancouver, British Columbia, V5Z 4E3 Canada.

C. P. Duncan, M.D., F.R.C.S.C.: Department of Orthopaedics, University of British Columbia, Vancouver, British Columbia, V5Z 4E3, Canada.

The radiographs should be carefully evaluated to recognize potential intraoperative difficulties. Inadequate bone stock to permit stable coaption and fixation of the femoral head to the acetabulum would be a contraindication to the procedure, without the use of more specialized techniques. Retained fixation hardware around the acetabulum or in the femur may require removal to successfully complete the technique. Extensive osteonecrosis of the femoral head, after debridement of unstable collapsing bone, may result in a greater leg length discrepancy. The patient would need to be aware of this before operation.

Ongoing infection, in most cases, would require debridement and control before the definitive procedure. Rotational or angular malunion of the femur would require appropriate modification of the position of arthrodesis to ensure that the final position of the limb is satisfactory.

Otherwise, the clinical and laboratory work-up is quite standard and similar to that used for any major reconstructive orthopaedic procedure.

SURGERY

Patient Positioning

The patient is positioned laterally on the operating room table with the affected side up (Fig. 1) and secured. A cross table anteroposterior radiograph is obtained to confirm the ex-

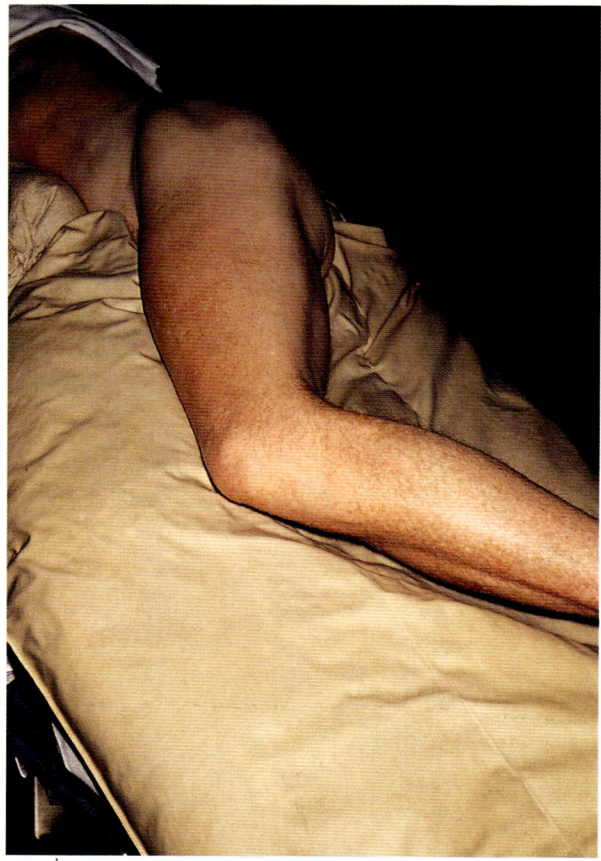

Figure 1. Patient in lateral position on operating room table, affected side up.

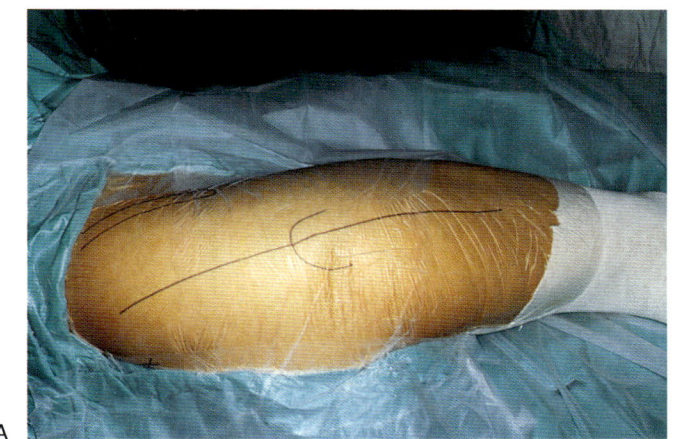

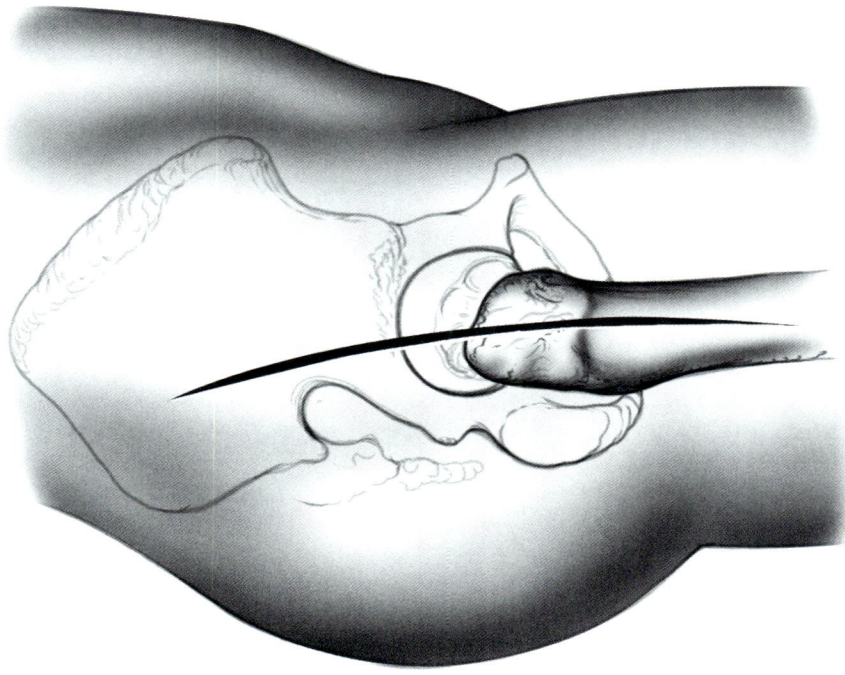

Figure 2 A, B. The incision is lateral, centered over the greater trochanter, extending somewhat posteriorly in its upper half.

act position of the pelvis. The underlying leg is placed in flexion to help reduce the degree of lumbar lordosis. This will assist precise positioning of the overlying leg in the desired final position of flexion. Patient positioning is crucial. The leg is prepped and draped free, leaving the knee and as much of the leg exposed as possible.

A straight lateral incision that curves slightly posteriorly proximally is made (Fig. 2 A, B). The fascia lata is divided and vastus lateralis is reflected (Fig. 3 A, B). The greater

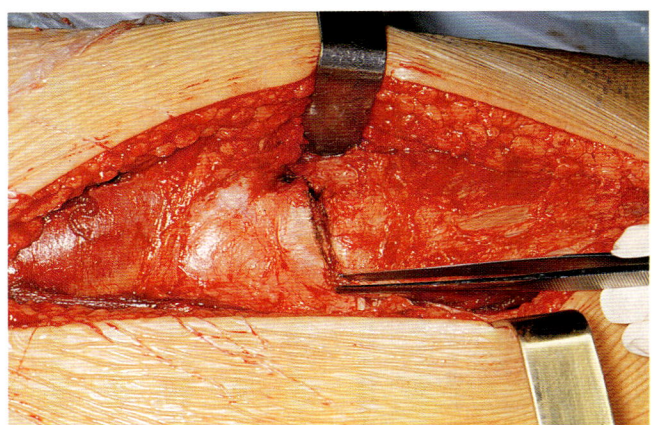
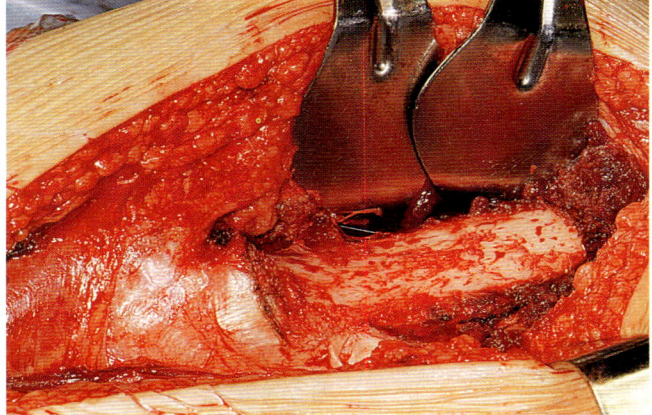

Figure 3 A, B, C. The femoral shaft is exposed by elevating the vasti.

trochanter is osteotomized and the abductor mass is elevated and retracted (Fig. 4 A, B). Great care is taken to protect the superior gluteal bundle. A generous capsulectomy is carried out and the hip is dislocated (Fig. 5 A, B). The acetabulum is then exposed. Medialization of the arthrodesis site is obtained by removing the medial acetabular bone to the inner wall of the pelvis (Fig. 6 A, B). The femoral head is shaped with a variety of instruments to remove osteophytes that would otherwise interfere with concentric reaming. An over-

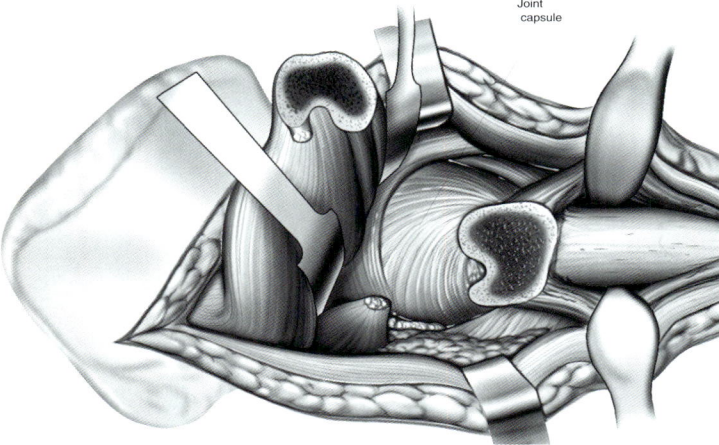

Figure 4 A, B. A standard trochanteric osteotomy is completed.

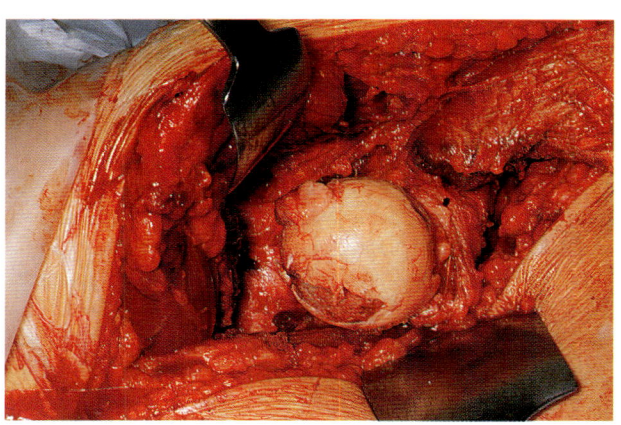
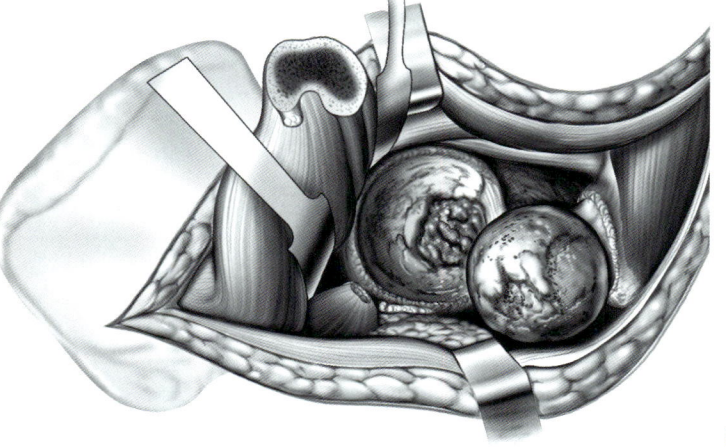

Figure 5 A, B. After a generous capsulectomy, the hip is dislocated anteriorly. The leg is placed in a drape-bag over the side of the table.

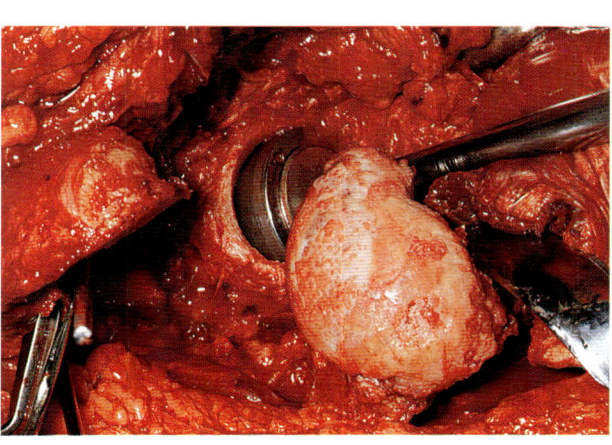
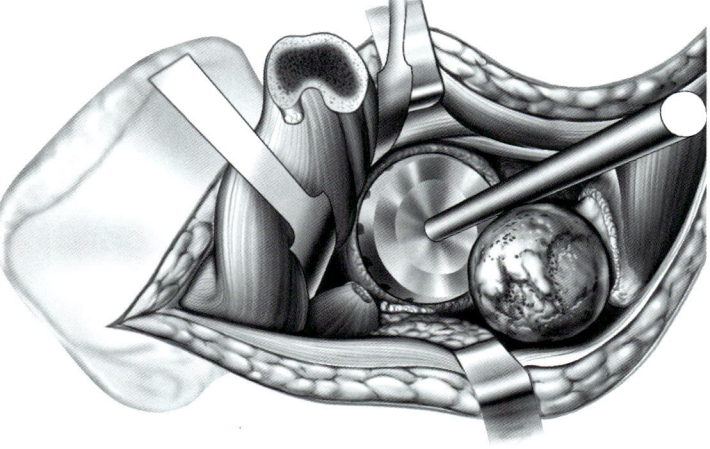

Figure 6 A, B. The acetabulum is reamed and modestly medialized.

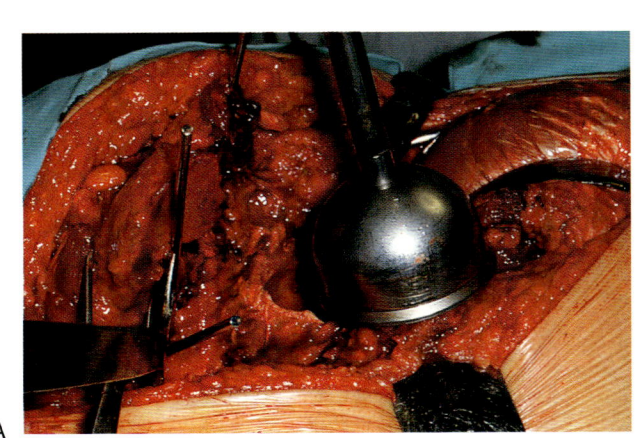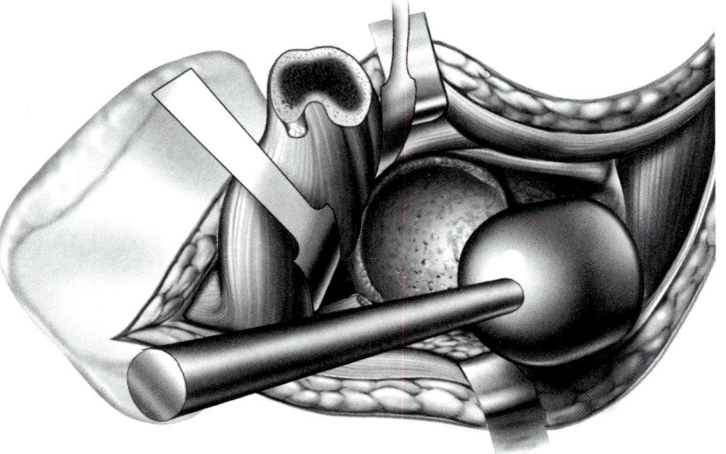

Figure 7 A, B. The femoral head is reamed with a matching concave reamer.

sized female reamer is used to shape the femoral head (Fig. 7 A, B). The reaming devices are selected in this manner in order to create a spherically congruent arthrodesis site (Fig. 8 A, B). The hip is reduced and the contact area is assessed. Usually this will result in a very tight cancellous-to-cancellous approximation (Fig. 9 A, B).

The leg is then carefully positioned and the cobra plate is affixed in the described fashion with one screw proximally. The desired final position is 20 degrees flexion, 5 degrees external rotation, and neutral duction (normally the femur is in 5 to 10 degrees of adduction with reference to the pelvis). As the application of compression tends to abduct the femur slightly, the initial application of the plate is applied with the leg adducted 10 degrees more than the desired final position (Fig. 10 A, B). The application of the compression plate begins with the central proximal screw through the roof of the acetabulum and the distal compression screw in the femoral shaft. Initial compression is applied and a check radiograph is taken to confirm that the femur is in the desired degree of adduction. This should measure 10 to 20 degrees so as to achieve the desirable final position when compression is

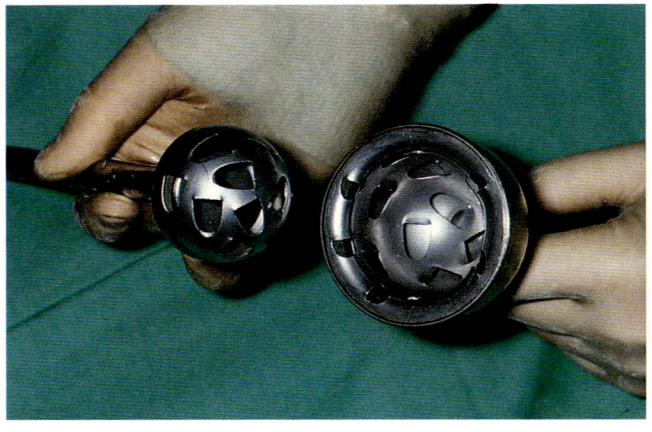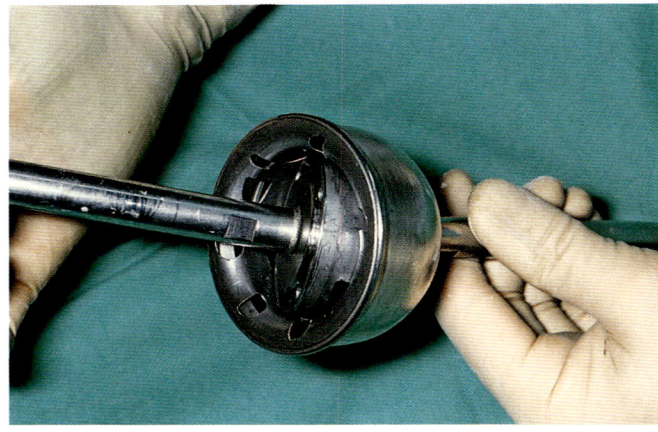

Figure 8 A, B. Matching reamers, formerly used for resurfacing arthroplasty of the hip joint.

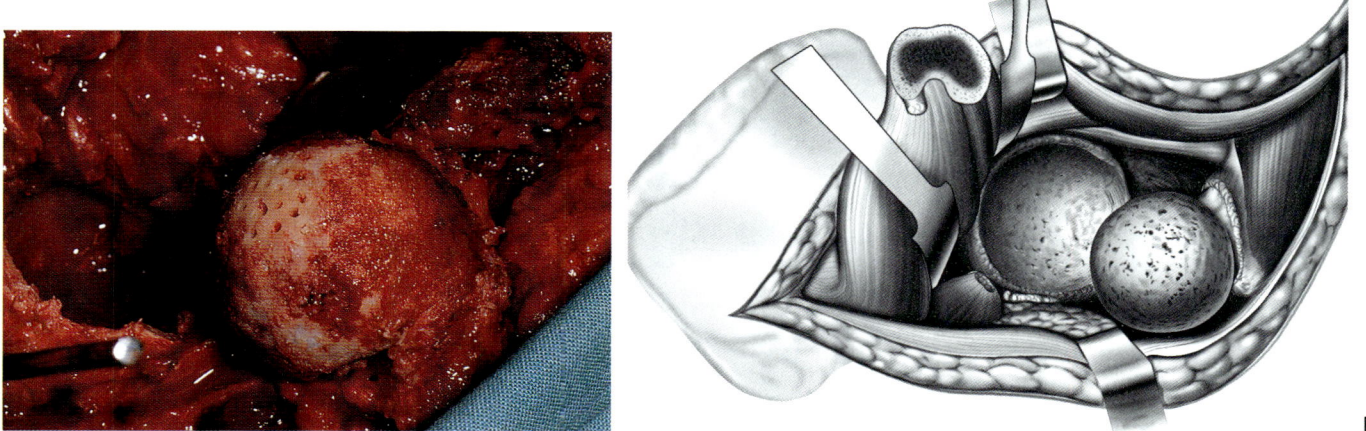

Figure 9 A, B. Prepared surfaces result in a very tight cancellous to cancellous approximation.

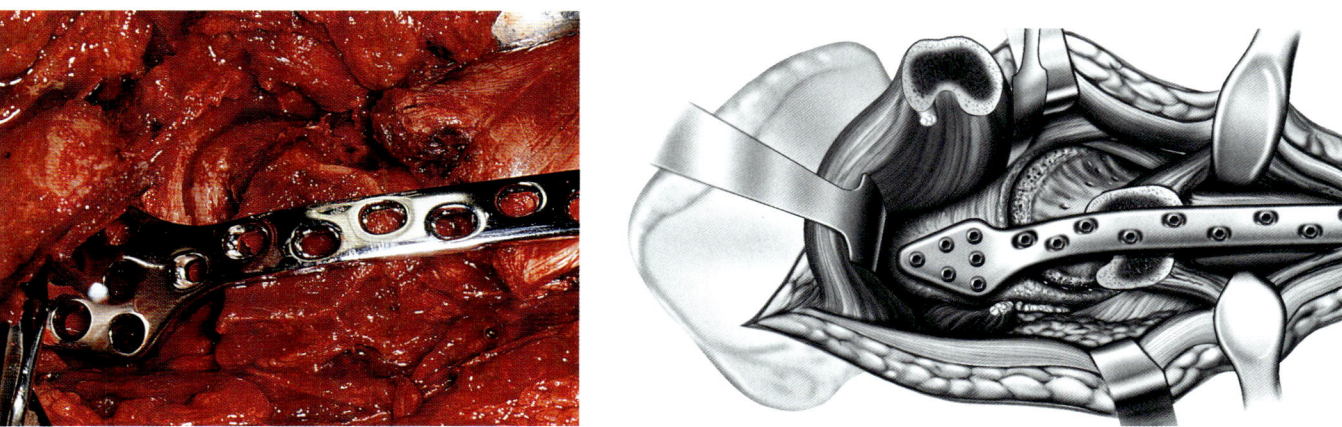

Figure 10 A, B. Application of the cobra plate after it has molded to the shape of the acetabulum and femur, and initial fixation with one proximal and the distal outrigger compression screw.

complete. If satisfactory, the remaining proximal screws are inserted, compression is completed, and the remaining screws are inserted into the femoral shaft. If there is any concern about position, another check radiograph is performed before the final screws are inserted. It is crucial to ensure that the correct degree of flexion is present before the proximal screws are inserted and the correct degree of rotation has been achieved before the distal screws are placed. Bone removed from the acetabulum and any additional bone from the greater trochanter region that was trimmed is used as a bone graft. The greater trochanter is reat-

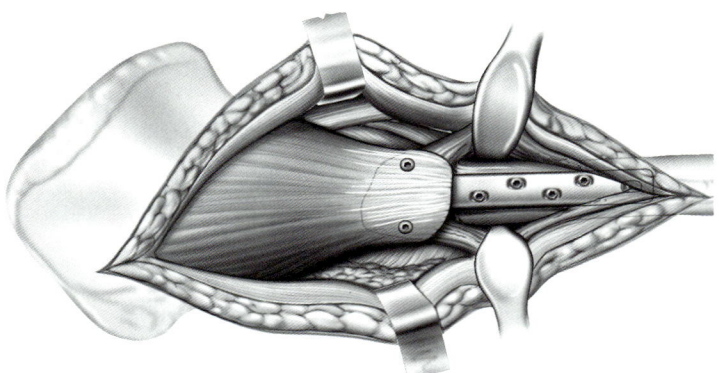

Figure 11. Replacement of the greater trochanter in the anatomic position.

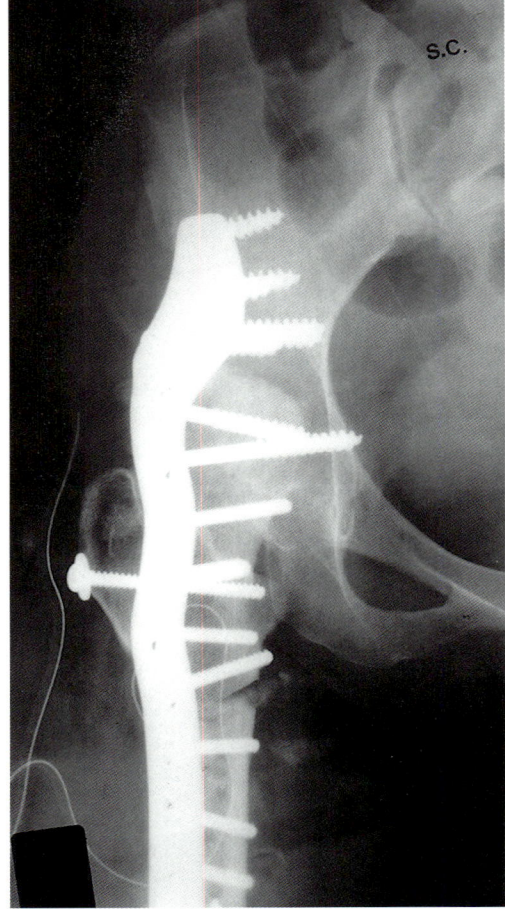

Figure 12. Final intraoperative radiograph.

tached in its normal position to preserve abductor muscle length (Fig. 11). A repeat radiograph is obtained (Fig. 12). The wound is closed in a routine manner.

POSTOPERATIVE MANAGEMENT

The patient is transferred to a standard orthopaedic bed and made comfortable with pillows. Mobilization begins on the first postoperative day. The drains, if used, are removed between 24 and 48 hours following surgery. Feather-touch weight bearing is permitted from the outset. The patient is discharged from hospital 5 to 7 days following surgery.

The patient is advised to use crutches at all times for three months following the surgery. With excellent coaptation and rigid internal fixation, partial weight bearing can begin at 3 weeks and gradually increase to full weight bearing by 12 weeks. The average time to independent, full weight bearing is 12 weeks.

In the straightforward case, union is expected at 3 to 4 months. The patient is followed up at 6 to 12 weeks. The persistence of pain, the presence of motion, and the failure of the joint space to become obliterated on the radiographs at six months would strongly suggest nonunion. This is particularly so if the screws are loose or if there is a halo of osteolysis around the screw tips.

If the patient received adequate education before the procedure and the technique is completed with precision, complete relief of hip pain is expected in every patient and a satisfactory level of function in the majority. It is wise to have the patient meet previous patients functioning well on a hip arthrodesis, before the operation. Return to work can be expected 6 to 12 months after the operation.

COMPLICATIONS

Malposition

Malposition can be avoided if the technique is followed precisely. Intraoperative radiographic monitoring will detect malpositioning, especially in difficult cases such as a previous femoral osteotomy.

Nonunion

Nonunion is very uncommon. Nonunion following this technique has been treated successfully by a precise repetition of the technique with bone graft and supplementary internal fixation.

Patient Dissatisfaction

Patient dissatisfaction may occur in spite of a successful arthrodesis. This outcome can be avoided by astute patient selection and appropriate preoperative education of the patient and family.

Unrelieved Pain

Continued pain in an apparently successful arthrodesis may necessitate the later removal of the internal fixation device.

ILLUSTRATIVE CASE FOR TECHNIQUE

A 36-year-old male presented with posttraumatic osteoarthritis of the left hip joint. He had been involved in a motor vehicle accident 18 years earlier at which time he sustained fractures of the left tibia and left femur. There was no obvious injury to the left hip joint. The left femur was treated by open reduction and intramedullary rod fixation. The left tibia fracture was treated closed. Both fractures healed, but on extraction of the intramedullary rod, the patient developed a wound infection. The infection resolved without surgical treatment and did not reoccur. At the time of presentation, the patient complained of constant left hip pain aggravated by activity and incompletely relieved by rest. The pain interfered with his sleep. His walking, sitting, and standing tolerance was all markedly limited.

The patient was employed as a computer programmer. He had essentially abandoned all former leisure activities. The patient expressed a desire to resume a wide range of physical activities without restriction.

On examination, the patient presented as a cooperative man (height 170 cm, weight 90 kg). His gait was characterized by a short left stance phase with associated trunk shift. There was a full range of pain-free spinal motion. No abnormality was noted in the right hip, right knee, or left knee. In the left hip the range of motion was 10 to 50. There was a fixed 35-degree external rotation contracture with a fixed adduction of 15 degrees. There were no neurovascular abnormalities. There was 2 cm of left thigh atrophy.

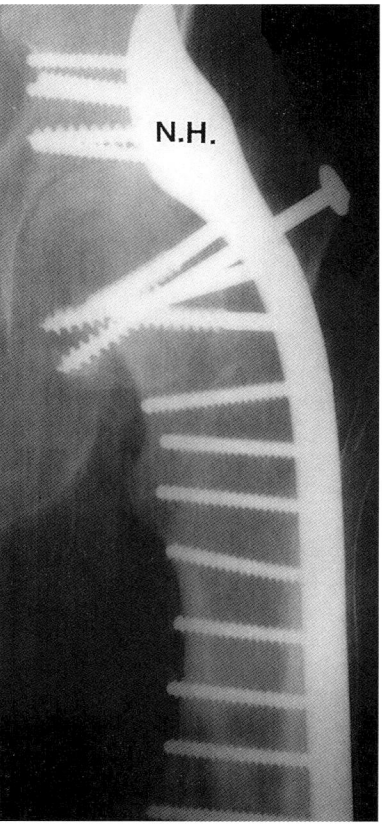

Figure 13. Radiograph of left hip arthrodesis in the illustrative patient.

Radiographs revealed end-stage, posttraumatic osteoarthritis of the left hip without evidence of infection. A healed ipsilateral femoral fracture was noted. Radiographs of the right hip, right knee, left knee, and lumbar spine were normal.

Arthrodesis was selected as the method of choice in view of patient age, patient expectation, body habitus, absence of low-back pain or ipsilateral knee disease, and history of a resolved local wound infection. After appropriate education, the patient and his partner demonstrated an understanding of the expected outcome.

The operation was performed by the described method (Fig. 13). The immediate postoperative course was uneventful. At three months following the surgery the patient was fully weight bearing, pain free, and walking without support. When seen and examined 10 years later, the patient said he did not consider himself to have any significant functional limitation. He had not developed any new musculoskeletal symptoms. Radiographs revealed a solid hip arthrodesis (Fig. 14 A, B). He continues to work as a computer programmer. In his leisure time he enjoys jogging, golf, and weight training. He continues to be pleased with the outcome of the surgery at 10 years and is aware of the possibility of conversion to total hip arthroplasty should he develop a problem in his low back and/or ipsilateral knee.

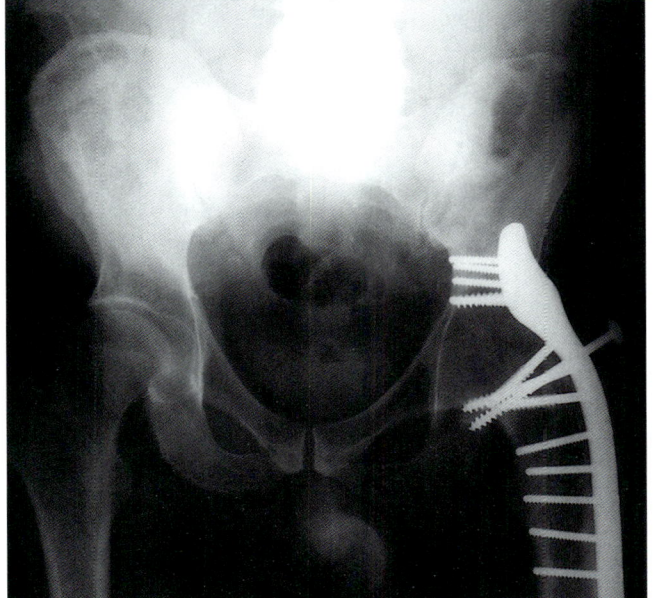
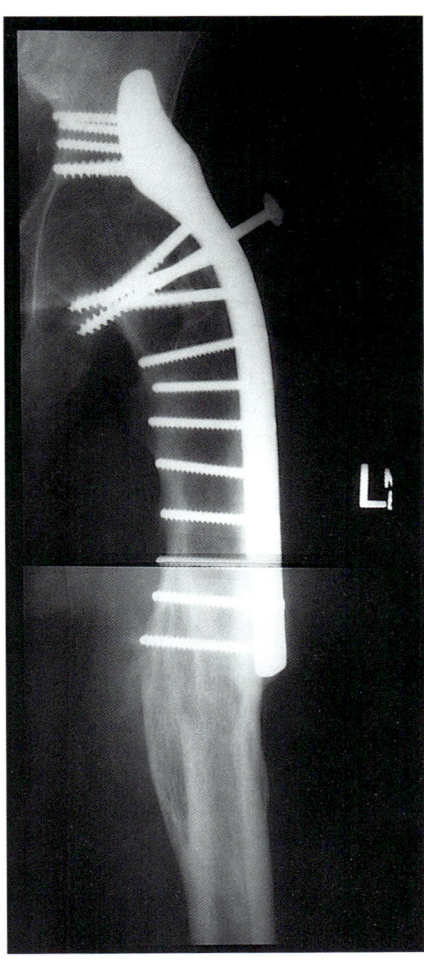

Figure 14 A, B. 10-year follow-up radiograph in the illustrative patient.

RECOMMENDED READING

1. Barmada, R. Abraham, E., and Ray, R. D. Hip fusion utilizing the cobra head plate. *J. Bone Joint Surg.*, 58(4):541–544, 1976.
2. Beauchamp, C. P., Duncan, C. P., and McGraw, R. W. Don't throw away the reamers - a new technique of hip arthrodesis, *J. Bone Joint Surg.*, 67-B(2):330, March 1985.
3. Fulkerson, J. P. Arthrodesis for disabling hip pain in children and adolescents, *Clin. Orthop. Re. Res.* 128:296–302, 1977.
4. Kostuik, J. and Alexander, D. Arthrodesis for failed arthroplasty of the hip. *Clin. Orthop. Rel. Res.*, 188:173–82, 1984.
5. Schneider, R. Hip arthrodesis with the cobra head plate and pelvic osteotomy, *Reconstr. Surg. Traumatol.*, 14(0):1–37, 1974.
6. Sponseller, P. D. McBeath A. A., and Perpich, M. Hip arthrodesis in young patients. A long-term follow-up study, *J. Bone Joint Surg.*, 66:853–859, 1984.

PART IV

Primary Total Hip Arthroplasty

11

Templating

Clement B. Sledge and John B. Sledge

PREOPERATIVE MANAGEMENT

Preoperative hip templating allows the surgeon to choose appropriate implants and anticipate unusual needs such as special devices, allografts, or a different surgical approach, e.g., transtrochanteric, transfemoral. This preoperative planning greatly facilitates accomplishment of the surgical goals of restoration of hip mechanics and leg length equality.

Restoration of hip mechanics is accomplished by establishing the appropriate relationship between the abductor moment arm and the moment arm through which body weight acts. In patients with osteoarthritis, this normally requires deepening the acetabulum that has migrated upward and outward. In patients with rheumatoid arthritis, by contrast, there is often an element of protrusio, and the acetabulum must be restored to its normal, more lateral position. The second aspect of restoration of hip mechanics is to restore the offset between the greater trochanter and center of the rotation of the head (Fig. 1). Because this is the moment arm through which the abductor muscles act, this moment arm must be restored, or abductor weakness will result. Restoration of the moment arm is accomplished by choosing a femoral implant with the appropriate offset.

In the absence of pelvic obliquity or, less commonly, hip contractures, discrepancy in *true* leg lengths and in *apparent* leg lengths on the two sides will be the same. Because of the usual age of patients needing total hip arthroplasty, pelvic obliquity is often fixed and related to degenerative changes in the lumbar spine with scoliosis or to arthritis involvement of the lumbosacral junction. In such cases, it is important to recognize that restoration of equality of the true leg lengths will result in the patient's feeling that the newly operated leg is either too long or too short. It is important, therefore, to use restoration of equality of *apparent* leg lengths as the appropriate goal of preoperative planning. One way that we find most reliable to assess differences in apparent leg lengths is to ask the patient to stand with the shorter leg on a wooden block. Varying thicknesses of block can be chosen until the patient feels that leg-length equality has been restored. The thickness of the block is the ad-

---

C. B. Sledge, M.D. and J. B. Sledge, M.D.: Department of Orthopedics, Brigham and Women's Hospital, Boston, Massachusetts 02115.

ditional length that should be added to the hip at the time of surgery. If there is no fixed pelvic obliquity, this amount will equal the difference between the true leg lengths.

Once the leg-length difference is determined by clinical evaluation, measurements are made on the patient's AP pelvic radiograph. Confirm that the hip to be operated on is short secondary to the intraarticular pathology. First determine a reference point for measurements; the "U body" or tear drop at the medial inferior aspect of the quadrilateral plate is useful for this purpose (Fig. 2). Draw a line connecting the bottom of the teardrop on the right with the bottom of the teardrop on the left. This "teardrop line" provides the reference point for further measurements. Next, find a readily reproducible landmark on the lesser trochanter. Sometimes this is the apex of the convexity of the lesser trochanter, and sometimes it is easier to identify the flat shoulder where the proximal portion of that lesser trochanter meets the femoral shaft. Locate the identical point on the opposite hip. Measure the vertical height from the teardrop line to the point chosen on the lesser trochanter. The difference between the measurement of this height on the two sides should equal the difference in true leg lengths. If it does not also equal the height of the block used to give the patient a sensation of leg length equality, there is a fixed pelvic obliquity. Because most elderly patients will not be able to correct their fixed pelvic obliquity, apparent leg length should be equalized using the thickness of the block as the target amount to be restored. If the pelvic obliquity is determined to be mobile, true leg lengths can be equalized.

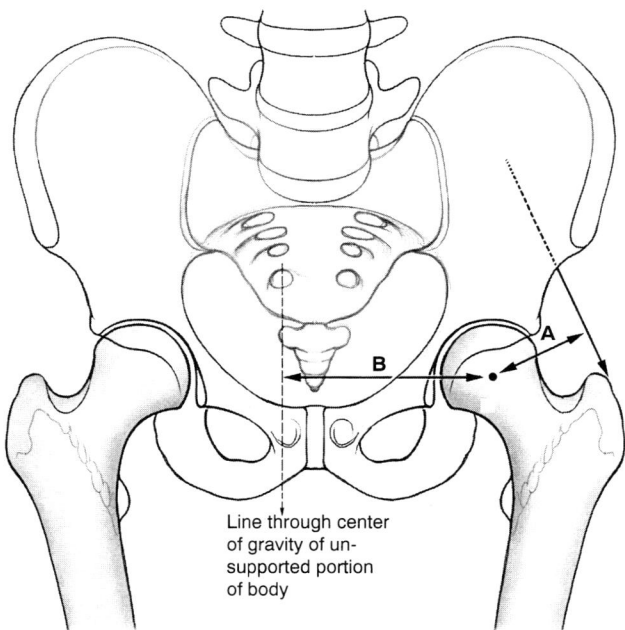

Figure 1. Drawing of an AP radiograph of the pelvis. Distance "A" is hip offset measured from the abductor muscle (or greater trochanter) to the center of the femoral head and represents the offset or moment arm through which the abductors exert force. "B" is the moment arm of body weight and is the distance between the center of the femoral head and the center of gravity of the body in single-leg stance on the opposite leg.

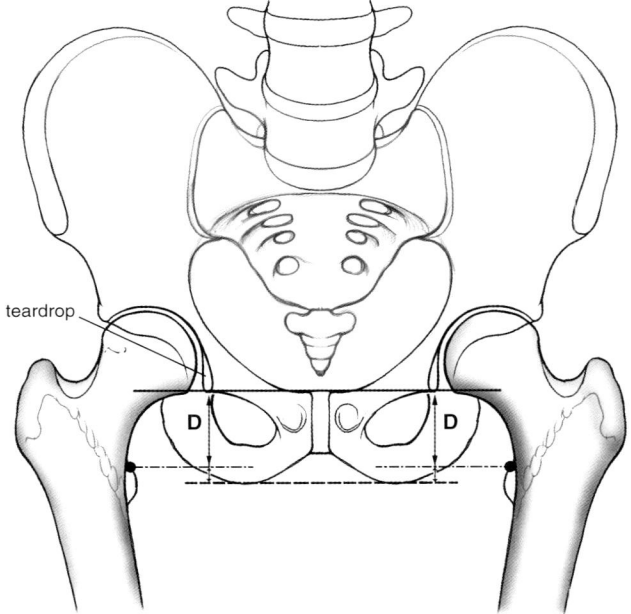

Figure 2. As in Fig. 1, "D" is the distance from the tear drop to an arbitrary point on each lesser trochanter. In situations where the tear drop is indistinct, a line connecting the ischial tuberosities can be used as illustrated by the dashed line.

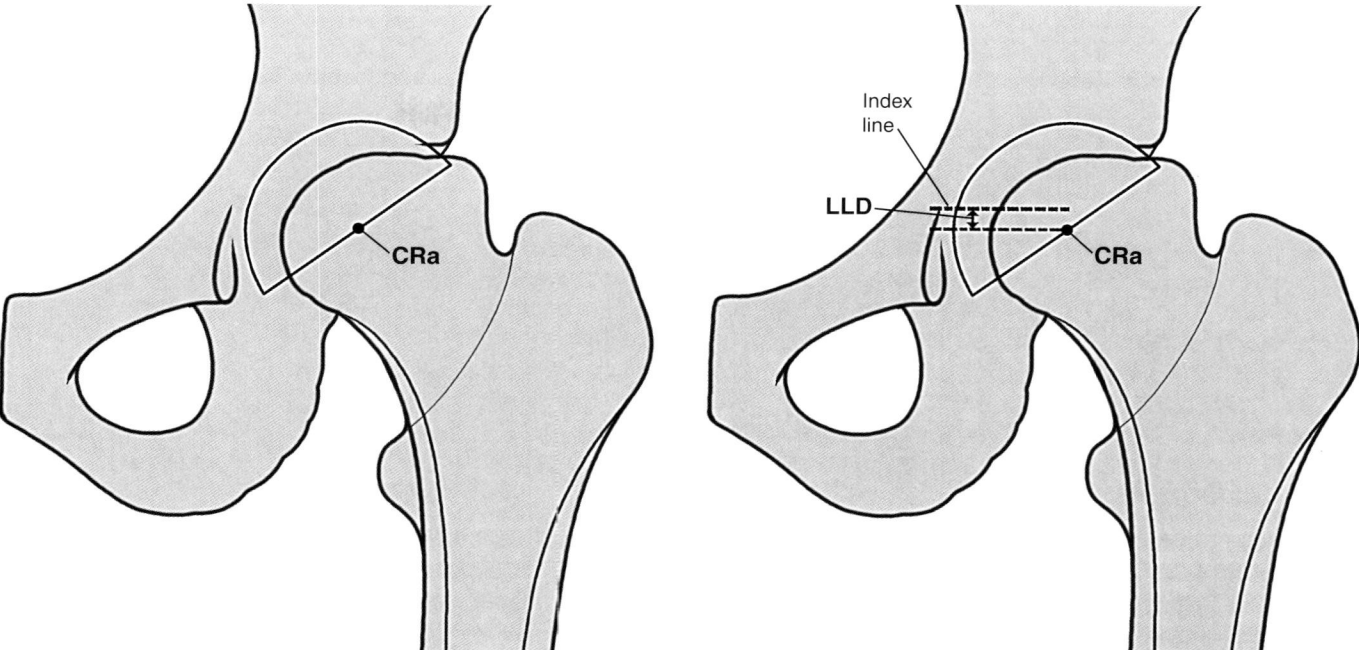

Figure 3. An acetabular template has been superimposed on the pelvic radiograph, maximizing bony containment of the component. The center of rotation of the acetabulum, CR$_a$, is marked on the radiograph.

Figure 4. The amount of additional length desired (LLD) is measured *above* the CR$_a$ and the "index line" is added to radiograph.

Using prosthesis x-ray templates, locate the desired position of the acetabular component, medializing to decrease the body moment arm and placing the template in a position to maximize bony containment of the component (Fig. 3). Mark the center of rotation of the acetabular component in this new location (CR$_a$). Next make an index mark (I) above the acetabular center of rotation at a distance equal to the amount of additional leg length desired (thickness of the block used to equalize the legs) (Fig. 4).

Choose a femoral component template of a sufficient size to fit the canal and with appropriate offset to restore the abductor moment arm (Fig. 5). The template will have a mark designating the center of rotation of the femoral head (CR$_h$) with various neck length/head sizes. Choose one that will lie on the index mark above the center of rotation of the acetabular component. There are usually two or three neck lengths that can be chosen; choose one that optimizes offset and places the femoral component in the femoral canal with 10 to 15 mm of inferior femoral neck remaining after resection. Mark the neck resection on the radiograph and measure the distance of the neck cut above the top of the lesser trochanter. This length should be written on the x-ray and referred to at the time of surgery when choosing the appropriate location for the neck cut. In addition, measure from the top of the lesser trochanter to the CR$_h$ chosen and mark that distance on the radiograph (Fig. 6). This will provide an additional measurement at the time of surgery, with a trial femoral component in place, that appropriate restoration of leg length has been achieved.

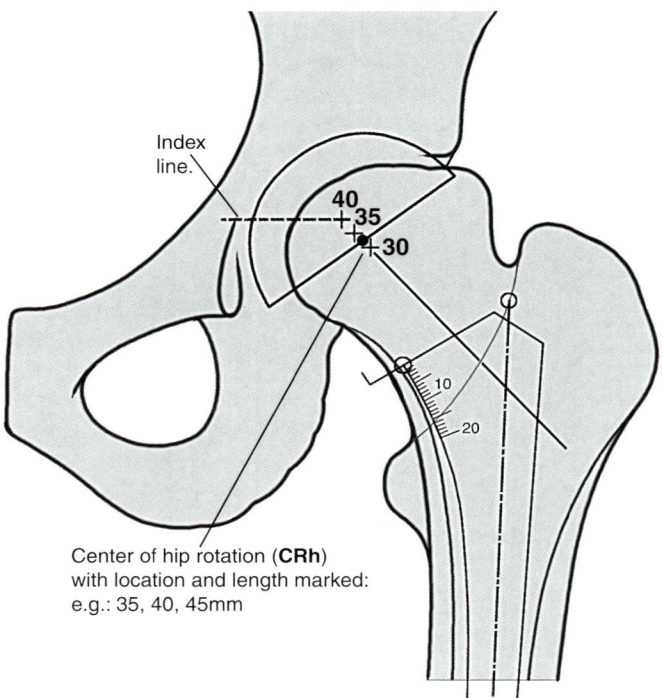

Figure 5. The femoral template is superimposed on the radiograph so that one of the available neck lengths (30, 35, or 40—representing heads of 0, +5 or +10 mm) is at the level of the index line.

ILLUSTRATIVE CASE FOR TECHNIQUE

A 70-year-old male presented with chronic left groin, thigh, and knee pain that had become progressively more severe over a 2- to 3-year period. Despite using two canes for support, he was able to walk less than 100 yards without being stopped by pain. In addition, he

Figure 6. With the proper templates in place, two additional measurements can be made: The level of neck resection (15 mm in this case) and the final neck length as measured from the top of the lesser trochanter to the index line. During surgery the final neck length is checked with trial components in place by measuring from the top of the lesser trochanter to the center of rotation of the trial femoral head.

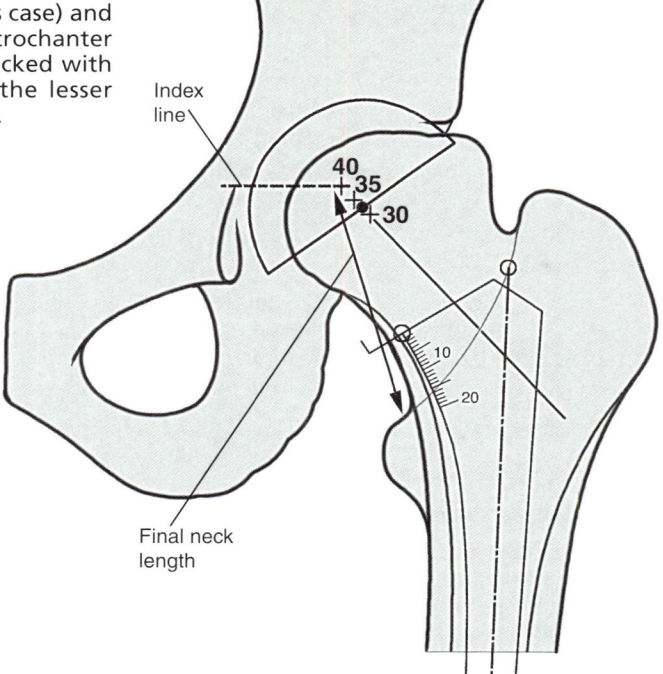

experienced night pain that awakened him from sleep each night, and he was unable to reach his shoes and socks or trim his toenails. He was not able to do stairs reciprocally even with his canes and a hand rail and had difficulty arising from a chair and getting in and out of a car. He was otherwise in good health and was retired from the military.

On physical examination, it was found that left hip flexion was limited to an arc of 70 degrees from a 20-degree flexion contracture with further flexion to 90 degrees. He had essentially no internal or external rotation and attempts to carry out rotation of his hip resulted in spasm and pain about the hip.

When he was standing, his left pelvis was low and produced a subjective sensation of a short left leg. By placing varying thickness blocks under the left foot while he was standing, it was found that a height of 9.5 mm produced a subjective feeling of leg length equality, although the left pelvis remained low because of his fixed pelvic obliquity. Radiographs of his pelvis revealed lumbar scoliosis and pelvic obliquity secondary to osteoarthritic disease at the lumbosacral junction (Fig. 7). Measuring from the apex of the lesser trochanter to the tear drop gave measurements of 50 mm on the right and 33 mm on the left for a true descrepancy of 17 mm (Fig. 8). His hip was templated by first establishing the center of rotation for the acetabular component, then drawing a line 9.5 mm above that for the desired leg length correction. A femoral template was then chosen and placed over the radiograph so that a +5 head (the 40 mm mark on the template) overlay the index line. This indicated a neck cut of 12 mm and an overall neck length of 55 mm. This plan was executed at

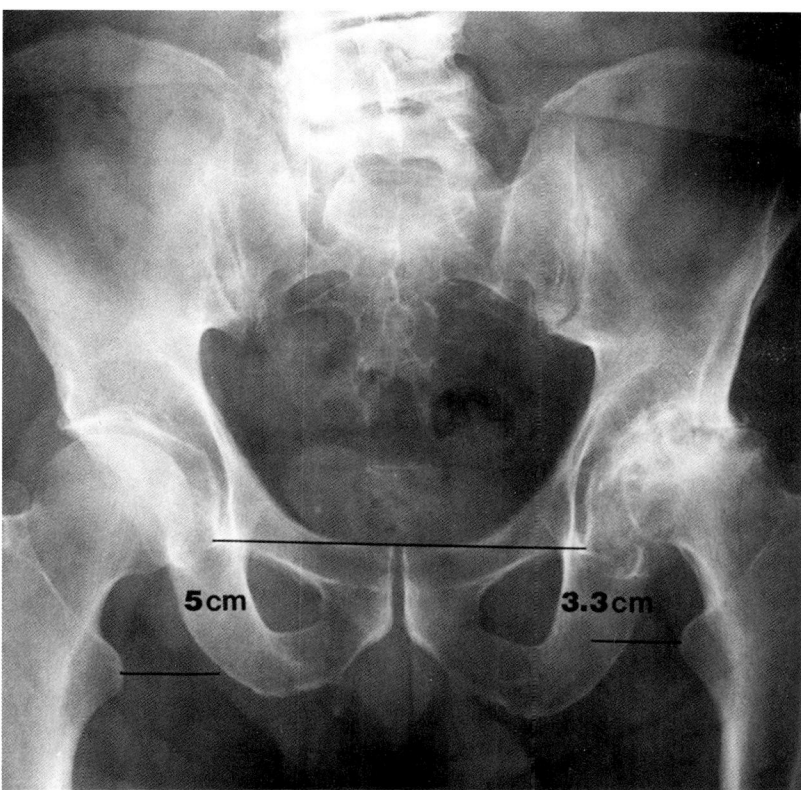

Figure 7. Preoperative radiographs of the patient showing measurement of the distances from the midpoint of the lesser trochanter to the tear drop on each side. The measurements indicate a true discrepancy of 17 mm.

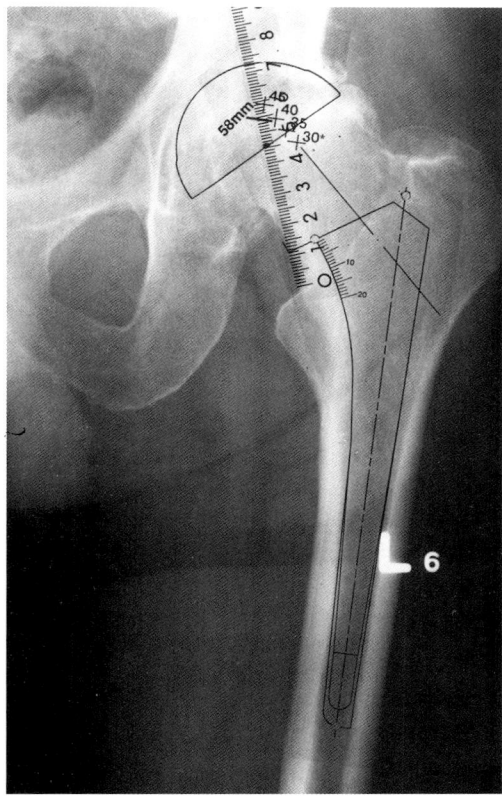

Figure 8. With both acetabular and femoral templates in place, a component neck length of 40 is indicated (plus 5 head), a femoral resection level of 12 mm, and a final neck length of 58 mm are indicated.

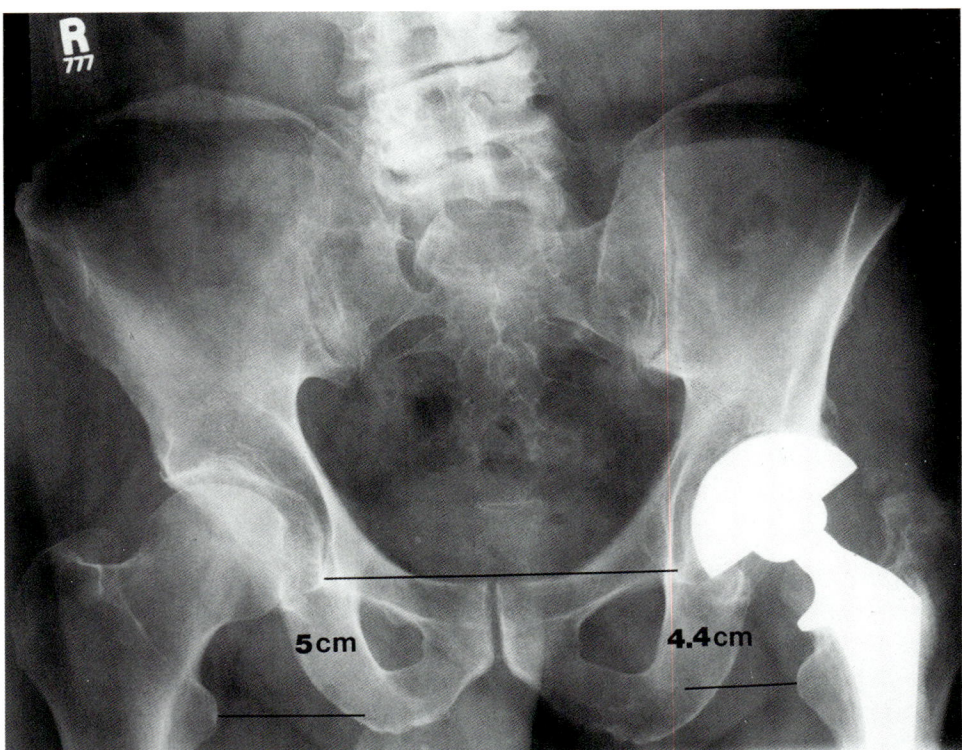

Figure 9. Postoperative radiographs reveal good placement of components with addition of 11 mm of length to the short leg, providing restoration of relative leg lengths, recognizing the fixed nature of the pelvic obliquity.

surgery (Fig. 9) and the post operative radiographs show excellent reproduction of the desired goals. The length added to the short side was 11 mm vs. the measured 9.5 mm discrepancy).

RECOMMENDED READING

1. Charnley, J.: *Low-friction Arthroplasty of the Hip: Theory and Practice.* Springer-Verlag, Berlin, 1979.
2. Ranawat, C. S., Dorr, L. D., and Inglis, A. E.: Total hip arthroplasty in protrusio acetabuli of rheumatoid arthritis. *J. Bone Joint Surg.*, 62:1059, 1980.

12
Cemented Primary Total Hip Arthroplasty

Chitranjan S. Ranawat, Michael J. Maynard, and Rajiv G. Deshmukh

INDICATIONS/CONTRAINDICATIONS

The orthopedic community has extensive experience with the use of surgical cement for bonding a prosthesis to bone in the human body—dating back over 25 years. Although alternative methods of bonding an implant to the bone have been developed, none has yet been shown to be as good as or better than cement for either short- or long-term fixation of total hip arthroplasty prostheses.

Cemented fixation is most durable when a perfect microinterlock between bone and cement is achieved at the time of primary implantation. Formation of an optimal bond is the challenge faced by each surgeon's technical competence.

Our indications for selecting cemented fixation in primary total hip arthroplasty (THA) include:

1. Patients who are 65 years old or older and those patients whose projected remaining life span is 15 years or less.
2. Patients whose bone quality is poor and would therefore not support the use of noncemented fixation.
3. Patients with past history of infection who require reimplantation where a local high level of antibiotic delivered by mixing with the cement would be beneficial.
4. Patients who have a neoplasm affecting the hip.
5. Patients who desire cemented fixation based on informed consent.

C. S. Ranawat, M.D.: Department of Orthopedic Surgery, Cornell University Medical Center, Lenox Hill Hospital, New York, New York 10021.

M. J. Maynard, M.D.: Cornell University Medical Center, Hospital for Special Surgery, New York, New York 10021.

R. G. Deshmukh, M.B., M.S., F.R.C.S.: Comprehensive Arthritis Service, Hospital for Special Surgery, New York, New York 10021.

We are unaware of any absolute contraindications to cemented fixation in primary total hip arthroplasty. However, scrutiny of patient demographics with respect to long-term survivorship data for cemented primary hip arthroplasty has indicated that the following attributes are associated with shorter survival of cemented fixation:

1. Age below 55 years
2. Weight above 80 kg
3. Active lifestyle (e.g., occupation requiring heavy labor)
4. Male gender

Therefore, for patients with two or more of these risk factors, we often choose alternative fixation methods such as porous ingrowth or hybrid techniques.

PREOPERATIVE PLANNING

Physical Examination

The differential diagnosis of primary hip pain is beyond the scope of this discussion. Our comments will be limited to the evaluation and management of patients clearly indicated for total hip arthroplasty because of severe arthritic involvement of the hip joint.

Patients with significant arthritic involvement of the hip may present with a variety of clinical symptomatology including pain, tenderness, gait disturbance, decreased range of motion, leg-length discrepancy, synovitis, and bursitis.

Adult patients usually present with pain, typically in the groin, as their chief complaint. The pain may persist at rest and may be present at night. Decreasing functional range of motion is commonly only a secondary complaint, and leg-length discrepancy is often unrecognized by the patient. Pain interfering with sleep or with routine activities of daily living or recreation is the most common symptom motivating patients to seek surgical relief.

Physical examination of a patient with hip pathology should, as a minimum, include the appraisal of:

1. Hip range of motion
2. Gait and motor power of hip abductors, extensors, flexors, and adductors
3. Relative leg lengths
4. Neurovascular status of both lower extremities
5. Status of the ipsilateral knee, ankle, and foot
6. Status of the lumbar spine

The evaluation of range of motion should be aimed at the detection of significant soft-tissue contractures that may need to be addressed at surgery.

Motor weakness of the abductors or extensors, when present to a moderate degree, may significantly affect the expected functional outcome. In these cases, patients should be informed that a limp requiring use of a cane may persist indefinitely after arthroplasty. In severe cases, such as may occur with long-standing ankylosis, consideration for the use of a constrained prosthesis to avoid the risk of dislocation may also be warranted.

Leg length discrepancy, if severe, may not be surgically correctable and this fact should be addressed in preoperative discussions with the patient.

The neurovascular status of both lower extremities should be documented preoperatively. Any obvious skin infections or areas of impending skin breakdown constitute an absolute contraindication to proximal implantation of an arthroplasty. An accurate preoperative examination is also important to the diagnosis and treatment of problems which may arise postoperatively. Complications involving the opposite "downside" leg have been reported during hip surgery performed in the lateral decubitus position.

The status of the ipsilateral knee, ankle, and foot are important to the success of postoperative rehabilitation. The foot and ankle must be stable, plantigrade, and free from skin problems. The knee must be stable. When all joints of the lower extremity are affected by arthritis to the extent that surgical intervention is indicated, we proceed by first achieving a satisfactory foot and ankle, followed by treatment of the hip and later the knee. In cases of severe knee deformity or instability, it may receive treatment before the hip.

The status of the lumbar spine should be determined preoperatively. Symptomatology attributable to lumbar spine pathology will not be relieved, and in some cases may be exacerbated, by the treatment of an arthritic hip, and the patient should informed of this possibility.

Long-Range Surgical Preparation

Proper surgical technique begins with appropriate preparation. Good quality roentgenograms, standardized to allow accurate estimation of magnification and templating, are the first necessity. We routinely obtain the following radiographs on all of our total hip arthroplasty patients:

1. AP of the pelvis and both hips
2. Frog-leg lateral of the affected hip
3. AP of the lumbar spine
4. Lateral of the lumbar spine

Roentgenograms of hips affected by arthritis reveal loss of joint space due to destruction of the articular cartilage. Osteophyte formation is common in most forms of degenerative arthritis but may be absent in rheumatoid arthritis. Cyst formation may also be apparent. Patients presenting with avascular necrosis may demonstrate collapse of the femoral head.

Protrusion deformity of the acetabulum may be present in a significant portion of patients with inflammatory arthritis. The appearance of this problem represents significant bone loss in the pelvis and presents difficult technical problems to the reconstructive surgeon.

Scrutiny of preoperative films should seek to answer three questions:

1. Can reconstruction be performed using an available off-the-shelf prosthesis, or should ordering of a specially sized, modified, or custom-made implant and associated bone-working tools be considered?
2. Is there significant superior and/or medial protrusion deformity, and will bone grafting be required to make up for bone loss in order to restore the hip center of motion to the proper position?
3. Is cemented or noncemented fixation likely to be the optimal choice for best long-term performance?

To answer the first question, templates of the intended implant system must be available for comparison with the radiographs (templating). Standard sizes of off-the-shelf prostheses will be appropriate for the vast majority of patients. In these cases, templating should be aimed at estimating the required implant sizes to ensure their availability in the operating room. On the AP pelvis radiograph, the distance from the lesser trochanter to the anatomic center of rotation of the hip should also be determined. This is most easily done on the opposite hip if it is uninvolved with arthritis. This distance gives an estimate of the length that must be recapitulated by the prosthetic joint reconstruction in order to achieve satisfactory leg-length equality.

Juvenile rheumatoid arthritis patients with their small bone size and frequently excessive anteversion, valgus, and protrusion deformities and acromegaly patients with their large bone size are the most likely patient groups to require fabrication of custom implants, or modification of existing implants, in order to achieve proper prosthetic fit. If a custom implant appears indicated, computed tomography (CT) scanning of the hip joints and proximal half of the femurs will be required to provide the detailed anatomical information required by the design engineers.

Several reports have described methods for the roentgenographic evaluation of protrusion. The primary significance of the magnitude of a protrusion deformity is that it reflects the amount of bone loss in the direction of the protrusion. This bone loss must either be replaced with bone graft or effectively offset by the prosthetic implants in order to achieve a successful reconstruction. The movement of the center of rotation of the joint off the proper anatomic position also disrupts the balance of the muscle forces across the hip joint by changing their directions of pull and the lengths of their moment arms. Over time, this leads to the development of soft-tissue contractures. These contractures must be ameliorated during joint reconstruction in order to achieve restoration of the center of rotation to the proper position and restore muscle balance.

Once the surgeon has located the proper anatomic position of the acetabulum on the roentgenogram, the relationship of this position to the actual bony acetabular limits will help define the technical requirements for acetabular reconstruction. If there is medial protrusion, a medial bone graft will likely be indicated in all but the mildest cases. Small to moderate amounts of superior bone loss can often be treated by surgically opening the mouth of the acetabulum and using a larger prosthesis. In cases where superior migration has enlarged the acetabulum by more than 15 to 20%, as estimated on the A/P view, bone grafting will be required. The best sources of bone graft, if available, are the resected femoral head and neck, and the iliac crest. Otherwise, femoral head allografting may be necessary and should be anticipated. Depending on the shape of the defect, the type and shape of the graft, and the quality and quantity of the supporting pelvic bone, fixation of the graft may be by interference fit or with screws. In some cases, the use of a protrusion ring may also be beneficial. The surgeon tackling a large protrusion deformity should be familiar with the preparation and fixation of bone grafts and the use of protrusion rings and should have these devices available to him or her in the operating suite.

The question of whether to use cemented or noncemented fixation involves the assessment of several variables including the patient's age and remaining life expectancy, activity level, bony deformity, and bone quality. Improvements in cementing technique have rendered cemented fixation extremely reliable and durable for both femoral stem fixation and socket fixation in the presence or absence of bone grafting. Therefore, the advantages of using noncemented fixation in a particular patient should be clear cut if cement fixation is to be eschewed.

As a final aspect of long-term surgical preparation, the surgeon should consider alternative courses of action if intraoperative technical complications, such as femoral fracture or perforation of the medial wall of the acetabulum, occur—as can easily happen when one is dealing with the osteoporotic bone of rheumatoid arthritis. The prudent surgeon will provide for solutions to these problems in the form of additional bone graft, wire mesh, long-stem implants, cerclage wires, and other devices available to the knowledgable professional.

Immediate Preoperative Patient Preparation

If possible, total hip arthroplasty patients, especially those with inflammatory arthritis, should be admitted to the hospital no later than the night before surgery. This allows time for adequate last-minute patient instruction and physical preparation and the assembly of all essential preoperative evaluations. Most standard protocols include a patient shower with Phisohex or Betadine and a bowel-cleansing enema on the night before surgery. In addition, most anesthesia protocols require that the patient ingest nothing by mouth after midnight of the night before surgery as a precaution against aspiration of stomach contents during anesthesia. Hospital admission on the day before surgery facilitates the accomplishment of these precautions.

Intravenous antibiotic prophylaxis is started just prior to surgery, with completion of infusion of the first dose just prior to the incision. It is continued for 48 hours postoperative.

Our first choice drug is cefazolin, vancomycin is administered to those patients with known or suspected allergy to penicillin and its analogues.

SURGERY

Selection of the Prosthesis

Our preferred cemented acetabular prosthesis is fabricated of ultra-high molecular weight polyethylene, non-metal-backed, with a combination of inner and outer diameter, which allows, for wear considerations, at least an 8-mm thickness of polyethylene at all points. Thus, a 22-mm inside diameter should be chosen when the outer diameter of the polyethylene socket is 50 mm or less. A 28-mm inside diameter may be used for outer diameters between 50 and 60 mm. A 32-mm inside diameter may be chosen, if desired, for outer diameters greater than 60 mm—especially if use of a -5 neck length option, usually available in this head size, would optimize the reconstruction.

The design of the cemented stem prosthesis and broaching system should provide for a uniform cement mantle at least 3 to 6 mm thick at all points, without significant stress risers. The prosthesis should be able to reproduce the anatomic geometry of the hip with respect to leg length, offset, and abductor moment arm. The ideal cemented prosthesis provides torsional stability with flat anterior and posterior surfaces and has a rounded medial surface. Furthermore, the design should allow easy access to all surfaces of the proximal stem, should revision surgery become necessary. The need for a collar on the prosthesis is controversial. Currently the preferred material for fabrication of the femoral stem implant is chrome-cobalt alloy and the surface finish should be roughened appropriately for a good mechanical bond with cement.

Chrome-cobalt femoral heads are preferred over titanium because use of titanium femoral heads has been associated with significantly accelerated wear of the polyethylene compared with the performance of the same diameter head using a cobalt-chrome alloy.

Anesthesia

In our experience, epidural anesthesia, with controlled hypotension, is the optimal anesthesia method for the performance of total hip arthroplasty. With this method there is reduced bleeding from all sources, which leads to significantly shorter operative time by direct lessening of the time the surgeon is occupied with hemostasis. Furthermore, cemented fixation of implants is improved by weakening of the hydraulic barrier formed by the blood in bone. This effectively lessens the resistance to cement intrusion into the bone as has been demonstrated by improvement of the roentgenographic appearance of the acetabular cement–bone interface achieved at surgery using this anesthetic technique.

Operative Technique

After preparation of the patient by the anesthesiologist has been completed, the patient is placed in the lateral decubitus position on an operating table, which has been fitted with anterior and posterior bolsters to hold the patient securely about the pelvis. The longitudinal position of the patient is adjusted so that the anterior bolster is positioned at the level of the symphysis pubis. The posterior bolster is directly opposite the anterior one, covering the top part of the gluteal crease in a properly positioned patient. With the patient held in a lateral position that is perpendicular to the floor, the bolsters are adjusted toward each other to form an effective "clamp," which holds patient securely. After tightening of the bolsters, the "downside" lower extremity should be observed for a few minutes to detect significant obstruction of venous return if it should occur. If this is noted, the bolsters should be adjusted until this problem is resolved (Fig. 1). We also place a pulse oximeter on one of the toes of the downside extremity for continuous monitoring during the operation. We then place soft cloth and foam-rubber padding around the lower extremity to avoid pressure sores. Proximally, we place a very soft "jelly-roll" bolster under the patient's axilla to prevent pressure on the brachial plexus. Both of the patient's arms and the patient's head are supported on pillows.

The performance of a proper hip arthroplasty requires a wide exposure (Fig. 2). We use a postero-lateral approach to the hip joint without trochanteric osteotomy most of the time. However, in cases where there is a severe distortion of the femoral or acetabular anatomy—as is often the case in congenital hip dysplasia, protrusio, posttraumatic arthritis, and revision arthroplasty, one should not hesitate to use a transtrochanteric approach. Under these conditions, a trochanteric osteotomy is definitely advisable and is often clearly superior in providing wide exposure.

At the time of the skin incision, the subcutaneous tissues are also sharply divided to expose the fascia. Then, palpation of the greater trochanter will aid the surgeon in choosing the proper position for the fascial incision. An appropriately placed fascial incision will course approximately 1 cm anterior to the insertion of the gluteus maximus onto the lateral femur (Fig. 3). The fascial fibers are divided sharply, and the fibers of the gluteus maximus are separated bluntly or with electrocautery, in line with the muscle bundles. The tendinous insertion of the gluteus maximus onto the shaft of the femur is divided with electrocautery. At this point, attention is given to hemostasis and installation of protective moist sponges and a Charnley retractor at the wound edges.

The short external rotators of the hip and the posterior one-third of gluteus minimus are now detached from their insertions on the posterior edge of the greater trochanter and are allowed to retract posteriorly (Fig. 4).

The hip capsule is opened first along its insertion onto the posterior femoral neck. A trapezoidal capsular flap is then formed by cutting the capsule radially near the superior border of the insertion of the piriformis tendon superiorly and near the inferior border of the inferior gemellus muscle insertion inferiorly. A narrow bent Hohmann's retractor is

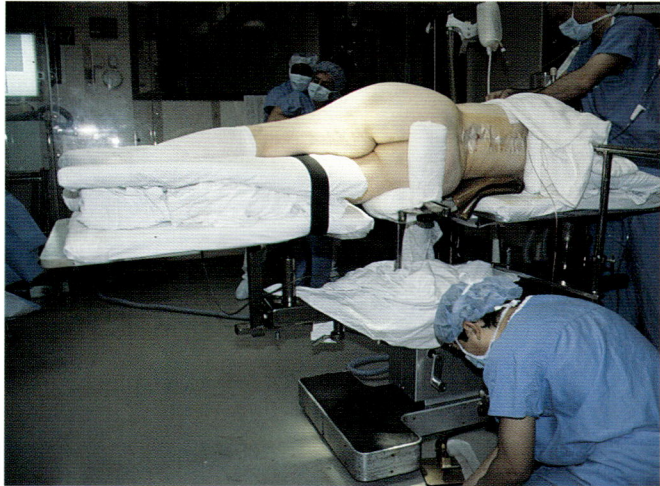

Figure 1. Patient positioned for left hip arthroplasty. The table is specially equipped with bolsters, which act as a "clamp" on the pelvic region. Note the thick padding under the right hip and the soft "jelly-roll" pad in place under the right axillary and chest region. The right leg is thoroughly padded. The left leg is free of restraint.

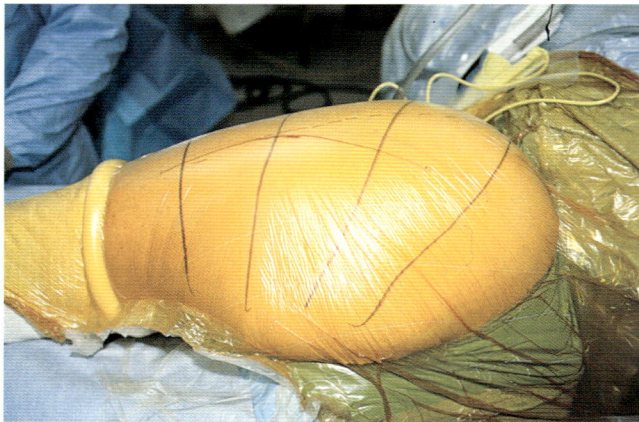

Figure 2. The left hip after prepping and draping. Transerve lines are drawn across the intended incision site for use as landmarks during final skin closure.

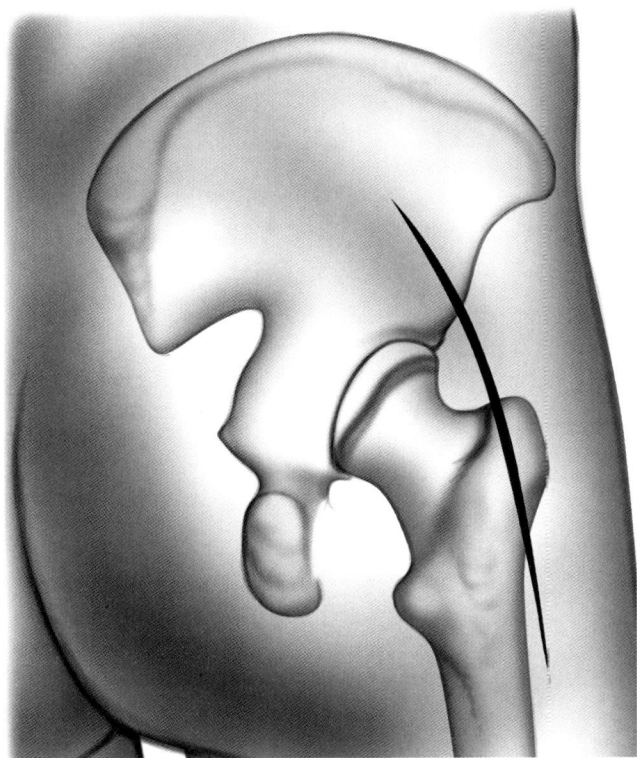

Figure 3. The skin incision is centered over the greater trochanter and extends distally over the shaft of the femur. It extends proximally with a slight posterior curve.

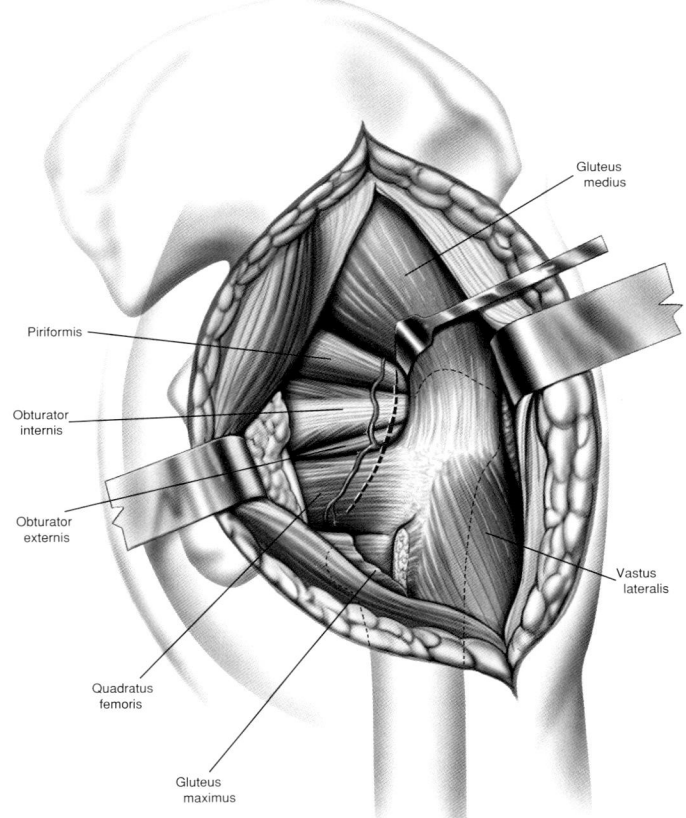

Figure 4. The short external rotators are detached near the insertion onto the greater trochanter.

then placed under the gluteus minimus, and the capsulotomy is extended superiorly and anteriorly. An Aufranc retractor is placed inferior to the femoral neck. The quadratus femoris is detached all along its femoral insertion down to the level of the lesser trochanter, and then the inferior part of the hip capsule is released as far inferiorly as can be easily viewed.

The hip can then usually be dislocated posteriorly with gentle adduction, flexion, and internal rotation. The center of rotation of the femoral head is now estimated and marked. Measurements are made and recorded from this point to the tip of the greater trochanter and the top of the lesser trochanter. The femoral neck cut is then performed at a 45-degree angle to the shaft of the femur at the level where the lateral end of the cut lies at the intersection of the superior cortex of the femoral neck and the greater trochanter (Fig. 5). The cut neck is sealed with bone wax to reduce the bleeding during acetabular preparation and fixation.

Attention is turned to the exposure of the acetabulum. A C-retractor is placed over the anterior lip of the acetabulum in front of the cut femoral neck. An Aufranc retractor is placed beneath the transverse acetabular ligament. The ligament is left intact, if possible, to act as a cement dam. A broad, bent Hohmann's retractor is placed into the bone just above the midpoint of the posterior wall. A Steinmann pin is placed superiorly to retract the gluteus medius and minimus.

The femur is mobilized anteriorly by releasing the reflected head of the rectus femoris muscle and the anterior hip capsule. Hip flexion and rotation are adjusted to provide the best exposure.

The labrum and synovial tissues obscuring the mouth of the acetabulum are removed sharply. The soft tissues in the acetabular fossa are also removed to allow a view of the true medial wall of the acetabulum.

The guiding principle of socket positioning is the normalization of the center of rotation of the hip in terms of superior inferior, anteroposterior, and medial lateral directions. Once adequate bony and soft-tissue exposure has been achieved, preparation of the acetabular bed should begin with progressive reaming—keeping this principle in mind—while attempting to provide at least 80%, and preferably 100%, coverage of the socket with viable bone (Fig. 6). One should also preserve as much hard subchondral bone as possible. In most cases the reaming is initiated with a 44-to-46-mm reamer directed medially until the true

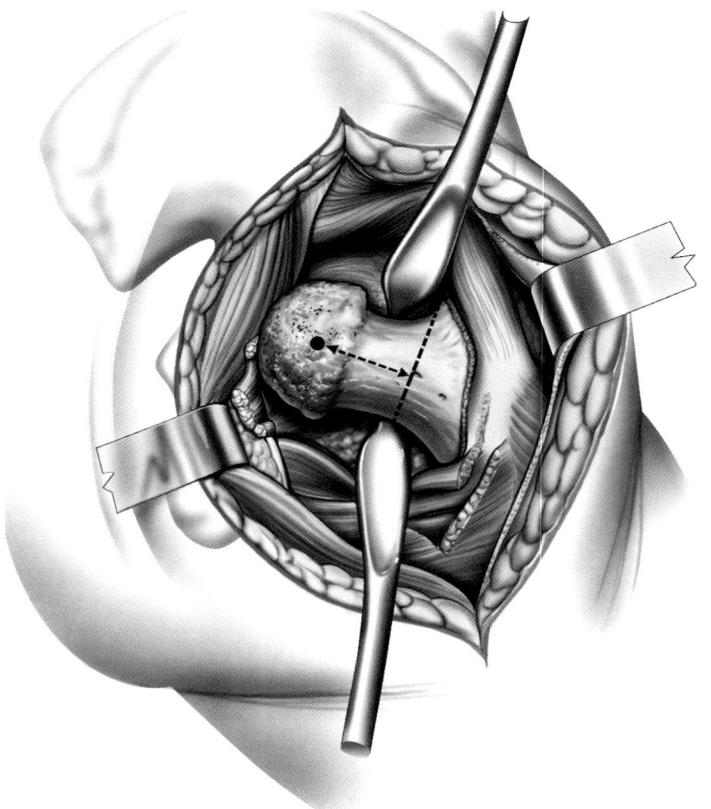

Figure 5. The femoral neck cut is made at a 45-degree angle to the shaft of the femur. The lateral point of the cut is at the junction of the femoral neck and the shaft.

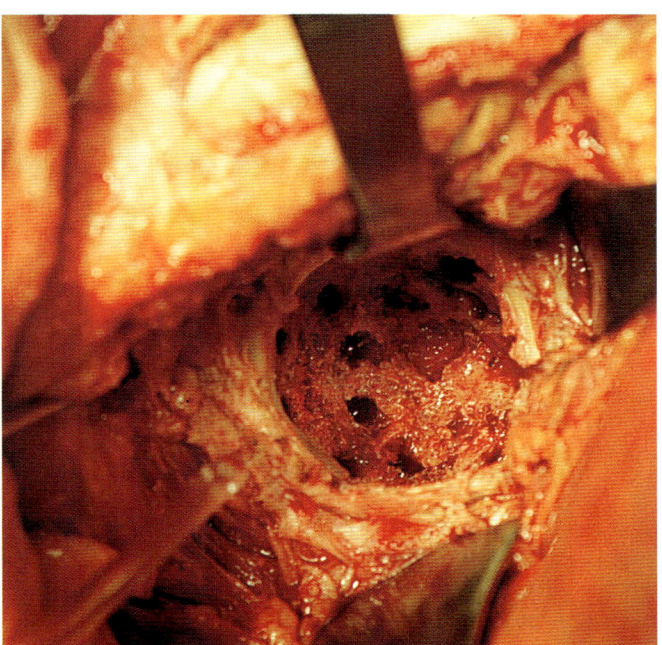

Figure 6. A properly prepared acetabular bed. Note the cement fixation holes.

medial wall of the acetabulum is reached. Progressive reaming should then ensue to enlarge the bony bed. Once the acetabular bed has been properly prepared, the size of the prosthesis to be implanted should be chosen to allow a uniform cement mantle of at least 2 to 3 mm thickness. The appropriate trial device may be used to assess the acetabulum and ensure provision for a homogeneous cement mantle of adequate thickness. During this maneuver one should form a mental picture of the proper position for implantation of the socket.

Next, maximize the surface area of the cancellous bone available for interlock with cement by fashioning multiple cement-fixation holes. A high-speed air-driven tool can facilitate the efficient creation of these anchoring holes. Place three relatively large (5 to 8 mm diameter, 8 to 10 mm depth) holes, one each in the ilium, ischium, and pubis, and several smaller holes in the superior aspect of the prepared bed. *Technical note:* in a properly reamed socket, the position for placement of the large holes is usually obvious because bleeding cancellous bone, revealing the medullary portion of the ischial and pubic bones, is often exposed—this is where the holes should be placed.

After reaming is complete and the anchoring holes have been prepared, the next step is to clean the bone thoroughly with a water pick. Then, perform a careful drying maneuver. This is done by packing the end of a clean, dry sponge individually into each of the large fixation holes and then pressing the rest of the roll into the acetabulum and holding it there for several seconds. The timing if this maneuver is crucial. The cement should already be mixed and within approximately one minute of the proper consistency for implantation at the time of final lavage and drying. In this way, as soon as drying is complete, the sponge can be removed and cement can be immediately pressed into a bed of clean, dry bone.

Presented evidence suggests that mixing the cement under vacuum (Fig. 7) and/or centrifuging the cement after mixing removes trapped air bubbles and improves the strength properties of the cement. We prefer to prepare the cement in the following manner:

The cement reagents are heated in a blanket warmer prior to surgery. This has the effect of speeding up the rate at which the cement cures after mixing. It also seems to aid in the release of air trapped in the cement during mixing—by causing it to bubble out.

The powdered and liquid forms of the cement are prepared in a mixing machine, which allows vacuum to be applied to the reagents during mixing.

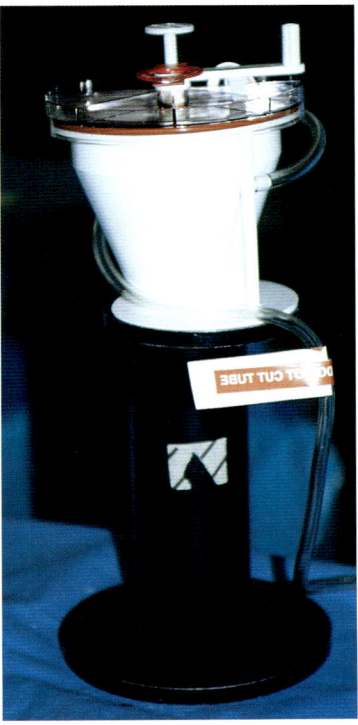

Figure 7. The vacuum mixing apparatus for acrylic cement.

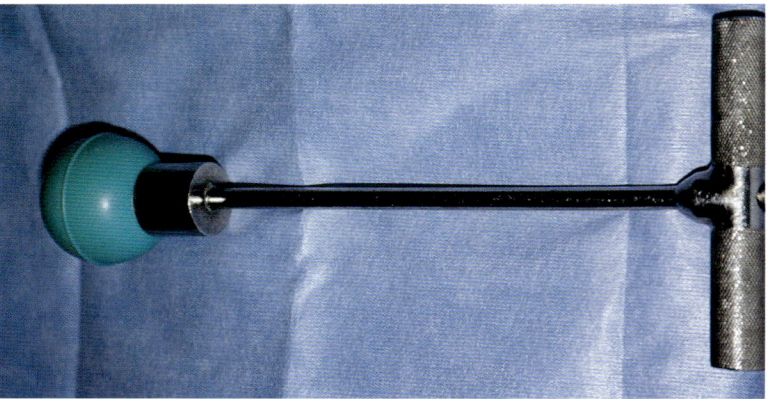

Figure 8. A hard rubber balloon on a handle, used to pressurize the cement into the acetabular bed.

Cement at 3 to 5 minutes of setting, which is slightly firmer than toothpaste consistency, can be rolled into a doughy ball. At this consistency, part of the cement should be coated over the outer surface of the acetabular prosthesis while it is on the holder. The rest of the cement is placed into the acetabulum and swiftly digitally pressurized into each of the large fixation holes. Then, this mass of cement is uniformly pressurized using a sturdy rubber balloon (Fig. 9). With this tool, pressure is applied for two to three minutes (Figs. 10, 11).

Next, immediately prior to implantation (Fig. 12) of the socket, any blood that has collected on the cement is cleaned off with suction and/or dry sponge. Then, using a curette, clean the cement away from the transverse acetabular ligament and nearby inferior margin of the acetabulum for a distance of about 5 mm—this is to avoid pushing cement into the obturator foramen when the socket is placed. Excess cement is removed from the periph-

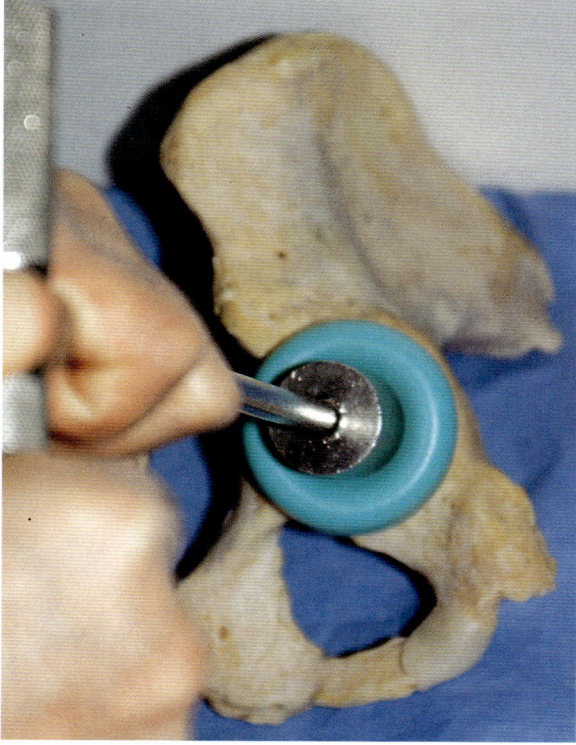

Figure 9. Demonstration of the balloon device on a cadaver model.

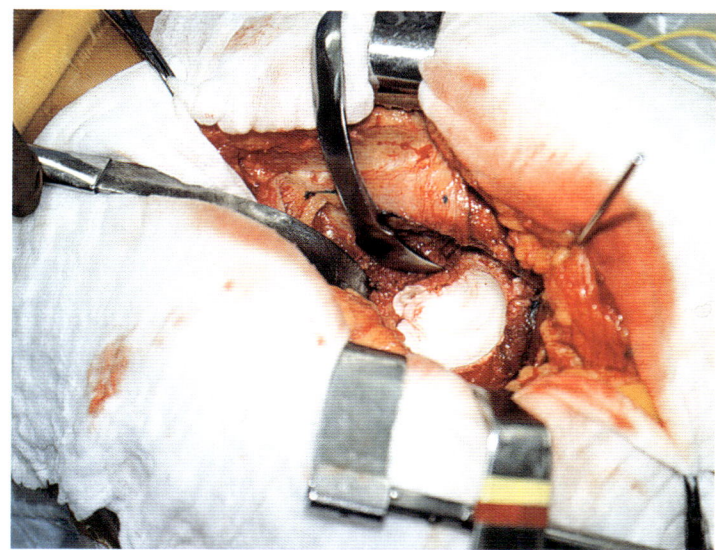

Figure 10. The ball of cement placed into the acetabular bed.

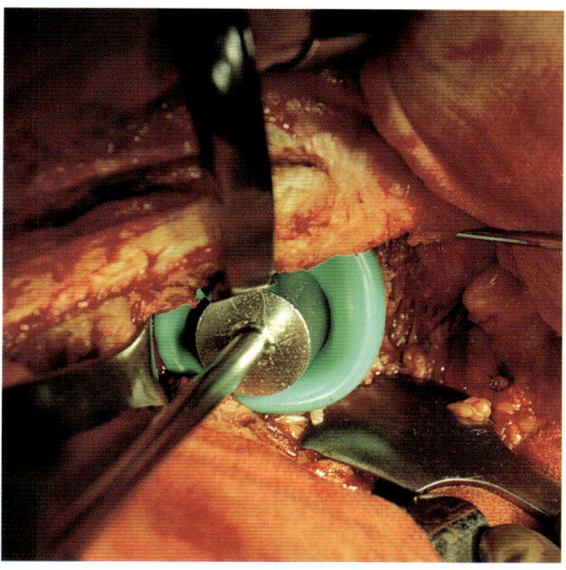

Figure 11. The balloon in use pressurizing cement in the acetabular bed.

ery of the acetabulum. The prosthetic socket, using the appropriate holder, is inserted into the cement, positioned, and pressed or impacted down into the properly medialized position. Meanwhile, it is also positioned at approximately 40 degrees of lateral opening and 15 degrees of anteversion. A "pearl" to remember at this point is that, in the absence of severe pelvic deformity, when properly positioned the prosthesis will completely occlude both of the large cement fixation holes placed in the ischial and pubic bones. If one or both is not completely occluded, recheck the socket position with respect to anteversion and lateral opening.

Pressure is maintained on the prosthesis while the cement hardens (Fig. 13). During this time, excess cement is removed from the periphery. Very often a portion of the prosthesis is left uncovered by bone superiorly. Digital pressure should be maintained, during the cement curing process on any part of the superior and posterior cement mantle that is left uncovered by bone.

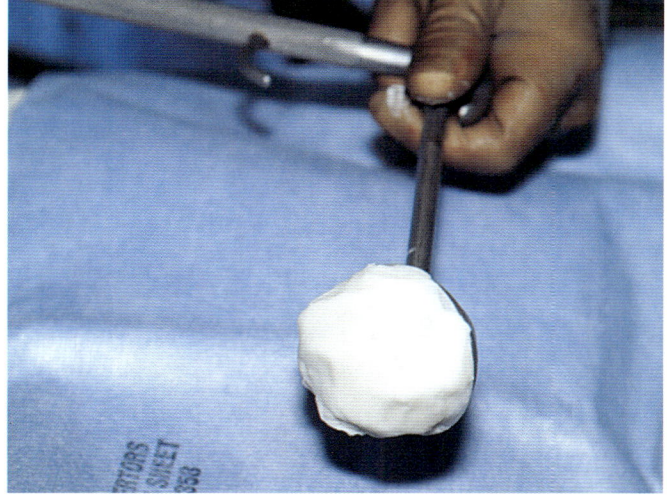

Figure 12. Cement is placed onto the prosthetic acetabular component prior to implantation.

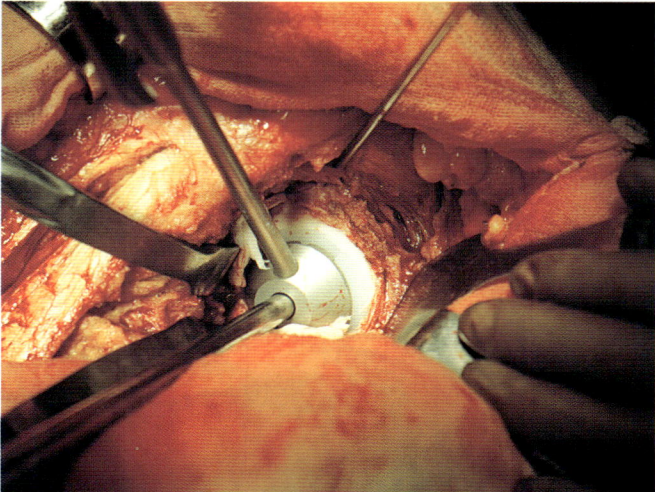

Figure 13. The acetabular component as it is pressed into place.

Once the cement has hardened, palpate the edges of the acetabulum searching for osteophytes and excess cement. Remove these, if present, using osteotomes and rongeur (Fig. 14).

Attention is now turned to the femur. The acetabular retractors are removed and a moist sponge is placed to protect the socket.

A large posterior femoral neck retractor is placed under the proximal femur and the leg is flexed and internally rotated to allow easy access to the femoral canal. An Aufranc retractor is placed to retract the soft tissues at the inferior margin of the femoral neck, and a narrow-angled Hohmann's retractor is placed under the gluteus medius superiorly to gain further exposure of the femoral canal and greater trochanter.

A "canal finder" or a straight intramedullary reamer with a pointed leading end is used to locate the medullary canal of the femur. The optimal starting point for this maneuver is at the piriformis fossa—located at the posterior corner of the intersection of the femoral neck and the greater trochanter (Fig. 15). The first reamer should be passed to a distance of approximately 150 mm. The medullary canal should then be prepared with progressively larger reamers (Fig. 16). Excessive reaming is not advisable, however, since this may remove the cancellous bone required for adequate cement interdigitation. Preoperative plan-

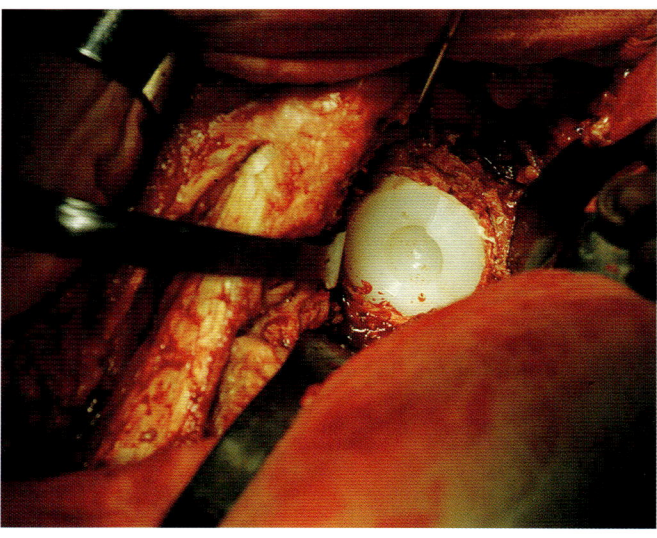

Figure 14. Acetabular component after implantation is complete.

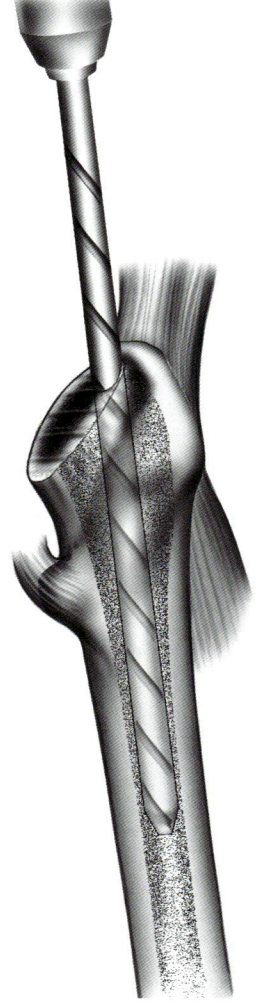

Figure 15. Femoral medullary reaming is begun at the posterolateral corner of the cut, in the region of the piriformis fossa.

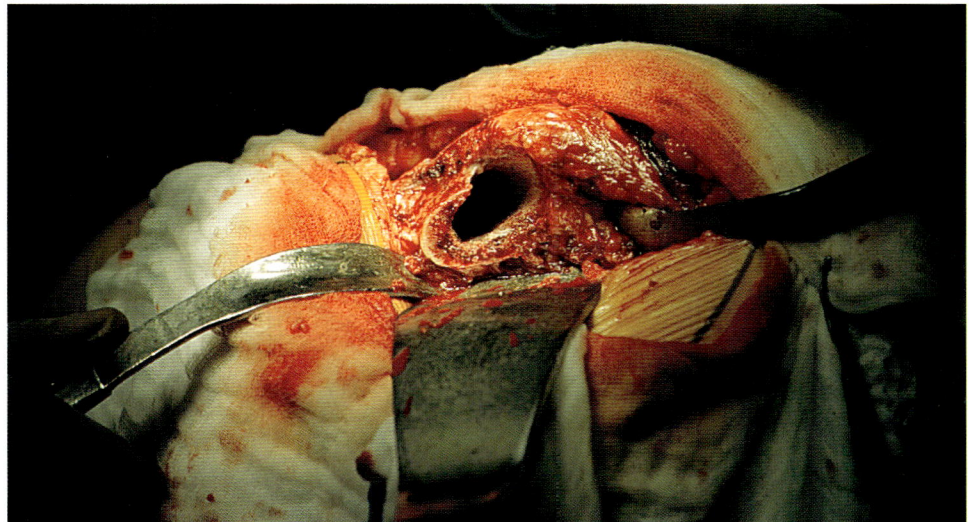

Figure 16. A properly prepared femoral canal.

ning using appropriate radiographs and templates can give the surgeon an estimate of the appropriate reamer size required.

The proximal femur is then broached up to the appropriate size using the broaches provided by the manufacturer of the prosthesis intended for implantation. During broaching, the desired amount of femoral anteversion should be maintained with each broach. The appropriate amount of femoral anteversion is determined by the patient's anatomy and gender and the position of the just-implanted socket. In general, this falls into a range of 0 to 15 degrees. The objective is to achieve a total anteversion of 25 to 45 degrees when the total anteversion of the socket and stem are considered together. Females fare better with combined anteversion closer 45 degrees while males require only around 20 to 30 degrees of anteversion for satisfactory function.

A trial implant of the appropriate size should now be placed into the medullary canal and impacted to the position desired for the actual implant. If using a modular system, the appropriate neck and head trials should be attached, and a trial reduction should be performed. Prior to trial reduction, it is a good idea to measure the distances from the center of rotation of this reconstruction to the greater trochanter and the top of the lesser trochanter. This will help the surgeon in the critical assessment of the trial reduction, the surgeon should assess the total anteversion, anterior capsule tension, leg length, and position required to dislocate the hip.

The total anteversion is judged by rotating the hip. while at neutral flexion/extension, to the position where the prosthetic neck is perpendicular to the face of the socket. At this point, the total anteversion is the amount of internal rotation of the hip. Two factors may confound this determination. First, the use of an elevated posterior rim on the socket (which is recommended) may make the perpendicular position a little more difficult to judge. Second, if the patient and/or the operating table have been tilted during the procedure, it may be difficult to determine frontal plane of the patient—the plane of reference for internal rotation—unless the tilt is corrected.

Anterior capsule tension should be assessed by palpation with the hip in neutral flexion/extension and complete external rotation. With a finger palpating the anterior capsule, the surgeon should use the other hand to rotate the femur externally. A small amount of external rotation should produce a palpable tightening of the capsule. If the capsule does not develop tension, consideration should be given to increasing the femoral neck length in order to tighten the anterior capsule and lessen the probability of anterior dislocation. If, on the other hand, the capsule develops excessive tension, consideration should be given to either reducing the neck length and/or offset or releasing the capsule (essentially an internal rotation contracture). It is usually prudent to release the anterior capsule in favor of preserving offset and neck length.

Leg length is judged by assessment of soft tissue tension and the measurements previously described. Position of the hip at dislocation is seen by internally rotating the hip while at approximately 10 degrees adduction and 30 degrees of flexion. The goal is a minimum internal rotation of 65 degrees in males and 75 degrees in females.

After trial reduction, the trial implants are removed, and the retractors are re-placed in the previously described positions. A cement restrictor should now be placed in the femoral canal. The distance at which it is to be placed should be measured directly off of the actual prosthesis which should, by now, be available in the sterile field. It should be placed deep enough to allow approximately 2 cm of cement distal to the tip of the prosthesis when fully seated. Cement preparation is now done as previously described, with the additional step of placement of the cement into a plastic cement "gun."

After the cement restrictor is placed, the medullary canal should be thoroughly lavaged with a water pick and suction. When the cement is within a minute of the proper consistency (toothpaste-like), a final lavage should be performed, followed by a drying maneuver with a clean, dry sponge. The sponge is packed into the canal and removed immediately prior to cement implantation. As soon as the sponge is removed, a final quick suction of the bottom of the canal is performed, and the cement is swiftly placed into the canal in a retrograde fashion—filling from distally to proximally (Fig. 17). The cement is digitally pressurized by placing the thumb of the distal hand to occlude the medial side of the top of the medullary canal while pushing a finger of the proximal hand (usually the index finger) into the cement (Fig. 18). More cement is placed to fill the detect created by the pressurizing finger and the procedure is repeated two or three times. Sufficient pressurization (Fig. 19)

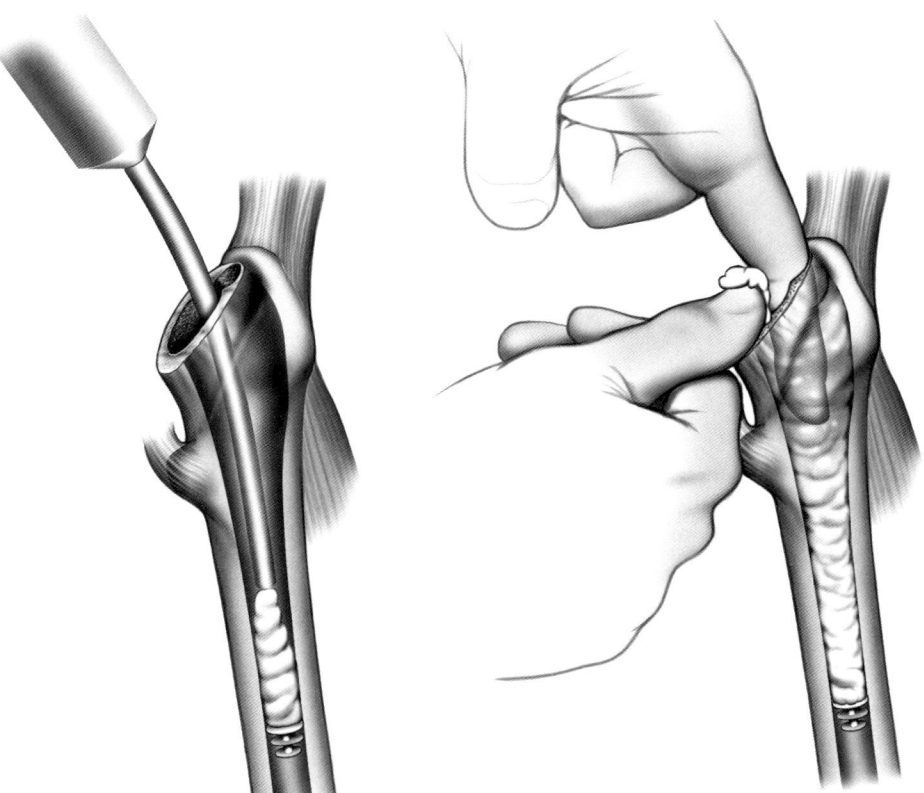

Figure 17. Cement is introduced in a retrograde fashion.

Figure 18. The cement is pressurized by occluding the entrance with the thumb while a finger presses the cement distally.

is signaled by the emergence of displaced fat and blood seen at the proximal femur. A doughy consistency of the cement optimizes the effectiveness of this technique. Final pressurization for half a minute is done with a wet lap pad occluding the cement at the cut neck.

The prosthesis is prepared for implantation by cleaning and drying, if necessary, and coating the proximal metaphyseal area circumferentially with cement. This eliminates the chance introduction of water, blood, and other material between the cement and the prosthesis during implantation (Fig. 20). Along with the textured surface found in modern implants, it ensures an improved mechanical bond of the cement to the prosthesis. A centralizer fitted onto the distal end of the femoral prosthesis is optional. After the cement column

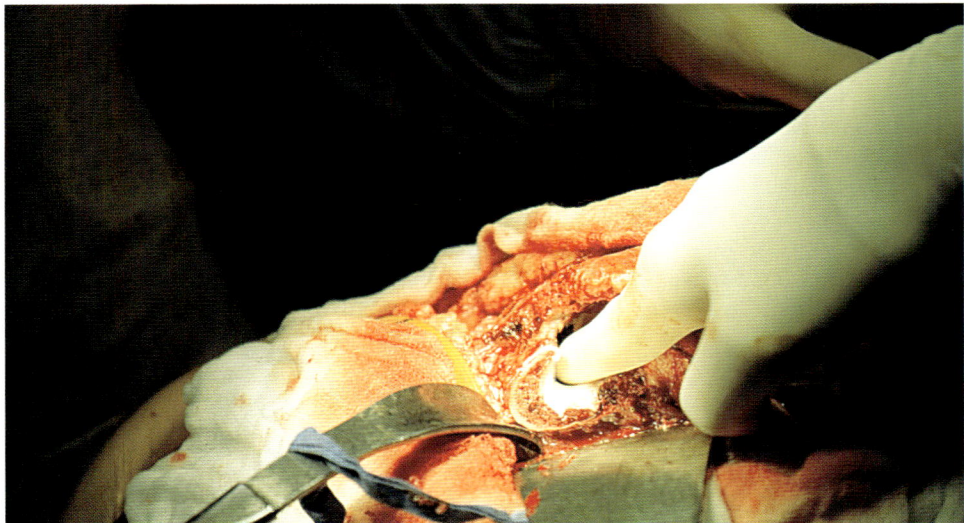

Figure 19. View of the cement column ready for pressurization.

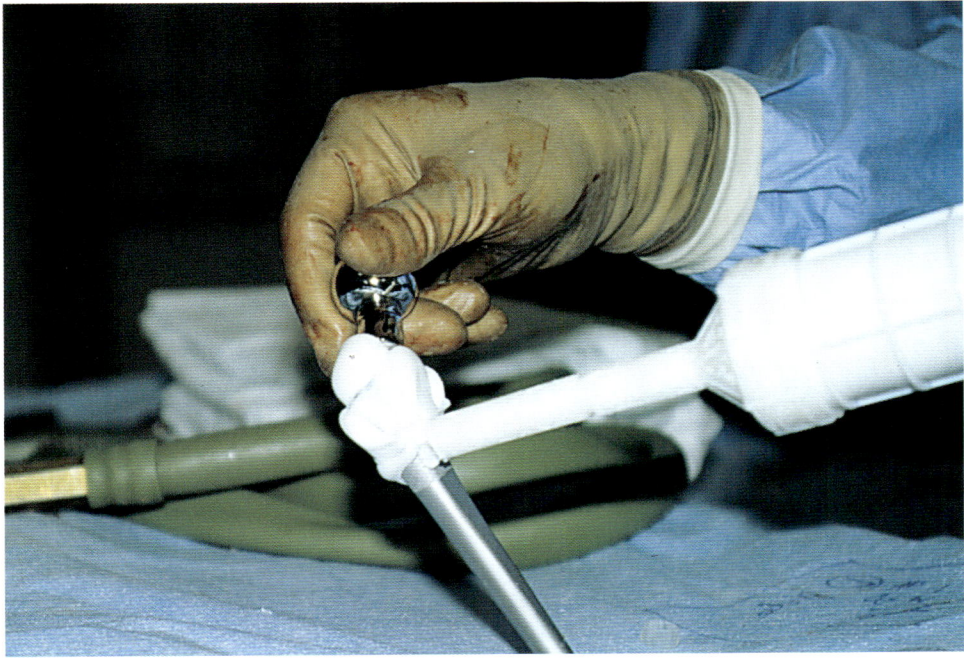

Figure 20. Cement is coated onto the prosthesis prior to implantation to preclude blood in the cement–prosthesis interface.

has been prepared (see Fig. 19), the prosthesis should be manually pressed down into the cement in a slow, steady fashion with the help of an axial pusher. This maneuver should be controlled to achieve neutral or slightly valgus position of the stem, the desired anteversion, and the proper proximal/distal position in one smooth movement. Occasionally, impaction of the prosthesis with a few blows from an impactor and mallet may be necessary to achieve an appropriately distal position. Gentle pressure should be used to maintain the position of the prosthesis while all excess cement is cleaned away and the cement is allowed to harden. During cement curing, the surgeon should compact any exposed cement using forceps and a moist sponge. Once the cement has hardened, the appropriate femoral head prosthesis, if not already attached, may be fitted to the trunnion with standard technique.

Two drill holes are now made in the posterior edge of the greater trochanter for use in reattaching the posterior soft tissues. A loop of suture is placed through each hole, using a straight needle, for later use. The hip is now reduced. A last check of position and soft-tissue tension is performed. The short external rotators of the hip and the posterior one-third of gluteus minimus and the posterior capsular flap are secured to each other with two nonabsorbable sutures, which are then drawn through the holes made in the greater trochanter using the suture loops previously installed for this purpose (Fig. 21). Then, with the hip placed in an abducted and externally rotated position, the sutures are used to draw the posterior soft tissues up snugly against the posterior surface of the greater trochanter, and they are then securely tied. The insertion of the gluteus maximus is repaired (Fig. 22).

The entire wound is now thoroughly irrigated with an antibiotic-saline solution. Two large suction drains are placed in the joint and are brought out through the fascia and skin anteriorly and distally. The fascia lata and fascia over the gluteus maximus are repaired

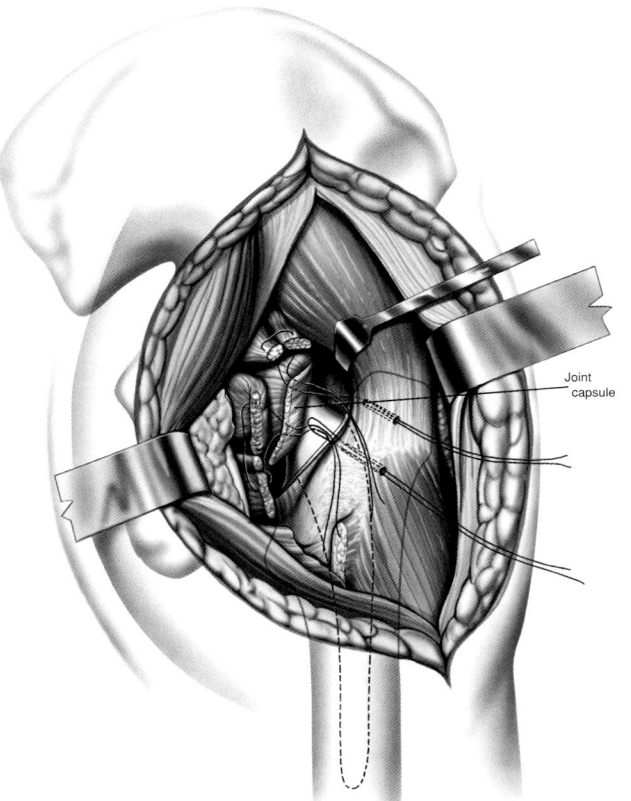

Figure 21. Sutures are placed through the external rotators and brought out through drill holes in the greater trochanter.

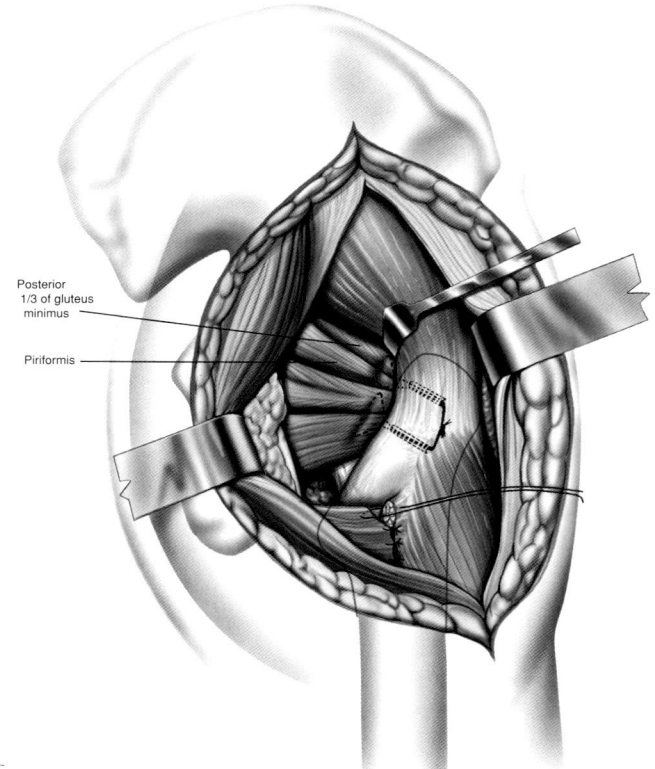

Figure 22. The capsule and short external rotators have been repaired. The gluteus maximus insertion is repaired.

with interrupted sutures. The subcutaneous tissues are also closed with a single layer of interrupted sutures, and the skin is closed with running nylon stitch. The wound is dressed with silk soaked in Betadine, covered with sterile gauze, and held in place with an elastic bandage that surrounds the hip, upper thigh, and pelvis.

POSTOPERATIVE MANAGEMENT

Typical Hospital Course and Rehabilitation

Primary total hip arthroplasty generally requires from 1 to 3 hours of operative time to complete. Surgical blood loss concomitant to a primary hip arthroplasty results in a requirement for 2 to 4 units of blood transfusion during and/or after surgery. Autologous predeposit of blood by the patient for his or her own use is available at many centers and, in combination with hypotensive epidural anesthesia, often avoids nonautologous transfusion.

The suction drains placed in the hip at surgery are usually removed after 24 to 48 hours. Abduction slings or an abduction pillow are applied to the operated limb for a few days after surgery to protect the hip from dislocating forces. Prophylactic antibiotics, as previously mentioned, are begun before surgery and continued intravenously for 24 to 48 hours postoperative. Anticoagulant therapy is usually started immediately after surgery.

Our rehabilitation protocol calls for the patient to begin standing up at the bedside by the second postoperative day. Progressive ambulation usually begins by the third postoperative day. In cases where cement fixation has been used, full weight bearing is allowed immediately. If a trochanteric osteotomy has been performed, special precautions and limited weight bearing on the hip are ordered. Ambulatory assistive devices for rehabilitation are tailored to the patient's needs. Patients with rheumatoid involvement of the upper extremities may require a special walker with platforms, which avoids weight bearing on the hands and wrists.

Most patients progress to discharge after a hospital stay of 7 to 10 days. Some patients with inflammatory arthritis may require further supervised rehabilitation, and, based upon individual needs, these patients are transferred, if possible, to a rehabilitation facility that is geared to accommodate their personal requirements.

Outpatient Rehabilitation

In most cases, an unsupervised program of ambulation at home is all that is necessary for a successful outcome after total hip arthroplasty. Our long-term total hip arthroplasty rehabilitation protocol requires the use of some type of ambulatory aid for at least two months after surgery. A walker or two crutches are prescribed for the first month. This may progress to a single crutch for an additional month and then to a cane, as necessary, thereafter. If necessary, the patient may be instructed in progressive resistance exercises to strengthen the hip abductors if they have difficulty weaning from a cane. Full benefit from the arthroplasty is usually realized by the end of twelve months.

The performance of a total hip arthroplasty requires the patient to observe special precautions to avoid dislocation of the prosthetic joint. These precautions are aimed at avoiding extremes of motion at the hip while the soft tissues violated by the surgery are allowed to heal. After a posterior surgical approach, acute flexion and internal rotation of the hip must be avoided. In this regard, the patient are carefully instructed in proper leg and body positioning as part of the rehabilitation protocol. They should use an elevated toilet seat and avoid soft or low chairs for several months after surgery. They should not lean forward from a sitting position and should not bend over from a standing position. Special assistive reachers and other devices are provided and should be utilized for dressing and other activities of daily living. A pillow held between the legs while sleeping is also prescribed for the first few months.

Long-term Results

Nearly 100% of patients experience dramatic, immediate, and complete relief of their arthritic hip pain after cemented total hip arthroplasty. Functional improvement is also apparent in the vast majority of patients. The ultimate functional level is usually determined by the preoperative functional status and the presence of comorbidities.

The main conclusion to be derived from the long-term experiences with cemented hip arthroplasty reported in the orthopedic literature is that longevity of fixation of a cemented implant is directly related to the quality of the initial surgical technique, the quality and quantity of bone available to support the prosthesis, and patient-related variables such as age, activity level, and body weight.

Surgical technique is perhaps the single most important determinant. Current standards require thorough bone preparation and careful cement handling and pressurization to achieve satisfactory cement-bone microinterlock. Improvements in prosthetic design have made durable cement-prosthesis bonding relatively easy to achieve.

COMPLICATIONS

The overall intraoperative surgical complication rate in primary total hip arthroplasty is less than 5%. The prevalence of neurologic complications related to total hip arthroplasty is approximately 1%–3%, and the majority of these resolve without treatment within the first six months after surgery. Although the exact prevalence of vascular complications is not known, they probably occur in less than 1% of cases. Significant malpositioning of the prosthetic components manifesting as postoperative joint instability and dislocation occurs in less than 3% of cases. The incidence of infection attributable to the surgical procedure itself after primary hip arthroplasty is than 1%. The osteoporosis commonly present in patients with inflammatory arthritis should make gentle manipulation of the limb and careful utilization of bone-working tools a constant priority of the operating surgeon in order to avoid occasional bony complications such as femoral perforation or fracture, and perforation of the medial wall of the acetabulum in these patients.

Deep Vein Thrombosis

Various reports in the literature have placed the incidence of deep vein thrombosis (DVT) (all sites) following THA at up to 50% to 80%—although not all are symptomatic. Based on clinical suspicion and V/Q scan, the incidence of related pulmonary embolism (PE) is estimated to be 6% to 19%. Fatal PE associated with THA has been reported to be as high as 1% to 3% in unprophylaxed patients. Thus, because of the obvious potential for significant morbidity and mortality in this regard, prophylaxis and surveillance are important components of perioperative and postoperative management.

Epidural anesthesia during the operative procedure and aspirin therapy in the immediate postoperative period are utilized for most patients according to our current DVT prophylaxis protocol. All patients receive venographic evaluation of the affected extremity on or about postoperative day five. If thrombosis is demonstrated, warfarin therapy is started. All patients undergoing bilateral arthroplasty, and those with a prior history of pulmonary embolism, are begun on warfarin therapy on the night after surgery—in lieu of aspirin therapy.

The incidence of DVT or PE may affect the function of the arthroplasty itself to the degree with which the event interferes with the course of postoperative rehabilitation. Otherwise, long-term effects upon durability and function are neglible.

Infection

The incidence of early infection, defined as that appearing within six months of surgery, is similar for all diagnoses and is less than 1%. The overall long-term infection rate for total hip arthroplasty performed using routine antibiotic prophylaxis and modern surgical technique is approximately 2%. The long-term rate for various subgroups of patients varies significantly, however. The infection rate for osteoarthritic patients is approximately 0.3%, while rheumatoid arthritis patients have a risk of 1.2%. The risk for psoriatic patients has been reported to be 5.5%, and for diabetic patients 6.6%. Patients in these groups also have a higher incidence of infection at other sites, such as lung, urinary tract, and skin, than do nonaffected patients. This is thought to be due to immune suppression caused by the disease processes themselves and related medications that degrade the effectiveness of a patient's immune response.

Established infection within a prosthetic joint is a devastating complication. The treatment of an established infection is removal of the implants and all associated fixation, and debridement of all locally infected soft tissue and bone. This is usually followed by a minimum of six weeks of appropriate intravenous antibiotic therapy. Reimplantation of a new prosthesis may then be performed if the infectious source has been identified and removed and diagnostic testing demonstrates the eradication of the infectious organism. Occasionally, especially in cases of infection involving a particularly virulent pathogen, it may be prudent to delay reimplantation until after a period of observation (sometimes up to a year), while off of antibiotic therapy.

Reimplantation after infection is technically more demanding than primary arthroplasty and always requires a surgeon experienced in its planning and execution, who also has all of the necessary tools and implants available. Occasionally, it may require the fabrication of custom tools and implants, and bone grafting.

Dislocation

Dislocation of the prosthetic femoral head from within the prosthetic acetabulum averages 0.5% to 3% in most reports and may occur at any time after total hip arthroplasty but is most common during the first several postoperative weeks. During this period, soft-tissue and muscle weakness about the hip are least able to resist any dislocating forces that may be applied.

Poor surgical technique may be a factor in dislocation. However, the vast majority of dislocations occur as a result of patient error—usually noncompliance in the observance of prescribed precautions. As mentioned previously, appropriate precautions usually involve the avoidance of certain body positions and activities. These will vary according to the details of the surgical technique as it relates to the weakening of various anatomical structures. Rehabilitation after THA should always include thorough instruction in these precautions and should provide, if possible, various aids such as long shoe horns, hand-extension devices for putting on hosiery, elevated toilet seats, and other related devices that help the patient to avoid the extremes of hip motion in the early postoperative period.

If dislocation occurs, it should be considered a surgical emergency. Injury to neural and vascular structures may acutely accompany the dislocation or the relocation event. A patient with suspected dislocation should be promptly transferred to a facility where roentgenographic evaluation and manipulative or operative treatment is available. The vast majority of dislocations are easily reducible with mild pain relief and/or muscle relaxation and gentle manipulation by an experienced physician. A few of these may, however, require open reduction under anesthesia and sterile technique in an operating room.

Our treatment protocol after an acute dislocation includes hospital admission for observation, fitting of an abduction brace, and reinforcement of physical therapy and precautions. We insist that the patient utilize the brace at all times, except when lying flat in bed, for a period of six weeks. The brace must be put on while lying flat prior to getting out of bed and must be removed while lying flat after returning to bed. After six weeks, some of the restrictions are removed, but brace usage is continued, sometimes up to several months.

Trochanteric Complications

Trochanteric nonunion is reported to occur in 3% to 9.5% of cases where a trochanteric osteotomy is performed as part of the surgical procedure. The rate is increased in patients with repeat osteotomies and in those with osteoporosis or other conditions that are associated with poor bone healing. It has been reported to be as high as 24% in one series of patients with rheumatoid arthritis. Nonunion may be painful but is rarely disabling because a fibrous union usually develops. Approximately 50% of patients with nonunion or fibrous union will demonstrate abductor weakness and a limp. These patients are usually comfortably ambulatory with the aid of a cane. Complete nonunions have a higher rate of dislocation and painful limp and may require surgical repair.

Heterotopic Ossification

Heterotopic ossification (HO) is a complication that may appear clinically with redness, low-grade fever, and aching pain around the affected hip. The diagnosis can be made roentgenographically when a hazy appearance can be seen in the soft tissue surrounding the hip. Males are affected 2 to 3 times more often than females, and the incidence in osteoarthritis is higher than in rheumatoid arthritis. Patients with ankylosing spondylitis, Paget's disease, and diffuse idiopathic skeletal hyperostosis (Forrestier's disease) carry a higher risk. Though overall, heterotopic ossification of varying degree has been reported in up to 30% of all patients after total hip arthroplasty, the incidence of significant HO compromising function of the joint is probably less than 5%.

For patients at particular risk, postoperative indomethacin has been shown to decrease the risk of HO. Low-dose postoperative irradiation has also been shown to be very effective. If severe heterotopic ossification does occur, it can significantly compromise joint function and may require surgical excision.

Leg-Length Discrepancy

Leg-length discrepancy is an occasional complication of hip reconstruction that may be quite annoying to the patient. Excessive lengthening is most often associated with a posterior surgical approach to the hip joint since lengthening may be required to achieve proper joint stability after this exposure. On the other hand, limb shortening may be required to achieve joint stability in cases where severe soft-tissue contractures are present. In most cases, leg-length discrepancy that is deemed clinically significant postoperatively can be satisfactorily treated with the use of a shoe lift. Revision surgery is rarely indicated.

ILLUSTRATIVE CASE FOR TECHNIQUE

A 65-year-old woman presents with pain in her left hip at rest and pain that limits her daily activities. She describes the pain by pointing to her left inguinal crease and indicating that it radiates into her upper left thigh. She says the pain causes her to limp after several blocks of walking and at the end of the day.

Radiographs reveal osteoarthritic changes in the left hip with complete loss of the joint space superiorly, marginal osteophyte formation, and minimal shortening of the limb (Fig. 23). Physical examination reveals pain and restriction of motion in the hip. The patient ambulates with a coxalgic gait.

Total hip arthroplasty was performed under hypotensive epidural anesthesia using cemented components. The patient convalesced normally in the hospital and was discharged after six days. Three months postoperative she was ambulatory without the use of a cane (Fig. 24A). At six months postoperative she returned to Florida and her golf game (Fig. 24B).

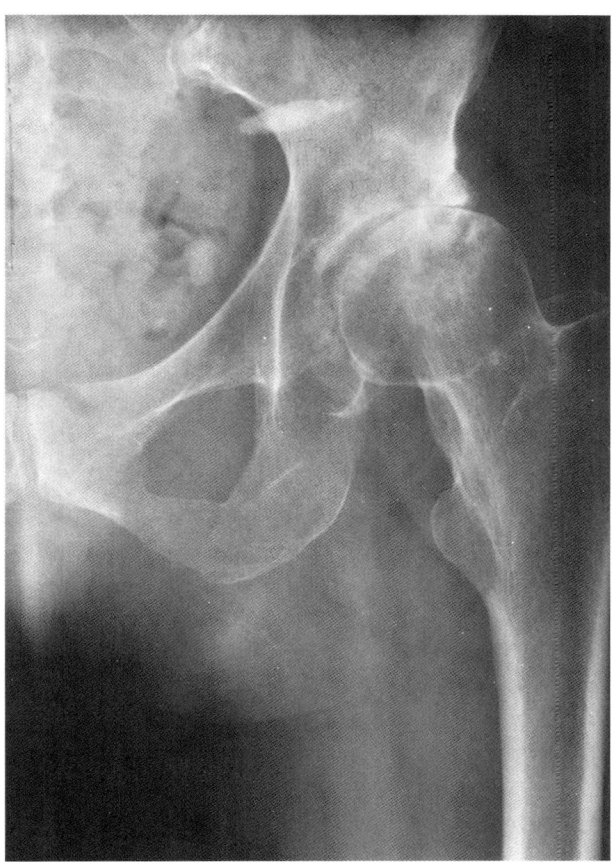

Figure 23. Radiograph of left hip involved with osteoarthritis.

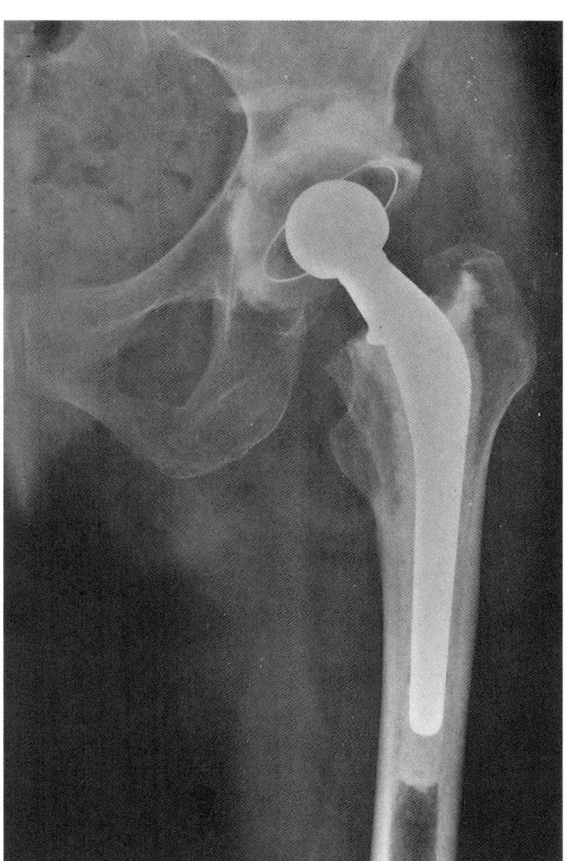

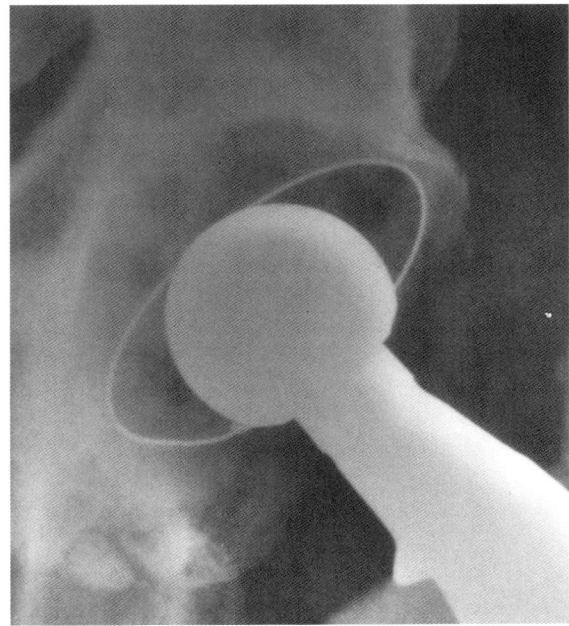

Figure 24 A, B. Radiographs of left hip after cemented arthroplasty.

RECOMMENDED READING

Bannister, G. C., Young S. K., et al. Control of bleeding in cemented arthroplasty. *J. Bone Joint Surg.* [Br.], 72-B:444–466, 1990.

Benjamin, J. B., Gie, G. A. et al. Cementing technique and the effects of bleeding. *J. Bone Joint Surg.* [Br], 69-B:620–624, 1987.

Cupic, Z. Long term follow-up of Charnley arthroplasty of the hip. *Clin. Orthop.*, 141:28–43, 1979.

DeLee, J. G., and Charnley, J. Radiological demarcation of cemented sockets in total hip replacement. *Clin. Orthop.*, 121:20–32, 1976.

Eftekhar, N. S., and Nercessean, O. Incidence and mechanism of failure of cemented acetabular component in total hip arthroplasty. *Ortho. Clin. North Am.*, 19:57–66, 1986.

Gruen, T. A., McNeice G. M. et al. "Modes of Failure" of cemented stem-type femoral components—a radiographic analysis of loosening. *Clin. Orthop.*, 141:17–27, 1979.

Krause, W. R., Krug, W. et al. Strength of the cement–bone interface. *Clin. Orthop.*, 163:290–299, 1982.

Maynard, M. J., and Ranawat, C. S. Linear and volumetric polyethylene wear in total hip arthroplasty. Rheumatoid Arthritis Surgical Society meeting, New York, 1990.

Ranawat, C. S., and Rose, H. 1985. Clinical and radiographic results of total condylar knee arthroplasty. A three to eight year follow-up. In: *Total Condylar Knee Arthroplasty.* C. S. Ranawat, editor. Springer-Verlag, Berlin, Heidelberg, Tokyo.

Ranawat, C. S., Rawlins, B. A., et al. Effect of modern cement technique on acetabular fixation in total hip arthroplasty: A retrospective study in matched pairs *Orthop. Clin. North Am.*, 19:599–603, 1988.

Ranawat, C. S., Beaver, W. B. et al. Effect of hypotensive epidural anaesthesia on acetabular cement bone fixation in total hip arthroplasty. *J. Bone Joint Surg.* (Br), 73-B:779–782, 1991.

Sharrock N. E., Mineo, B. et al. "Is hypotensive anesthesia safe in treated hypertensive patients?" *Anesth. Analg.*, 68S:256, 1989.

Thompson, G. E., Miller R. D. et al. Hypotensive anesthesia for total hip arthroplasty: a study of blood loss and organ function (brain, heart, liver and kidney). *Anesthesiology*, 48:91–96, 1978.

Vazeery A. K., and Lunde, O. Controlled hypotension in hip joint surgery: an assessment of surgical hemorrhage during sodium nitroprusside infusion. *Acta Orthop. Scand.*, 50:433–441, 1979.

13

The Hybrid Total Hip Replacement

William H. Harris

INDICATIONS/CONTRAINDICATIONS

The decade of the eighties provided crucial information concerning patient selection for total hip replacement (THR), with specific clarification of two important issues. The first is the resolution of the major dichotomy of the eighties in THR, namely "cement versus cementless." We learned that this is the wrong way to pose the question. The critical observation is that the decisions of what type of acetabular reconstruction to use in primary total hip replacement must be made completely independently of decisions for the femoral component. To be committed blindly to "cement" or "cementless" is inappropriate. Second, concerning femoral components, the decade of the eighties clearly established that modern cement techniques are preferable to cementless fixation, regardless of age, sex, or diagnosis. The overriding reason for this is the high and rising incidence of lysis of the femur around cementless femoral components.

Both the *clinical course* of loosening of femoral and acetabular components and our studies of autopsy-retrieved femoral and acetabular components established that the mechanisms of loosening are entirely different. On the femoral side, loosening of cemented components is mechanical in origin and occurs primarily by debonding at the cement–metal interface, the exact opposite of the traditional thought that failure initiated at the cement–bone interface.

Conversely, the mechanism of both cemented and cementless failure of acetabular components is biologic in origin, specifically the ingress of particulate debris followed by macrophage invasion. The lytic effect of enzymes and cytokines released as a result

---

W. H. Harris, M.D.: Department of Orthopaedic Surgery, Massachusetts General Hospital, Boston, Massachusetts 02114, Harvard Medical School, Boston, Massachusetts 02115.

of the particulate ingestion by the macrophages leads to bone resorption and loss of fixation.

Decisions should not be made on the basis of "I always cement" or "I never cement." Decisions should be made on the basis of the long-term data indicating the optimum results. In this regard, the decade of the eighties made it quite clear that the optimum femoral fixation is the modern use of modern cement. Eleven-year data show that with contemporary cementing techniques, femoral revisions are 2% and total femoral loosening (revised and not revised) is 3%. Fifteen- and twenty-year data show that with excellent cementing, femoral revision and lysis rates can be under 10%.

Strikingly, similar results apply for the young, as well. In our series of patients aged 50 and under (average age, 41) with contemporary femoral cementing, the femoral loosening rate at 12 years was 2% and the femoral revision rate was zero. In the younger group, the lysis incidence was zero. In the older age group (average age, 57) femoral lysis occurred in only 7% by 11 years, and this was all focal lysis in areas of defects in the cement mantle or a very thin cement mantle, all of which occurred in patients without loosening.

In contrast with these figures, are the *high and rising* incidence of lysis on the femoral side in association with all cementless femoral components after 5 to 7 years. This dominating adverse response, taken in conjunction with increased thigh pain, increased loosening, increased heterotopic ossification, and increased pain and limp in cementless components compared to cemented components, makes the decision quite clear. The femoral component is optimally fixed using contemporary bone cementing techniques.

On the acetabular side, the decision is somewhat less clear. Setting aside those components that have been shown to have a high incidence of failure at just 5 to 7 years such as screw-ring devices and the PCA socket, both cemented and cementless acetabular components function well over the first 5 to 7 years. There is no significant difference, clinically or radiographically, between a cemented and a well-designed cementless acetabular component at five years. The critical issue, of course, will be the difficulties that occur by 10 years or by 15 years. But such data are not available. Therefore, the decision to cement or use cementless implants on the acetabular side is based on expectations.

Most series of cementless acetabular components have shown loosening rates in the neighborhood of 40% or 50% by 10 years. Our expectation is that the hemispherical cementless titanium acetabular component with a fiber mesh will have a lower loosening rate by 10 years than will cement. At five years they function very well but the 10-year data are not available.

This belief is augmented by the observations that press-fitting this type of acetabular component significantly reduces the radiolucent zones at the cement–bone interface at five years and, it is hoped, will protect against the polyethylene invasion. Our experimental studies in dogs show that the press-fit enhances bony ingrowth and peripheral stability. These features appear to be positive in terms of reducing the lytic process that leads to loosening. For these reasons, we use a cementless acetabular component.

However, the decade of the eighties has also shown us that certain design features are essential for success of cementless acetabular components. There must be excellent fixation of the polyethylene in the metal shell. Optimum coaptation against the host bone is important for maximizing bone ingrowth, particularly at the periphery of the socket. Minimum thickness of polyethylene should be about 6 mm and whenever possible, more. As a consequence, the 32-mm head should rarely be used. Our preference is for a 26-mm head except for small patients, who require a 22-mm head.

In short, we recommend a cementless hemispherical acetabular component made of titanium and covered with titanium fiber mesh combined with a cemented femoral stem of contemporary design using modern cementing technique—a hybrid THR—for all primary THR regardless of age, sex, or diagnosis. The acetabular component is preferably press-fit, but if conditions are not optimum for press-fit, the shell should be fixed with screws. The femoral component should be of forged chrome cobalt with a broad, rounded medial border without sharp corners and should have a collar. The surface should be precoated proximally and distally and rough in texture.

The cementing should be the third-generation technique, including the use of a medullary plug, cement gun, pressurization, porosity reduction, and strong cement, and the implant should be centralized to create a cement mantle that has a minimum thickness of 2.5 mm.

PREOPERATIVE PLANNING

The assessment of the patient includes a detailed history and physical examination concerning the orthopaedic complaint, medical evaluation, ECG, BUN, SGOT, PT and PTT, blood count including platelet count, and urinalysis. Other tests are done if specific features of these interrogations suggest the need for additional evaluation. We obtain the following x-ray films: AP hips and pelvis centered over the pubis, frog and true lateral of the involved hip, and, if indicated, scanograms to evaluate leg lengths. Other films may be required in special circumstances such as developmental dislocation of the hip. Whenever possible, we have the patients donate their own blood preoperatively, the amount depending on the complexity of the case.

For most primary patients, the preoperative planning is not complex. The size of the acetabular component most likely to be used is determined from templating the hemispherical shape of the acetabular component on both the AP and true lateral view. Unless there is major deformity of the acetabulum, this is not a complex task. The largest socket possible should be used and coverage should be complete or nearly so. The socket should be medialized to the medial wall. The dome should be more craniad than the lateral lip.

Once the acetabular template has been positioned, the femoral template is used. In the cemented femoral component series that I use, the templates contain a dotted line indicating the location of the cement mantle. This is a valuable feature.

The alignment of the femoral component, its height relative to the centering of the femoral head in the acetabular recess, the offset of the prosthesis relative to the offset of the femur, and the size of the medullary canal determine the optimum size and location of the prosthesis to be used.

We avoid long head–neck pieces because of the decreased range of motion that results from the flange necessary for the long head-neck piece.

SURGICAL TECHNIQUE

The major advantages of avoiding trochanteric osteotomy are reduced operating time, reduced blood loss, more rapid rehabilitation, and the absence of trochanter complications.

The Incision

The patient is positioned in the true lateral position with the involved hip up, in the true lateral position, using the Maquet pelvic support system. The skin is prepared in the usual way, and the lower extremity is draped free.

The optimum approach is a Langenbeck or Kocher incision with subsequent excision of both the posterior and the anterior capsule. Curve the distal portion of the incision posteriorly to enhance mobilization of the posterior flap (Fig. 1).

When the fascia has been divided, the skin and subcutaneous tissue are protected by sewing a sponge to the lateral edges of the fascia lata throughout the full extent of the wound.

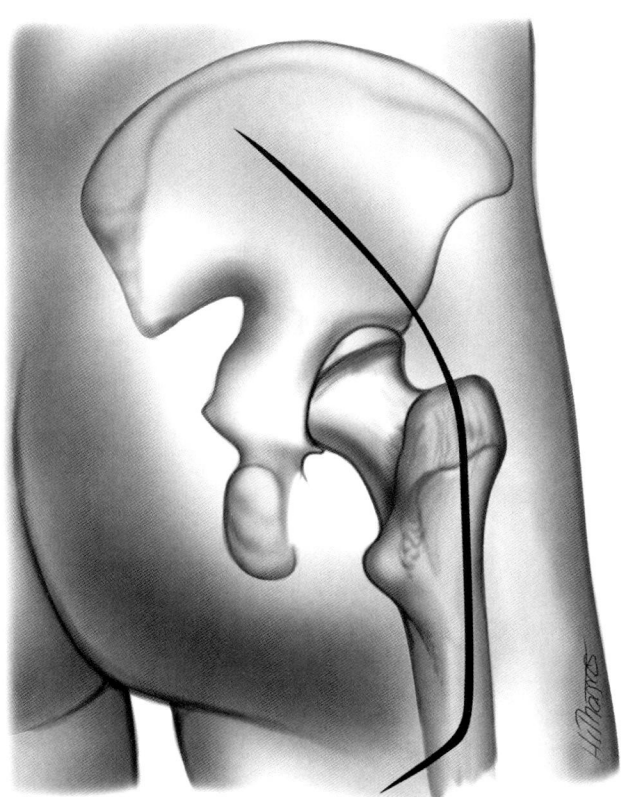

Figure 1. The skin incision is a modification of the posterolateral incision described by Kocher. The modification is that the distal end of the incision turns posteriorly. This modification helps a great deal increasing the quality of the exposure posteriorly. The proximal limb should lie just craniad to and parallel to the craniad border of the muscle belly to the gluteus maximus.

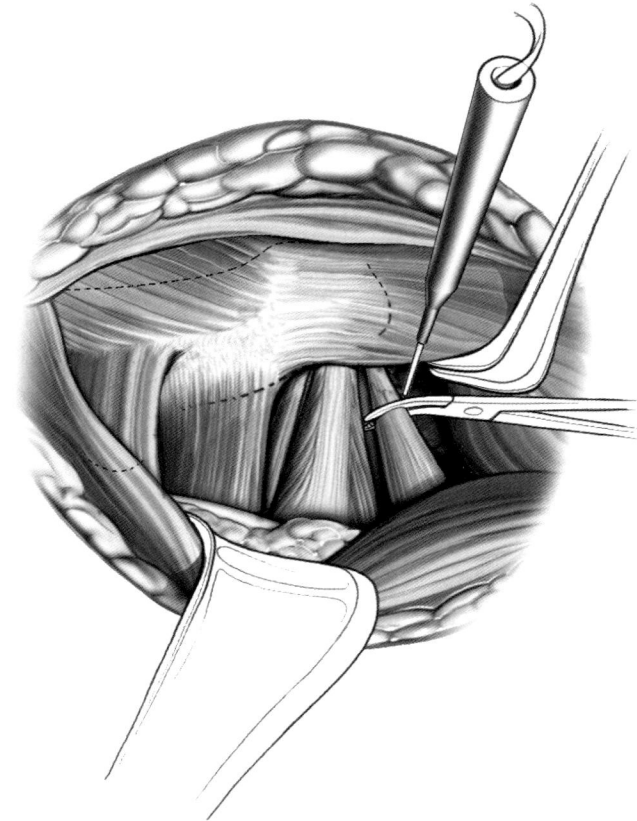

Figure 2. The insertions of the short external rotators into the femur are divided, including the piriformus, gemellus superior, obturator internus, obturator inferior, and obturator externus. The proximal half of the quadratus femoris is also divided.

Exposure of the Hip Joint

The key landmark for division of the short external rotators is the identification of the tendon of the piriformis muscle (Fig. 2). This tendon runs parallel to the posterior border of the gluteus medius and can be readily palpated as it approaches the posterior superior portion of the greater trochanter. The gluteus medius is retracted superiorly and the tendon of the piriformis is divided. The remaining short external rotators are divided including division of the gemelli and obturator internus. The proximal two-thirds of the quadratus femoris is divided. The tendon of the obturator externus is identified, isolated by passing a curved clamp deep to it, and cut.

The tendon of the gluteus maximus is isolated by passing a clamp deep to it, to protect the sciatic nerve, and is divided (Fig. 3).

Capsulectomy

With the leg in maximum internal rotation, the posterior capsule is excised (Fig. 4).

While the operation can be done without further capsular excision, I prefer to excise the anterior capsule. With the leg in 45 degrees of hip flexion and maximum external rotation, the anterior wound flap is retracted anteriorly and the leading edge of the anterior portion of the gluteus medius muscle is identified.

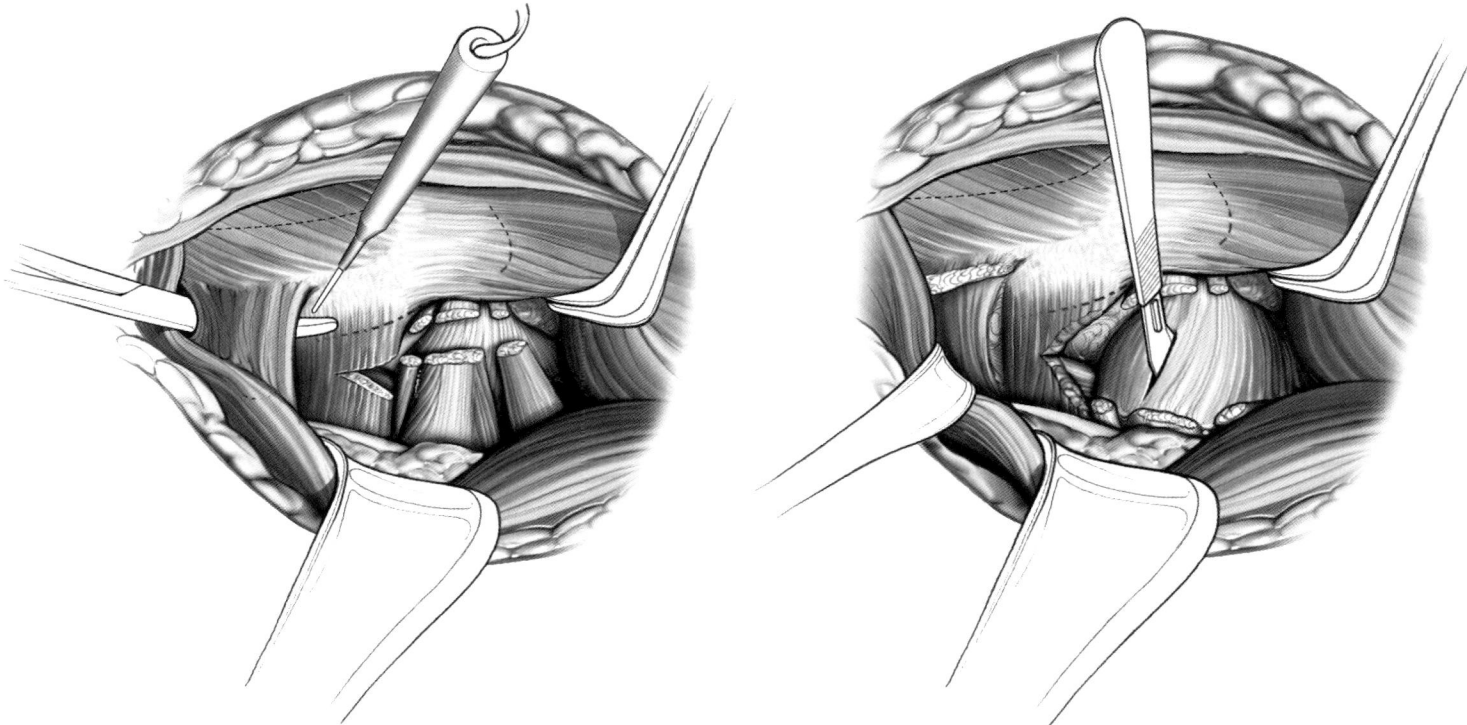

Figure 3. The insertion of the gluteus maximus into the femur is also released. It is usually quite vascular.

Figure 4. Deep to the short external rotators, the posterior capsule is excised.

A Cushing elevator is passed underneath the tendon of the gluteus minimus protecting both the gluteus medius and minimus (Fig. 5).

Exposure of the anterior capsule is completed by passing a cobra retractor across the front of the hip joint into the pelvis, underneath the origin of the rectus femoris tendon from

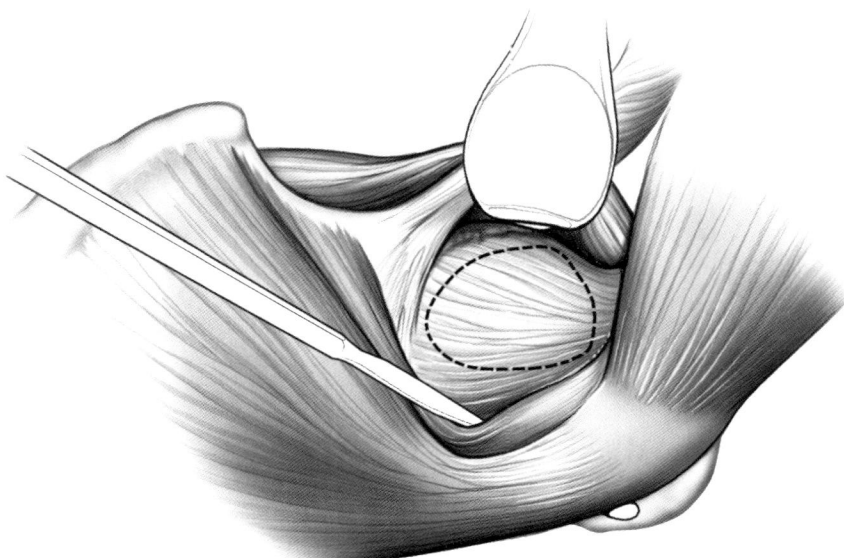

Figure 5. The anterior capsule is exposed by first placing the lower extremity in flexion and external rotation. A Cushing elevator is passed underneath the gluteus medius and minimus craniad to the superior capsule. A cobra retractor is placed across the front of the joint into the iliac fossa, over the capsule and under the iliopsoas. Then the remaining capsule is excised in two stages. First the anterior capsule is removed. Then the iliopsoas tendon is separated from the inferior capsule, and the inferior capsule is excised.

the anterior inferior iliac spine (Fig. 5). The landmark for this channel is a theoretical line bisecting the femoral neck, aiming toward the anterior inferior iliac spine. This retractor must not stand erect but must be at a 45-degree angle, with the handle pointing distally.

The anterior capsule is then excised in two steps, first the major portion of the anterior capsule and then the medial inferior aspect, since the latter is the area most likely to contain major blood vessels. Bleeding is minimized by separating the medial inferior portion of the capsule from the iliopsoas tendon. Making this separation both reduces the amount of bleeding associated with excision of the medial inferior portion of the capsule and creates better access to that region for control of any bleeding that does occur.

To assure that a complete capsulectomy has been achieved, the index finger of one hand should be able to pass freely, from the front, around the femoral neck inferiorly and make contact with the other index finger coming in from behind the greater trochanter.

Similarly, the index finger should pass freely from front to back across the superior portion of the femoral neck.

Determination of Leg Length

The optimum way to determine leg length is to drive the reference jig for the leg-length caliper into the wing of the ilium, just below the anterior inferior iliac spine (Fig. 6).

The leg-length caliper is then positioned from the reference pin to measure the distance from the reference pin to the vastus tubercle. The position of the leg is marked on the drapes with a marking pencil. For all subsequent measurements, the limb is replaced in that same position.

Dislocation is carried out in maximum internal rotation and adduction using the bone hook (Fig. 7).

Osteotomy of the Femoral Neck

In making the first cut, it is preferable to leave the neck longer than desired, to allow flexibility in the final determination of leg length. If necessary, a second osteotomy cut can be

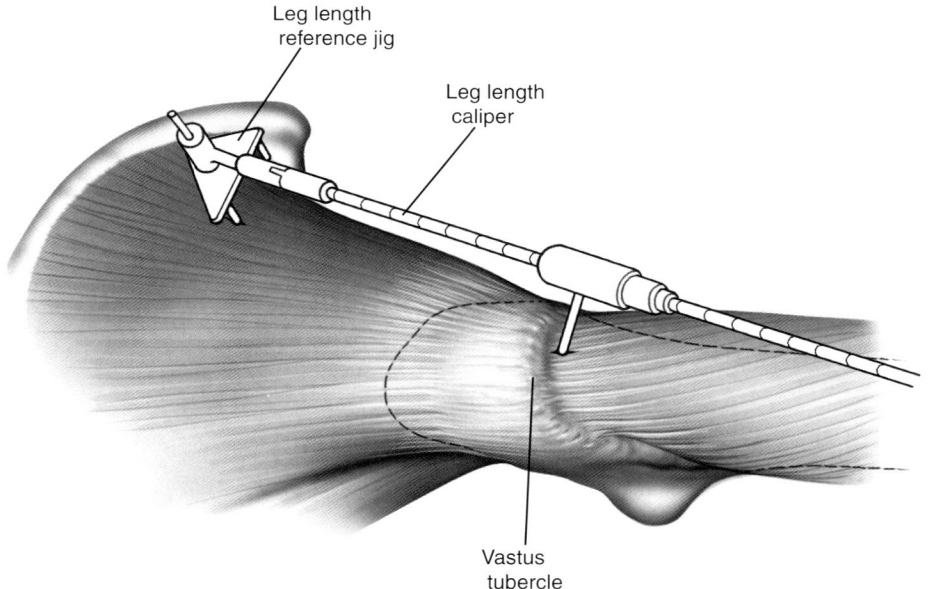

Figure 6. The reference marker for the leg length caliper is driven into the wing of the ilium at the anterior superior iliac spine. The leg length caliper then attaches to the reference marker and the movable length indicator is adjusted to touch a fixed point on the greater trochanter. The position of the lower extremity is marked on the drapes so that it can be reproduced for subsequent measurements.

made subsequently, after the acetabular component has been inserted and the trial reduction has been carried out.

With the tibia pointing directly toward the ceiling, the neck osteotomy guide is aligned over the femur (Fig. 8) with the posterior surface of the flag abutting the femoral head and its stem exactly in line with the midline of the medullary canal. There is one guide for each size of femoral component. The size chosen for use is based on the preoperative templating. Each neck osteotomy guide has three horizontal slots, one for use with a 32-mm head,

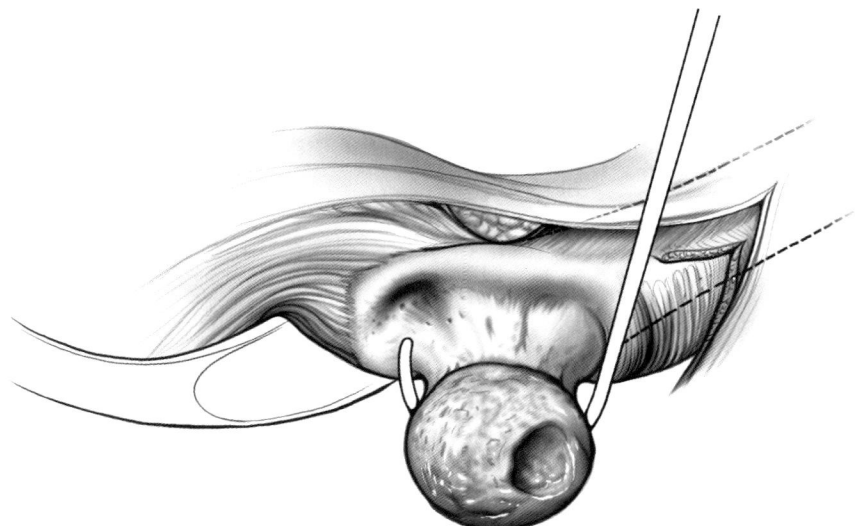

Figure 7. Dislocation takes place in internal rotation, delivering the head posteriorly with the aid of the bone hook.

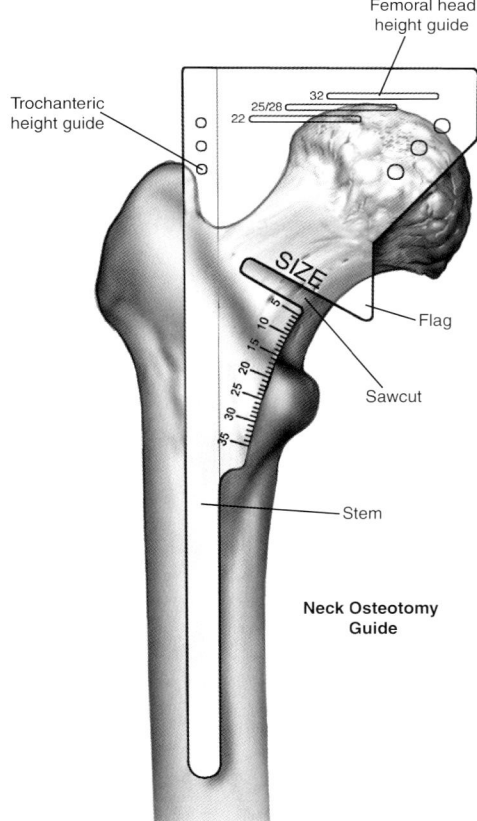

Figure 8. The neck osteotomy guide is positioned over the proximal portion of the femur so that the stem of the guide is in direct alignment with the midline of the shaft of the femur. If the aim of the reconstruction is to reproduce the length of the existing femur, the neck osteotomy guide is advanced in a craniad fashion until the tip of the femoral head can be seen through the chosen horizontal slot in the neck osteotomy guide. There is one slot for the 32-mm head size, one for the 26 to 28-mm head size, and one for the 22-mm head size. If the leg is to be lengthened, the neck osteotomy guide is subsequently advanced further craniad by an amount equal to the desired increase in the leg length. In either case, it is wise to advance the neck osteotomy guide slightly higher so that extra length is left on the neck at the time of the first cut. This allows for any necessary correction in length and also allows bone to be reamed away with the calcar reamer.

one for a 28 or 26-mm head and one for a 22-mm head. The neck osteotomy guide is superimposed over the femoral shaft. The height of the neck osteotomy guide relative to the head of the femur is determined by moving the guide craniad or caudad until you can look through the horizontal slot (corresponding to the head diameter you plan to use) and see the superior surface of the femoral head. The slot in the inferior margin of the flag portion of the neck osteotomy guide indicates the position for the osteotomy.

Once this position of the osteotomy guide has been determined, move the guide 5 mm further craniad before marking the cut, to add extra length to the remaining femoral neck after the head is removed, by sawing along the mark to, but not into, the trochanter (Fig. 9). If necessary, the cut is completed by bringing the saw from the superior neck to the oblique cut parallel to the medial border of the trochanter (Fig. 10).

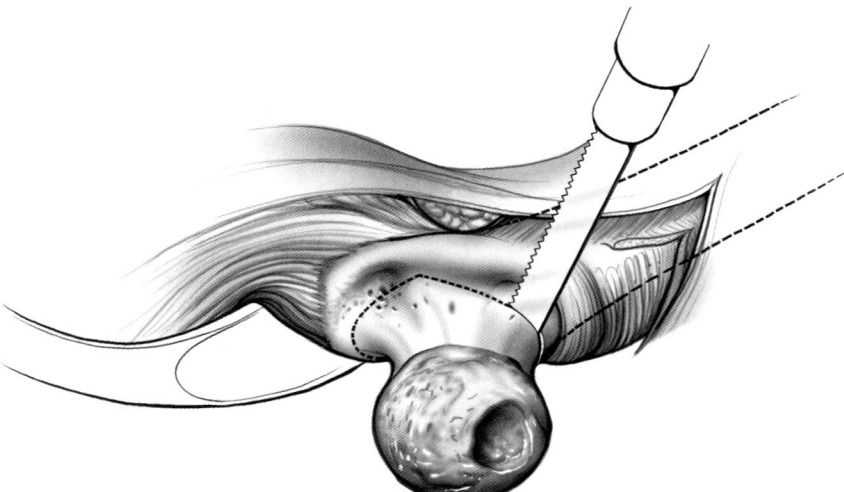

Figure 9. The femoral neck is cut along the line determined by the neck osteotomy guide back to the base of the greater trochanter.

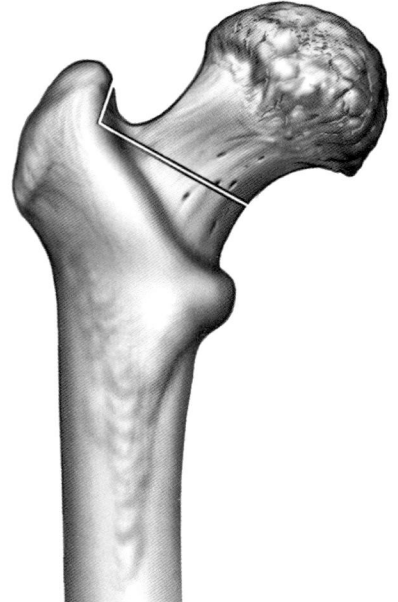

Figure 10. If the osteotomy does not divide the neck completely when the saw reaches the greater trochanter, the saw is withdrawn and brought from craniad to caudad along the base of the trochanter as indicated by the vertical dotted line.

Exposure and Preparation of the Acetabulum

The key issue in obtaining wide exposure of the acetabulum is the retraction of the femur anteriorly, made possible by the anterior capsulectomy.

The cobra retractor is placed underneath the femur at the level of the remaining femoral neck, and the tip of the cobra retractor passes up over the anterior margin of the acetabulum (Fig. 11). Retracting the cobra medially reflects the femur anteriorly, exposing the acetabulum.

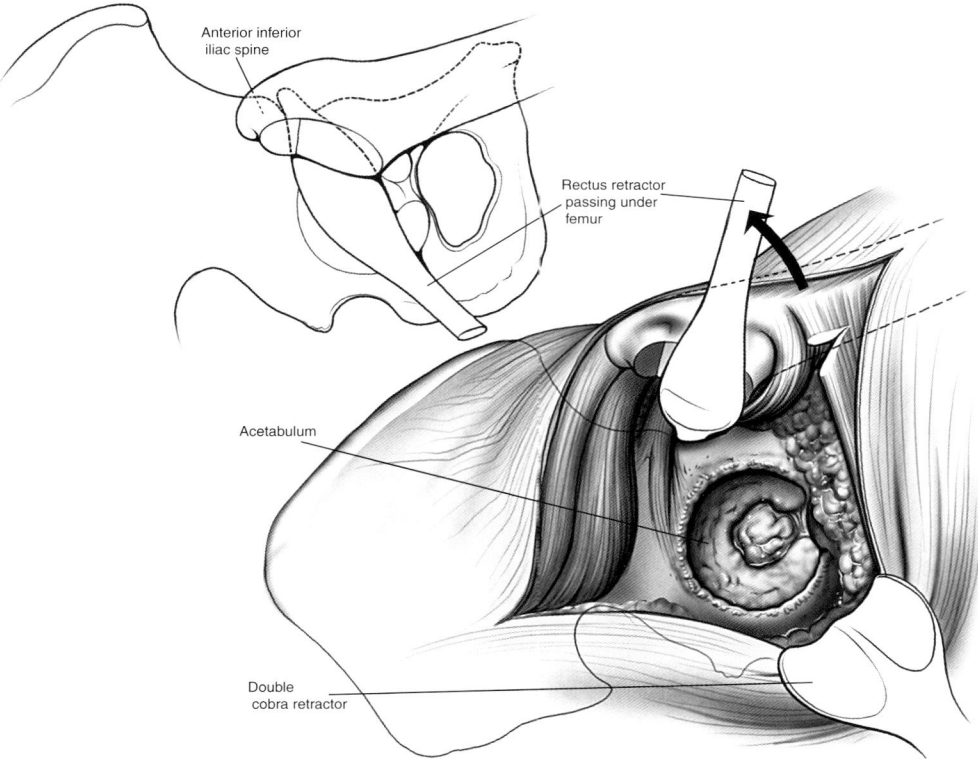

Figure 11. Exposure of the acetabulum is carried out by passing a cobra retractor underneath the femur and over the edge of the anterior column as shown. The cobra retractor is then reflected medially, carrying the femur medially and exposing the acetabulum. Further enhancement of the exposure of the acetabulum is created by using the double cobra, which retracts the inferior and lateral soft tissues out of the way.

The acetabulum is reamed to as large a diameter as possible. All articular cartilage and soft tissue are removed down to bleeding bone. The apex of the reamed socket must be more craniad than the lateral lip.

Reaming is carried down to but not into the medial wall of the acetabulum at the depth of the Haversian notch (Fig. 12).

When possible, we press-fit the acetabular component, but in instances of bone deficiency or fragile bone stock, we do not use press-fitting. The acetabular component is fixed with screws. In the press-fit cases, we use the design of this acetabular component, which has a solid backing without holes.

It is important to appreciate that recommendations about the amount of press-fitting are design specific. A recommendation to use a 3- or 4-mm press-fit for one design may not apply to other implant designs. Similarly, the amount of press-fit will differ between very large and very small acetabular components.

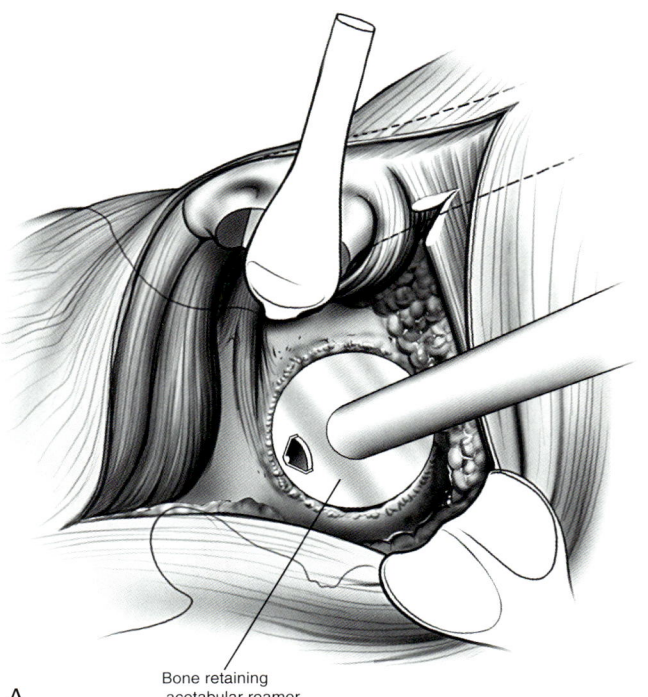
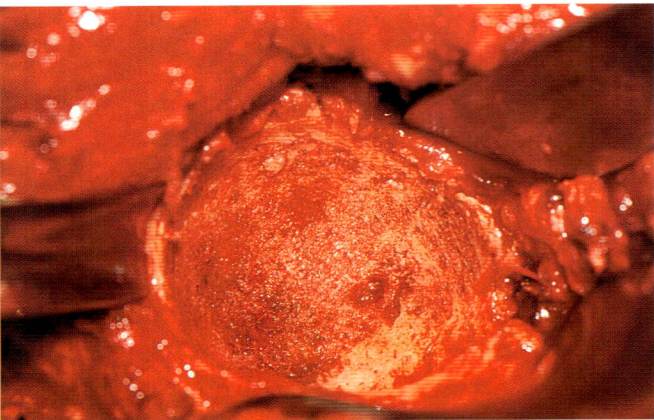

Figure 12. (A) The acetabulum is reamed in a hemispherical manner. It is important that the apex be higher than the lateral lip. It is important that all soft tissue be removed from the periphery of the acetabulum. (B) The acetabulum after reaming. This shows both the exposure achieved by this approach and the appropriate reaming down to cancellous bone in a hemispherical contour.

Optimum Position and Insertion Technique of the Acetabular Component

After reaming the acetabular recess to its optimum dimension (Fig. 13), insert the reamer head as a trial implant. If it slides easily to the bottom of the recess, it will not provide sufficient press fit. Then insert the reamer head that is 2 mm larger. If it cannot be forced to the bottom and sits about 2 mm proud (Fig. 14), there will rarely be difficulty in inserting that size as a press-fit component.

Bone stock is the next consideration. The key issues are fragile bone, dense or sclerotic bone, and defects in the rim. With normal elasticity of the periacetabular bone, the risk of

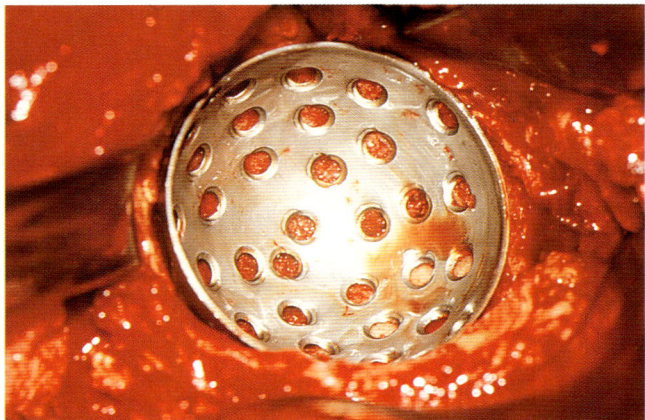

Figure 13. The reamer head can be used as a trial for the press fit size to be used. In this illustration, the same reamer head was inserted as had been used to ream the socket. It fit in easily and touched the bottom of the acetabulum.

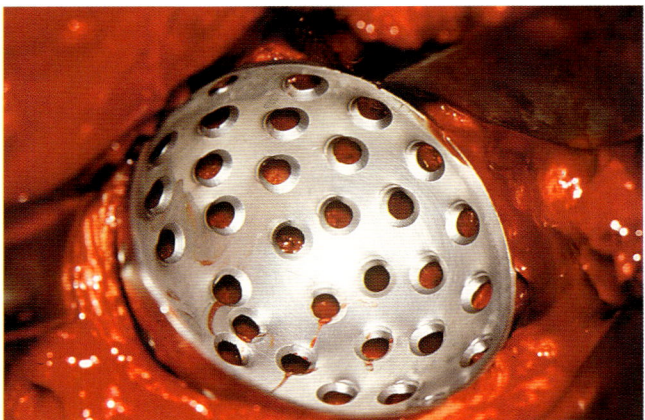

Figure 14. In this illustration the reamer head, which is 2 mm larger, has been inserted. It does not fit all the way to the bottom of the acetabulum and stands proud about 2 mm around the periphery. For some sockets a 2-mm press fit may be satisfactory. More press fit may be needed at times. Keep in mind that the issue of the magnitude of how much press fit is optimum is design specific. It varies from one design of acetabulum component to another.

fracture of the acetabulum in doing a 2-mm press fit is small. Some cases require a 3-mm or 4-mm press-fit. However, if the bone is fragile, as in some cases of rheumatoid arthritis, or if there is a defect in the rim of the acetabulum, press-fitting may be inappropriate.

It is also important to remove all soft tissue from the *entirety of* the rim of the acetabulum.

The third major consideration is this: the optimum situation is to have full contact of the fiber mesh against bone throughout the acetabular component, but a small gap at the dome is apparently not a detriment. Small gaps at the dome (0.5 mm) generally disappear.

In the early experience with these techniques, two things are helpful. Start by using a 2-mm press-fit with a shell that contains holes for screws. You gain experience with 2 mm of press-fit, and if it is not stable, you can add screws. Then, as your experience expands in getting good press-fit with full seating at the dome, progress to a press-fit socket without screw holes.

In driving the acetabular component into the acetabular recess, multiple strikes but not massive blows are used. Usually 30 to 50 blows will be applied to make the press-fit socket "bottom" in the dome of the acetabulum.

The optimum position of the acetabular component is 45 degrees of abduction (lateral opening), and 20 or 30 degrees of forward flexion (anteversion or anterior opening). The press-fit cup positioner (Fig. 15) is designed so that if you place the vertical arm of the guide triangle vertically, it automatically positions the acetabular component in 45 degrees of abduction or lateral opening.

Then if the appropriate horizontal arm of the guide triangle (right or left horizontal arm as is appropriate for the side being operated on) is brought into the coronal plane of the patient, the cup is automatically put in 20 degrees of anteversion or anterior opening. If 30 degrees of anteversion is desired, the cup positioner is moved 10 degrees further forward. The press-fit cup positioner has a threaded end onto which the polar hole of the acetabular component attaches. The proper alignment is achieved by placing the short arm of the cup positioner to the vertical position and by bringing the appropriate (right or left) anteversion arm of the positioner into the coronal plane of the patient.

If you use a shell with screw holes in it, you can see whether you have "bottomed" and can check for any gaps using the depth gauge. If a gap exists, further impaction will often reduce or eliminate it.

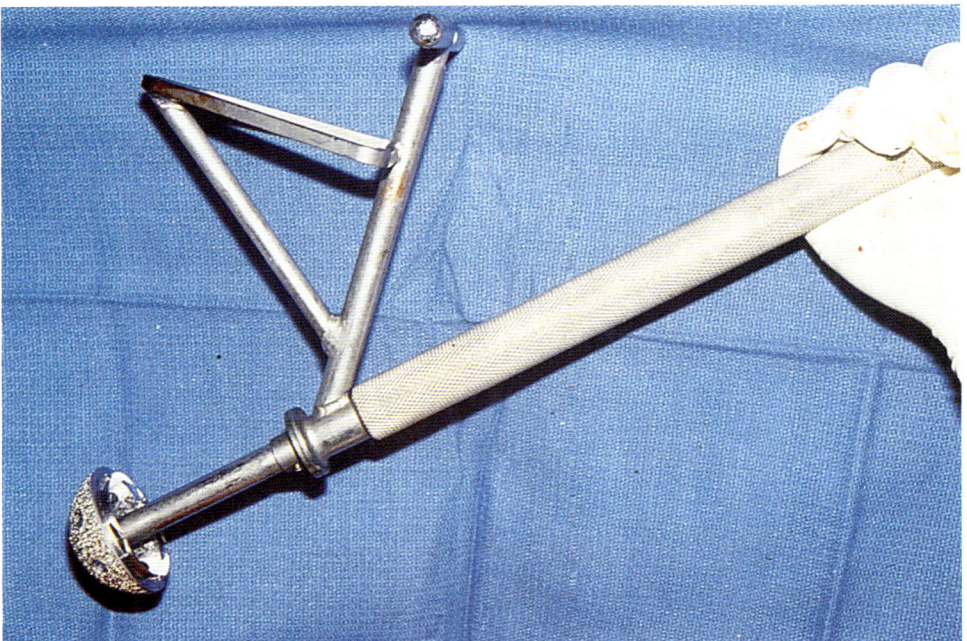

Figure 15. The press-fit acetabular cup positioner allows accurate determination of the optimum position of the acetabulum, namely 45 degrees of abduction and 20 degrees of forward flexion and at the same time permits impaction of the press-fit acetabular component.

Preparation of the Femur

With the leg in internal rotation, the tibia pointing toward the ceiling, and the antler retractor underneath the femur (Fig. 16), a Charnley awl is used to start the track down the medullary canal (Fig. 17). The bone at the base of the trochanter laterally is removed with the box osteotome (Fig. 18) and/or the router (Fig. 19). Then, successively, rasps of increasing sizes are inserted (Fig. 20). The largest rasp that will comfortably fit into the medullary canal is driven fully home. In contrast with cementless femoral components, fit and fill are not important concepts, but having a complete cement mantle is. It is better to use a smaller rather than a larger implant if the issue is in doubt.

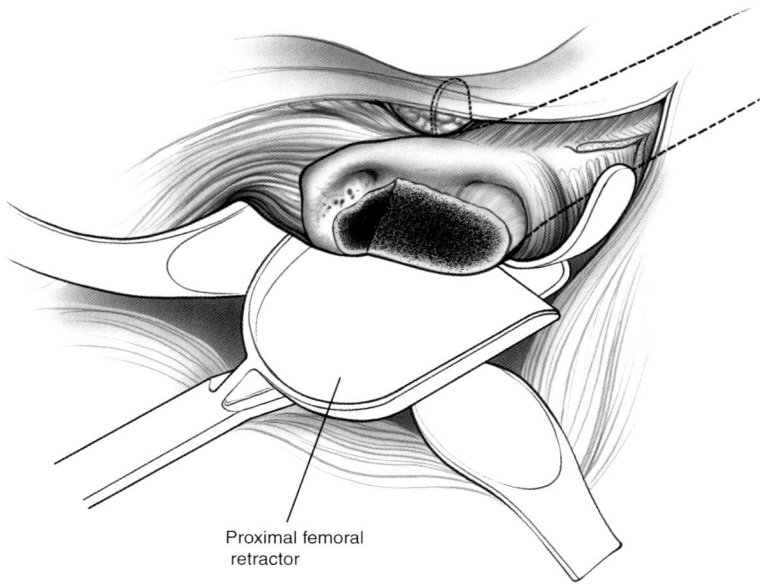

Figure 16. The proximal part of the femur is brought well out of the wound by using the proximal femur or "antler" retractor.

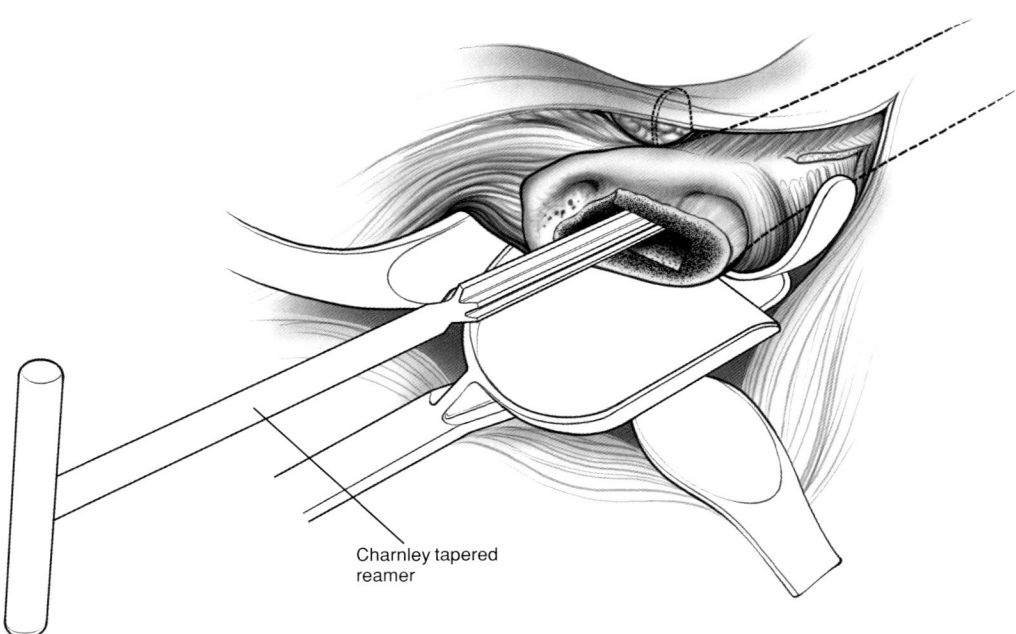

Figure 17. The medullary canal is "sounded" using the Charnley tapered reamer.

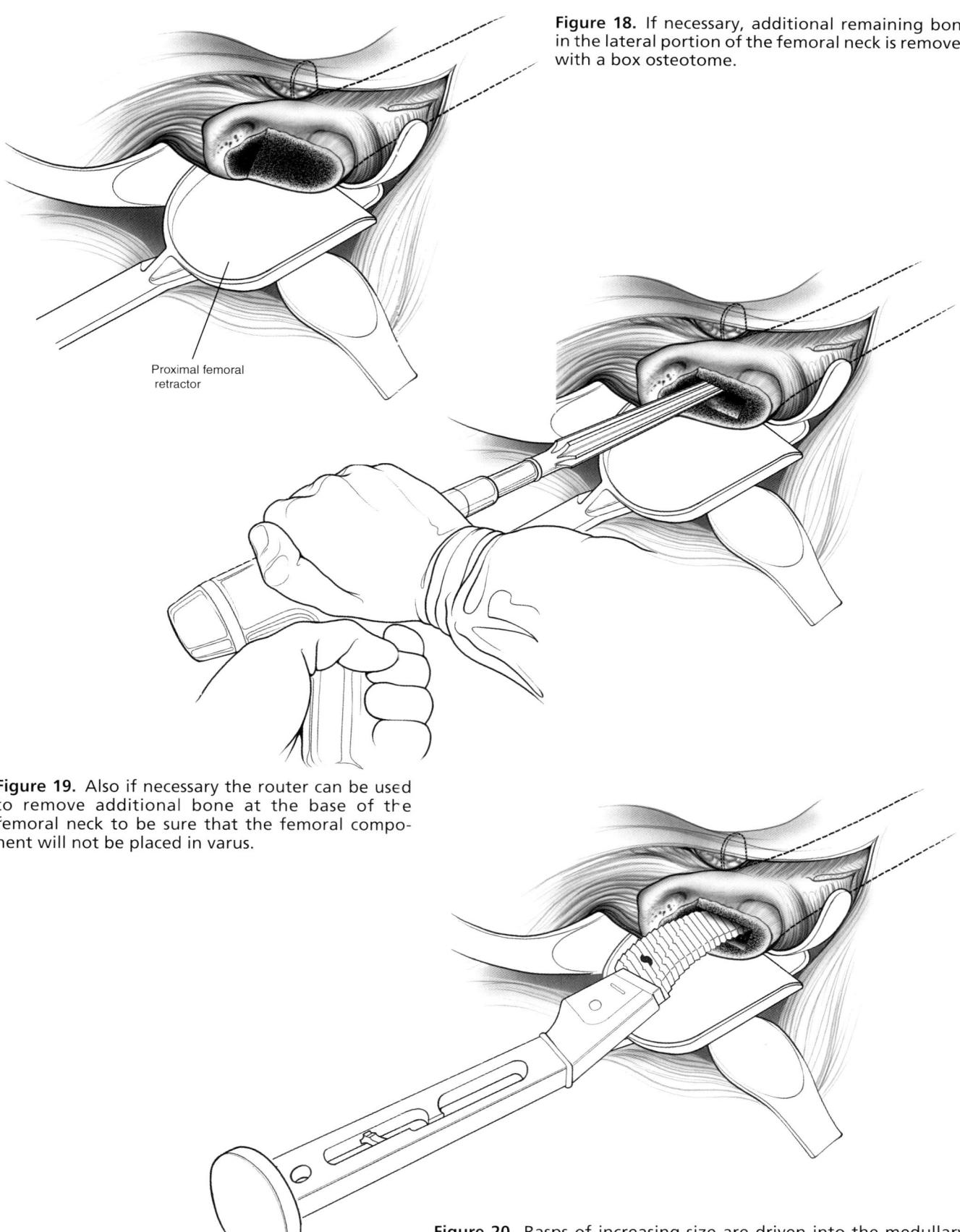

Figure 18. If necessary, additional remaining bone in the lateral portion of the femoral neck is removed with a box osteotome.

Figure 19. Also if necessary the router can be used to remove additional bone at the base of the femoral neck to be sure that the femoral component will not be placed in varus.

Figure 20. Rasps of increasing size are driven into the medullary canal. The attitude of the rasps should be in neutral varus-valgus position and 15° of anteversion.

The femoral rasp is anteverted by 15 to 20 degrees. Once the largest rasp that will fit has been driven fully home and countersunk into the bone 3 or 4 mm, the rasp handle is removed (Fig. 21), exposing a trunnion. This trunnion is the guide for the calcar rasp. The calcar rasp machines the medial neck area for a precise fit of the collar (Fig. 22).

The same trunnion also is the center post of the provisional collar-neck piece (Fig. 23). The trial reduction allows determination of range of motion, leg length, and stability.

At the time the trial reduction is made, adjustments of leg length can be arranged. If more length is needed, a longer head-neck component is used. If less length is needed, more femoral neck is cut off.

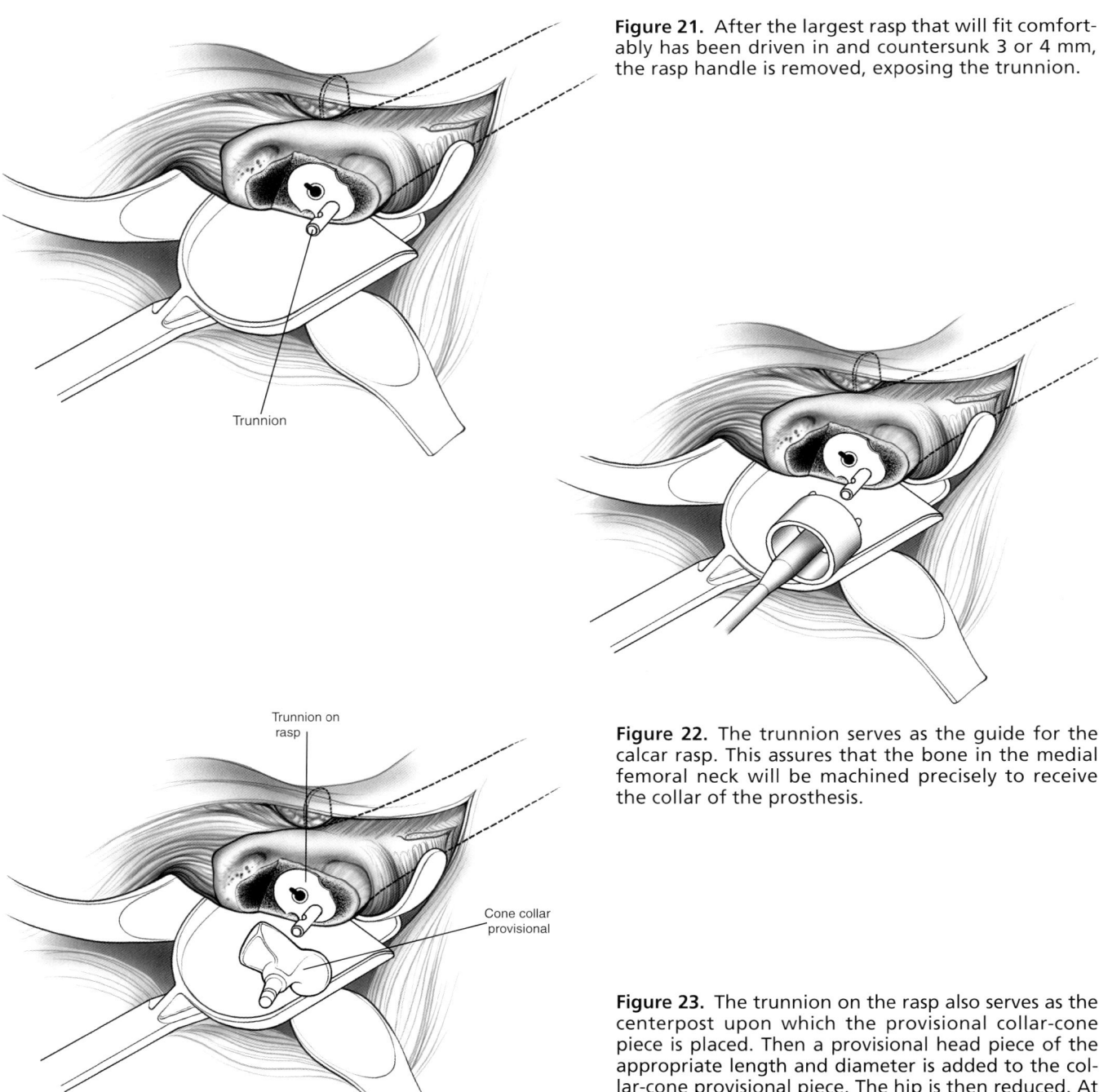

Figure 21. After the largest rasp that will fit comfortably has been driven in and countersunk 3 or 4 mm, the rasp handle is removed, exposing the trunnion.

Figure 22. The trunnion serves as the guide for the calcar rasp. This assures that the bone in the medial femoral neck will be machined precisely to receive the collar of the prosthesis.

Figure 23. The trunnion on the rasp also serves as the centerpost upon which the provisional collar-cone piece is placed. Then a provisional head piece of the appropriate length and diameter is added to the collar-cone provisional piece. The hip is then reduced. At this point an assessment is made of leg lengths, range of motion, and stability.

In checking stability of the hip joint, the two most likely positions for dislocation (extension with external rotation and flexion with internal rotation) are carefully assessed. If there is impingement, the necessary steps are taken to correct it.

The handle is reattached to the rasp and the rasp is removed from the medullary canal.

A curette is used to remove firmly all weak cancellous bone.

Cementing the Femoral Component

The experience of the past 30 years has proven without any doubt that the technique used in femoral cementing is critical to long duration of fixation. The key elements are (a) plugging the canal, (b) use of a cement gun, (c) pressurization, (d) porosity reduction of the cement, (e) precoating and/or a rough surface on the stem, and (f) centralization in order to provide a uniform cement mantle.

I prefer a PMMA plug because it is the most reliable, better than either polyethylene or bone plugs. To limit the distal extent of the cement plug, I first place a polyethylene plug 3 mm distal to the locus where the tip of the stem will be and then layer 1.5 cc of doughy cement on top of it, using the medullary plug syringe (Fig. 24).

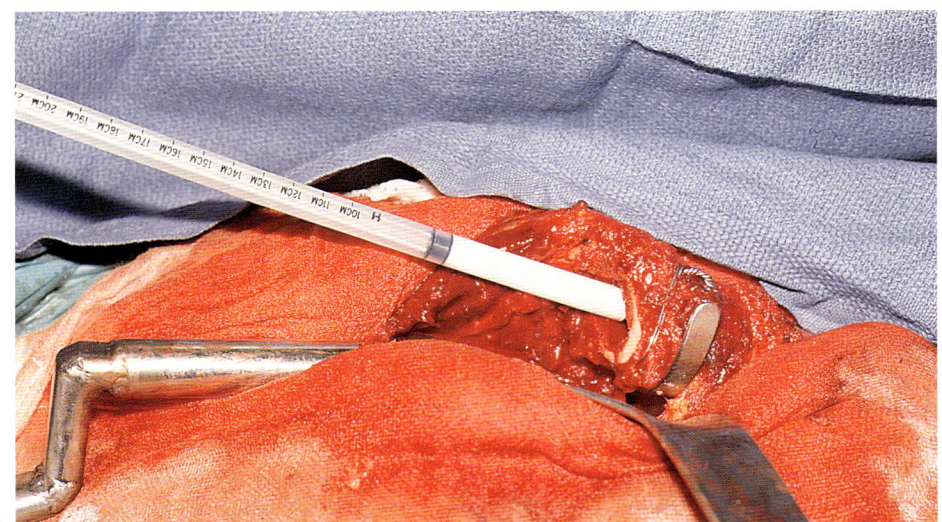

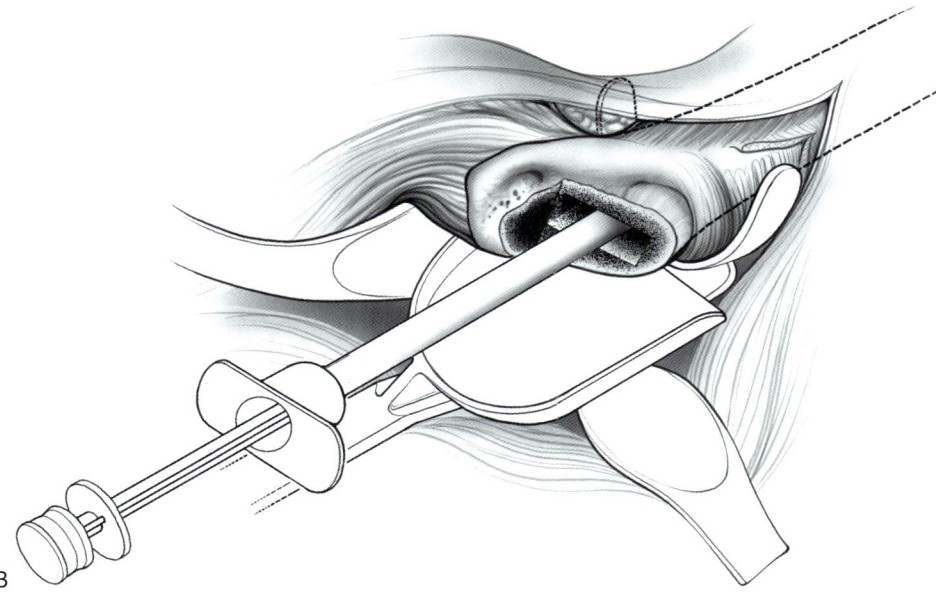

Figure 24. (A) The medullary plug syringe filled with a bolus of doughy bone cement at its tip, to be inserted down the femoral medullary canal and injected at a location 3 cm distal to the locus that the tip of the femoral component will occupy. (B) After a plastic plug has been inserted, 1.5 to 2 ccs of doughy PMMA is delivered to the top of the plastic plug using the medullary plug syringe to insure optimum occlusion of the medullary canal. This is important in optimizing pressurization of the cement. The plastic plug should be placed 3 cm below the location where the tip of the stem will come to lie.

Porosity reduction of the cement is essential to increase the fatigue strength of the cement. Centrifugation and vacuum mixing are both useful, but centrifugation is preferable.

It is important to start with a strong cement and then to strengthen it further by removing the voids by porosity reduction.

The loosening of cemented femoral components begins as debonding, failure at the cement–metal interface. For that reason it is crucial to precoat and/or roughen the surface of the femoral component, especially at the two areas of maximum interfacial strain, namely prox-

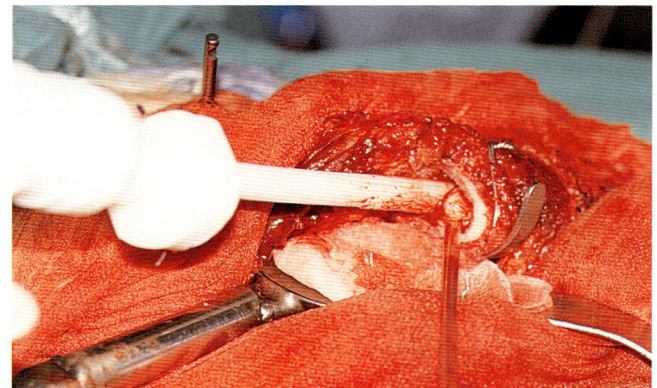
A

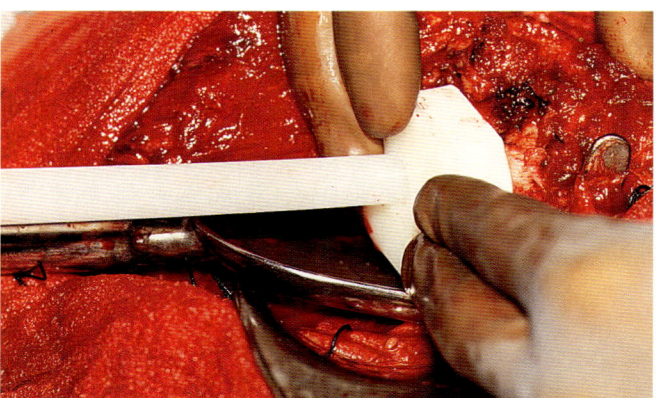
B

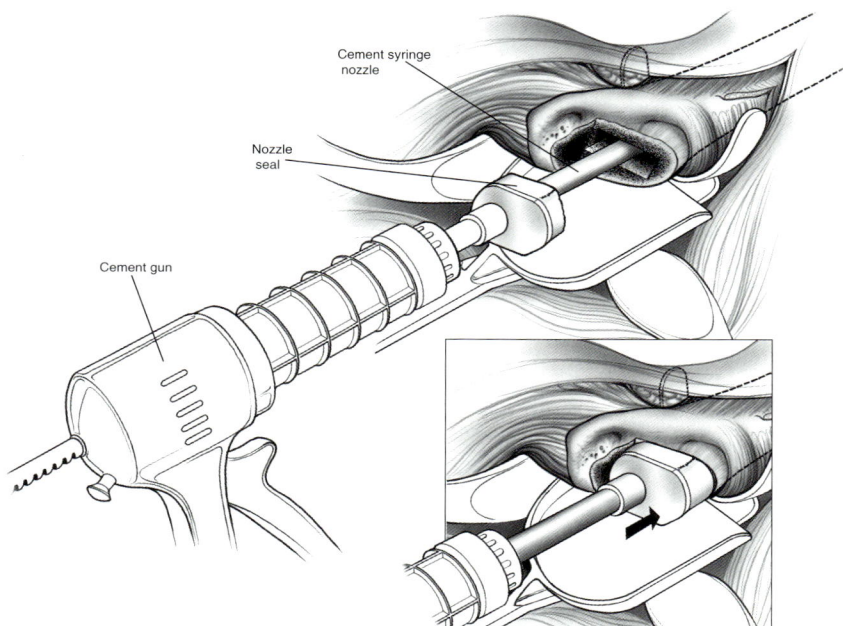
C

Figure 25. (A) The nozzle seal is placed over the nozzle of the cement delivery system and pushed up toward the cement cartridge as far as possible. The nozzle is then introduced down the medullary canal to the plug and the cement is injected into the medullary canal.

When three-fourths of the nozzle has been forced out of the medullary canal by the pressure of the injected cement, the nozzle seal is moved into position over the cut edge of the femoral neck and provides a seal while the remaining cement is injected into the medullary canal. (B) The cut surface of the femoral neck has been occluded by the nozzle seal. Further cement is injected through the nozzle as the nozzle is withdrawn out of the medullary canal and out of the femoral neck seal. This pressurizes the cement during the injection of the cement into the femoral medullary canal. (C) The nozzle of the cement gun in the femoral medullary canal with the nozzle seal retracted back against the cement cartridge. Note that the medullary canal has been filled with cement up to the level of the lesser trochanter, and a small amount of cement has reached the area of the femoral neck osteotomy. At this point, the nozzle seal can be brought into position against the cut surface of the femoral neck.

imally and distally. Pressurization of the cement is best done using a series of seals to block off the femoral neck, both during ingestion and after the medullary canal has been filled with cement. The first step is to plug the medullary canal to restrict the flow of bone cement and to enhance cement pressurization. As noted above, I plug the medullary canal with a combination of a polyethylene plug with a cement plug on top of it. After the plastic plug of the appropriate size is placed 30 mm below where the tip will reside, 1.5 cc of doughy cement is delivered on top of the plastic plug using the medullary plug syringe (Fig. 25).

For cementing a small stem, two packs of cement will be required, but for larger stems, four packs are prepared. To strenghten the cement to five times the strength obtained with normal mixing, the cement is centrifuged while the medullary canal is being cleaned and dried. Standard cement is used, but early, while it is in a lower viscosity state but just doughy.

The chrome cobalt head is impacted onto the stem. The medullary canal is cleaned using a pulsating water lavage and then dried using a dry sponge followed by a sponge soaked in dilute (1:500,000) epinephrine.

The cement is introduced in a retrograde fashion from the plug upward with the cement gun.

The nozzle seal improves the cement distribution during the process of withdrawing the nozzle. This nozzle seal resides high on the nozzle near the cartridge, when the nozzle is first inserted (Fig. 25). When the nozzle has been driven up out of the canal by the pressure of the injected cement until the nozzle is 4 to 6 cm in the canal, the nozzle seal is pushed down the nozzle until it occludes the opening in the femoral neck. As more cement is injected, it pressurizes the cement and also eliminates laminations and voids that are commonly the result of drawing the nozzle out of the cement.

Then the femoral neck seal is used (Fig. 26). Additional cement is injected for further pressurization of the entire cement mass.

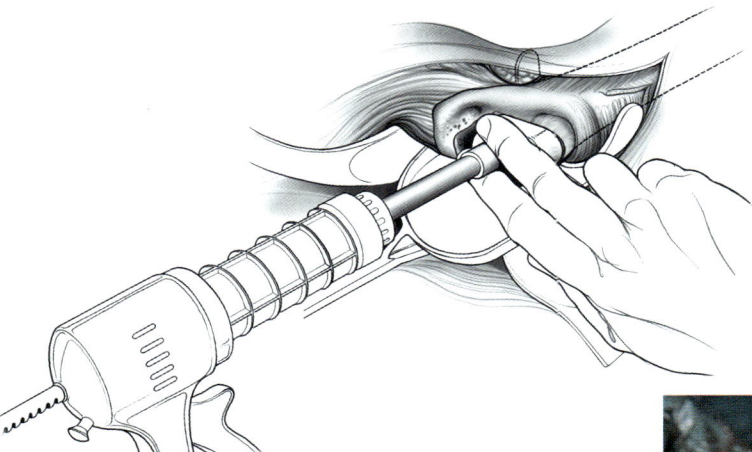

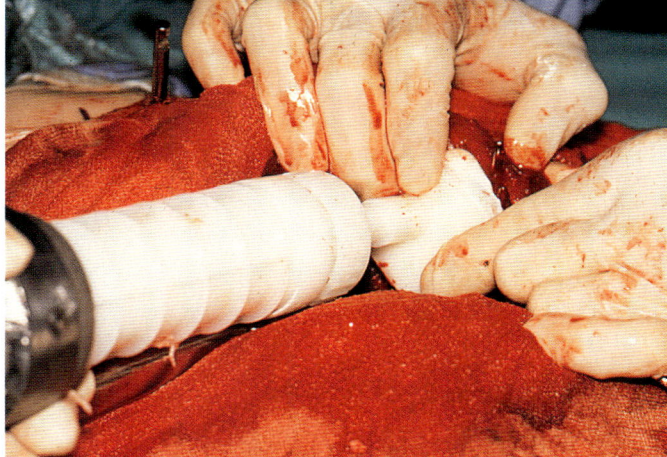

Figure 26. (A) Once the medullary canal is completely filled with cement and the nozzle has been withdrawn, the femoral neck seal is used to occlude the femoral neck further, and the final pressurization takes place. (B) Once the femoral medullary canal is filled with cement, the entire cement mass is pressurized once again using the femoral neck seal, shown in Fig. 27 B.

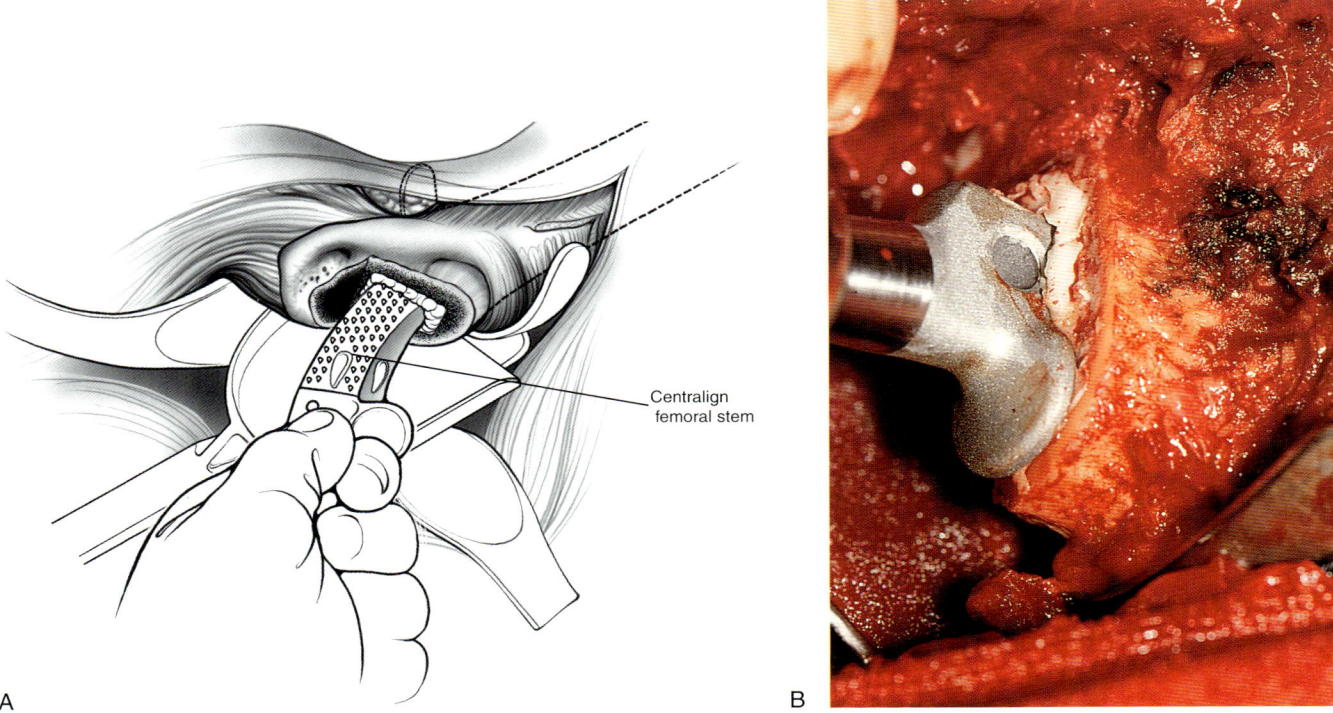

Figure 27. (A) The femoral stem is introduced in neutral varus-valgus position and 15° of anteversion with a single steady motion that delivers the collar precisely on the machined portion of the femoral neck. Remaining extraneous cement is removed. The femur is held still and the femoral component is held still until the cement has polymerized. (B) Close-up photograph of the collar resting solidly on the milled surface of the medial portion of the femoral neck. The contact is broad and intimate. This permits direct stress transfer from the collar to the medial portion of the femoral neck.

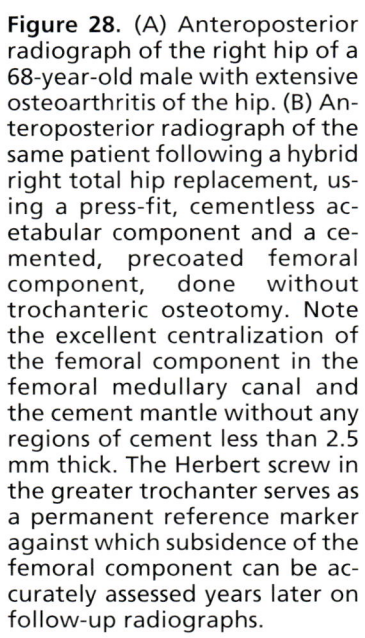 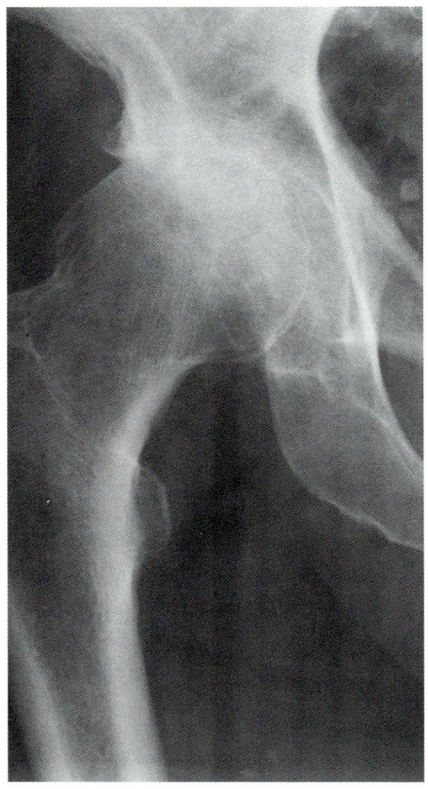 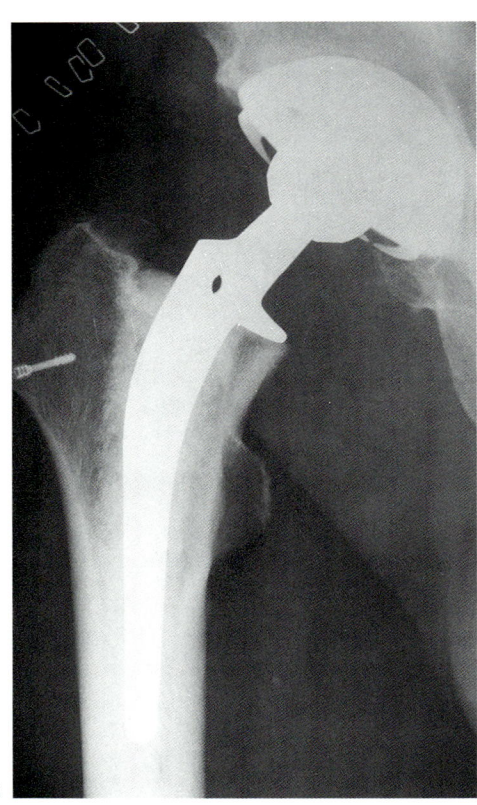

Figure 28. (A) Anteroposterior radiograph of the right hip of a 68-year-old male with extensive osteoarthritis of the hip. (B) Anteroposterior radiograph of the same patient following a hybrid right total hip replacement, using a press-fit, cementless acetabular component and a cemented, precoated femoral component, done without trochanteric osteotomy. Note the excellent centralization of the femoral component in the femoral medullary canal and the cement mantle without any regions of cement less than 2.5 mm thick. The Herbert screw in the greater trochanter serves as a permanent reference marker against which subsidence of the femoral component can be accurately assessed years later on follow-up radiographs.

The femoral component is introduced (Fig. 27) in neutral varus–valgus alignment with 15 to 20 degrees of anteversion. Careful positioning of the prosthesis leads to intimate contact between the femoral collar and the machined surface of the medial neck region.

While the femoral component is held motionless until the cement has polymerized, excess cement is removed.

Centralization of the femoral component is a critical issue. The optimum cement mantle has a minimum thickness of 2.5mm. There should be no cement thinner than this, if possible, and voids or defects in the cement mantle should be avoided.

The PMMA centralizers built onto the stem (Fig. 28) play an important role in this, aided by the fact that the rasps are larger than the stem by an amount necessary to create this thicker mantle.

The femoral component is then reduced. Stability, range of motion, abductor tension, and leg lengths are checked. If satisfactory, the hemostasis is obtained, the suction drains are inserted, and the wound is closed in layers. The extremity is kept in abduction and 30 to 40 degrees of flexion initially to assure stability of the hip.

Figure 28, A and B, show the preoperative and postoperative anteroposterior radiographs of the right hip of a patient who has had such a hybrid primary total hip replacement.

POSTOPERATIVE MANAGEMENT

The patients are generally out of bed bearing full weight when standing with both feet on the second postoperative day. They progress rapidly from a walker to crutches, partial weight bearing. Discharge is usually at about seven days.

They shift from two crutches to one when they can do so with a normal gait and without pain, commonly four to five weeks postoperatively.

Three or four weeks later, they may shift to a cane and are free to discard the cane when they can walk with a normal gait without pain.

Patients with trochanteric osteotomy are advised to continue using their two crutches for three months or, rarely, longer.

RESULTS

Ninety percent of the patients have good or excellent results, being pain free or having at most slight occasional pain. The average range of motion is over 90 degrees of flexion. Eighty-five percent can put on their shoe and sock and cut their toenails.

We caution against high-impact activities such as tennis, volleyball, and jogging. Golf, swimming, and bike riding are recommended sport activities.

REHABILITATION

With the exception of those patients who have specific deformities or contractions, the postoperative rehabilitation is not complex. Patients are taught to manage crutches and climb stairs. They are instructed in getting to their shoe and sock in flexion and external rotation to reduce the likelihood of postoperative dislocation. After two or three months, sidelying abduction and extension against gravity are instituted. During the first three months we advise patients not to rise from a chair or to climb stairs using their recently operated hip.

COMPLICATIONS

The major complications associated with the surgery itself are dislocation, nerve damage, postoperative wound hemorrhage, heterotopic ossification, and leg-length discrepancy.

The prevention of dislocation is multifactoral. The optimum position of the components is 45 degrees of abduction and 20 degrees of anteversion of the acetabular component and

15 degrees of anteversion of the femoral component. Offset and abductor tension play important roles. It is optimum to match or increase the offset of the patient's own joint. If the offset is reduced, the abductors become lax, leading to an increased incidence of limp and dislocation.

If the offset cannot be matched by the prosthesis itself, one can advance the trochanter or lengthen the limb. Neither of these corrects the offset, but both can correct the abductor laxity. Obviously, in the instance of a limb that is short, lengthening the limb restores both the appropriate leg length and abductor tension. The decision in a patient with equal leg lengths to advance to trochanter or to lengthen the limb must be made on the basis of local factors. Women very much dislike having the leg made too long. Men are less concerned about it. Generally we would recommend advancing the trochanter rather than lengthening the limb, but there are circumstances in which increased leg length is an appropriate move. For example, if the opposite leg must be operated on subsequently and it can be lengthened an equal amount in a subsequent operation, then it is preferable to lengthen the limb on the first hip rather than advancing the trochanter.

It is easier to dislocate a total hip replacement than it is a normal hip. As a result, all patients need to be cautioned against positions of danger, which with this surgical approach are predominantly external rotation in extension and internal rotation in flexion. Both positions are made worse by adduction.

Nerve damage is most commonly partial damage to the sciatic nerve, usually the peroneal branch, produced by pressure on the sciatic nerve with a retractor or stretching the sciatic nerve in an effort to lengthen the limb. Usually, it is unwise to try to lengthen the limb more than 2 or 2.5 cm, unless special circumstances exist. Nerve lesions can also be produced by postoperative hematomas. In most instances, conservative management is the optimum course. There is a high probability of resolution of the nerve injury, if, indeed, it is neuropraxia. The femoral nerve can also be compromised by unusual retraction, hematoma formation, or dislocation. Again, conservative management is generally optimum.

The functional deficit of a severe femoral palsy is worse than that of a severe peroneal palsy. The management of both generally requires the use of an orthosis. The appropriate orthosis for a femoral palsy is a long leg brace (groin to ankle) that has a drop lock.

RECOMMENDED READING

1. Barrack, R. L., Mulroy, Jr., R. D., and Harris, W. H.: Improved cementing techniques and femoral component loosening in young patients with hip arthroplasty. A 12 year radiographic review. *J. Bone Joint Surg.*, 74-B:385–389, 1992.
2. Charnley, J.: *Low Friction Arthroplasty of the Hip*. Springer-Verlag, Berlin, 1979.
3. Harrigan, T. P., Harris, W. H.: A three-dimensional non-linear finite element study of the effect of cement-prosthesis debonding in cemented femoral total hip components. *J. Biomech.* 23:1047–1058, 1991.
4. Harrigan, T. P., Kareh, J. A., O'Connor, D. O., Burke, D. O., Harris, W. H.: A finite element study of the initiation of the failure of fixation in cemented femoral total hip components. *J. Orthop. Res.*, 10:134–144, 1992.
5. Harris, W. H.: A new approach to total hip replacement without osteotomy of the greater trochanter. *Clin. Orthop.*, 106:19–26, 1975.
6. Harris, W. H., Davies, J. P.: Modern use of modern cement for total hip replacement. *Orthop. Clin. North Am.*, 19:581–589, 1988.
7. Harris, W. H., and Sledge, C. B.: Medical progress: total hip and total knee replacement (first of two parts). *N. Engl. J. Med.*, 323:725–731, 1990.
8. Maloney, W. J., Jasty, M., Burke, D. W., O'Connor, D. O., Zalenski, E. B., Bragdon, C., and Harris, W. H.: Biomechanical and histologic investigation of cemented total hip arthroplasties. A study of autopsy-retrieved femurs after *in vivo* cycling. *Clin. Orthop.*, 249:129–140, 1989.
9. Mulroy, R. D. Jr., Harris, W. H.: The effect of improved cementing techniques on component loosening in total hip replacement. An 11-year radiographic review. *J. Bone Joint Surg.*, 72-B:757–760, 1990.
10. Schmalzried, T. P., Harris, W. H.: The Harris-Galante porous-coated acetabular component with screw fixation: radiographic analysis of eighty-three primary hip replacements at a minimum of five years. *J. Bone Joint Surg.*, 74-A: 1130–1139, 1992.
11. Schmalzried, T. P., Kwong, L. M., Jasty, M. et al.: The mechanism of loosening of cemented acetabular components in total hip arthroplasty. Analysis of specimens retrieved at autopsy. *Clin. Orthop.* 274:60–78, 1992.
12. Schmalzried, T. P., Wessinger, S. J., Hill, G., Harris, W. H.: The HGP acetabular component press fit without screw fixation: A 5 year radiographic analysis of primary cases. *J Arthroplasty*, 9:235–242, 1994.

14

Cementless Primary Total Hip Arthroplasty

Ajai Cadambi and Charles A. Engh

INDICATIONS/CONTRAINDICATIONS

The authors use extensively porous-coated implants for primary surgery in cases of (a) primary or secondary arthritis, (b) rheumatoid arthritis, (c) idiopathic avascular (osteo) necrosis of the femoral head, and (d) displaced femoral neck fractures with underlying arthritis. Adequate bone stock must be present in order to seat the prosthesis in a cementless fashion. Candidates for cementless hip arthroplasty should be carefully selected with regard to activity level. Before surgery the patient should be instructed thoroughly on the planned therapy and activity regimen. Contraindications for cementless total hip arthroplasty include (a) history of local infection; (b) inadequate or absent bone stock, which precludes rigid cementless fixation of components; (c) paralysis or neuromuscular disease; (d) Charcot arthropathy; and (e) poor patient compliance with the initial limited weight bearing restrictions.

PREOPERATIVE PLANNING

The patient is examined preoperatively to determine the extent of limb length discrepancy present, as equivalent limb length is one of the goals of arthroplasty. This is done by using both standing blocks and direct measurements (anterior-superior iliac spine to medial malleolus). In addition, the range of motion of the hip is recorded, since this may influence the procedure planned. For example, if an adduction contracture is present, an adductor tenotomy may be indicated as part of the arthroplasty.

A. Cadambi, M.D.: The Texas Hip and Knee Center, Fort Worth, Texas 76104.
C. A. Engh, M.D.: Department of Orthopaedics, University of Maryland School of Medicine, Baltimore, Maryland 21201; and Anderson Orthopaedic Research Institute, Alexandria, Virginia 22307

Templating

Implant sizing is dependent on an accurate radiographic technique. Templating in most cases is performed on two radiographs, an anteroposterior (AP) view of the pelvis and a lateral view of the proximal half of the femur. The appearance of the AP pelvis radiograph should be similar to that illustrated in Fig. 1. Both acetabula and at least eight inches of both femora are included on the radiograph. The femora should be internally rotated so that the femoral neck is parallel to the plane of the film (0 degrees of anteversion). If it is not possible to obtain an internal rotation view due to a severely arthritic hip, then the contralateral hip (if normal) is used to plan the procedure. In this case, the surgeon makes the as-

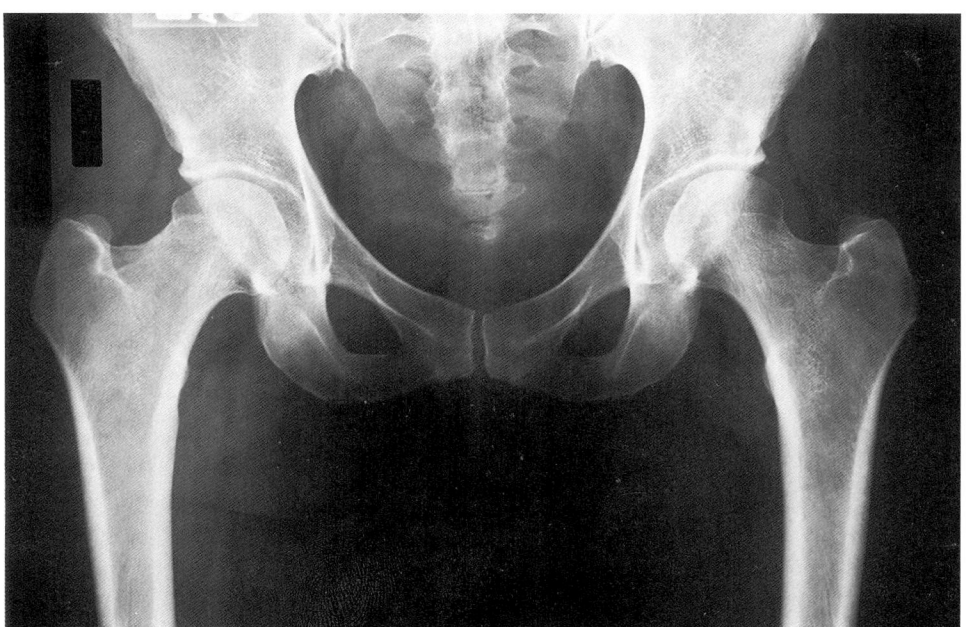

Figure 1. AP pelvic radiograph used for preoperative planning, both femora are internally rotated.

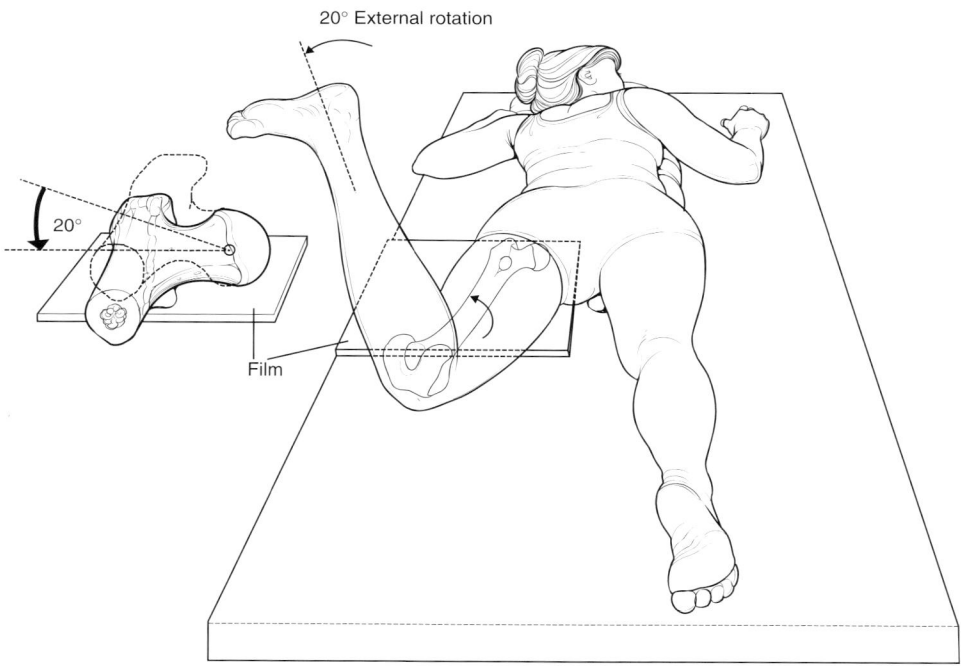

Figure 2. Patient positioning for PA radiograph of the femur, which is sometimes needed for preoperative planning.

sumption that the shape of the malrotated arthritic femur is similar to that of the normal one. If both hips are involved with disease and cannot be internally rotated, then another radiographic method is necessary to determine the shape of the proximal femur in 0 degrees of femoral neck anteversion. We use a posterior to anterior view of the femur in the desired amount of internal rotation. Appearance of the pelvis is not important on this view. It therefore can be tilted in order to achieve the desired femoral rotation. (Figs. 2, 3).

In our preoperative planning sequence, a lateral radiograph of the femur is also used (Fig. 4). The rotation of the femur is controlled by having the greater trochanter of the proximal femur, the lateral condyle of the distal femur, and the lateral malleolus of the ankle

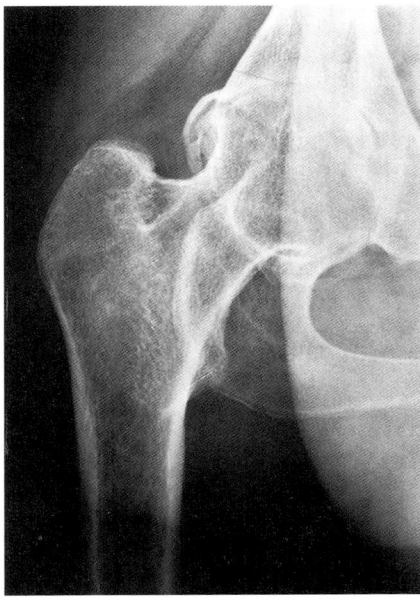

Figure 3. Radiographic appearance of proximal femur when the posterior to anterior technique illustrated in Fig. 2 has been used.

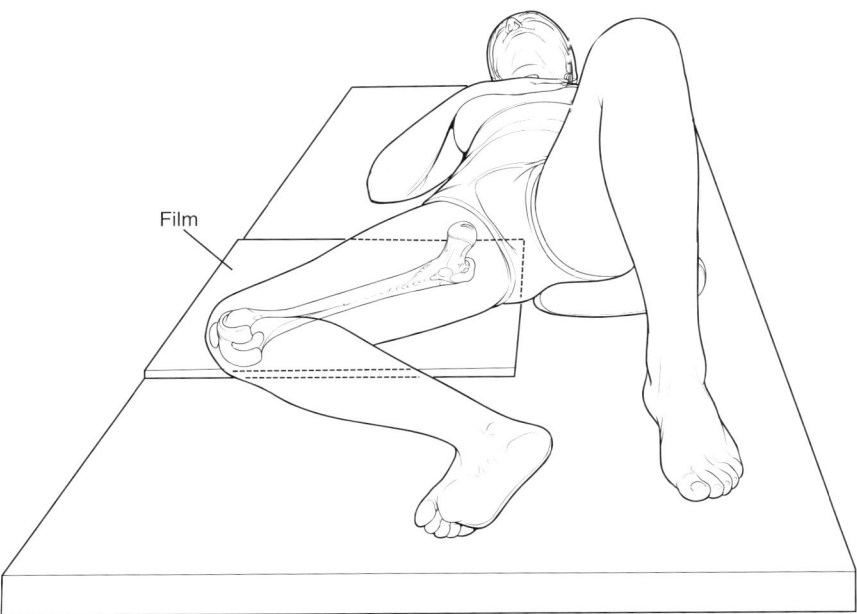

Figure 4. Radiographic technique recommended for the table-down lateral radiograph of the proximal femur. The long axis of the femur is parallel to the film cassette and perpendicular to the radiographic beam.

touch the table top. The radiographic beam is directed at a 90-degree angle to the femoral shaft (Fig. 5).

Once adequate radiographs are obtained, the surgeon can proceed with determining implant size and position. The majority of this planning is performed on the AP pelvis radiograph. Steps involved in the templating process include (a) determining the acetabular cup size and positioning, (b) determining the femoral stem type and diameter, and (c) determining the level of the femoral neck cut and the correct neck length for the femoral implant.

Determining the Size and Position of the Acetabular Component. The acetabular components used by the authors range in size from 46 to 76 mm in outer diameter. The acetabular templates correspond to these sizes. Templating is performed on the AP pelvis radiograph. If there is only minimal acetabular damage, planning is not difficult (Fig. 6). The selected template should be large enough to contact the acetabular subchondral bone over the entire porous coated area. The cup should be large enough to span the distance from the teardrop (inferomedially) to the acetabular rim (superolaterally). The template should be placed at an angle of inclination of from 40 to 60 degrees with reference to the transverse teardrop line. Holes are present in the template so that the superior and inferior aspects of the cup can be marked on the film. The planned center of rotation of the acetabular component is also marked through the template. Horizontal and vertical slots in the template are used to mark the horizontal and vertical position of the component.

Femoral Templating. The prosthesis used by the authors is a modification of their initial fixed-head prosthesis. In 1984, it was changed to a modular design with a 32-mm femoral head and a Morse Taper. In 1986, a second stem was developed for small-sized patients, generally females less than 64 inches in height. Recently, a third stem shape has been made for extremely large-boned patients. The neck of these three stem designs has also been changed. The implant used in small patients has a neck-shaft angle of 125 degrees.

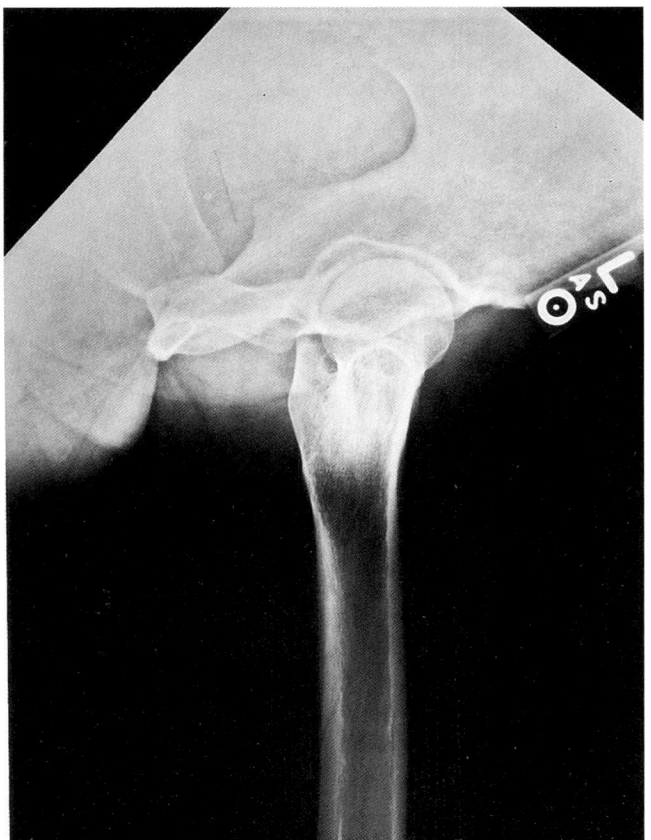

Figure 5. Appearance of lateral femoral radiograph obtained by the table-down lateral technique.

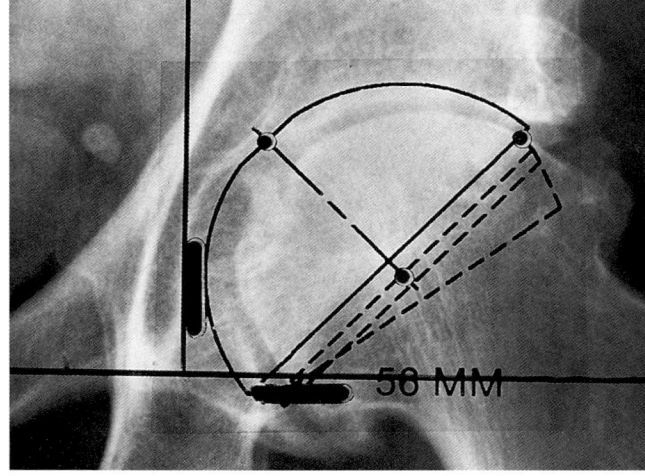

Figure 6. Authors' recommended acetabular templating technique.

The neck design of the original prosthesis, now termed the large design, has retained a 135-degree neck-shaft angle but the position of the neck on the collar of the prosthesis has been modified to increase the femoral head offset. The neck for the stem used for extra large-boned patients is similar, but proportionally larger. The stem portion of the three designs remains nontapered and cylindrical with a porous-coated surface extending to within 2 cm of the tip of the stem. Each design is made in incremental cylindrical sizes. Since the femoral neck of the stems is anteverted, templates for a left and a right design exist.

The template should be placed in line with the center line of the proximal femur. The template is of the correct distal diameter if it appears slightly larger than the patient's femoral isthmus. The porous coating should contact a distance of at least 3 cm of the medial and lateral walls of the femoral isthmus. The correct proximal implant design (small, large, or extra large) must also be selected. The proximal shape of the implant is considered to be correct if the curvature on its medial side parallels the calcar. After templating the femur, the surgeon should be able to determine the correct stem diameter, proximal stem design, and expected area of porous coating to contact cortical bone.

Determining the Neck Cut and Implant Neck Length that Will Restore Limb Length and Maintain Femoral Offset. Ideally, the femur should be displaced laterally away from the pelvis at a distance equal to or greater than that present preoperatively, in order to maintain proper abductor tension (1,2). In addition, equal leg length should be restored. Once the position of the acetabular component has been fixed, increasing the neck length of the femoral component is the only method to increase lateralization of the femur. Limb length can be adjusted by changing the neck length of the prosthesis or by changing the seating level of the prosthesis. The authors, therefore, first determine the neck length that will maintain lateral offset and then adjust the femoral template along the femoral center line until leg length is correct (Fig. 7).

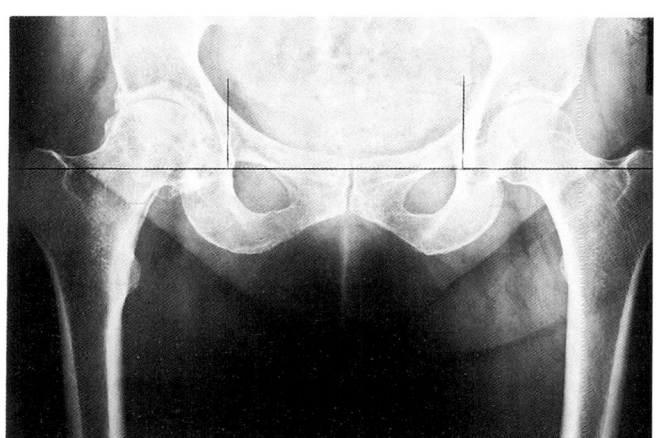
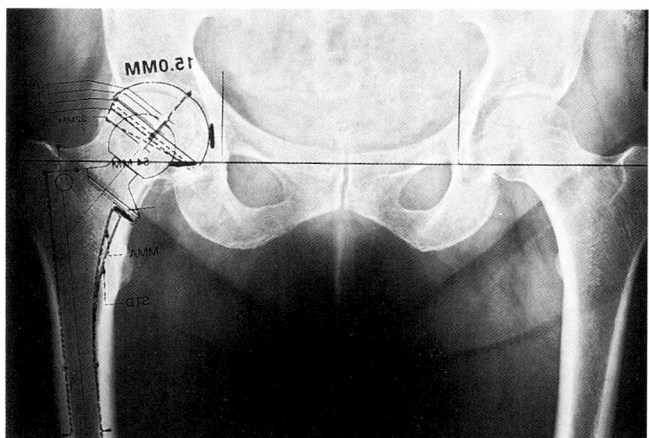
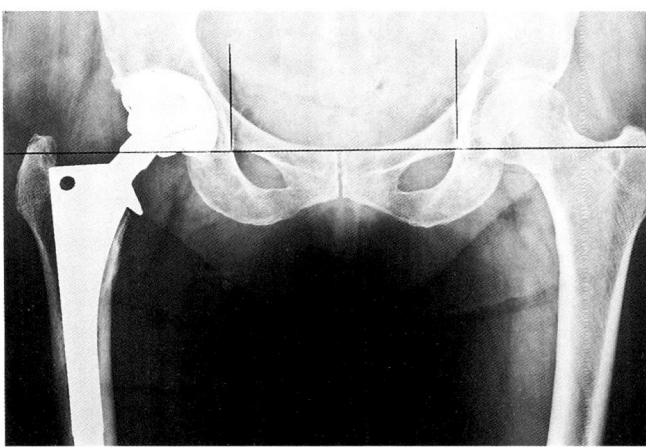

Figure 7. (A) Preoperative radiograph of a case with unilateral hip disease on the right side. The right femur is properly rotated for templating, and no leg-length discrepancy exists. The templating is done only on the right side. (B) Because there is no deformity or leg-length difference, no correction of femoral offset (lateralization) or leg length is required. The femoral template is therefore positioned so the center of the prosthetic femoral head lies directly over the center of the acetabular component. (C) Postoperative radiograph of the same case. Femoral offset and leg length are unchanged. Shenton's line remains unbroken.

When leg-length discrepancy exists, the amount of leg-length correction must be factored into the preoperative planning (Fig. 8A). After determining the position for the new acetabular component, the objective is to select a neck cut and a neck length that will maintain the femoral offset already present, but restore equal leg length (Fig. 8 B, C).

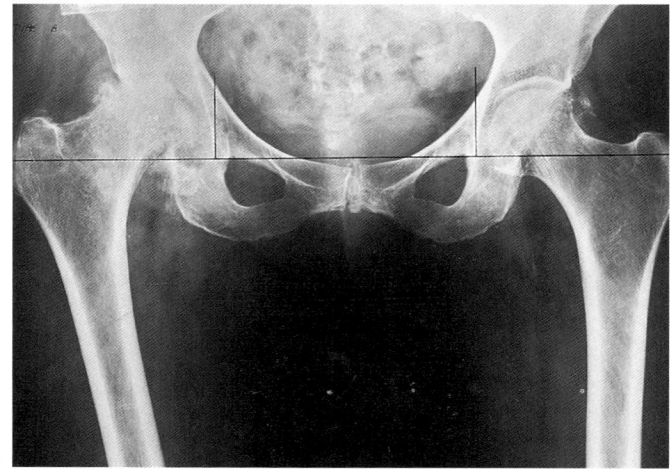

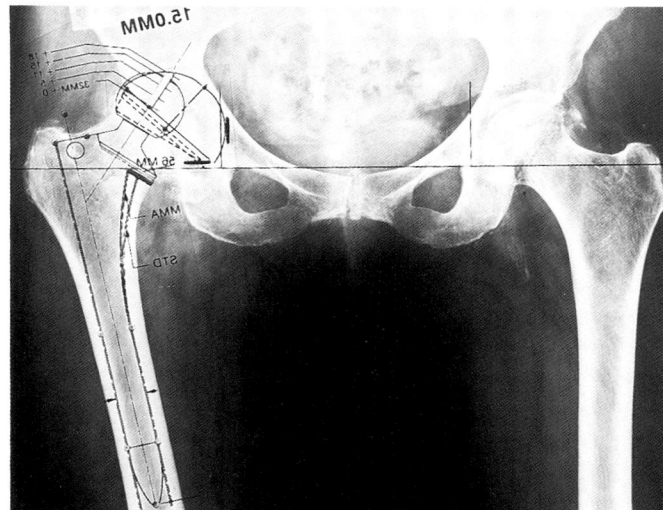

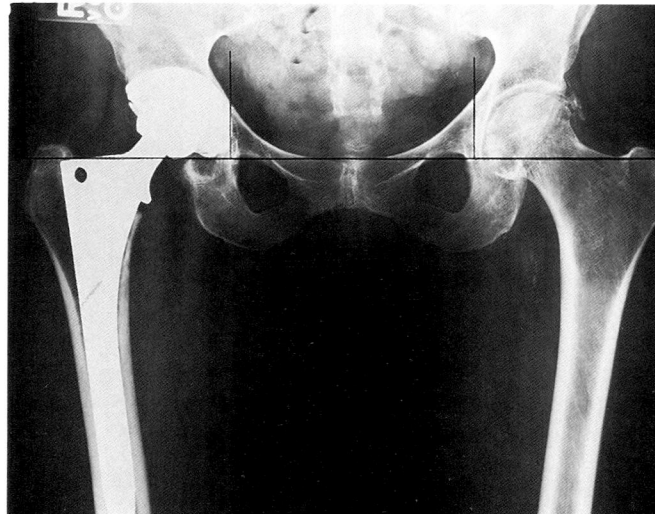

Figure 8. (A) Preoperative radiograph of a case of unilateral hip disease on the right in which there is a broken Shenton's line and shortening of the right leg. The objectives are to maintain the existing lateralization of the right femur and to restore leg length. The right femur is properly rotated for templating, so templating is done on the right side. (B) Preoperative radiograph with templates in place. The authors have selected a prosthetic neck length that will maintain femoral lateralization. The femoral template has been positioned so that the selected prosthetic head center is above the acetabular template center the distance required to restore leg length. Once the femoral neck resection level is marked, the best proximal and distal stem size can be determined. (C) Postoperative radiograph.

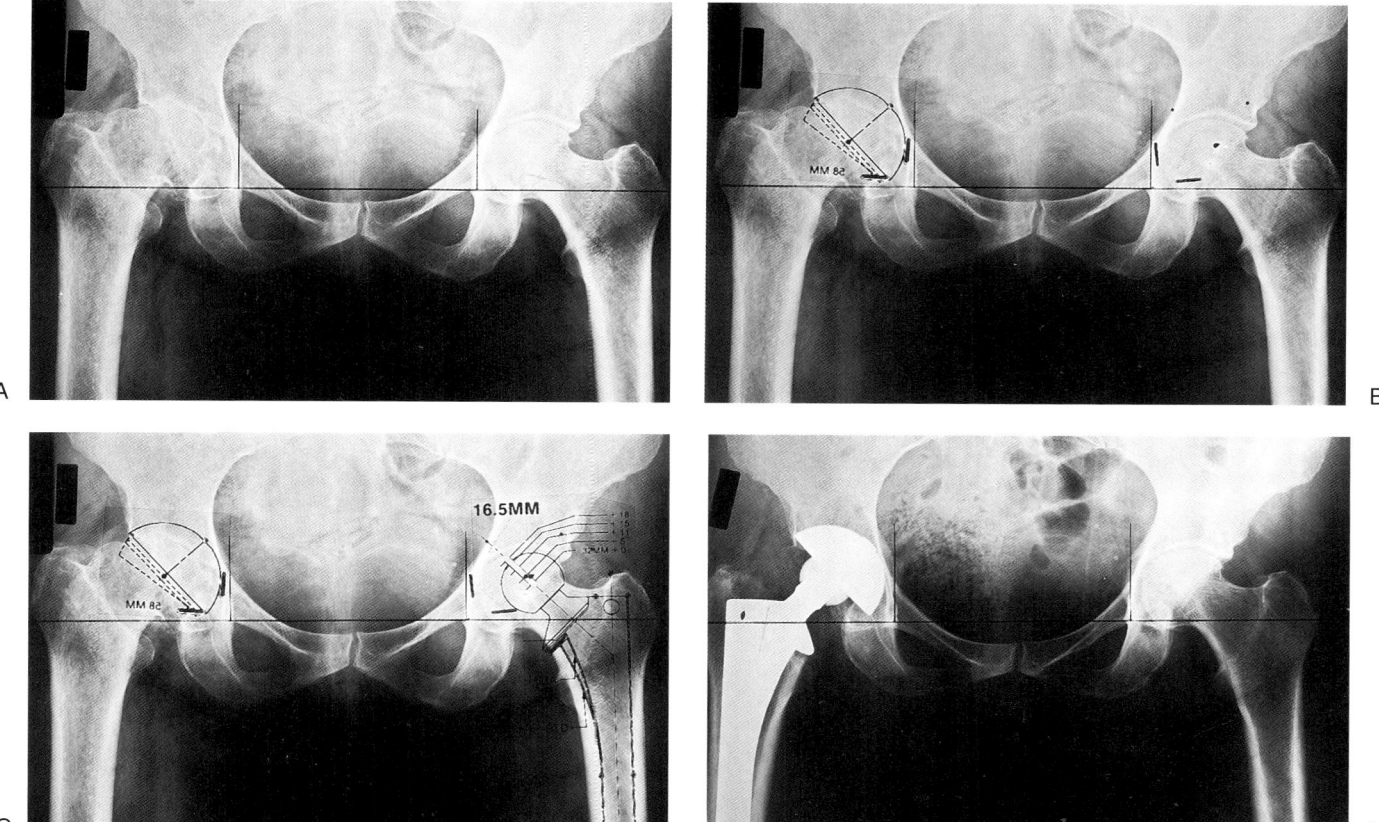

Figure 9. (A) Preoperative radiograph of a case of unilateral hip disease with deformity. The right hip is not correctly rotated for templating, so the templating must be done on the contralateral left side, which is correctly rotated. (B) The first step in templating involves selecting the acetabular component. The relationship of the slots in the template to the horizontal and vertical teardrop lines facilitates transfer of this template position to the left side of the radiograph. (C) Neck resection level and neck length are determined on the normal left side. If at surgery the right femoral neck is cut at this level and the neck length which was selected from the left side is also used, the vertical and horizontal distances separating the right femur from the pelvis should be similar to those existing on the left. (D) Postoperative radiograph showing that the horizontal and vertical distances separating the femora from the pelvis are similar.

In many cases, deformity and stiffness of the arthritic hip make it impossible to obtain an AP radiograph of the involved hip that is suitable for templating. If the patient has unilateral hip disease, the opposite side of the same x-ray can be used for the planning (Fig. 9). Planning when the rotation of the arthritic hip cannot be controlled is more complicated, but careful study of the steps shown in Fig. 9 should clarify this method.

SURGICAL TECHNIQUE

Exposure

The patient is placed in the lateral decubitus position on the operating table, and pelvic clamps, which are attached to the operating table, are used to hold the patient rigidly in this position. All bony prominences and the axilla are padded. Standard draping techniques are used with careful exclusion of the groin and perineum from the operative field. The lower (non-operated) leg is strapped to the table with the hip flexed 30 degrees and the knee at a 90-degree flexed position. If the upper leg is placed directly on top of the lower leg and both

Figure 10. The authors' method for positioning the patient for surgery through a posterior lateral hip incision.

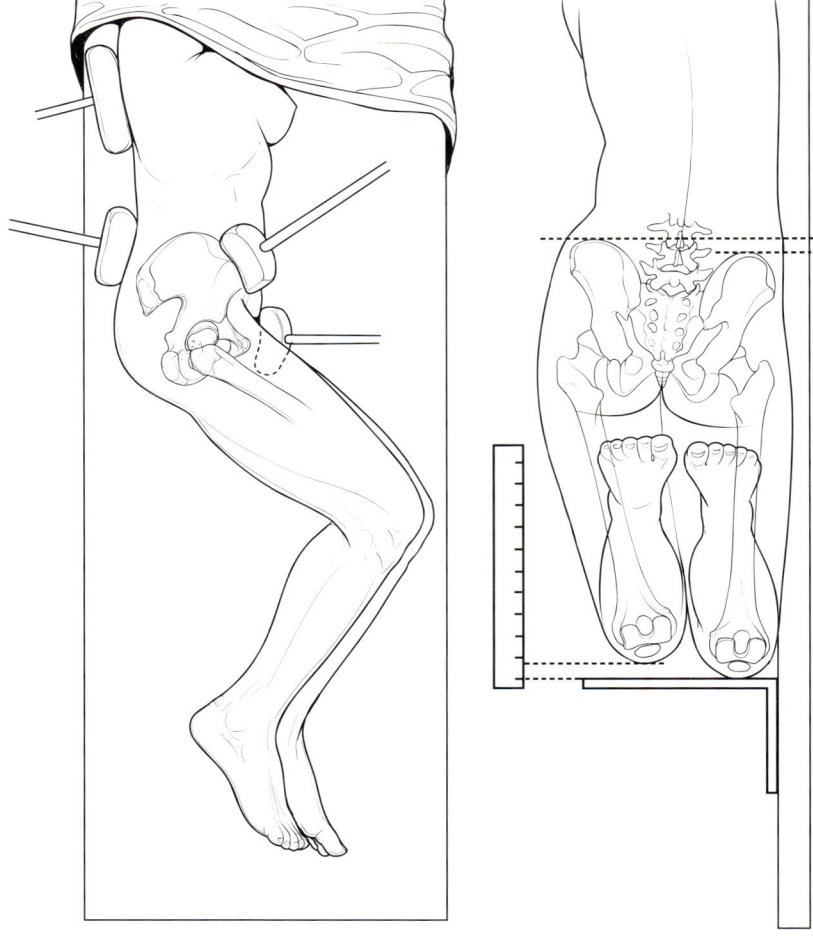

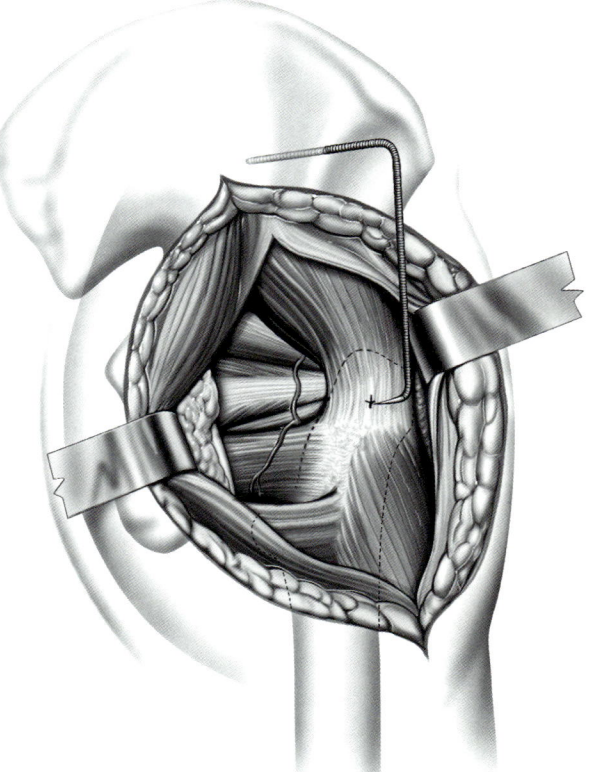

Figure 11 A, B. A threaded Steinmann pin fixed to the ileum just above the acetabulum is bent to contact the greater trochanter. This is the authors' technique for measuring the position of the femur relative to the ilium prior to femoral head resection.

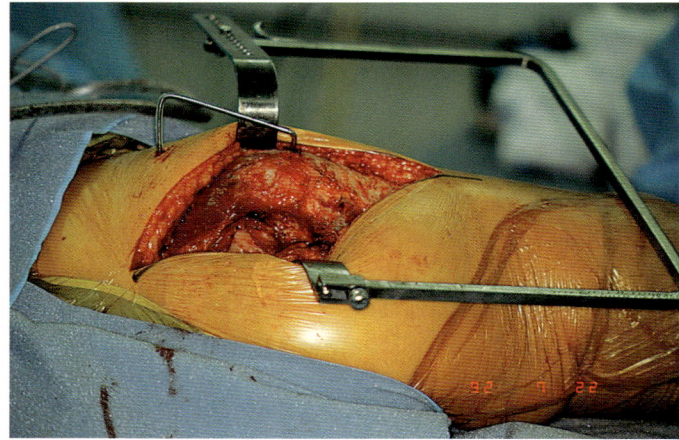

A

B

knees are flexed 90 degrees, it is possible to compare leg lengths. When the patient lies on the operating table in the lateral position, a pelvic tilt occurs. This creates an apparent leg-length discrepancy with the upper leg appearing shorter than it actually is. We use a right angle and a ruler to measure (at the knees) the apparent difference in femoral lengths (Fig. 10).

The posterior approach is used by the authors on all primary hip arthroplasties (3, 4). This approach allows for adequate exposure of both the acetabulum and proximal femur.

Once the superficial dissection is complete, the short external rotators are released from the posterolateral femur, and a posterior capsulectomy is then performed. Prior to dislocation of the hip and resection of the femoral head, a 5/32-inch threaded Steinmann pin is placed through the gluteus medius muscle into the ileum. The pin is then bent twice at 90 degree angles so that the exposed tip touches the greater trochanter (5). This point is marked with a stay stitch so that offset and length can be monitored after placement of the trial implants (Fig. 11). It is important to always place the upper leg back in the same position prior to measuring limb length using either of the above techniques.

The hip is dislocated by flexing, adducting, and internally rotating the femur. The femur can be delivered into the surgical field by using a retractor placed under the lesser trochanter. The femoral head is resected with the provisional cut. We routinely complete the capsulectomy by resecting the remaining anterior capsule. (Fig. 12). With resection of the thickened, contracted anterior capsule, patients are able to regain external rotation postoperatively, thus allowing them to perform routine activities such as putting on socks and shoes.

Anterior capsulectomy is accomplished by having a surgical assistant extend and internally rotate the hip joint while a second assistant applies lateral traction to the proximal femur with a bone hook (placed at the level of the lesser trochanter). This places the anterior capsule under tension so that it can be released from the anterior femur with the cautery. A curved Mayo scissor can be placed into the sheath of the psoas tendon in order to protect it and the underlying anterior musculature.

Once the capsule is released from the femur, a retractor can be placed over the anterior acetabular rim on the pubis, thus displacing the femur anteriorly. This anterior displacement can be facilitated by detaching a portion of the gluteus maximus tendon from its insertion on the posterolateral femur. The remaining capsule, the labrum, and transverse acetabular ligament are then easily resected. The pulvinar (fatty tissue) is then removed from the cotyloid notch (acetabular fossa), and a blunt retractor is placed into the obturator foramen. This retractor rests on the inferior edge of the acetabular fossa. This point corresponds

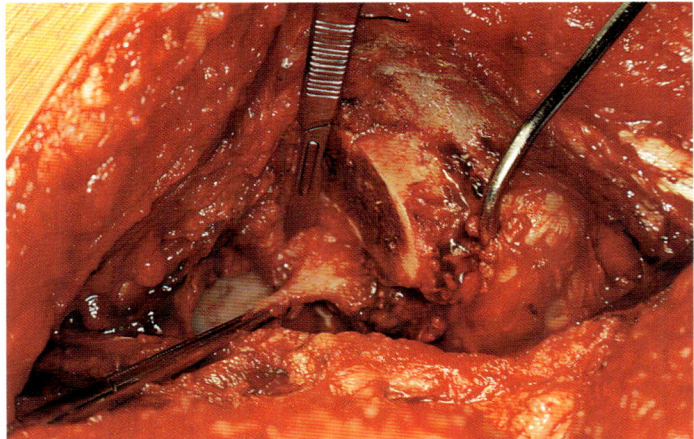

Figure 12. The femoral head and the posterior capsule have been surgically removed. A hook beneath the lesser trochanter is used to apply traction to the femur and to "tent-up" the anterior capsule. This illustration shows the capsular attachment to the anterior femoral neck being cut.

with the lower edge of the acetabular teardrop on radiographs. The floor of the acetabular fossa corresponds with the lateral edge of the teardrop. A special posterior retractor is placed with its point in the obturator foramen (Fig. 13). The exposure obtained using this technique is necessary as the entire acetabular rim must be visualized in order to place the cementless component.

Acetabular Preparation and Component Insertion

The acetabulum is prepared using spherical reamers of increasing diameter. We use cutting reamers with outside diameters measuring from 36 to 75 mm. The reamers sizes progress in 1-mm increments. The reamers should be oriented in approximately 45 degrees of abduction and 25 degrees of anteversion. In this orientation, the flat posterior surface of the reamer should be in the same plane as the rim of the acetabulum (Fig. 14). Reaming is continued with progressively larger reamers until all articular cartilage is removed. The subchondral plate is partially removed so that punctuate bleeding is present. However, excessive reaming of the subchondral plate and the anterior and posterior columns should be avoided. We usually do not ream to the depth of the acetabular fossa, and reaming should not proceed medially past this inner table. In general, at least two-thirds of the subchondral plate should present a healthy bleeding surface.

Once a *hemispheric* acetabular bed is obtained with the debris-retaining reamers, an acetabular trial component is placed to assess the coverage and optimum position of the acetabular component (Fig. 15). The face of the trial component is also placed parallel to the acetabular opening. This usually corresponds to 45 degrees of abduction and 20 degrees of anteversion. The relationship between the inferior medial rim of the cup and the acetabular teardrop should be nearly identical to that recorded in the preoperative plan. This orienta-

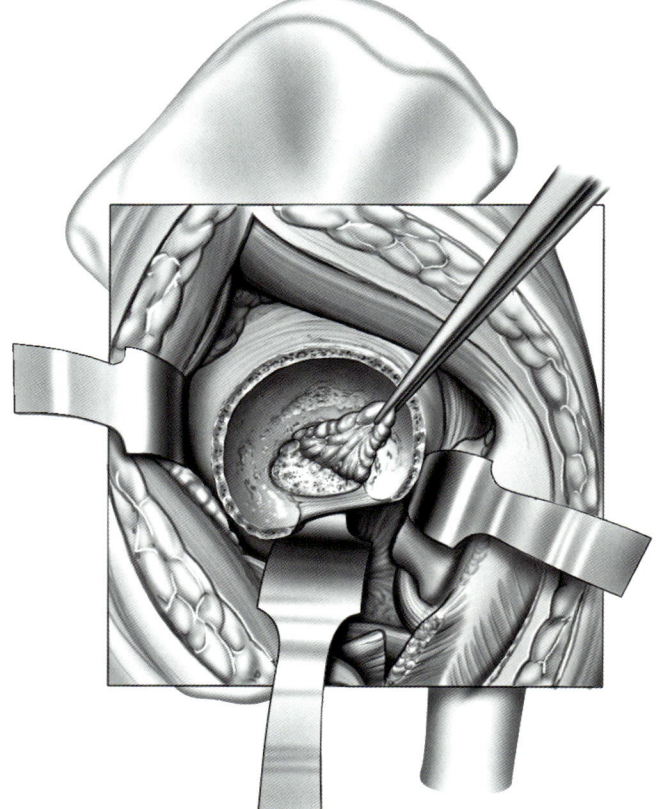

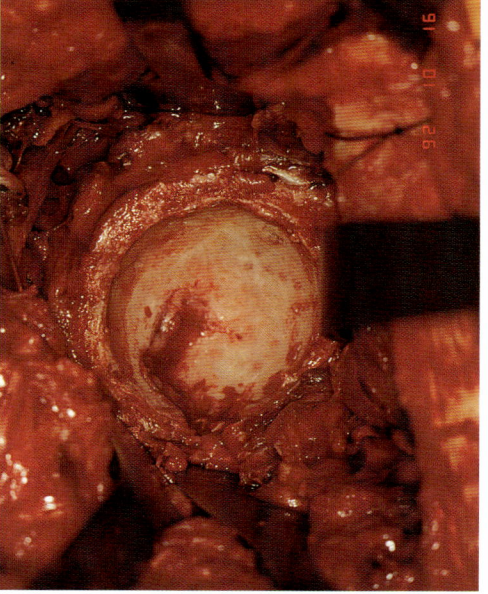

Figure 13 A, B. Acetabular exposure obtained after anterior and posterior capsulectomy. Osteophytes have been removed from the acetabular rim. The transverse ligament has not been resected. Retractors have been placed inferiorly on the origins of the ischeal and pubic rami. Another retractor placed over the anterior column has displaced the proximal femur anteriorly.

tion defines the vertical position of the acetabular component. The horizontal position is determined by the depth to which it has been placed within the acetabular fossa. The acetabular trial should fit snugly within the acetabulum. We use a trial that is the same diameter as the final reamer size. Surface contact between the component and the prepared acetabular cavity can be inspected through the perforations in the trial shell.

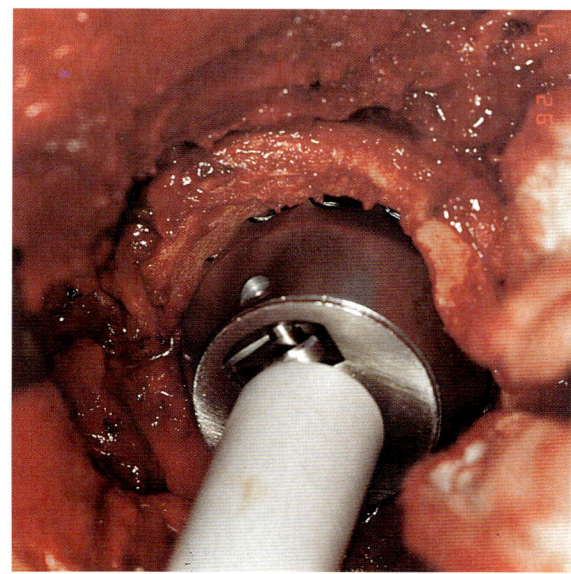

Figure 14. The acetabular "cheese grater" reamers are used with the base of the reamer parallel to the acetabular rim.

Figure 15 A, B. An acetabular trial shell is used to estimate how the porous surfaced component will fit in the prepared acetabulum.

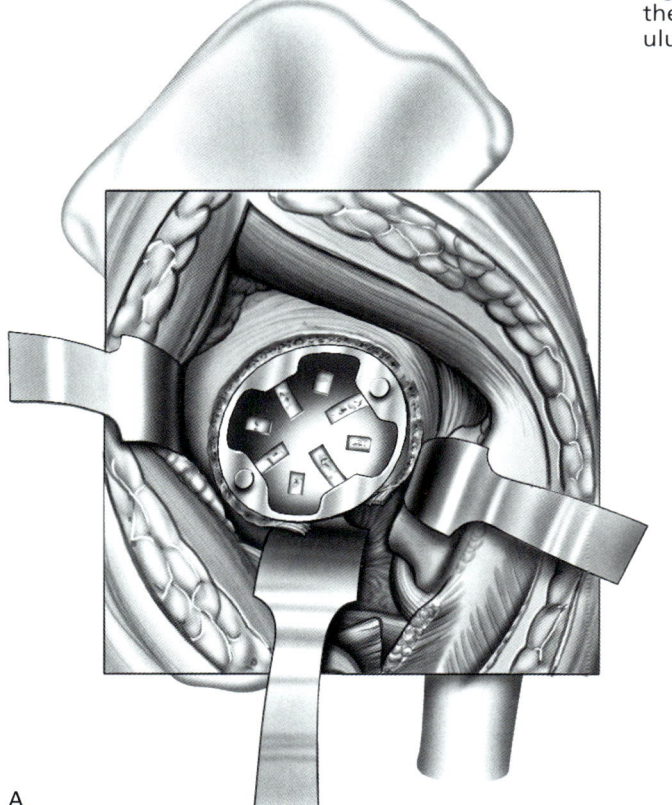

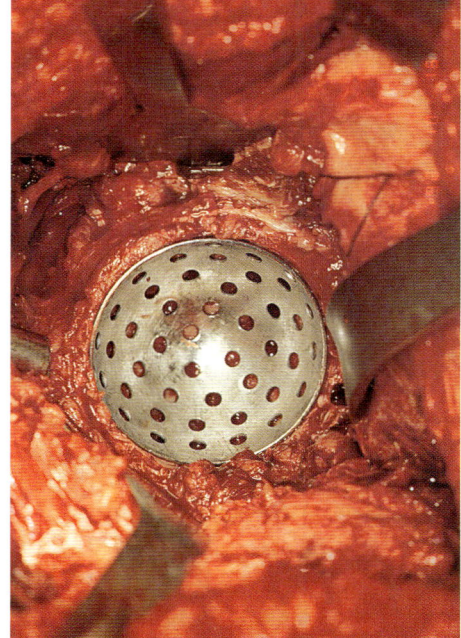

A

B

The acetabular component that is implanted has a diameter that is 1 mm larger than the final reamer used. Radius gauges are used to confirm the sizes of the acetabular trial, the final reamer, and the actual acetabular implant (Fig. 16). Different cup types can be used, but the authors prefer a cup without spikes or screw holes for most cases. The central apex hole in the cup is threaded and can be connected to an impactor. After the cup is inserted and the impactor is removed, the central hole can be filled with a threaded plug. With careful preparation of the acetabulum, excellent implant stability can be obtained without the use of screw fixation. The absence of screw holes eliminates cold flow of polyethylene and may diminish the egress of polyethylene debris into the ileum. This particulate debris has been implicated as a cause of periacetabular osteolytic lesions (6, 7). If the surgeon feels that ad-

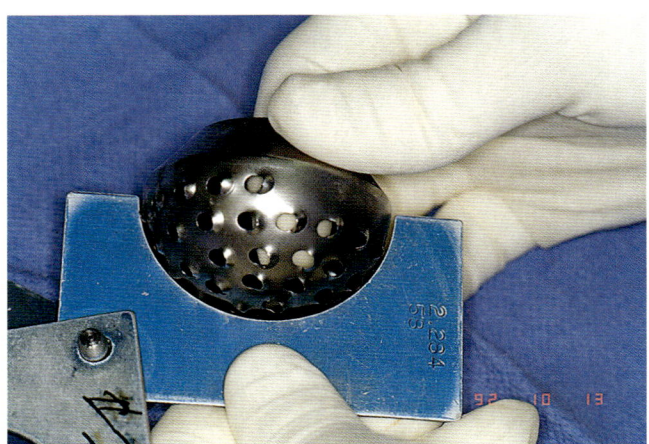

Figure 16 A, B, C. The "last" acetabular reamer, the trial cup, and the porous-coated component are all measured. The porous-surfaced component should be 1 mm larger in diameter than the acetabular trial shell.

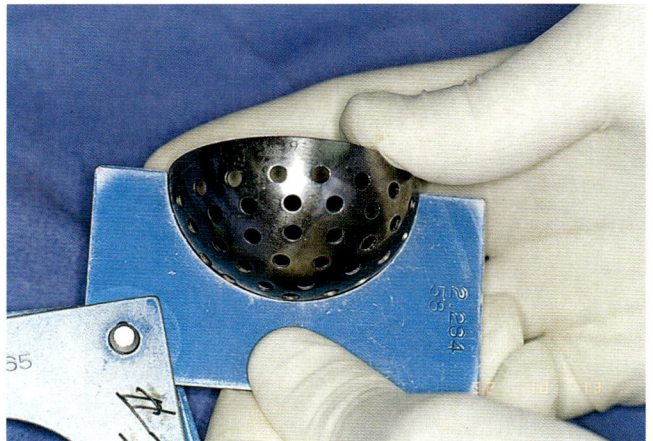

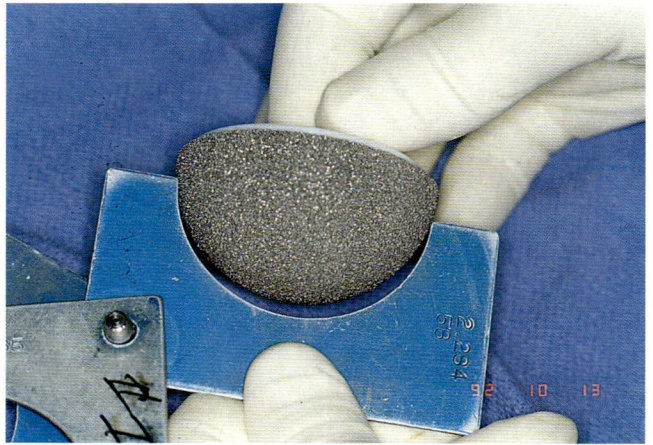

junctive fixation is necessary, then a cup with spikes or holes for screw fixation can be used. After the acetabular component has been seated, a polyethylene trial liner can be inserted prior to implanting the femoral component (Fig. 17).

Femoral Preparation

Correct pilot-hole positioning is critical for proper femoral component placement. We use a high-speed cutting instrument to make this hole just anterior to the pyriformis fossa. The pilot hole should be at least 2 mm larger than the size planned for the intramedullary canal. The position of the pilot hole can be estimated from the preoperative radiographs. When the pilot hole is made larger than the anticipated distal implant size, the possibility of eccentric reaming is reduced. As progressively larger drills are inserted into the medullary canal, these drills must not contact the pilot hole. If this occurs, the hole must be enlarged in order to prevent the proximally located pilot hole from influencing the direction of the drills distally. The goal is for the drills to enlarge the canal distally without proximal impingement (Fig. 18). A small drill fits loosely in the distal canal, but does not con-

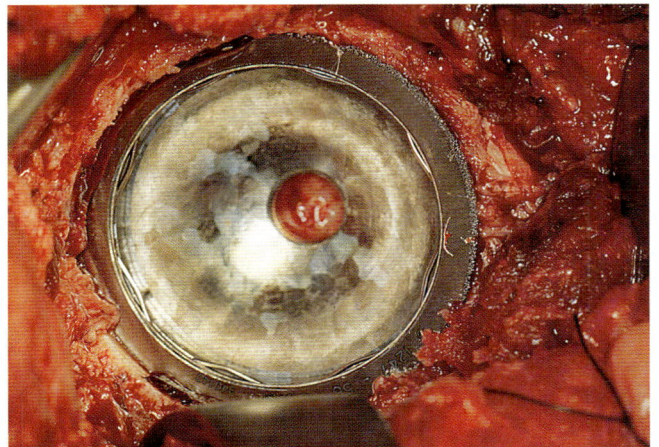
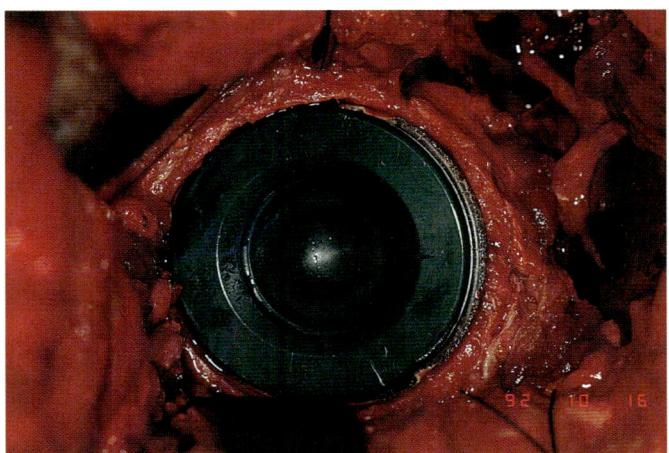

Figure 17. (A) The appearance of the porous shell in the acetabulum should be similar to that of the trial shell. (B) A trial acetabulum "poly" is used for the trial reduction in most cases.

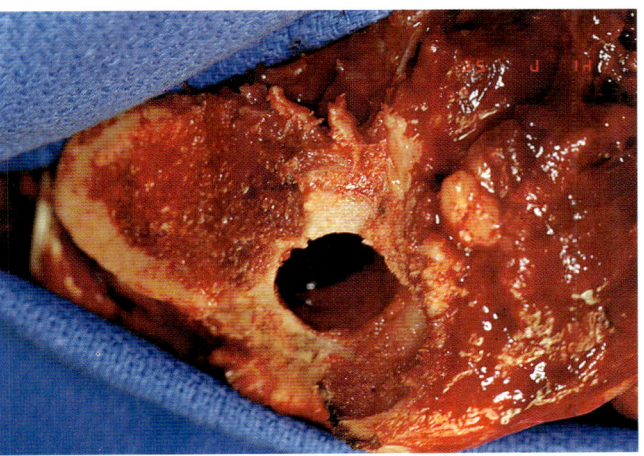
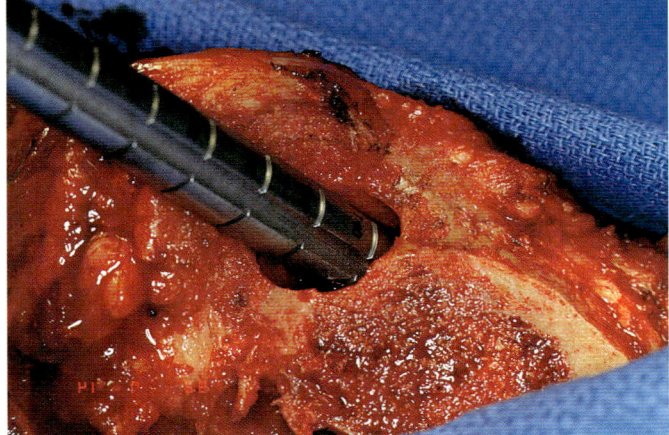

Figure 18. (A) The entry/pilot hole, used to drill the intramedullary canal, is placed as far lateral as possible in the femoral neck, so that it will be "in-line" with the intramedullary canal. (B) The femoral reamers should not contact the rim of the entry/pilot hole.

trol proximal drill position (Fig. 19A). However, when larger drills are used, the tight distal diaphyseal fit will control the position of the proximal part of the drill. To complete the drilling correctly, it is necessary to enlarge the pilot hole (Fig. 19 A, B; Fig. 20).

The distance drilled can be determined from the calibrations on the drill (1-cm increments). As the canal is reamed, the drill size that first begins to bite, as well as the drilling distance, should correspond relatively closely to the drill sizing from the preoperative plan. If this is not the case, this should serve as a warning that the drilling is not being performed correctly. In this case an intraoperative x-ray should be obtained to check the drill orientation. This problem may occur if the pilot hole is made incorrectly, thus influencing the distal path of the drill. In this scenario, a smaller than anticipated drill may impinge in a varus position distally. The drills should advance distally without manual pressure if reaming is concentric and centered. As larger drills are used, they will begin to bite over progressively larger distances. We prefer to have at least 3 cm of the intramedullary canal reamed in a cylindrical fashion, with this area corresponding with the circumferential porous coating of the femoral component.

Once the distal femur has been prepared, blunt-tip proximal reamers and rasps are used to prepare the metaphyseal bone. A blunt side cutting reamer can be used to shape the inside of the femoral neck (Fig. 21). The rasps are driven to a point just below the level of the neck resection, and the calcar is planed flat.

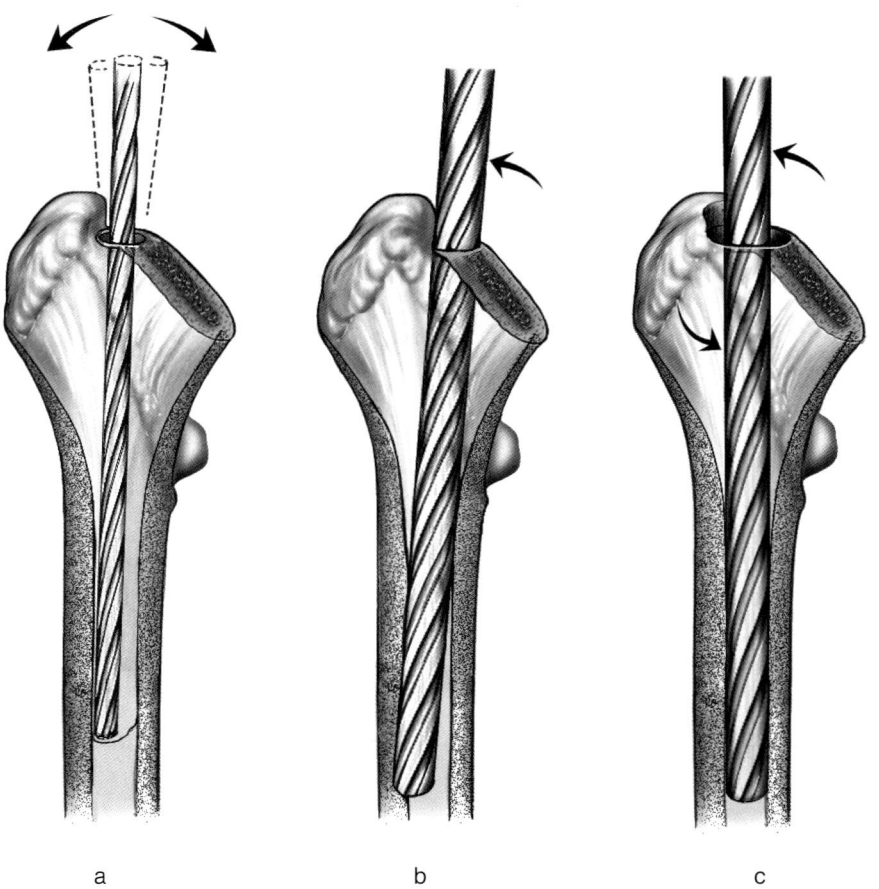

Figure 19 A, B, C. These three illustrations show why it is sometimes necessary to modify the pilot hole to accommodate larger-sized reamers.

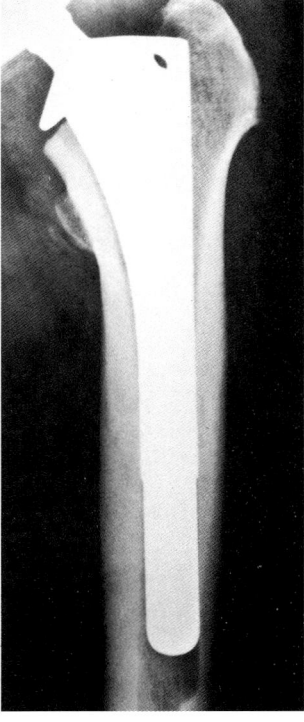

Figure 20. The postoperative radiograph of a case in which an incorrect pilot hole caused eccentric canal reaming and a suboptimal position of the femoral prosthesis.

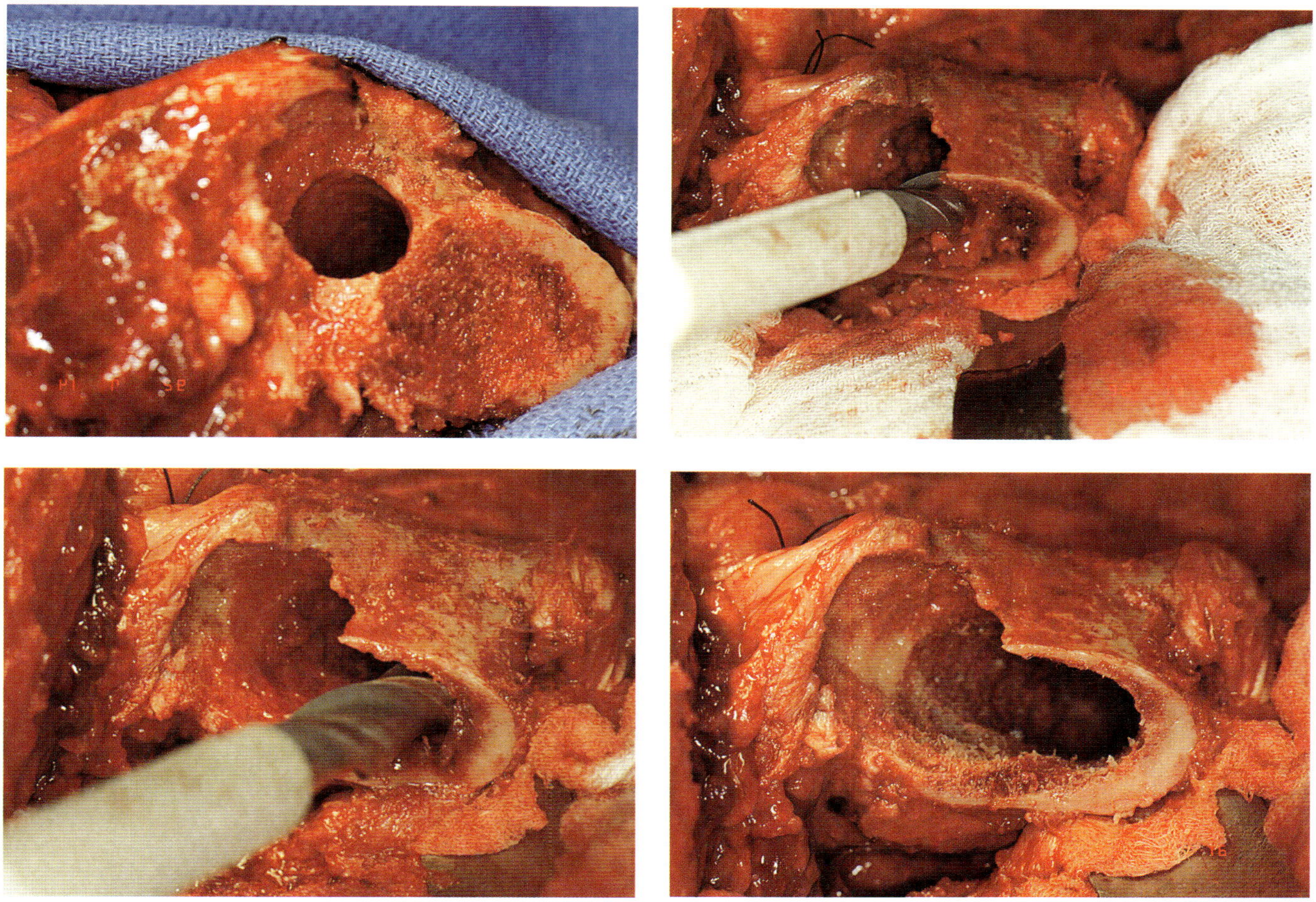

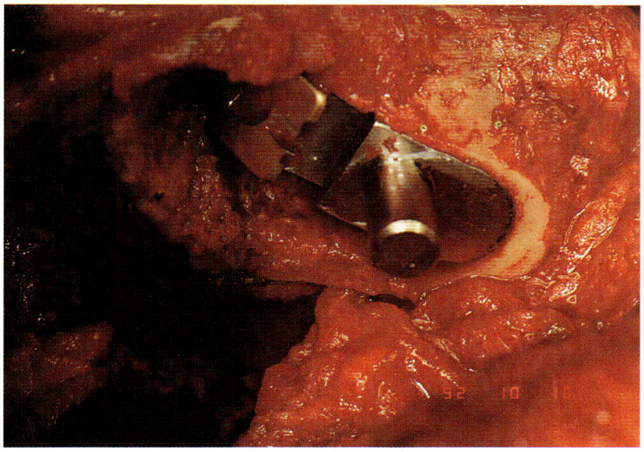

Figure 21 A, B, C, D, E. A sequence of intraoperative photographs illustrating the use of a blunt-nosed side-cutting reamer instead of a rasp to prepare the femoral neck. After the inside of the femur has been prepared to match the shape of both the rasp and the porous-surfaced prosthesis, the rasp is then countersunk to the correct level for "facing" the femoral neck for the collared prosthesis.

Trial Reduction

With the trial rasp in place, a trial reduction can be performed using the corresponding left or right (anteverted) neck segment. Limb length and offset can both be assessed using the Steinmann pin and stitch (Fig. 22). Leg length should also be checked with measurements at the knees. Adjustments can be made in the femoral offset and limb length by changing the neck length, the implant seating level (by recutting the femoral neck and driv-

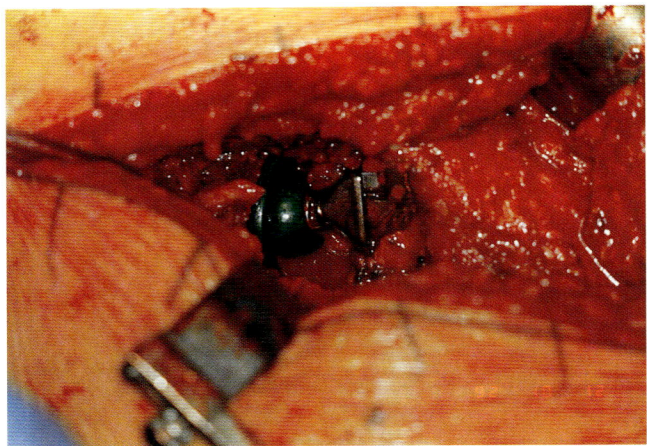
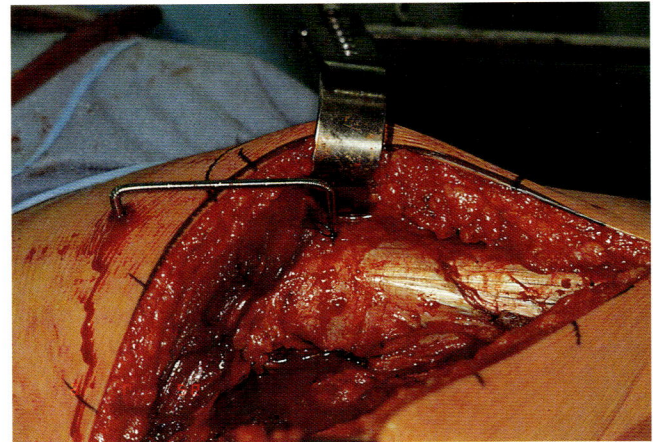
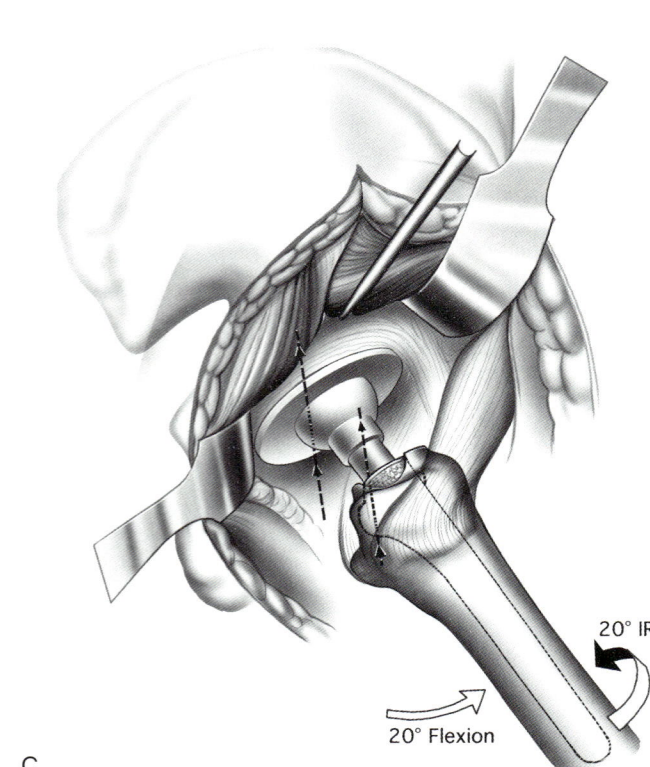
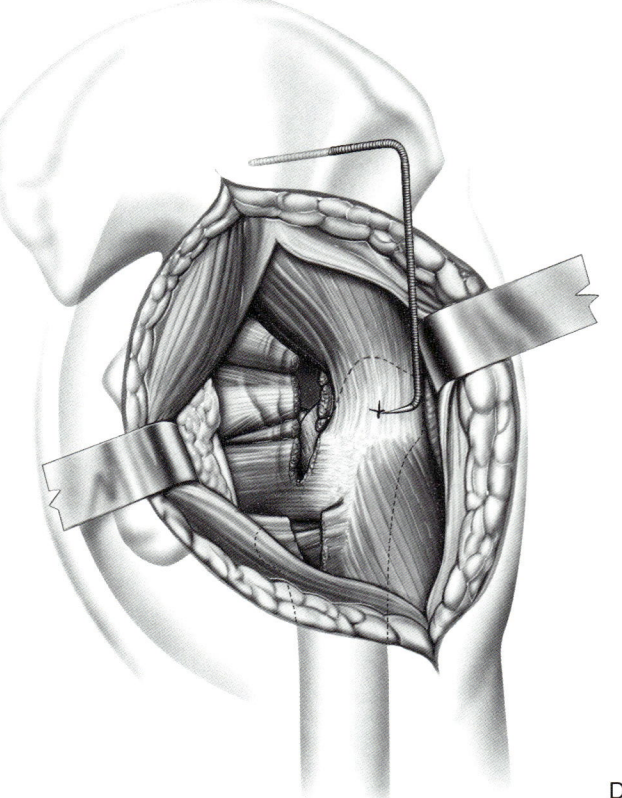

Figure 22 A, B, C, D. A trial head and neck are applied to the rasp and the hip is reduced. As a general rule, the alignment of the two components is correct if the face of the acetabular component and the collar of the trial neck are in the same plane when the femur has been flexed 20 degrees and internally rotated 20 degrees. The distance separating the femur from the pelvis is then measured by checking the relationship between the end of the iliac pin and a stitch previously placed in the greater trochanter.

ing the implant further distally), the neck-shaft angle (change from the 135-degree to the 125-degree neck-shaft angle implant), or a combination of the above. These options are discussed at length in the preoperative planning section.

Our goal is to restore limb length while maintaining or increasing femoral offset. Decreased femoral offset results in poor hip abductor tension and power, increased joint re-

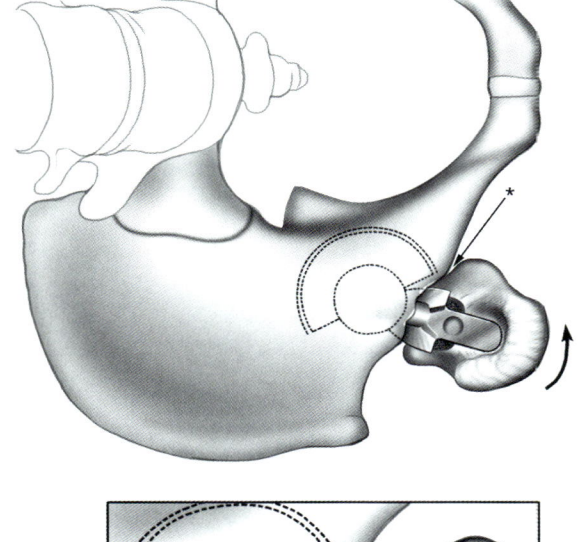
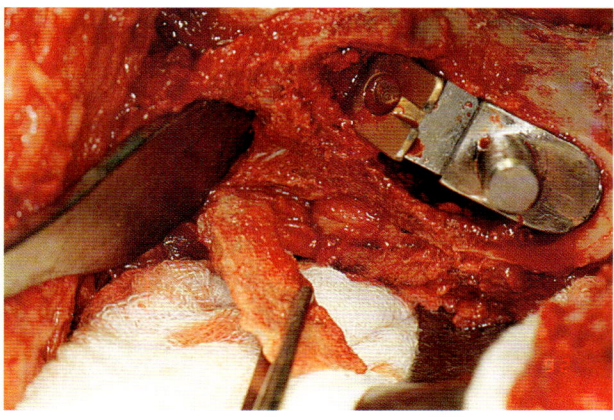

Figure 23 A, B. Posterior hip stability can often be improved by resecting the anterior portion of the greater trochanter or part of an abnormally prominent anterior femoral neck.

active forces, and, most importantly, an increased likelihood of postoperative hip dislocation (1).

The stability of the hip can be assessed with the trial components in place. Posterior stability is assessed with the hip in flexion, adduction, and internal rotation. In most instances, the hip should be stable when flexed 90 degrees, when adducted 20 degrees, and when internally rotated at least 50 degrees. In addition to assessing posterior stability, it is necessary to confirm anterior stability by placing the hip in full extension and external rotation. This is critical when an anterior capsulectomy has been performed.

When evidence of hip instability is present, the cause must be determined. Component malalignment may be a source of instability. Once the drills and rasps have been placed, the rotation of the femoral component is essentially fixed. If excess anteversion is present, femoral head anteversion can be reduced by 20 degrees by using a left trial neck on the right femur or vice versa. Frequently, posterior instability is produced by bony impingement between an abnormally prominent anterior portion of the greater trochanter and the pelvis. This problem can be solved by resecting a portion of the anterior trochanteric prominence (Fig. 23). Impingement can also be decreased by displacing the femur a greater lateral distance away from the pelvis (increasing the offset). This is done by using a longer neck segment on the prosthesis. We prefer not to rely on build-up polyethylene acetabular liners to increase hip stability. A build-up area that is placed posteriorly (to improve posterior stability) may actually cause anterior instability if the neck of the femoral implant impinges on the polyethylene build-up when the hip is placed in extension and external rotation.

Femoral Component Insertion

After limb length, offset, and stability are confirmed, the trial components and broach are removed, and the final polyethylene acetabular liner is impacted into place. At this point, a decision has to be made as to the ideal amount of interference fit for the femoral compo-

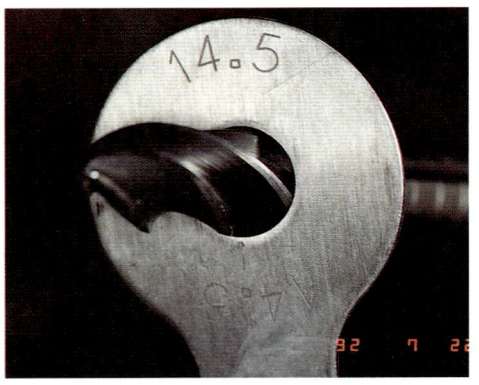 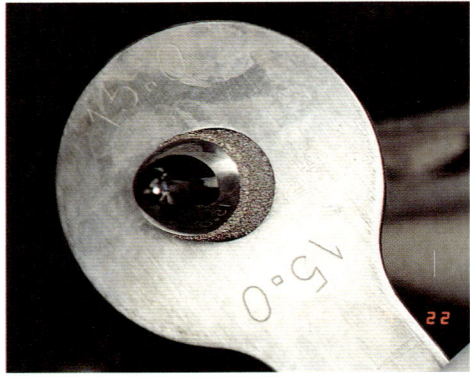

Figure 24 A, B. The distal size of the largest reamer and the prosthesis are checked with hole gauges.

nent. We recommend that the femoral component and final drill both be measured with a series of hole gauges (Fig. 24). In most cases, we insert a stem that has a distal diameter that is 0.5 mm larger than that of the last drill. In this manner a tight initial "scratch fit" is obtained in the cylindrically machined femur; however, there are exceptions. In some young patients with very hard cortical bone, the drill will bite firmly over a distance greater than 5 cm. To avoid difficulty in stem insertion in these patients, the femoral canal is drilled to the same diameter as that of the final implant (i.e., in a "line-to-line" fashion). The important point is that the porous-coated component must be large enough in diameter so that it cannot be manually pushed down the canal farther than the level shown in Fig. 25. Forceful impaction should be necessary to drive the prosthesis down the last 4 to 5 cm of the canal. With the components in place, final reduction is performed after the head segment has been impacted in place. A 28-mm ceramic ball is used in younger, more active patients.

Wound Closure

The wound is lavaged using pulsatile irrigation (4 liters) and closed with absorbable Vicryl suture in layers. The gluteus maximus tendon, pyriformis tendon, and short external rotators are sutured to their insertions on the posterolateral femur, and two one-eighth-inch drains are placed deep to the iliotibial band.

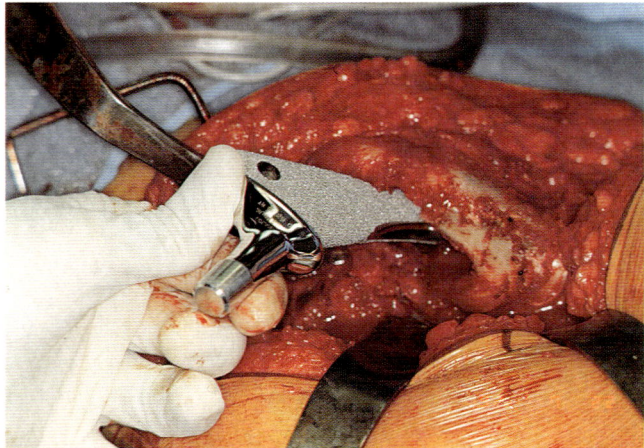

Figure 25. Forceful impaction with a two-pound hammer is needed to seat the implant. It should not be possible to push the implant by hand past the point shown in this illustration. Forceful impaction should be required beyond this point

POSTOPERATIVE MANAGEMENT

Patients are given prophylactic IV antibiotics for 48 hours postoperatively (cefazolin 1 gm every 8 hours) unless the drains are maintained for a longer period. The drains are left in place for the first two postoperative days unless drainage is greater than 50 cc per 8 hours. An abduction pillow is used (when the patient is in bed) for the first six weeks postoperatively.

We use an aggressive DVT (deep venous thrombosis) prophylaxis protocol. Patients undergo pre- and postoperative (at the six-week checkup) venous ultrasound studies in order to detect the presence of thrombi. Knee-high thromboembolitic deterrent hose and sequential pneumatic compressive stockings are also used during the hospitalization. Unless contraindicated, all patients receive Coumadin based on daily prothrombin times obtained during the hospitalization. The target prothrombin time is 1.25 to 1.5 times the control. After the patient is discharged, the Coumadin dosage is adjusted as needed based upon weekly prothrombin times. Therapy is discontinued after six weeks unless there is evidence of venous thrombosis.

On the first postoperative day, patients sit at the bedside. On the second postoperative day, patients transfer to a chair, and on day three, ambulation is started in the therapy gym.

Since minimal motion at the bone-implant interface is essential for ingrowth and biological fixation, a protected weight-bearing protocol is used for the first three months postoperatively. This includes a month of ambulation with two crutches, followed by a month using one crutch, and finally one month using a cane. This duration of protected weight bearing is dependent upon three factors: (a) the patient's bone quality, (b) the tightness of the fit of the femoral and acetabular components at the time of operation, and (c) the appearance of the immediate postoperative radiographs. In patients with poor cancellous bone quality, particularly female patients over 60 years of age, ingrowth fixation of the femoral component often requires a longer interval. If thigh pain on full weight bearing occurs, a longer interval of partial weight bearing is indicated.

In terms of range of motion and muscle strengthening, patients undergo a two-phase protocol. Phase I occurs during the first six weeks, as patients perform hip flexion (less than 70 degrees) and abduction exercises on the therapy mat. The phase II protocol starts at the six-week postoperative visit and includes active abduction against gravity, active assisted flexion past 90 degrees, and exercises to increase external rotation. Throughout the protocol, the patient is instructed on posterior dislocation precautions (avoid flexion combined with adduction and internal rotation). After six weeks, the patient while sleeping is allowed to discontinue the use of the abduction pillow. Exercise such as swimming and stationary bicycling is allowed at this time.

COMPLICATIONS

Intraoperative Femoral Fractures

A recent study from this institution (8) discusses our experience with the etiologies and management of this problem. After primary hip arthroplasty using the Anatomic Medullary Locking (AML) stem (DePuy, Warsaw, Indiana), a 3% incidence of intraoperative fracture has been noted. Fractures occur in two locations: proximally, and, more, commonly, distally at the tip of the prosthesis. The fractures are classified as incomplete or complete and are usually not discovered until the immediate postoperative radiographs are examined. Causes of intraoperative femoral fracture include: (a) eccentric distal reaming of the femoral canal due to improper pilot hole placement, and (b) impingement of the broaches or femoral implant due to incorrect orientation or incomplete bone preparation.

The treatment goal for intraoperative femoral fractures should be to provide stability for both bone ingrowth and fracture healing. Stable, incomplete proximal fractures need no additional treatment if rigid distal stability is obtained with the implant. Complete, displaced proximal fractures require cerclage wire fixation if the fracture is noted intraoperatively. A longer, fully coated implant is used to bridge the defect, thereby obtaining stability distally.

Nondisplaced and minimally displaced, incomplete distal femoral fractures (linear fissure at the tip of the implant) are managed nonoperatively with toe-touch weight bearing until fracture consolidation is seen. In these cases, the thicker, stronger posterior femoral cortex is usually intact. Complete displaced distal fractures require open reduction and internal fixation with compression plating.

In our experience, patients sustaining an intraoperative fracture have had similar clinical and radiographic outcomes as patients without fracture. Careful preoperative planning and operative technique should reduce the risk of this problem. Intraoperative stability of the femoral component must be achieved in order to obtain bone ingrowth and fracture healing.

Nerve Palsy

Nerve palsy is a rare complication of primary total hip arthroplasty. Palsies can occur due to stretch injury or direct trauma from compression or transection. Femoral, obturator, and sciatic nerve palsies have been reported in the literature. Acetabular retractors must be placed carefully so that the sciatic nerve is protected by the short external rotators. The anterior acetabular (pubic) and inferior acetabular retractors must be placed carefully also to avoid injuring the femoral and obturator nerves, respectively. The leg should be supported when the hip is dislocated in order to avoid excessive tension on the sciatic nerve. The amount of limb lengthening obtained [especially in cases of developmental dysplasia of the hip (DDH)] should be carefully monitored to prevent a sciatic stretch palsy. Limb lengthening of greater than 4 cm has been associated with a higher incidence of sciatic nerve injury (9). In the event that a sciatic nerve deficit is noted postoperatively in the recovery room, the patient is immediately returned to the operating room for exploration in order to rule out any compressive lesion or direct injury to the nerve.

Early Postoperative Dislocations

Early postoperative dislocations occur in approximately 3.5% of our cases. These are usually posterior dislocations. Our protocol for treating these dislocations is as follows: Closed reduction is performed either in the emergency room or in the operating room under light general anesthesia. Hip stability and the position at which dislocation occurred are recorded. The patient is then treated in a commercially available hip brace. Usually the hip is maintained in a slightly abducted position, and hip flexion is limited to 70 degrees. The brace is usually worn for six weeks. During this time, the patient is encouraged to perform isometric exercises and is allowed to be fully weight bearing. When the brace is removed, the patient is instructed on how to avoid future dislocations. For example, if the dislocation had been a posterior one, the patient would be advised to reach toward the floor only if both hips are abducted and externally rotated. The patient would also be advised to reach toward his or her feet only with both arms between the legs. If a second dislocation occurs, reoperation is usually indicated. At reoperation the acetabular component is usually revised, bony prominences on the trochanter or around the acetabular cup are removed, and the prosthetic neck is lengthened. Postoperatively the patient is again treated with a six-week interval of bracing followed by instructions regarding ways to avoid dislocation.

Heterotopic Ossification

Although radiographic signs of mild heterotopic ossification are a frequent occurrence (found in more than 15% of our cases), ossification resulting in impaired hip function rarely occurs (less than 0.1% of our cases). Surgical removal of this heterotopic bone has been, in our experience, successful in improving patients' hip motion. This surgery is usually performed more than one year after the hip replacement. Patients whom we consider to be at a high risk of forming heterotopic ossification are treated either on the day of surgery or on the day after surgery with irradiation (10). The periprosthetic area is shielded. We have not experienced an increased incidence of failed prosthetic osseointegration in our irradiated patients.

Expected Outcome

The authors have been performing primary total hip replacement by the method discussed in this chapter for 15 years. Information on each hip replacement patient is entered into a computerized database. The data include a pre- and postoperative questionnaire completed by the patient and an evaluation completed by the surgeon. The surgeon's evaluation includes assessment of current function, a list of any interim complications, and a radiographic assessment. This information is used to inform new patients regarding the expected long-term outcome of their surgery.

Based on analysis of this information, we now inform our patients that osseointegration of the femoral component can be expected in more than 95% of our cases and that none of these osseointegrated femoral prostheses have ever required removal. Ten years after surgery, patients with an osseointegrated femoral prosthesis and a stable acetabular component can be expected to be free of hip pain and have normal or near-normal hip function. Patients whose postoperative radiographs show signs of failed osseointegration of the femoral prosthesis or signs of instability of the acetabular component can be expected to have a less satisfactory clinical result. Less than 0.5% of the patients operated on by us more than 10 years ago have required revision of their femoral prosthesis, and less than 10% have required revision of their acetabular component.

Acetabular revisions are most frequently performed for component malposition causing recurrent hip dislocations or for excessive wear of the polyethylene-bearing surface. In the latter cases, the revision procedure has usually involved only exchange of the polyethylene within the acetabular shell. We also inform our patients that there is a 15% probability that their 10-year postoperative radiographs will show problems that may require surgical treatment after 10 years, the most frequent problem being osteolytic cysts either in the greater trochanter or in the pelvis adjacent to the rim of an acetabular component.

Fortunately, to date, all of these complications have been correctable. As a result, patient satisfaction and current functional outcome have been no different for those patients who have gone more than 10 years without treatment of a complication from those who have required some interim treatment.

ILLUSTRATIVE CASE FOR TECHNIQUE

The case of a 38-year old businessman with avascular necrosis illustrates the authors' typical primary total hip replacement case. This patient, whose pain became resistant to analgesics, experienced difficulty putting on his right shoe and sock. He also needed to use a handrail for stair climbing and a cane for walking distances.

The patient's Trendelberg sign was negative; he had restricted abductor and internal rotation in his right hip and a 0.5-cm leg-length discrepancy. To correct the patient's problems, the authors performed a total hip arthroplasty involving AML femoral and acetabular components. Postoperatively he was maintained on restricted weight bearing for three months, but was allowed to return to work on crutches one month after surgery. Currently, he has a full range of motion in his hip and walks for unlimited distances without a detectable limp. He also has no difficulty putting on his right shoe and sock and can ascend and descend stairs normally. His two-year postoperative radiographs demonstrated signs of osseointegration of the femoral component and a stable acetabular component. His ten-year postoperative radiographs (see Fig. 8) have an appearance similar to that of his two-year postoperative radiographs.

RECOMMENDED READING

1. Steinberg, B., and Harris, W. H.: The "offset" problem in total hip arthroplasty. *Contemp. Ortho.*, 24: 556, 1992.
2. Johnston, R. C., Brand, R. A., and Crowninshield R. D.: Reconstruction of the hip: A mathematical approach to determine optimum geometric relationship. *J. Bone and Joint Surg.*, 61A: 6389, 1979.
3. Engh, C. A., Bobyn, J. D.: *Biologic Fixation in Total Hip Arthroplasty.* Slack, Thorofare, New Jersey, 1985.
4. Engh, C. A., Glassman, A. H., and Bobyn, J. D.: Surgical principles in cementless total hip arthroplasty. *Tech. Orthop.*, 1: 59, 1986.
5. McGee, H. M., and Scott, J. H.: A simple method of obtaining equal limb length in total hip arthroplasty. *Clin. Orthop.*, 194: 269, 1985.
6. Santavirta, S., Hoikka, V., Eskola, A. Konttinen, Y. T., Paavilainen, T., and Tallroth, K.: Aggressive granulomatous lesions in cementless total hip arthroplasty. *J. Bone and Joint Surg.*, 72-B: 980, 1990.
7. Schmalzried, T. P., Jasty, M., Harris, W. H.: Periprosthetic bone loss in total hip arthroplasty. *J. Bone and Joint Surg.*, 74-A: 849, 1992.
8. Schwartz, J. T., Mayer, J. G., and Engh, C. A.: Femoral fracture during non-cemented total hip arthroplasty. *J. Bone Joint Surg.*, 71A: 1135, 1989.
9. Kavanagh, B. F.: The hip. In: *Joint Replacement Arthroplasty.* B. F. Morrey, editor. Churchill Livingston, New York, 1991.
10. Gregoritch, S. J., Chadha, M., Pelligrini, V. D., Rubin, P., Kantorowitz, D. A.: Randomized trial comparing preoperative versus postoperative irradiation for prevention of heterotopic ossification following prosthetic total hip replacement: preliminary results. *Int. J. Radiat. Oncol. Biol. Phys.*, 30(1):55–62, 1994.

PART V

Revision Total Hip Arthroplasty

15

Secondary Total Hip Arthroplasty: After Infection

Eduardo A. Salvati and Jay R. Lieberman

INDICATIONS/CONTRAINDICATIONS

When pain develops after total hip arthroplasty and there is no clear explanation for persistent symptoms, the surgeon should include infection as part of the differential diagnosis. In general, the clinical presentation of an infected total hip arthroplasty falls into three categories. *First*, an acute early infection which may occur within the first three months after the initial total hip arthroplasty. The patient may be febrile and have a painful hip. The wound may appear erythematous, or spontaneous drainage may be noted. An infected hematoma may be present.

The second group is the late, acute, hematogenous infection, which usually develops after a pain-free interval. The patient usually presents with an acute onset of hip pain, which may be accompanied by a febrile episode.

The third group is the insidious latent infection. These patients usually never have had a pain-free interval after the original total hip arthroplasty. In these cases the diagnosis of infection versus prosthetic loosening may be difficult, since the white blood cell count, the differential cell count, and the sedimentation rate may all be within normal limits.

E. A. Salvati, M.D.: Cornell University Medical College, Hospital for Special Surgery, New York, New York 10021.

J. R. Lieberman, M.D.: Department of Orthopaedic Surgery, UCLA School of Medicine, Center for the Health Sciences, Los Angeles, California 90024.

The diagnosis of an acute infected total hip arthroplasty is not difficult in the face of a draining sinus or an inflamed wound. However, the diagnosis may be much more difficult in the case of a patient who appears with hip pain, normal wound healing, and unremarkable laboratory findings and radiographs.

We recommend joint aspiration as the procedure of choice for identifying an infected total hip arthroplasty. The aspiration is performed with local anesthesia and under strict antiseptic conditions. The procedure may be performed in the office, but fluoroscopic control is preferable. The hip is prepped and draped in a sterile fashion. The landmarks used to identify the hip joint are the femoral artery and a line drawn from the anterior superior iliac spine to the symphysis pubis. The hip joint is located approximately two fingerbreadths lateral and proximal to the femoral artery. One can tell that the joint has been entered by metallic contact between the tip of the needle against the head or neck of the femoral component.

The fluid aspirated must be sent immediately to the bacteriology laboratory for Gram stain, aerobic, anaerobic, and fungal cultures and sensitivities. It is important that the aspirate be inoculated as soon as possible into the appropriate broth and culture medium. We favor the use of a transport system with a culture medium to support the bacteria during the time of transport. Cultures may need to be incubated for one week to increase the chances of identification of an insidious organism of low virulence that may require a longer time to grow. The benefits of using a blood-culture bottle for synovial fluid cultures include an increased volume of inoculum and greater dilution of possible inhibitors of bacterial growth.

When enough fluid is aspirated, a complete cell count and differential may also provide valuable information. When the cell count shows more than 25,000 leukocytes per ml and a differential count reveals greater than 25% polymorphonuclear cells, infection should be suspected. Fluids should also be analyzed for glucose and protein levels. In normal synovial fluid, protein levels are about one-third serum levels, but with an infection they approach serum levels. Glucose values in normal synovial fluid are similar to those of plasma. However, in the presence of infection, the synovial glucose levels are lowered due to the presence of organisms and cells that utilize sugar in their metabolism. A low glucose and a high protein level are suggestive of an infection. A negative culture following an aspiration in which fluid was obtained should exclude the possibility of infection, provided adequate bacteriologic techniques were used without delay (2).

If no fluid is aspirated, we generally do not inject saline into the hip joint because of the questionable accuracy of this technique. In these cases, a hip aspiration may be repeated at a later date under fluoroscopic guidance. Cultures obtained from draining sinuses frequently grow mixed flora and the main pathogen causing the deep periprosthetic infection may not be identified.

We recommend the use of technetium bone scans to rule out other pathology (i.e., tumors, stress fracture) in those cases where the patient has enigmatic hip pain, despite normal radiographs and a negative hip aspiration. The specificity of a bone scan is not sufficient to make a diagnosis. We have developed an algorithm for the evaluation of a painful total hip arthroplasty (Fig. 1) (5).

In rare cases, after all these tests, the diagnosis may still be unclear, even though there is a strong clinical suspicion that there is an infection. In such cases, an arthroscopic or open biopsy may be appropriate. Multiple tissue specimens must be obtained from the joint. It is important that antibiotics not be given prior to the aspiration, biopsy, or surgical procedure to maximize the chances of isolating and identifying the infecting organism.

Occasionally, the surgeon is confronted with the dilemma of deciding whether an isolated positive culture is of pathological significance. This problem emphasizes the importance of obtaining multiple cultures. One positive culture might represent a contaminant if several other cultures fail to grow the same organism. This is particularly true if the growth occurs in the broth only. Growth in plates is less likely to represent contamination. The organisms usually encountered as contaminants are those mostly found in the perioperative environment which include *Staphylococcus epidermidis*, diphtheroids, and *Lactobacillus*.

PLAIN RADIOGRAPHS

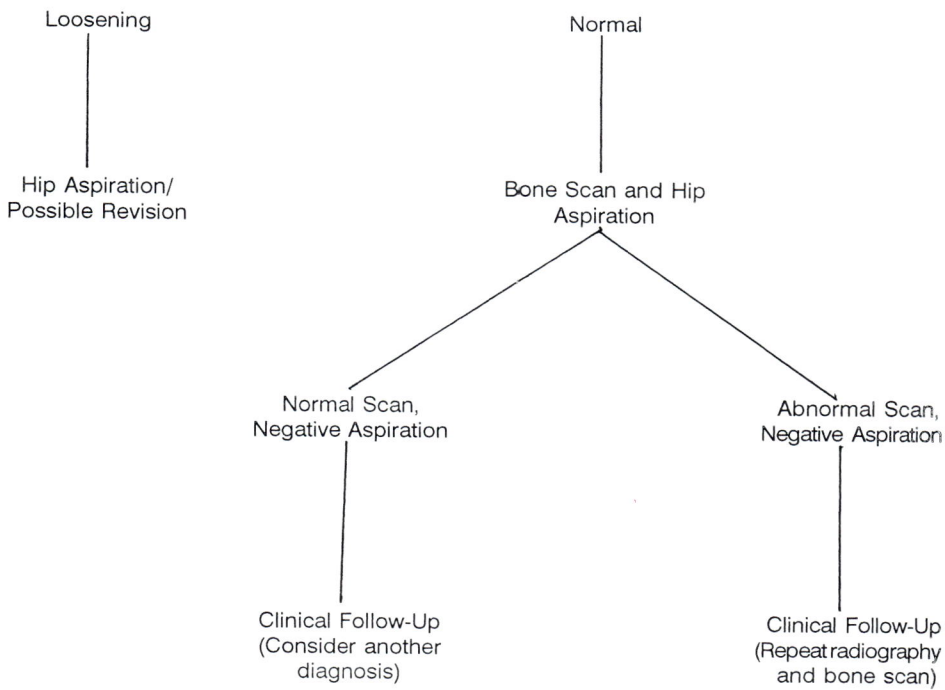

Figure 1. Algorithm for evaluation of a painful total hip arthroplasty.

PREOPERATIVE PLANNING

Once an infection has been diagnosed, a decision must be made regarding the treatment of choice and the removal of the prosthetic components. The management of each individual infected hip arthroplasty is determined by the time and mode of presentation, the virulence of the infecting organism, the medical and immunological status of the patient, and the condition of the hip.

An acute early infection (less than three months after implantation) may be treated by immediate incision, debridement, and primary closure over drainage tubes. The drainage tubes are left in for approximately 2 days. In these early infections, the bone–cement interface or the bone–implant interface is most likely still intact and not compromised by the septic process. When such an infection is recognized early, there is a limited chance of salvaging the total hip arthroplasty, particularly if the bacterium is highly sensitive to antibiotic therapy, and the diagnosis and intervention are prompt.

Late infections are generally treated by removal of the components and a thorough debridement and either a one- or two-stage reimplantation. A one-stage reimplantation is possible only in those cases where there is mild inflammation of the periprosthetic tissues at the time of incision and debridement, and the bacterium is exquisitely sensitive to antibiotics. At the present time we favor a two-stage reimplantation protocol. This protocol not only allows the soft tissue to heal, but enables one to attain appropriate serum bactericidal titers, which are essential for the successful eradication of an infection in a total hip arthroplasty.

Suppression of a periprosthetic infection with antibiotic therapy alone is rarely indicated. It may allow prosthesis retention in the elderly patient, provided the infection is acute and there are no signs of systemic involvement or prosthetic loosening. In addition, the bacteria must be exquisitely sensitive to oral antibiotic therapy, which must be well-tolerated by the patient. Few patients are able to satisfy the above criteria to be treated with antibiotic suppression. A review of 19 patients with an infected total hip arthroplasty treated at The Hospital for Special Surgery with antibiotic suppression revealed no deterioration in approximately half the patients at four year follow-up (3). The remainder of the patients deteriorated or required removal of the infected prosthesis. In the last few years, we have combined arthroscopic irrigation and debridement with lifelong antibiotic suppression in several cases where the infection was acute, the patient was too frail to tolerate a major surgical procedure, the prosthesis was well-fixed, and the organism was extremely sensitive to oral antibiotics. The early results appear promising.

SURGERY

There are several important steps in the surgical exposure of any revision hip surgery. We generally employ a posterolateral approach with the patient in the lateral decubitus position. The incision is made to allow greater trochanteric osteotomy if necessary. The key elements include a meticulous exposure to identify the iliotibial fascia, and the vastus lateralis and the posterior borders of the gluteus medius; and an extensive capsulotomy and skeletonization of the proximal femur so that the hip can be dislocated in an atraumatic fashion (Fig. 2). A trochanteric osteotomy or an extended proximal femoral-type osteotomy is performed if increased exposure is necessary. This is often required if the bone and cement are well interdigitated or with a bone ingrown cementless prosthesis. When a trochanteric osteotomy is performed, the hip is dislocated by adduction and external rotation and then brought across the anterior aspect of the table. The knee is flexed to 90 degrees and the foot is secured to a stool placed at the proper height to avoid stretching the sciatic nerve (Figs. 3, 4). This position allows excellent visualization of the femoral canal, which is necessary when removing a well-fixed femoral component.

The identification of the infecting organism is one of the most important factors in the successful treatment of an infected hip arthroplasty. Therefore, in addition to the preoperative hip aspiration, at the time of the incision and debridement, multiple cultures are taken, prior to the administration of intravenous antibiotics. An intraoperative synovial fluid aspiration is performed, and tissue cultures are obtained from the femoral canal, the acetabu-

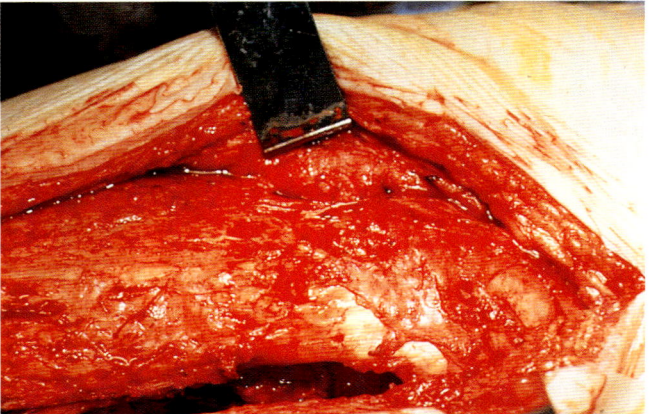

Figure 2. Photograph demonstrating posterolateral approach to the hip. The iliotibial fascia (behind retractor), vastus lateralis, and gluteus medius are well-defined.

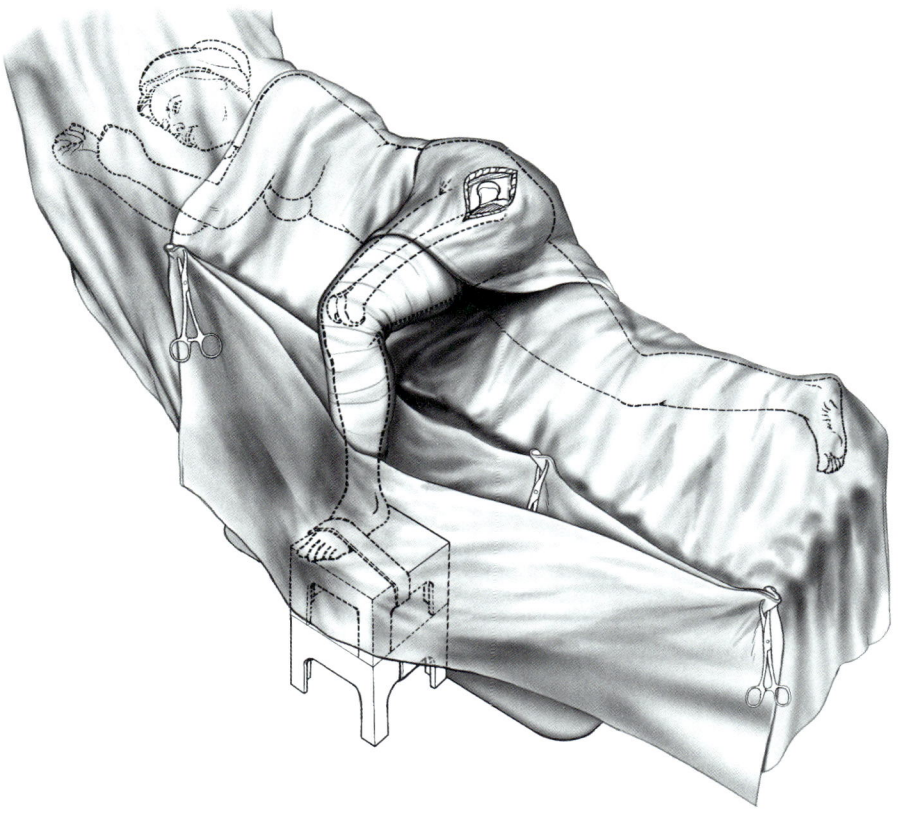

Figure 3. The hip is dislocated via adduction, external rotation, flexion, and longitudinal traction. The leg and foot are placed into a sterile bag.

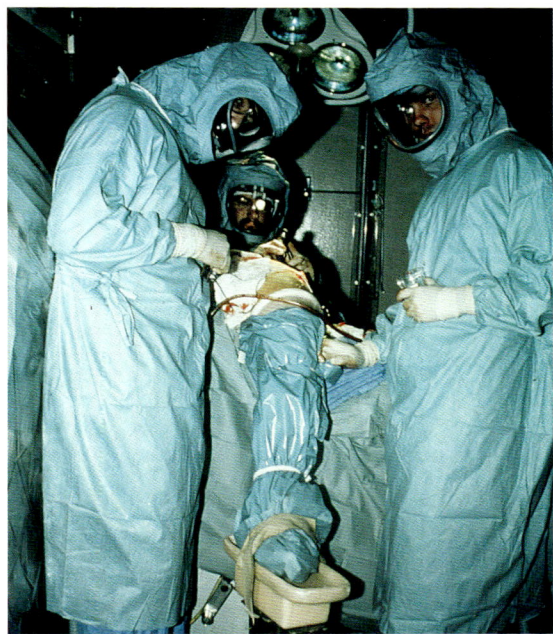

Figure 4. A photograph depicting position of the leg after dislocation of the hip. The knee is flexed 90 degrees and the foot is strapped to a stool. This position allows for excellent visualization of the femoral canal.

lar bed, and the pseudocapsule. These specimens are sent for Gram stain, aerobic, anaerobic and fungal cultures.

The removal of the prosthetic component and acrylic cement may be quite challenging, especially in those cases where the septic process is of recent onset. The prosthetic components may not yet be loose, and tight interdigitation between bone and cement or between the bone and a cementless implant may make removal of the component challenging. In general, this demands a laborious and meticulous technique to avoid unnecessary loss of bone stock. We recommend the use of a greater trochanteric osteotomy to provide better exposure in such cases in order to avoid a perforation of the femur. In extremely complicated cases an extended greater trochanteric osteotomy may be indicated. We favor the use of hand tools to remove the proximal cement or to disrupt the prosthetic bone interface in a cementless implant. We try to avoid femoral cortical windows when removing the cement. The technique can weaken and potentially devascularize the bone, and a longer femoral component is also required to bypass the defect. These are all important issues when dealing with an infected hip arthroplasty where there is obvious concern about recurrence of infection. Mechanical tools are used to remove the distal cement plug or remove a distal bone pedestal.

In cases where the infection has been of longer duration, the bone cement interface or the bone-prosthetic interface may be compromised, and removal of the prosthetic component and cement may be easier. In general, we attempt to remove all of the cement unless there is a serious risk of compromising bone stock, which could jeopardize future reimplantation.

After removal of all of the components and cement, if present, a thorough debridement is performed. The femoral canal and the acetabular bed are meticulously cleaned to remove all fibrous and inflamed tissue (Fig. 5). The hip is then irrigated with a saline solution containing polymyxin and bacitracin. The polymyxin destroys the osmotic properties of the bacterial cell membrane, and the bacitracin interferes with the second stage of cell-wall synthesis. We acknowledge that the use of antibiotics in the irrigation fluid is controversial.

The fascial layers are meticulously closed followed by the subcutaneous tissues and skin with interrupted sutures. In a rare case, where the tissues are extremely inflamed, the wound can be packed open and closure performed a few days later when the inflammation has subsided. If a trochanteric osteotomy has been performed, it is reattached to the femur with a single wire. Large-hole drains are employed for about 2 days. A continuous irrigation system is no longer used

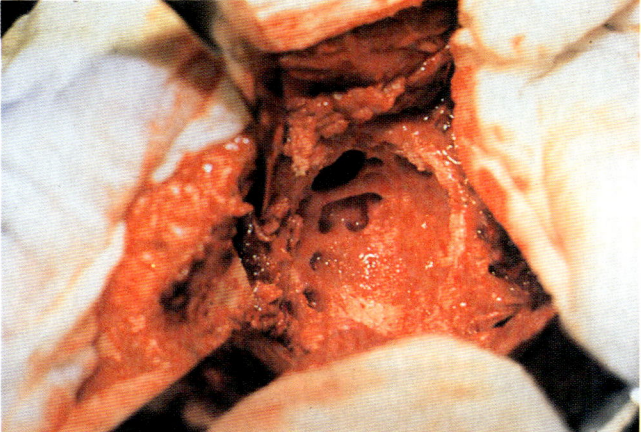

Figure 5. A photograph depicting the acetabular bed after debridement. All fibrous and inflamed tissue must be removed.

POSTOPERATIVE MANAGEMENT

The lower extremity is then placed in balanced suspension with tibial skeletal traction for approximately 2 weeks. Once acceptable stability of the hip is obtained, which is assessed by gentle push-pull, skeletal traction is removed and the patient is started on gentle, progressive active range of motion exercises. This is followed by dangling, standing, and partial weight bearing ambulation with a walker attended by a physical therapist. The patient progresses in his rehabilitation program as tolerated. Prophylactic anticoagulation is indicated to reduce the risk of thromboembolism, which is increased due to the long period of recumbency.

Antibiotic Therapy

Our protocol includes six weeks of intravenous antibiotics in doses sufficient to obtain a post-peak serum bactericidal titer (SBT) of at least 1:8. A tube dilution technique is employed in which the serum bactericidal activity of the antibiotic against the patient's own infecting organism is determined. Post-peak serum specimens are drawn one, one and one half, two, three, or six hours after the administration of antibiotics, depending on whether the dosage frequency was every four, six, eight, twelve, or twenty-four hours, respectively. The serum samples are then diluted from 1:2 to 1:2048 and are then added to the infecting organisms in culture. The serum bactericidal titer (SBT) is the highest dilution of serum, causing 99% killing of the infecting organism. The choice of drug and dosage is dependent on the quantitative sensitivity of the organism, with consideration given to the ability of the drug to penetrate and kill (minimum bactericidal concentration) as opposed to inhibit (6).

The six weeks of therapy is measured from the time that the prosthesis and all foreign bodies are removed. Our patients are treated by an infectious disease consultant who selects the antibiotics and monitors the post-peak serum bactericidal titers. Changes in the antibiotic regimen are made according to the results of the cultures and titers. Postreimplantation, the patient receives intravenous antibiotics until intraoperative cultures are reported as negative. If the cultures are still positive, intravenous antibiotic therapy with appropriate titers is continued for at least six more weeks.

We believe that the post-peak SBT is one of the key prognostic factors in determining the success of a reimplantation. The minimum bactericidal concentration (MBC) reveals the potential ability of the antibiotic to kill the organism, but it is the post-peak SBT that reflects the antibiotic concentration actually delivered to the blood stream. It may also reveal any synergistic effects that occur when multiple antibiotics are being used to treat an infection. Thus, the success of the antibiotic therapy is dependent on the MBC and SBT obtained rather than on the identity of the organism. Gram-negative organisms may be exquisitely sensitive to antibiotics and even bacteria of the same species can have variable sensitivities. A gram-negative infection may not be virulent (4).

In the past, authors have defined specific implantation guidelines based on the identity of the organism. Gram-negative organisms, especially *Pseudomonas*, were considered virulent. Mc Donald et al. recommended delayed reimplantation for total hip arthroplasty infected with a gram-negative organism (5). Since 1975, we have obtained minimum bactericidal concentrations (MBC) and post-peak serum bactericidal titers (SBT) to help determine whether an infected total hip arthroplasty should be considered for reimplantation. A post-peak SBT of at least 1:8 was necessary to consider reimplantation. In a recent study of 32 infected hip arthroplasties treated with a two-stage reimplantation protocol, a minimum post-peak SBT of 1:8 was achieved against all gram-positive organisms, except one Enterococcal isolate. A minimum 1:8 titer was obtained in seventeen of twenty gram-negative isolates (4).

In this series 29 of the 32 (90%) reimplanted hips received a full six-week course of intravenous antibiotics. Two patients received four weeks of antibiotics and one received 20 days. There were no recurrent infections in these three patients. The post-peak serum bactericidal titers obtained in these patients were 1:16, 1:512, and 1:2048 respectively. This suggests that in the presence of highly sensitive bacteria, a shorter course of intravenous antibiotics of perhaps 3 to 4 weeks may be sufficient. At an average of 40 months after reimplantation, infection recurred in three hips (9.4%). Minimum post-peak serum bactericidal titers of 1:8 were obtained in 28 of the 32 hips that were reimplanted, and only one of these hips (3.6%) had a recurrent infection. Two of the four hips, in which inadequate post-peak SBT levels were obtained developed a recurrent infection ($p = .035$). An inadequate post-peak SBT was noted to be statistically significantly more common in patients that had a recurrent infection (4).

Reimplantation

A decision to reimplant a new hip replacement depends on the general health of the patient, the potential for rehabilitation, the quality of the soft tissue and bone, the bone loss, and the ability to obtain appropriate antibiotic levels. In general, reimplantation is considered after the patients have received six weeks of intravenous antibiotics with a serum bactericidal titer of at least 1:8, no signs of infection, benign clinical course, and wound healing.

Adequate preoperative planning is essential in order to have available appropriate-sized components to facilitate a satisfactory biomechanical reconstruction when there is a bone-stock deficit. In addition, arrangements must be made to have allograft bone present if there are severe deficiencies of either the acetabulum or the femur. At the time of reimplantation, multiple cultures are obtained, as well as Gram stains and frozen sections. In addition, the tissues are carefully inspected and if there is still evidence of acute inflammation further debridement is performed, and reconstruction may be delayed. If the Gram stain is positive or if there are greater than five polymorphonuclear cells per high-power field at frozen section, the reimplantation may also be delayed. In these cases, the wound is closed and the patient is continued on skeletal traction and intravenous antibiotics. If the postoperative cultures are negative, the patient is considered ready for reimplantation. If the postoperative cultures are still positive, then the patient is treated again with six weeks of intravenous antibiotics.

We prefer to use antibiotic impregnated cement for reimplantation. Our previous work evaluating the joint fluid of total hip arthroplasties implanted with gentamicin-impregnated cement revealed high local antibiotic levels and low serum levels. Local antibiotic levels on postoperative day one averaged 14.9 μg/ml which was seven times higher than levels obtained in patients receiving intravenous gentamicin (2.2 μg/ml). The antibiotic level in the joint persisted and was measured to be 5 μg/ml at four weeks. In contrast, the serum levels averaged only 0.01 μg/ml on post-operative day seven (1,7). The high local concentration of gentamicin in these hips was effective against not only gram-negative but many gram-positive bacterial isolates including *Staphylococcus aureus* and *Staphylococcus epidermidis*. Thus, antibiotic-impregnated cement provides high local levels of antibiotic and low serum levels, which decreases the potential for systemic toxicity.

Commercially mixed antibiotic impregnated cement (i.e., Palacos) is unavailable in the USA and the surgeon must hand mix the antibiotics. We generally use Tobramycin-impregnated cement since Gentamicin is not available in powdered form. When mixing the antibiotic with the cement, it is important to create a homogeneous mixture in order to avoid regions of high antibiotic concentration that could be biomechanically weak. The addition of liquid antibiotics is contraindicated because it adversely affects the biomechanical characteristics of the cement. Although the addition of a species-specific antibiotic is appealing, the elution characteristics of some antibiotics are erratic and their effects on the biomechanical properties of the cement are unknown (9).

After the prosthesis is inserted, we treat the patient following our standard revision hip replacement protocol. Drains are usually kept in for approximately 24 to 48 hours. The patient is maintained on intravenous antibiotics until the intraoperative culture results are negative.

COMPLICATIONS

One of the most dreaded complications after the treatment of an infected total hip arthroplasty is recurrence of infection. The keys to avoiding recurrence include identification of the infecting organism, a thorough incision and debridement, and appropriate serum bactericidal titers. If there is a recurrence, one must aggressively treat the infection, and component removal is usually necessary. In this instance, the surgeon must have a frank discussion with the patient about the prognosis of this hip. Serious consideration should be given to leaving the patient with a resection arthroplasty, as the success of second reimplantations decreases.

ILLUSTRATIVE CASE FOR TECHNIQUE

The patient was a 57-year-old male, 16 months status post a revision right total hip arthroplasty, who complained of severe right hip pain. The patient had undergone a cementless right total hip arthroplasty three years before. During the course of this procedure a spiral femoral fracture was sustained, which was treated with cerclage wires. Fifteen months later, the patient underwent a cemented revision for loosening of the femoral component.

When the patient was referred for evaluation, he had pain with weight bearing and he was able to ambulate only three blocks with a pronounced limp. The patient attained some relief with antiinflammatory medications, but he found the decrease in his activity level unacceptable. Radiographs revealed a continuous radiolucent line surrounding the femoral bone cement interface. The position and fixation of the acetabular cup was good (Fig. 6).

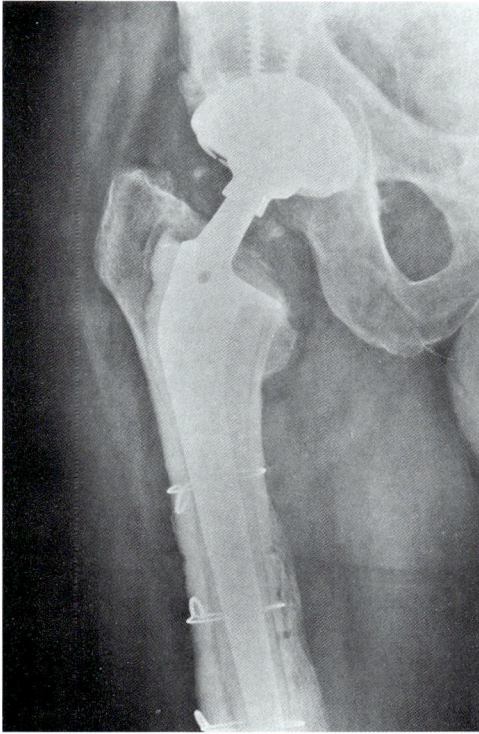

Figure 6. Radiograph 16 months status postrevision with a cemented femoral component demonstrates a continuous radiolucent line at the bone–cement interface.

The patient subsequently underwent revision of the femoral component. During exposure of the hip, inflammatory tissue was noted surrounding the hip joint. Multiple tissue specimens were sent for frozen section, Gram stain, and culture. The frozen section revealed both acute and chronic inflammation. Multiple polymorphonuclear leukocytes and gram-positive cocci were noted on the Gram stain. Accordingly, the hip was considered infected. A thorough incision and debridement was carried out. A trochanteric osteotomy was performed to facilitate removal of both components and cement. Two drains were placed in the hip and these were removed after 48 hours (Fig. 7).

The patient was started on intravenous cefazolin for a presumed gram-positive infection. The cultures grew out *Staphylococcus epidermidis*. Post peak serum bactericidal titers were 1:16 for cefazolin and 1:64 for clindamycin. The antibiotic regimen was then changed to clindamycin as a result of the higher SBTs. The patient received a six-week course of intravenous antibiotics. The hip wound and the postoperative course were benign.

The hip was subsequently reimplanted with a cementless acetabular component and a cemented femoral component. Two allograft femoral heads were morselized and impacted into the femoral canal. The femoral component was fixed with tobramycin-impregnated cement. Post-operatively, the patient remained on intravenous antibiotics until the intraoperative cultures were negative. The drains were discontinued at 48 hours.

The patient is doing well 8 years after the procedure. He has no hip pain and ambulates unlimited distances, without support nor limp. There has been no recurrence of infection (Fig. 8).

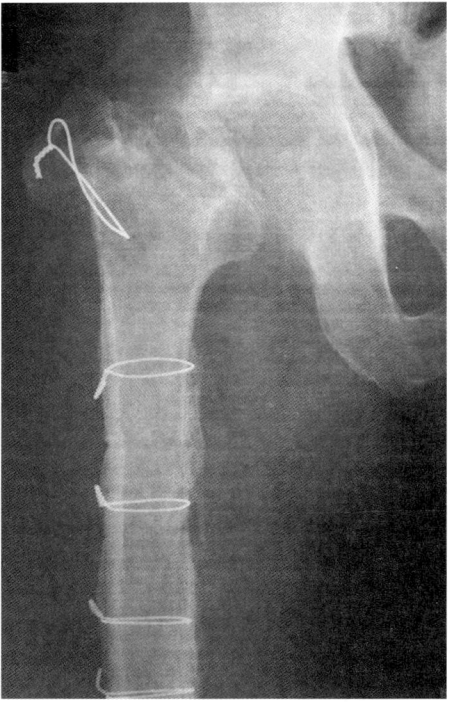

Figure 7. Radiograph after incision, debridement and removal of the components and cement. A trochanteric osteotomy was performed to facilitate cement removal.

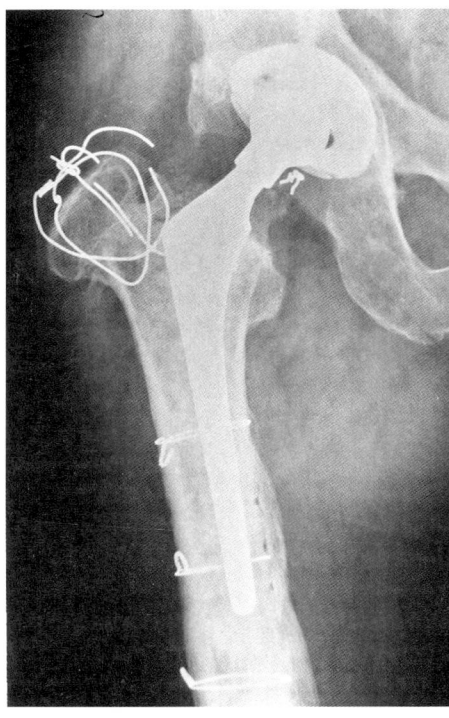

Figure 8. Radiograph 18 months after reimplantation with a hybrid total hip arthroplasty. The femoral component was implanted with tobramycin impregnated cement and impaction grafting of allograft bone. The trochanteric osteotomy has healed.

RECOMMENDED READINGS

1. Callaghan, J. J., Salvati, E. A., Brause, B. D., Rimnac, C. M., and Wright, T. M.: Reimplantation for salvage of the infected hip: rationale for the use of gentamicin-impregnated cement and beads. The Frank Stimidified Award of the Hip Society. In: *Proceeding Thirteenth Annual Meeting of the Hip Society.* CV Mosby, St. Louis, 1985, pp. 65–94.
2. Garvin, K. L. and Hanssen, A.P.: Infection after total hip arthroplasty. *J. Bone Joint Surg* 77A:1576–1588, 1995.
3. Goulet, J. A., Pellicci, P. M., Brause, B. D., and Salvati, E. A.: Prolonged suppression of infection in total hip arthroplasty. *J. Arthroplasty*, 3:109–116, 1988.
4. Lieberman, J. R., Callaway, G. H., Salvati, E. A., Pellicci, P. M., and Brause, B. D.: Treatment of an infected total hip arthroplasty with two-stage reimplantation protocol. *Clin. Orthop.*, 301:205–212, 1994.
5. Lieberman, J. R., Huo, M. H., Schneider, R., Salvati, E. A., and Rodi, S.: Evaluation of the painful hip arthroplasties. Are technetium bone scans necessary? *J. Bone Joint Surg.*, 73-A:475, 1993.
6. McDonald, D. J., Fitzgerald, R. H., Ilstrup, D. M.: Two stage reconstruction of a total hip arthroplasty because of infection. *J. Bone Joint Surg.*, 71-A:829–834, 1989.
7. Salvati, E. A., Callaghan, J. J., and Brause, B. D.: Prosthetic reimplantation for salvage of the infected hip. *AAOS Instruct. Course Lect.*, Volume XXXV:234, 1986.
8. Salvati, E. A., Callaghan, J. J., Brause, B. D., Klein, R. F., anc Small, R. D.: Reimplantation in infection. *Clin. Orthop.*, 207:83–93, 1986.
9. Wright, T. M., Sullivan, D. J. H., and Arnoczky, S. P.: Report on an investigation of the effect of antibiotic additions on the fracture properties of polymethylmethacrylate bone cements. *Acta Orthop. Scand.*, 55:414–418, 1984.

16

Acetabular Revision

Clement B. Sledge and Hugh P. Chandler

INDICATIONS/CONTRAINDICATIONS

Acetabular revision may be complex or simple. In a modular acetabulum with a well-fixed liner, simple liner exchange is indicated for wear or in conjunction with femoral revision for loosening to extend liner wear life. Simple liner exchange is not possible in a cemented component or in an uncemented component in which the polyethylene liner is not modular. In general, the indications for revision of a cemented or an uncemented acetabular component include: 1) pain in the groin and an acetabular component with a complete radiolucent line (RLL), 2) a progressive RLL with or without pain, and 3) a definite change in position of the component on radiographs, indicating loosening. The presence of bone loss from fracture or osteolysis is one of the more complex indications for revision. The location and amount of bone loss are critical elements to assess in preoperative planning for needed equipment and for the appropriate surgical approach.

It is useful to use some system of classifying bone loss to facilitate surgical planning (Fig. 1). The simplest classification includes four categories: *first,* contained defects with intact rim; *second,* rim deficiency; *third,* combined deficiency of socket and rim; and *fourth,* pelvic discontinuity.

Acetabular revision is contraindicated in patients not capable of undergoing an extensive surgical procedure or nonambulatory patients without pain. If an asymptomatic, nonprogressive RLL is present, or the rate of progression of wear, migration of the component, or bone loss are so slow that the patient can reasonably be expected to live out his life before revision becomes mandatory because of pain, loss of function or catastrophic mechanical failure, acetabular revision is not warrented.

C. B. Sledge, M.D.: Department of Orthopedic Surgery, Brigham and Women's Hospital, Boston, Massachusetts 02115.

H. P. Chandler, M.D.: Department of Orthopaedic Surgery, Massachusetts General Hospital, Boston, Massachusetts 02114.

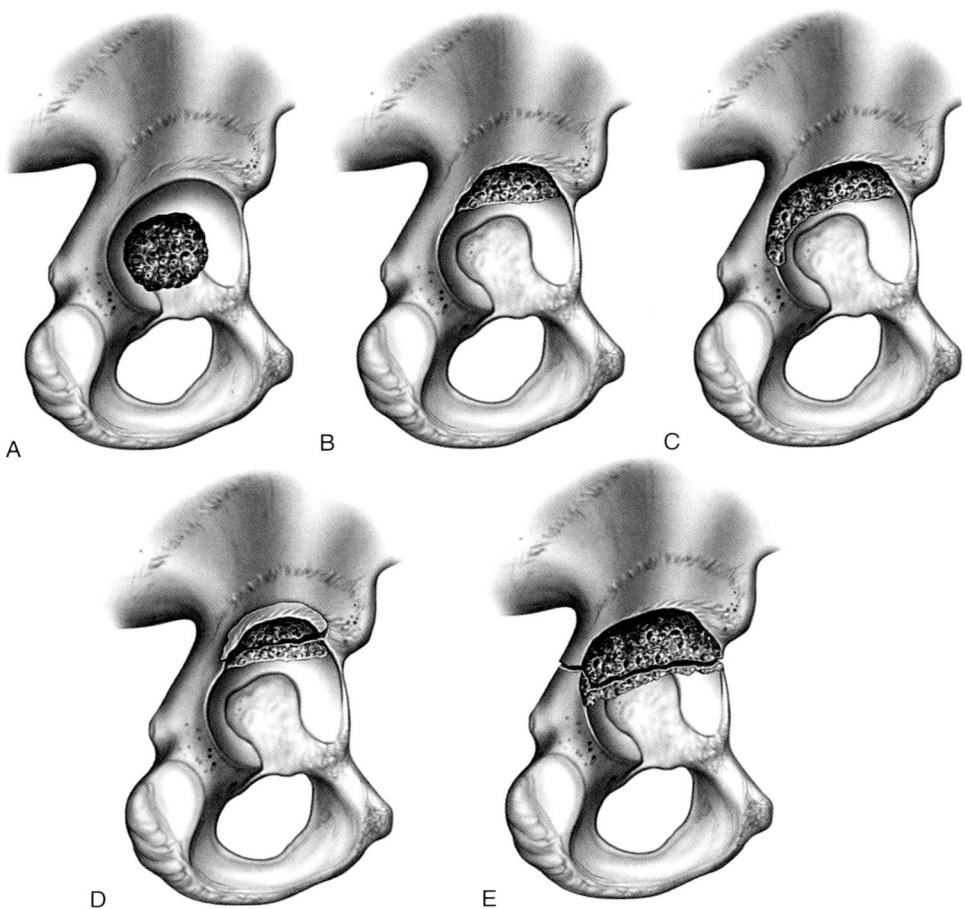

Figure 1. The four classes of bone loss that are useful for facilitation of surgical planning are: (A) cavitary defects with an intact rim; (B,C) rim deficiencies which may be in one or more quadrants of the acetabulum, such as (B) superior or (C) combined superior/posterior; (D) combined cavitary and rim defects; and (E) pelvic discontinuities in which the superior and inferior acetabulum has separated as a result of posterior and anterior column defects.

Sepsis is a relative contraindication. The first priority is to rule out infection; if infection exists, the organism and its antibiotic sensitivity should be determined. This information, along with the general condition of the patient and the nature and quantity of bone loss will determine whether single-stage or two-stage revision is appropriate. If the construct is otherwise stable and an organism sensitive and responsive to antibiotics is present, one-stage revision might be undertaken. However, if there is enough bone loss to require bone grafting or the use of reconstruction shells or plates, two-stage reconstruction is more prudent.

PREOPERATIVE PLANNING

It is important to understand the nature and extent of the bone deficiency before undertaking the revision operation so that special equipment can be obtained, if necessary. The type and amount of allograft, the type and size of protrusion shell, and the presence or absence or column defects should be anticipated. Standard radiographic views, supplemented by Judet views to evaluate the anterior and posterior columns, are usually sufficient. On oc-

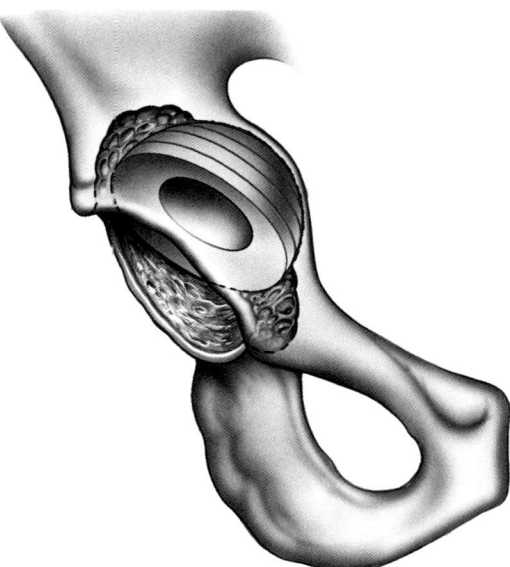

Figure 2. In the "monkey trap" defect, the shape of the protrusion is such that the cavity is larger than the entrance.

casion, if there is suspicion of more extensive bone loss, CT scans with correction for metal artifact will be necessary. If protrusion is extensive, either MRI or angiography can be utilized to demonstrate the location of the iliac vessels.

Contained defects without shift in component position can usually be managed by simple revision with an uncemented cup. If there is a protrusio, it may be a cylindrical intrapelvic migration that can be managed by bone grafting of the defect and insertion of a press-fit acetabular component into the intact rim. If, however, the shape of the protrusion is such that the cavity is larger than the entrance ("monkey-trap") (Fig. 2), the entrance is deficient, and supplemental fixation, such as a shell, will be required.

Rim defects and combined defects with rim loss and cavity loss will require restoration of the rim by a combination of bone graft and plate fixation as well as bone grafting of the contained defect, probably supplemented with a protrusio shell or cage. Pelvic discontinuity is usually best treated by means of a pelvic reconstruction plate that stabilizes one column, usually the posterior. An acetabular allograft into which the component is cemented can also be used. The composite of allograft and acetabular component is fixed into the prepared defect by screws into the adjacent intact pelvic bones.

This chapter will illustrate the treatment of massive protrusio defects utilizing a protrusio shell and particulate allograft. Several different types of protrusio rings or shells are available: the Burke-Schneider cage, the Mueller ring, and the Osteonics "gap cup™". The latter, being easily available in the United States will be utilized in the illustrative case.

Surgical Approach

A transgluteal (direct lateral) or a posterior approach can be used for simple loosening without significant bone loss, for cylindrical protrusio, and for minor posterior column defects. A transtrochanteric approach is useful for more extensive rim defects, especially if there is an intact femoral component that must be displaced to visualize the acetabulum.

If a ring, shell, or acetabular allograft will be required, an iliofemoral approach allows good visualization of the entire acetabulum and iliac wing to facilitate screw fixation of the proximal plates of the reinforcement shell or for secure fixation of an acetabular allograft

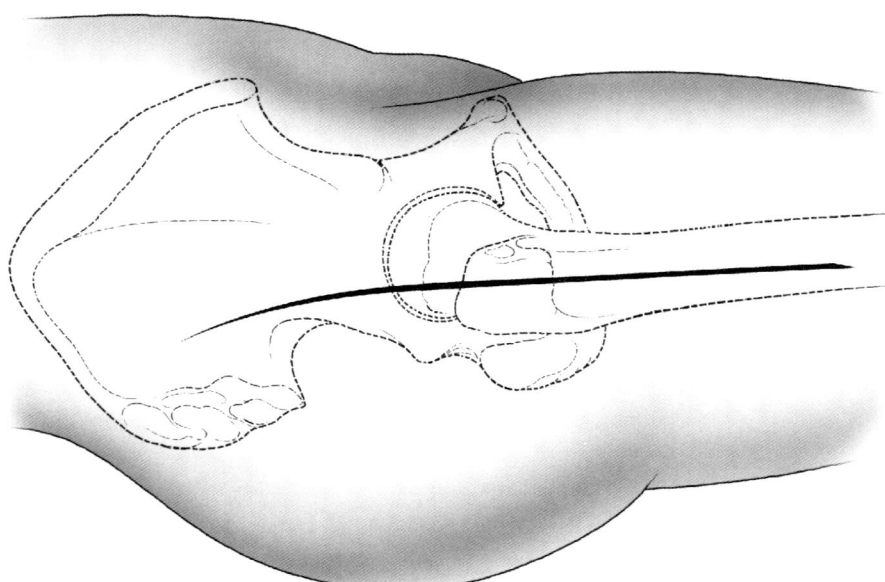

Figure 3. An extended ilio-femoral incision may be necessary to provide adequate exposure to the deficient acetabulum, including the pelvic columns and the iliac wing. In most instances, however, a standard transtrochanteric approach will suffice. The skin incision should be generous to allow proximal dissection of the abductors.

(Fig. 3). An alternative approach, if the anterior and posterior columns are intact, is to use a transtrochanteric approach and strip the iliac wing muscles proximally (Fig. 4). In thin patients, the standard iliofemoral approach can be modified; after a transtrochanteric approach to the acetabulum, a second incision is made over the iliac crest and the gluteal mus-

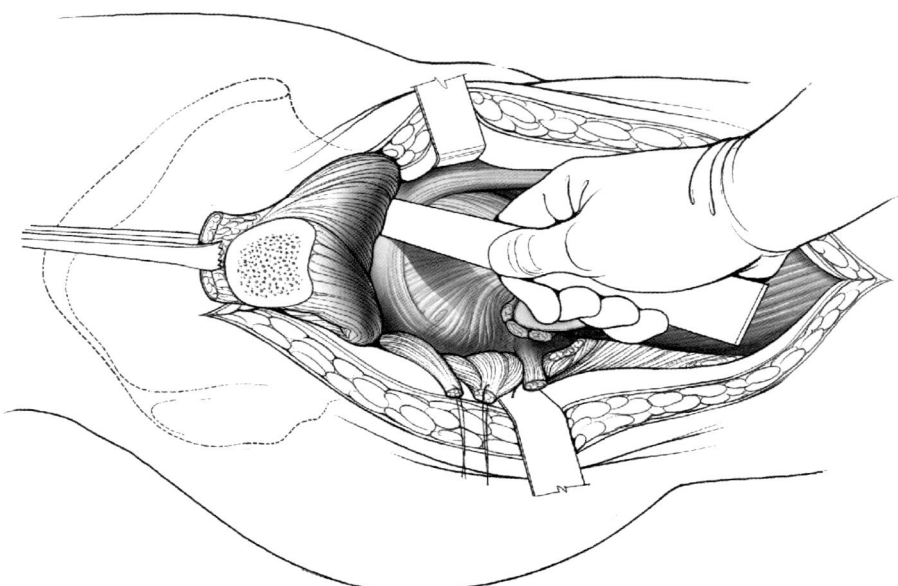

Figure 4. After trochanteric osteotomy, the abductors are stripped proximally to expose the iliac wing for supplemental fixation of the reinforcement shell and to allow adequate exposure of the superior rim. If the rim is deficient, allografting can be carried out with this enhanced exposure.

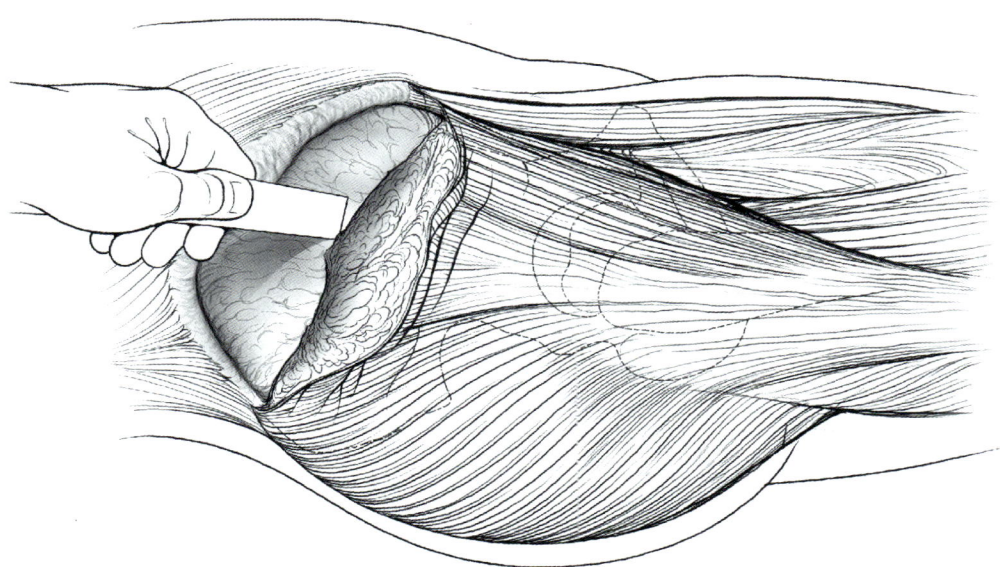

Figure 5. Adequate exposure of the iliac wing is accomplished by stripping the abductors from the ilium until the dissection joins the previous exposure shown in Fig. 4.

cles are stripped from the iliac wing (Fig. 5). Dissection is continued distally until it meets the subperiosteal dissection carried proximally from the acetabulum (Fig. 4). When the two dissections connect, it is easy to pass the arms of the reinforcement cup from distal to proximal against the surface of the ilium. The supplemental fixation screws can then be readily inserted through the proximal incision.

Preparation of the acetabulum depends on the amount and location of bone loss. If column support is lost, it must be restored by supplemental bone graft and flexible plates. Central defects are filled with solid sheets of allograft cut in shingle fashion from an allograft femoral head if there is no central floor, or they are filled with particulate bone if there is sufficient central support. Superior rim defects are augmented with particulate or solid allograft so that the acetabular implant can be placed in its proper anatomical location. When optimal bony integrity has been achieved, the acetabulum is reamed to a concentric shape and size consistent with the reinforcement shell chosen (Fig. 6). Additional particulate al-

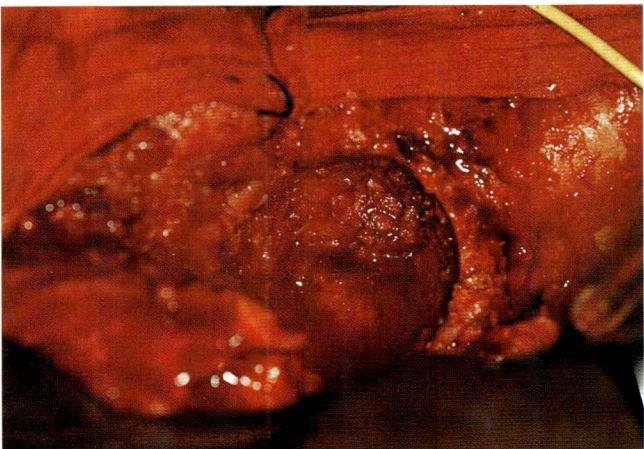

Figure 6. The loose acetabular cup as well as soft tissue and debris have been removed from the acetabulum revealing a deficiency in the rim in the 11 to 12 o'clock position.

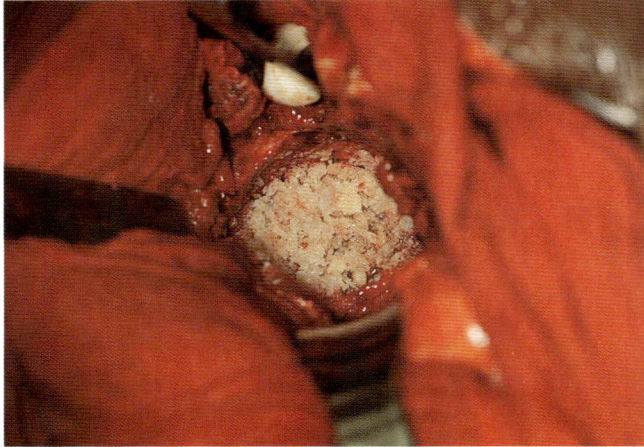

Figure 7. A large amount of particulate allograft bone was placed in the depths of the acetabular defect until the floor was restored to the proper level.

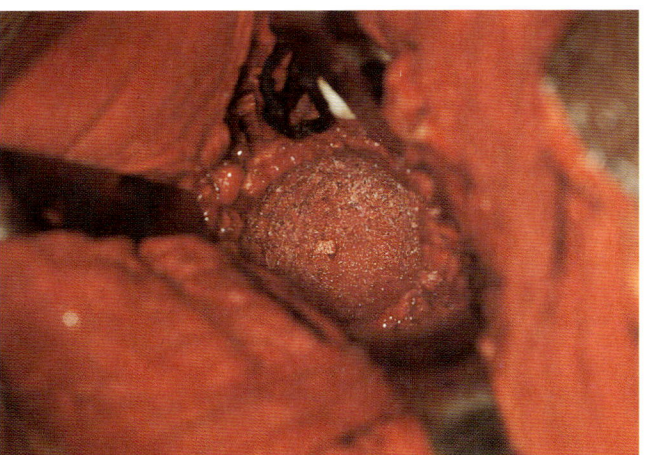

Figure 8. Reamers were used in reverse to shape the allograft and host bone to a concentric shape and size to match a 56-mm reinforcement shell.

lograft bone is added to the depths of the acetabulum and contured with reamers used in reverse to ensure mechanical support of the implant (Figs. 7, 8). The reinforcement shell is contoured to fit snugly within the prepared acetabulum so that the hook engages the inferior margin of the acetabulum (obturator foramen) and the proximal plates lie flush with the exposed iliac wing (Figs. 9, 10). Screws are inserted through the holes in the cup portion of the shell and through the extended arms (Fig. 11) and a polyethylene cup is then fixed to the shell with methylmethacrylate bone cement (Fig. 12). Orientation of the cup is obviously important to provide an adequate range of motion without dislocation. Because of the alterations in bony anatomy encountered in these revision procedures, orientation of the cup must be assessed carefully by using all available landmarks as well as positioning guides. If the femoral component is not being revised, the head may be simply exchanged for a new one or leg lengths and stability may be adjusted by changing neck length at this time. With motion and stability found to be satisfactory, closure is carried out in routine fashion.

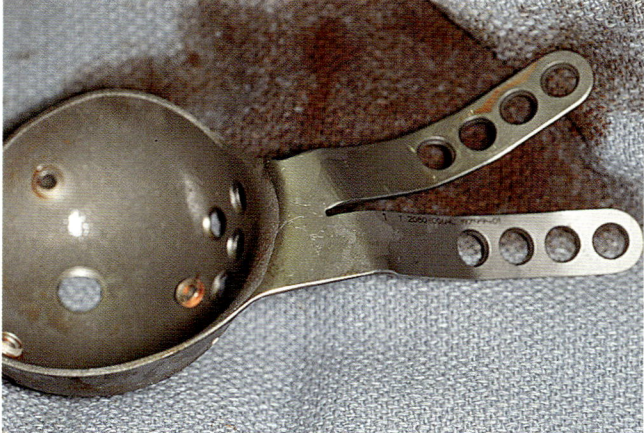

Figure 9. The iliac arms of the reinforcement shell have been contoured to match the iliac wing when the inferior hook is engaged under the inferior rim and the cup is firmly seated in the prepared acetabular bed.

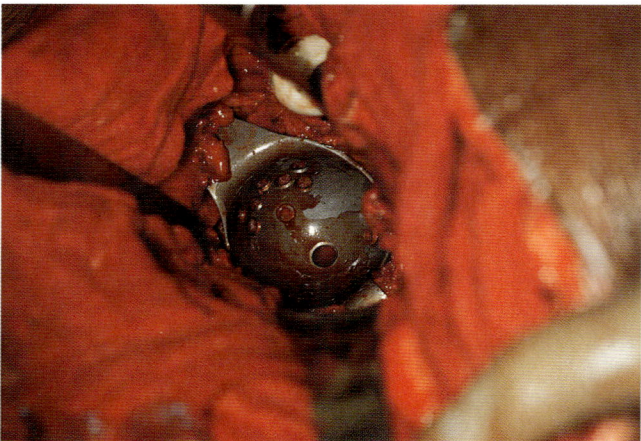

Figure 10. The shell is in place, and good stability is achieved. The iliac arms lie about 2 in. posterior to the anterior superior iliac spine.

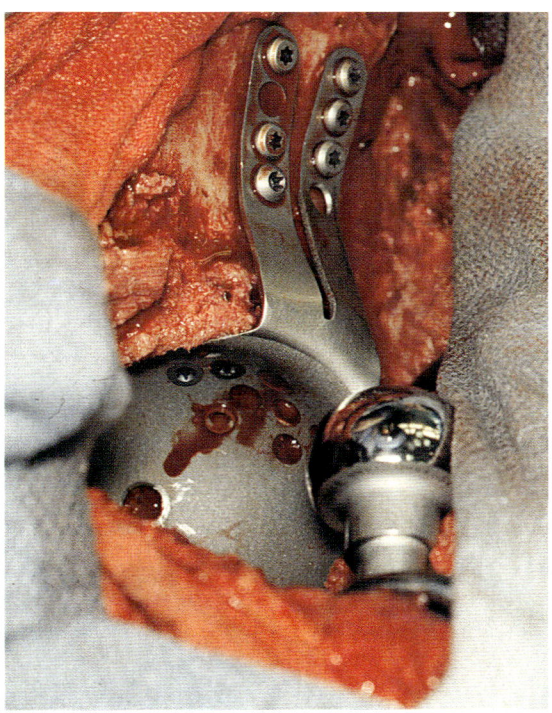 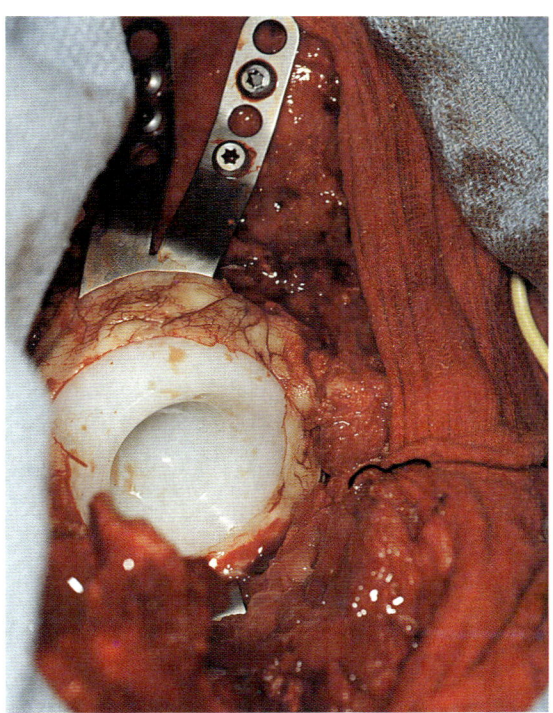

Figure 11. Screws are inserted through the dome of the shell and through its iliac arms.

Figure 12. A polyethylene cup is cemented into the acetabular shell with 30 degrees of flexion and 45 degrees of abduction.

POSTOPERATIVE MANAGEMENT

It is difficult to generalize regarding the postoperative management of patients undergoing acetabular revision. Their management must be dictated by several factors that vary from case to case—the integrity of the host bone, the quality of the surgical construct (including the stability of the implant and any bone graft used), and the ability of the patient to conform to the prescribed exercise and crutch program. In general, the exercise program can be instituted immediately. Abductor exercises must be avoided until healing of the trochanter if trochanteric osteotomy has been employed. If structural grafts are used, crutch/cane support should be maintained until there is radiographic evidence that grafts have begun to incorporate and the implant is stable, as demonstrated by the absence of migration on serial radiographs.

COMPLICATIONS

As with any massive revision operation involving foreign materials (metal, polyethylene, polymethylmethacrylate, and allograft), infection is the major concern. Unless careful attention is given to restoration of leg lengths and appropriate soft tissue tension, dislocation will occur. Reestablishment of posterior capsular and muscle integrity is useful in diminishing the likelihood of his dislocation.

Unless the reinforcement shell is well supported either by host bone or impacted allograft bone, mechanical failure is likely. Fixation of the shell and its support must be rigid at the conclusion of surgery.

Biological failure (nonunion of bone grafts and failure of incorporation of porous implants) is usually a consequence of mechanical failure. The incidence can be decreased by generous use of bone graft and stable fixation of the implant at the time of surgery. In addition to achieving stable fixation of the construct at the time of surgery, appropriate protection of the hip, through patient education and the use of crutch support, must be insured

ILLUSTRATIVE CASE FOR TECHNIQUE

A twenty-year-old woman presented with left hip pain. At the age of 12 she had undergone total hip replacement for a slipped capital femoral epiphysis. She did well until the age of 18 when she underwent revision of her index hip replacement with revision of a loose acetabular component utilizing an uncemented cup supplemented by central bone graft. Ingrowth of the uncemented cup did not occur and an intrapelvic dislocation ensued (Fig. 13).

Revision was undertaken utilizing the previous incision and a supplemental incision over the iliac crest (Fig. 14). A deficiency in the acetabular rim was identified, precluding the use of a press-fit acetabular component. It was elected, therefore, to utilize an acetabular shell with supplemental iliac fixation. A large amount of morselized allograft bone was utilized in the central defect under the acetabular cup. Excellent mechanical stability was achieved by the combination of allograft particulate bone and the reinforcement shell (Fig. 15). A polyethylene acetabular component was cemented into the acetabular shell in a position of 40 degrees of abduction and 30 degrees of flexion (Fig. 16). This provided a very stable hip. Immediate postoperative radiographs revealed good position of the component (Fig. 17).

Postoperatively she was started on an exercise program avoiding side-lying abduction to protect the trochanteric osteotomy until there was radiographic evidence of healing. At eight weeks she was walking on two crutches with a three-point gait. Radiographs revealed evidence of early union of the trochanter, good position of the acetabular shell, and begin-

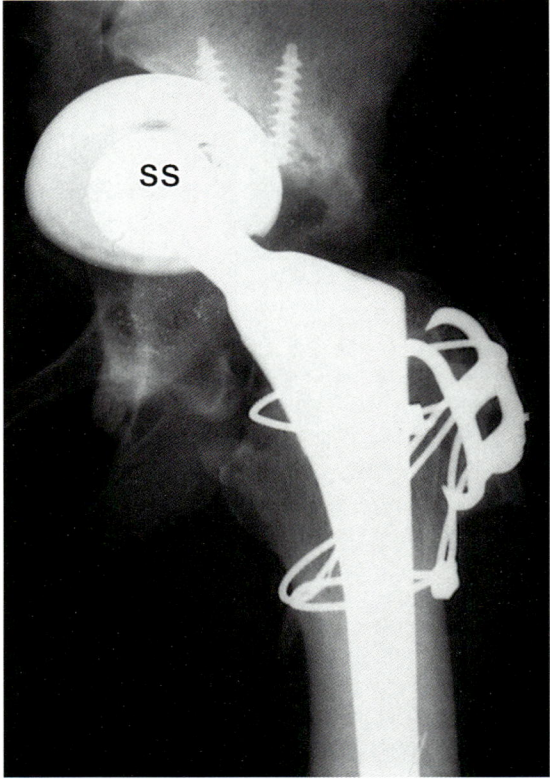

Figure 13. Preoperative radiograph showing central displacement of the acetabular component with disruption of the acetabular floor.

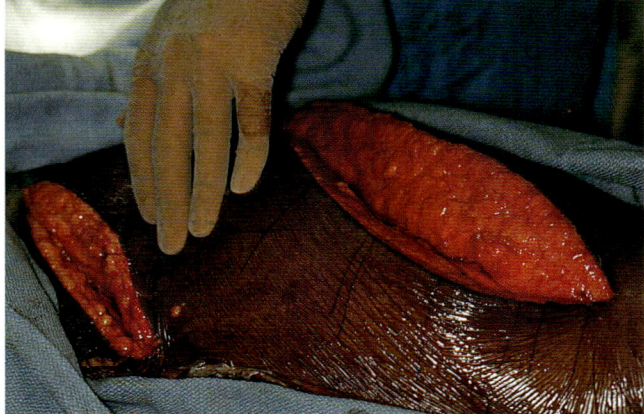

Figure 14. The previous incision, supplemented by an iliac crest incision, is utilized for exposure.

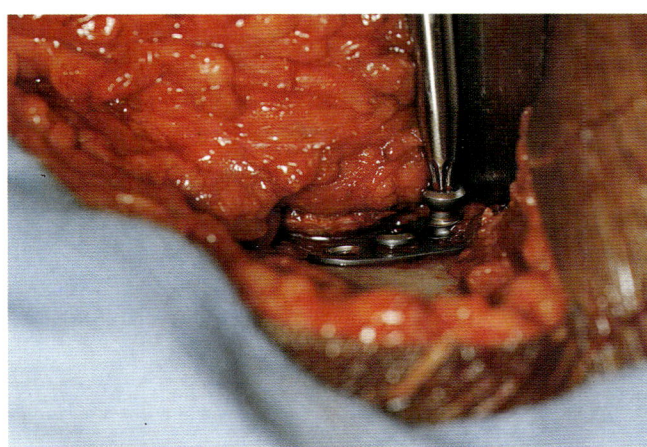

Figure 15. Screws are inserted into the fixation arms of the shell, utilizing the exposure provided by stripping the abductors through the proximal iliac incision.

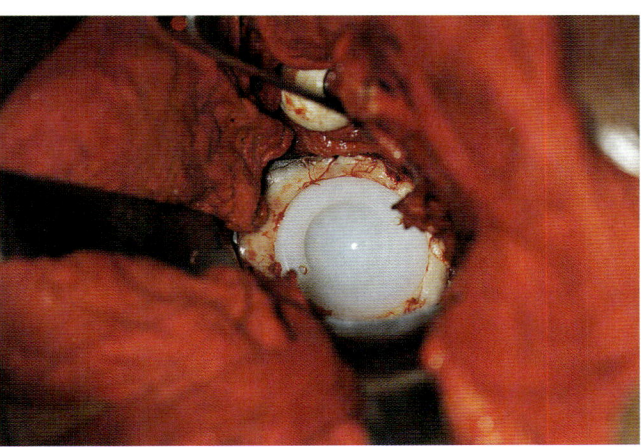

Figure 16. The shell is fixed into the acetabulum with screws, and the polyethylene cup is cemented into the shell.

ning incorporation of the allograft bone that had been placed centrally (Fig. 18). Range of motion was excellent with flexion to 115 degrees, internal rotation of 20 degrees, and external rotation of 40 degrees with strong abduction. She was allowed to progress to unsupported ambulation and return to sedentary work.

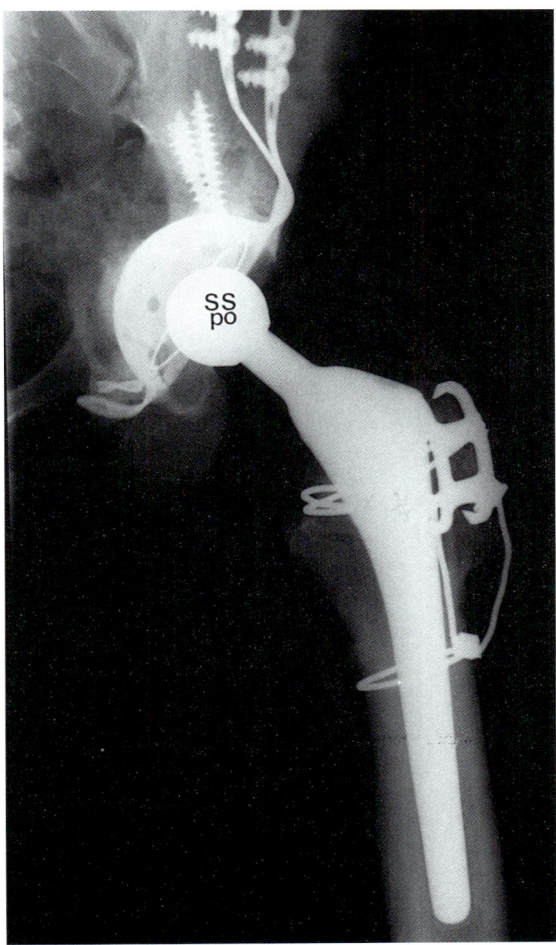

Figure 17. The immediate postoperative radiograph showing the position of the new acetabular construct.

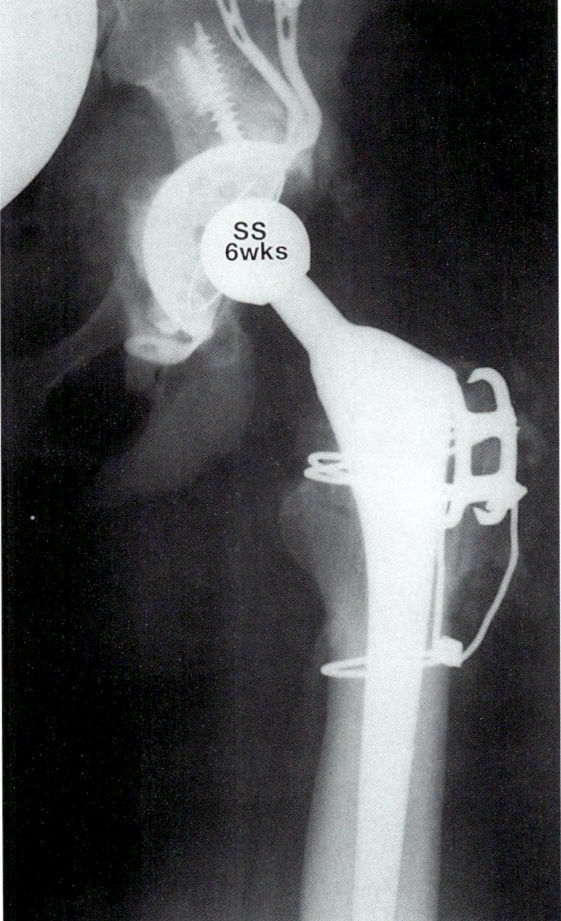

Figure 18. At 8 weeks, the trochanteric osteotomy is healing, early graft incorporation is evident, and the position of the implants is unchanged.

RECOMMENDED READING

1. D'Antonio, J.A., Capello, and W. N. Borden, L.S., et al. Classification and management of acetabular abnormalities in total hip arthroplasty. *Clin. Orthop.*, 243:126–137, 1989.
2. Trancik, T.M., Stulberg, B.N., Wilde, A.H., Feiglin, D.H., Allograft reconstruction of the acetabulum during revision total hip arthroplasty: clinical radiographic, and scinitgraphic assessment of the results. *J. Bone Joint Surg.*, (AM) 68-A 527–33, 1986.
3. Berry, D.J., and Muller, M.E. Revision arthroplasty using an anti-protrusio cage for massive acetabular bone deficiency. *J, Bone Joint Surg.*, (Br) 74 (5):711–715, 1997.
4. Zehnter, M.K., Ganz R. Midterm results (5.5–10 years) of acetabular allograft reconstruction with the acetabular reinforcement ring during total hip revision. *J. Arthroplasty* 9(5):469–479, 1994.

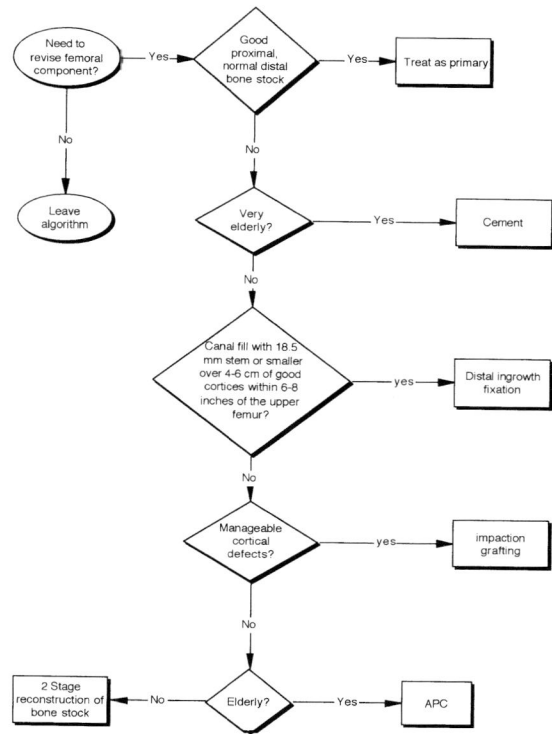

Figure 1. An algorithm for femoral component revision.

tween the bone and the ingrowth surface, and relative stability of the interface (minimal motion) to allow for the ingrowth to occur. Unfortunately, the revision femur rarely provides the appropriate environment for obtaining ingrowth proximally, and several clinical series of revision stems that provided for proximal ingrowth and utilized proximal stabilizing stem characteristics only revealed the inadequacy of this technique.

While some stems may take advantage of obtaining distal stability in order to achieve ingrowth proximally, in patients with good bone stock distally and the geometry to obtain good contact with a cylindrical stem over a 4 to 5 cm distance, an ingrowth type of stem with distal ingrowth fixation appears to be an effective choice. Several series in the literature document good results over a 5- to 10-year follow-up with this type of fixation. The main prerequisites of this technique include the ability to achieve appropriate intraoperative stem stability by virtue of the distal canal interference fit and the ability to limit postoperative weight bearing during the ingrowth phase of rehabilitation. This technique may be extended in cases of inadequate or patulous proximal bone stock by use of a "collapsing" osteotomy, using cerclage fixation to bring fractured proximal cortical remnants into contact with the upper portion of the stem.

The main long-term concern with this type of "distal" fixation is that it does nothing to restore upper femoral bone stock. Additional concern focuses on the fact that as stem stiffness increases (proportional to the increasing diameter of stem needed to obtain an interference fit in an expanded endosteal canal, a situation commonly encountered in the revision setting), severe stress shielding may take place proximal to the distal ingrowth region, and over time further proximal bone loss will occur.

Unfortunately the older patient with accompanying osteopenia and canal expansion tends to be the patient who has more significant stress-induced bone remodeling and is more susceptible to thigh pain than the younger patient, as noted in many cementless primary THA series. In addition, the ability to restore bone stock in the younger patient remains an attractive option.

Ling, Gie, Mckail, and Elting have explored the use of impacting allograft bone chips into the proximal femoral canal and then using cement fixation to fix the stem in the newly "created" allograft neoendosteal canal. This technique (at short- to intermediate term follow-up) appears to hold promise for obtaining better fixation at the endosteal surface by improving the quality of the bone present for cement interdigitation while allowing for bone stock restoration to the upper end of the femur. It would appear to be an appropriate technique in the patient who has substantially compromised endosteal bone stock or substantial endosteal expansion (the so-called patulous proximal femur). In particular, this technique may be used above long distal cement columns that may be difficult to remove and can be used to support the bone packing above.

Unfortunately the number of technical and biological variables that may influence the outcome in this technique are considerable, and as of yet have not been well investigated. Indeed the clinical reports are early and few. Nonetheless, there is great enthusiasm for this technique in many centers. It certainly would appear to be a highly technique-dependent procedure and should be used with caution, appropriate training, and preferably in the most reasonably well-suited candidates who do not appear to be most appropriate for alternative more established techniques.

Finally, in some circumstances, sufficient bone stock has been lost so as to require massive structural allografting for any reconstructive effort. This "court of last resort" technique was initially developed by orthopaedic oncologists, and, following its initial success, has been adopted for the multiple operated total hip revision candidate with overwhelming bone loss. While in some cases of massive proximal femoral bone loss it may be reasonable to use a "proximal one-third" femoral-replacement type of stem or even a modular oncology type of prosthesis (particularly in patients with limited life expectancy), these options do not allow for reattachment of the abductor mechanism and require violation of the distal femur for fixation. The allograft prosthetic composite (APC) allows for more consistent abductor reattachment and may allow for less violation of the distal femur. While carrying with it a unique set of technical requirements—as well as the biological variability inherent in structural bone grafting and the risk of disease transmission—it remains an essential part of the revision surgeon's armamentarium. However, as noted in the accompanying algorithm, in the younger patient who is not a candidate for the other techniques mentioned, due to massive bonestock loss and in whom bone-stock restoration is desirable, a two-stage procedure may be employed where bone stock is initially restored via auto- and allografting, setting the stage for a second procedure to implant and fix a stem into the improved femoral canal. This technique again appears to be one of last resort, and there is no literature support for this.

While multiple techniques are available to the revision surgeon, and he must be familiar with the technical requirements of each, his most significant task is to evaluate the patient's unique characteristics in an attempt to determine which specific procedure is most likely to provide the greatest benefit and fewest complications and to restore greatest function. The following description of these techniques will be of benefit in this regard.

17A

Revision with Cemented Femoral Component

Craig G. Mohler and Dennis K. Collis

INDICATIONS/CONTRAINDICATIONS

The reported results of revision of the femoral component utilizing cement were initially discouraging with relatively high failure rates at short follow-up periods (1,5,8). The introduction of modern cementing techniques and prostheses has dramatically improved the results of cemented femoral component reconstruction in revision hip surgery (4,6). The senior author (DKC), has utilized cement for femoral component reconstruction extensively since beginning practice and has reported 3.6 percent rerevision rate in a series of 110 hips with an average 4.1 years follow-up (2). The authors perform cemented femoral component revision in patients with reasonable femoral bone quality and prefer to use this technique in patients who are older than 60 years of age. Segmental femoral defects, extreme femoral bone loss, fractures around loose femoral components, and younger patients often require the use of other techniques, such as impaction femoral allograft reconstruction or extensively porous-coated femoral components, as discussed in the introduction to this chapter.

PREOPERATIVE PLANNING

When using cement for femoral reconstruction in revision hip surgery, preoperative planning is essential. Good quality anteroposterior radiographs and cross-table and frog-leg lateral views must be obtained, as the entire length or the femoral stem and cement column must be visualized in two planes. The central element of preoperative planning is the selection of the proper prosthesis. The surgeon must be thoroughly familiar with the prosthe-

---

C. G. Mohler, M.D. and D. K. Collis, M.D.: Oregon Health Sciences University, Portland, Oregon 97201.

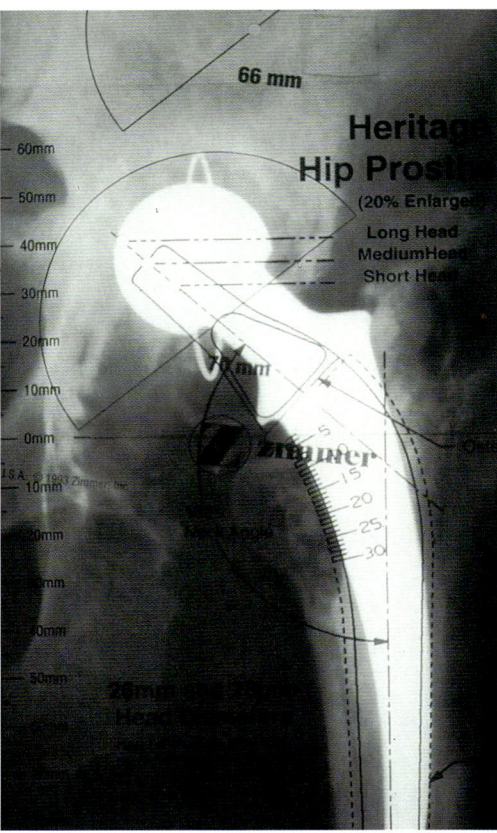

Figure 1. Templating should be an essential part of preoperative planning. Templating allows measurement of leg length, ensures selection of the proper size and length of the femoral component, and allows the surgeon to visualize the expected restoration of limb length and offset.

sis to be used and should ensure the availability of all stem sizes and lengths necessary to reconstruct the femur successfully. We use a polished forged chrome-cobalt stem of rectangular geometry with broad lateral borders, a distal centralizer, and a modular head. Preoperative templating aids the surgeon in determining what size implants will be necessary (Fig. 1) and in visualizing the results of revision, including restoration of limb length and offset. Templating also alerts the surgeon to the need for special prosthetic stems such as calcar replacement or extra-long (200 to 250 mm) stems. Another element of preoperative planning includes the visualization of potential pitfalls that could render femoral component revision with cement difficult or impossible to perform (such as severe femoral bone loss or periprosthetic femoral fractures).

SURGICAL TECHNIQUE

The patient is placed in a lateral decubitus position, with a vacuum-pack bean-bag or appropriate pelvic positioners to secure the torso. The down leg must be carefully padded to prevent contralateral limb problems such as compartment syndrome, which has been reported in hip revision surgery. Prior to making the incision, the location of previous inci-

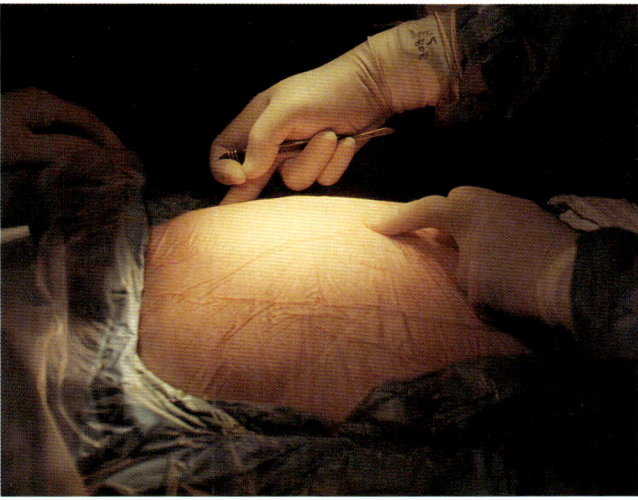

Figure 2. The location of previous incision is noted. If possible, one should use a straight lateral incision for revision hip surgery, unless a closely adjacent, slightly anterior or posterior incision exists.

sion should be noted (Fig. 2). Previous incision should be utilized if properly located, rather than creating a narrow skin bridge between the old and new incision, which may invite skin necrosis. For most revision hip surgery, a direct lateral incision is performed (Fig. 3). After exposure of the fascia lata, hemostasis with electrocautery is performed. The fascia lata is then opened and the interval between it and the underlying vastus lateralis fascia is developed. It can be helpful to begin distally in virgin tissues to develop this interval and then move proximally.

The greater trochanter is exposed, and previously placed wires, if present, are removed. Electrocautery dissection is utilized to isolate the adductor muscle mass anteriorly and posteriorly. A cobra-type blunt-tipped retractor is inserted posteriorly along the proximal fe-

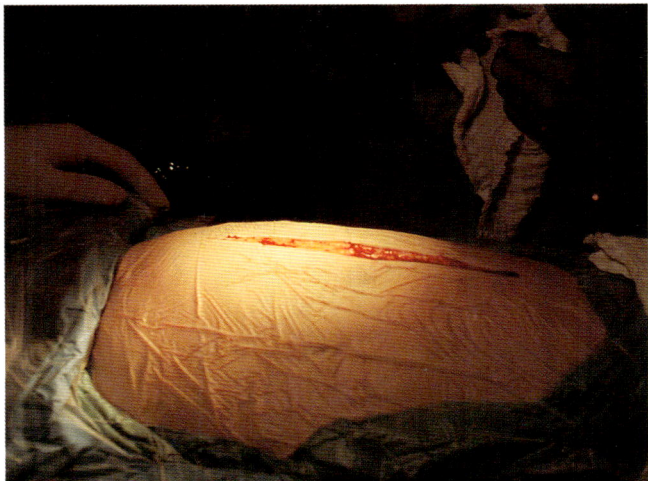

Figure 3. The incision should be adequate to complete the task at hand. Inadequate or poorly placed incision can lead to struggles in exposure. It is well to remember the old adage, "think twice, cut once."

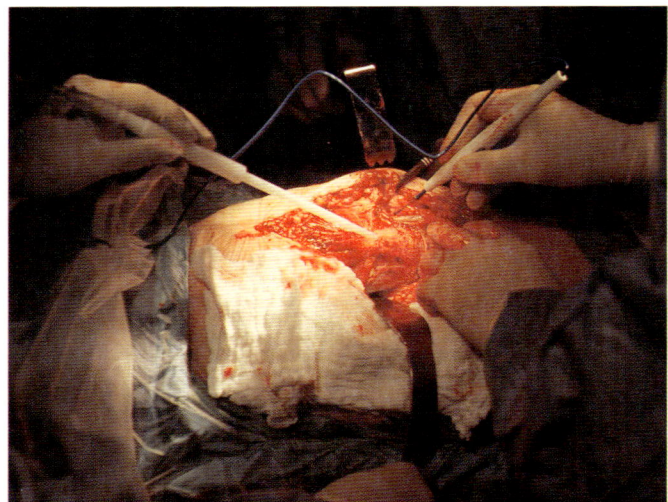

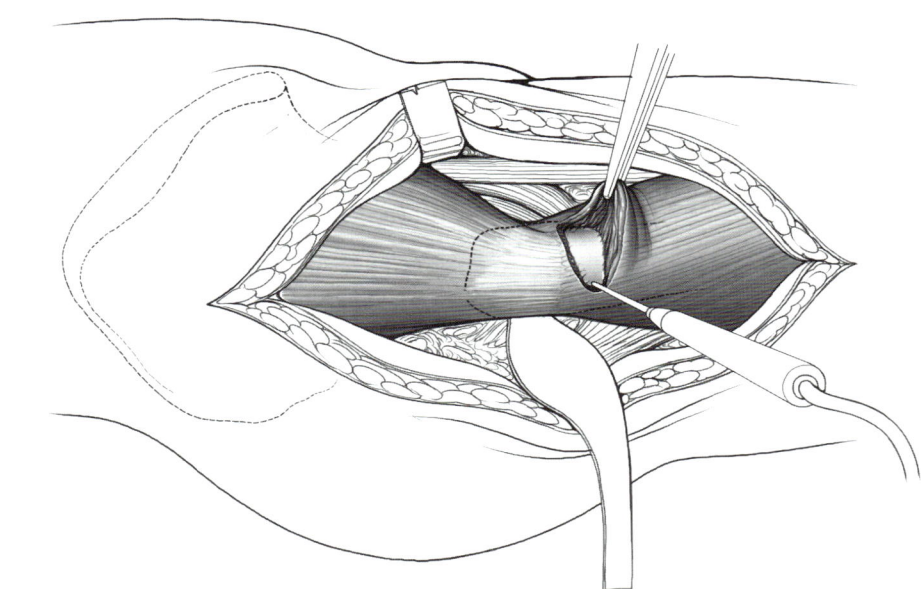

Figure 4 A, B. After the incision of the fascia lata, self-retaining retractors (such as the Charnley) may be placed. The senior author prefers a large, blunt-tipped cobra retractor (bottom of figure) during this portion of the exposure. The abductor muscle mass is isolated anteriorly and posteriorly and the origin of the vastus lateralis removed in preparation for trochanteric osteotomy.

mur to aid in exposure (Fig. 4). This retractor must be carefully placed directly on the bone to avoid injuring the sciatic nerve.

We routinely use trochanteric osteotomy in revision hip surgery because of the unparalleled exposure it offers. After elevation of the origin of the vastus lateralis, trochanteric osteotomy is carried out with a curved gouge (Fig. 5). Progressive mobilization of the greater trochanter, often requiring release of portions of the pseudocapsule, allows proximal retraction of the trochanter. The trochanter is then secured in place with a stout abductor retractor and fixed with two large, smooth Steinman pins inserted into the ilium. A preliminary leg-length measurement is carried out (Fig. 6) using the pins and the ilium as a reference point measured against a point on the proximal femur.

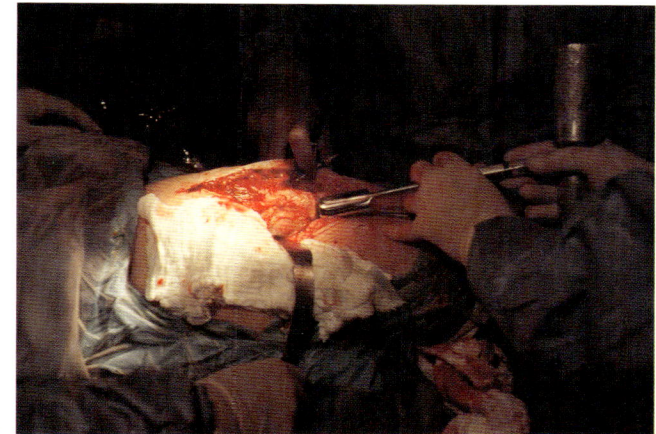

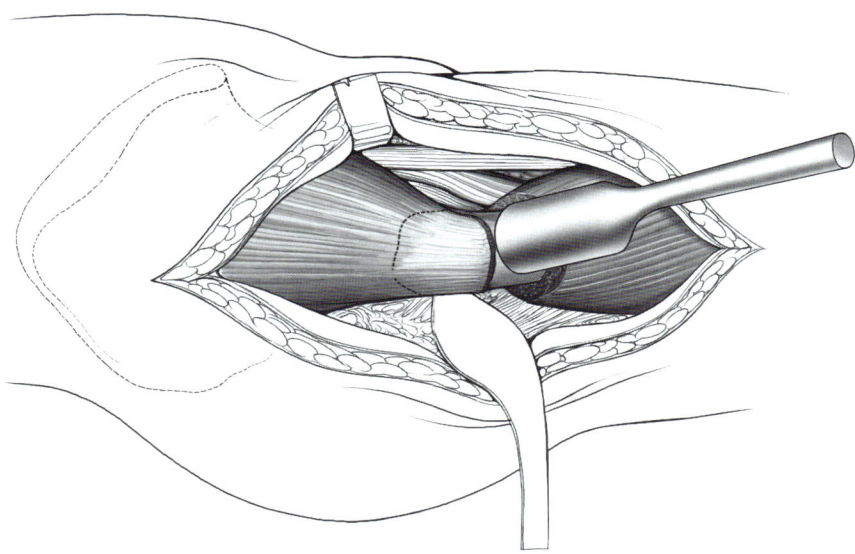

Figure 5 A, B. A curved gouge is used to osteotomize the greater trochanter. Care must be taken to remove a large enough fragment of bone to allow secure reattachment.

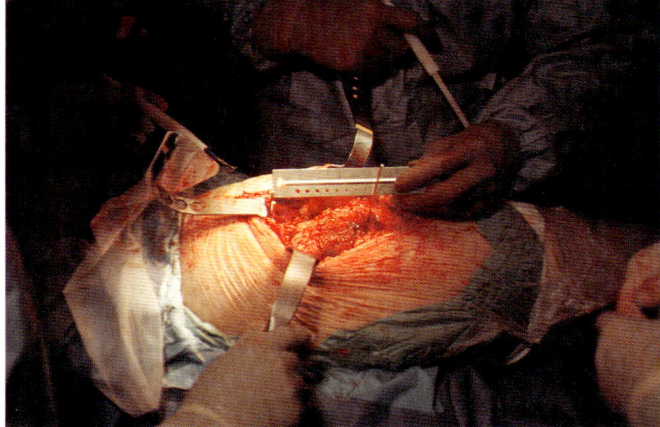

Figure 6. A large abductor retractor fixed with two stout, smooth Steinman pins is used to secure the trochanter. These pins serve as a reference point for leg-length measurements. A third pin is placed at a selected point on the lateral femur and a measurement obtained and recorded.

After the limb-length measurement, appropriate retractors are inserted for exposure of the hip. We prefer a blunt-tipped, double-pronged retractor placed anteriorly. Great care must be taken to insert this retractor on the bone of the anterior column to avoid injury to arterial and venous structures. A blunt-tipped cobra-type retractor is placed in front of the psoas tendon, and a second cobra retractor is placed posteriorly, again with care to place the retractor directly on bone. The retractors thus placed, excision of the pseudocapsule is carried out prior to dislocation of the hip (Fig. 7). Dislocation of the hip is facilitated by excision of as much pseudocapsule as is necessary essentially to skeletonize the proximal fe-

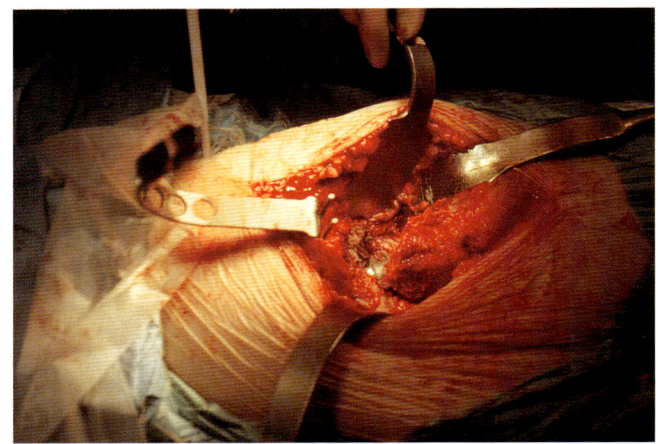

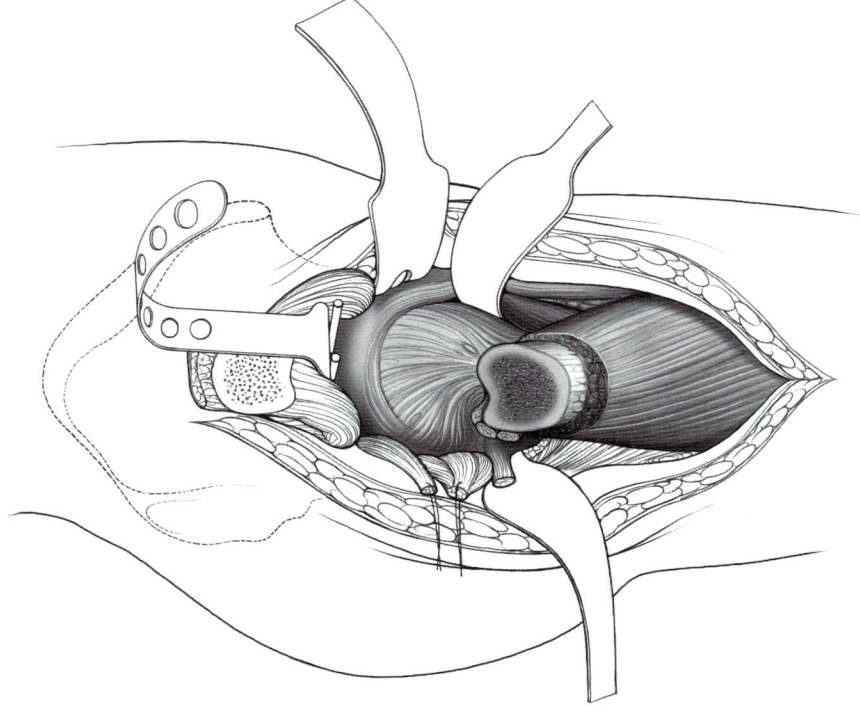

Figure 7 A, B. The placement of retractors for exposure and resection of the pseudocapsule is critically important. The upper right blunt-tipped, double-pronged retractor at the top of the figure is placed directly on anterior column bone. The abductor retractor is seen on the left. A blunt-tipped cobra posterior retractor is placed directly on the ischium.

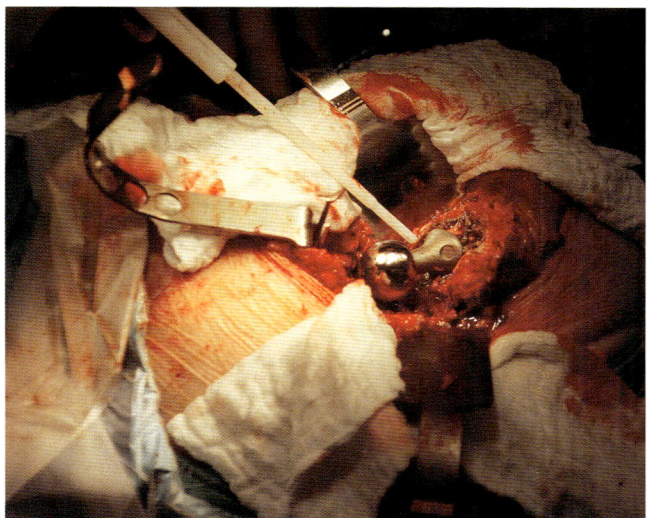

Figure 8. Hip dislocation is carried out only after enough pseudocapsule has been excised to allow easy dislocation with relatively little force. Note that in the figure the femoral component is grossly loose.

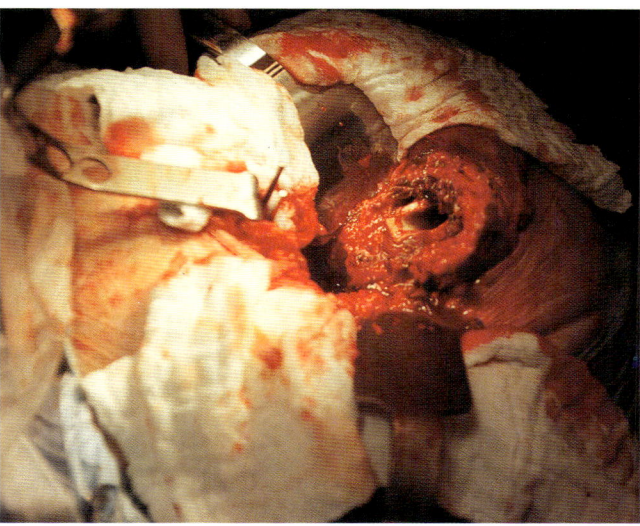

Figure 9. Femoral preparation begins with elevation of the proximal femur from the wound using a large "antler" or similar retractor. The hip is extremely rotated and the leg placed into the sterile leg pocket on the opposite side of the operating table.

mur (Fig. 8). The hip is externally rotated and adducted, and the leg is then placed into a sterile leg pocket and stabilized by an assistant. Femoral component extraction must be carried out carefully. Removal of small amounts of bone and cement may be necessary to completely expose the collar and shoulder of the implant. Great care must be taken to completely expose the implant proximally prior to its removal, as over zealous, forceful attempts at removal of the component without removing overlying cement and/or bone can lead to fracture of the proximal femur. If a monoblock stem is to be extracted, it can be removed by hand (if one is fortunate) or grasped with a commercially available stem extractor, which features a device that loops over the femoral head. A sliding hammer mechanism can then be used to extract the component. Modular stems may require more specialized instrumentation, such as a modular universal extraction device. Well-fixed components can be difficult to remove and require meticulous removal of proximal cement with hand or ultrasonic tools or a high-speed burr. Care must be taken when using even thin osteotomes to remove proximal canal cement with the prothesis in place, as osteotomes can act as a wedge and fracture the proximal femur. Occasionally, creation of an anterior window or even an extended femoral osteotomy is necessary to remove well-fixed textured or precoated femoral stems.

Once the femoral component has been removed, acetabular revision (if necessary) is carried out (see chapter 16). We prefer to leave cement in the femur undisturbed until after acetabular preparation. Early overzealous removal of femoral cement prior to acetabular preparation can lead to unnecessary blood loss from exposed femoral cancellous bone and should be avoided.

After acetabular preparation and component insertion is completed, the femur is exposed. A large, blunt proximal femoral retractor placed posteriorly beneath the proximal femur helps elevate the femur from the wound (Fig. 9). The leg is again placed into a sterile leg pocket and secured by an assistant. Cement removal is carried out in three areas of the femur: proximally, centrally, and distally. We prefer standard hand tools for femoral cement removal. Proximal cement removal is carried out with a variety of gouges and osteotomes. The cement is then grasped with a pituitary rongeur and removed. Curettes are utilized to remove pseudomembrane that can be grasped with a forceps or rongeur. Meticulous removal of all pseudomembrane is critical, as creation of a new cancellous bed for cement interdigitation is essential when using cement on the femoral side. Cement in the middle region of the femur must be carefully removed with hand tools to pry it away from the femoral canal wall. Again, loose, fibrous tissue and pseudomembrane must be thoroughly removed; this is facilitated by the use of hooked curettes or "crochet hooks." The use of a lighted canal irrigator, which simultaneously illuminates and irrigates the canal, is useful, as the distinction between cement and femoral cortical bone can be difficult to see. Removal of cement within the canal is also facilitated by the use of offset osteotomes to allow the surgeon to work while visualizing the canal.

Distal cement, including the plug, can be difficult to remove, particularly if solidly fixed. Occasionally the plug of cement can be grasped and removed, but often the plug must be drilled with commercially available drill guides and low-torque cement drills of varying diameters. Alternatively, an ultrasonic or thermal "plug puller" can be useful. Following plug removal, the canal is scraped with a variety of curettes to thoroughly cleanse the interior of the femur of all fibrous tissue and cement. At the conclusion of this procedure, the surgeon should be confident that a cleaned, well-prepared canal has been created to accept the insertion of cement. Following removal of the prosthesis and cement, it is common to find areas of sclerotic bone, which may be gently "freshened up" with a high-speed burr to expose cancellous surfaces, while care is taken to avoid perforating the femoral canal. During cement removal from the femur, we monitor the length of time that the leg is positioned in the sterile pocket. After 20 to 25 minutes of work on the femoral canal, we bring the leg back onto the table for 5 to 10 minutes to prevent prolonged compression of the "down leg."

The appropriate-sized trial prosthesis is selected and inserted, and a trial reduction is carried out. A leg-length measurement is again carried out, with the retractor pins in the ilium as a reference point. Stability is verified, although the absence of the trochanter makes assessment of stability somewhat difficult. At this time, the surgeon must assess the approximate neck length that will be necessary to restore limb length and stability.

Prior to insertion of cement, the surgeon notes the appropriate location of the collar of the femoral component in its relation to the calcar of the femur. In some cases, the stem will need to be cemented somewhat "proud" to restore limb length, and this should be noted prior to cement insertion. The surgeon must guard against excessive anteversion or retroversion of the component, using bony landmarks in the proximal femur, and rehearse insertion of the stem in the appropriate position prior to cementing.

The surgeon must note the position of the leg, and it is useful to ask the assistant securing the leg to keep it perpendicular to the floor as a reference point. After removal of the trial prosthesis, the proximal femur is again exposed. Pulsatile lavage irrigation is carried out with a canal irrigator and brush to clean the cancellous bone surfaces vigorously. After the appropriate prosthesis has been selected, the placement of the cement plug is carried out. A cement mantle that extends 2 cm distal to the tip of the prosthesis is essential for good cementing technique. The cement plug inserter is placed against the actual femoral component to be used (Fig. 10), and a mark is made on the inserter to insure insertion of the plug to the proper location. A long, thin sponge soaked in a 1:100,000 epinephrine solution is then packed into the canal, while cement mixing is commenced.

Cemented femoral component revision requires more cement than would be used in cementing a primary femoral component. Often up to four packs of cement are necessary to fill the canal successfully after pressurization. A powdered antibiotic (tobramycin 1.25 g) may be added to every 80 g of cement mixed.

A commercially available vacuum mixer or centrifugation device is used for porosity reduction for optimum cement fatigue strength. After one minute of mixing, the cement is placed into a gun. Most commercially available cement guns will hold only three packs of cement, and therefore, when planning to use four or more 40-g packs, a second gun should be utilized.

There is a tendency to insert cement early, but we feel that cement should be inserted in a fairly doughy stage to prevent back flow of blood from cancellous bone surfaces. Cement insertion is carried out when cement extruding from the tip of the cement gun resists gravity, and does not stick to a gloved hand. The canal sponge is removed, and a final suction-

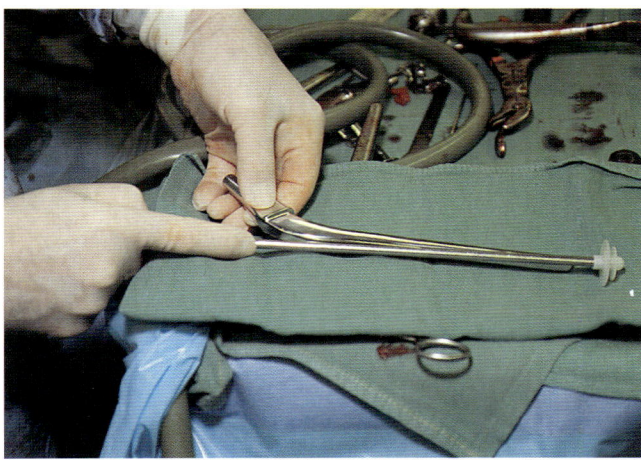

Figure 10. After the prosthesis has been selected, a plastic cement restrictor is inserted. Depth of insertion of the restrictor is checked by measuring against the component. One should aim for at least 2 cm of cement distal to the tip of the prosthesis and centralizer.

ing of the canal is performed. It can be useful to have the assistant on the opposite side of the table lift the leg at this stage to allow any remaining blood to flow out of the canal. The canal is further dried with a clean, dry, thin sponge packed into the canal. Insertion of cement into a clean, dry canal is essential for successful long-term reconstruction.

Cement insertion is carried out retrograde, with a long-tipped introducer and cement gun. Pressurization is then carried out using a proximal femoral pressurizer (Figs. 11, 12). The

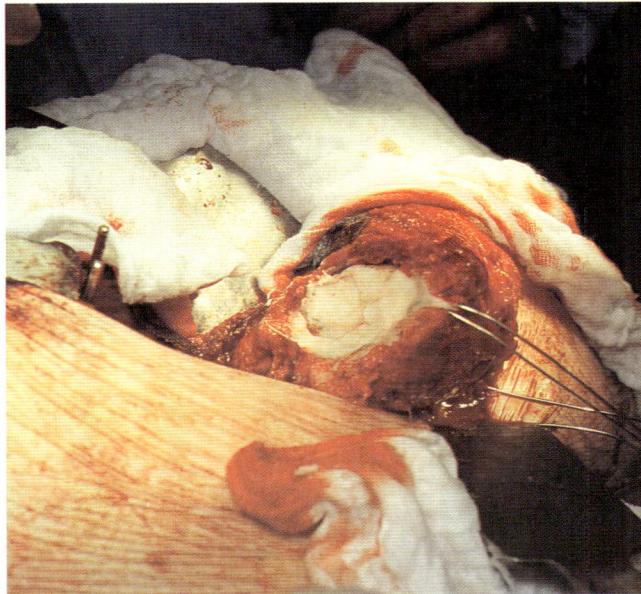

Figure 11. The canal must be completely filled with cement prior to pressurization.

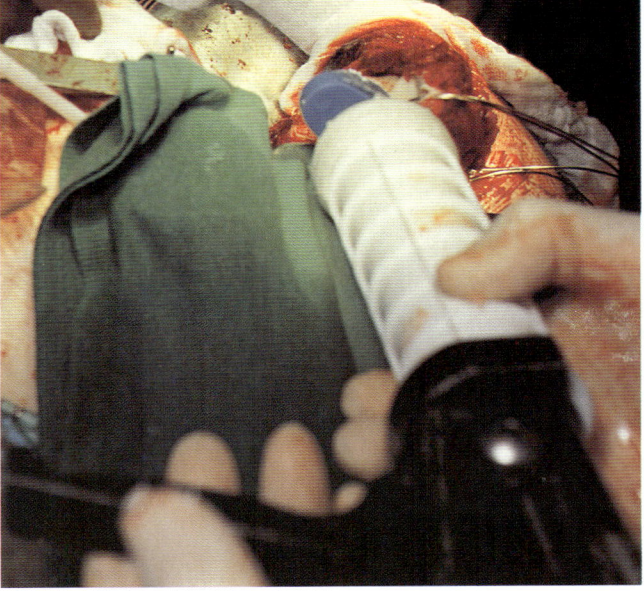

Figure 12. Cement pressurization is carried out for 30 to 60 seconds, and a rubber pressurizer is used to seal off the canal. If this is successful, one usually notes marrow contents extruding from venus sinusoids in the proximal femur.

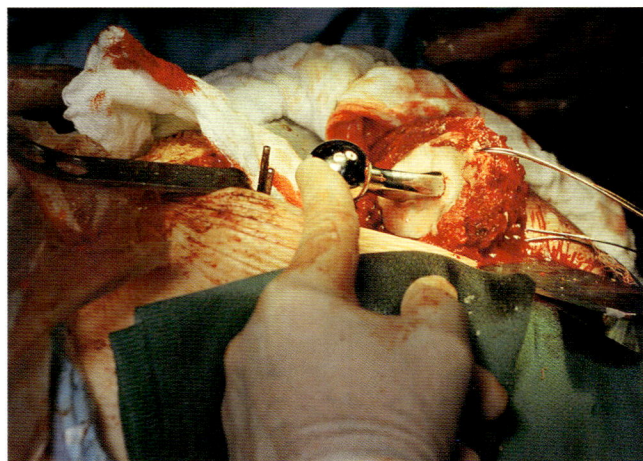

Figure 13. The surgeon must pay close attention as the final position of the stem is reached. The collar of the stem must be placed at the appropriate level noted during trial reduction.

stem is usually inserted by hand 6 to 8 minutes after cement mixing with great care to replicate the stem position noted during trial reduction (Fig. 13). Excess cement is cleansed from around the proximal femur while the stem is held in place by the surgeon. Strict attention must be paid at this time to avoid any stem movement while the cement cures. After cement curing, the appropriate cobalt-chromium femoral head may be inserted or a trial reduction carried out with a variety of trial heads. The appropriate head is then selected, the hip reduced, and a final leg length measurement obtained. Vigorous antibiotic irrigation of the wound is then carried out. The leg is abducted and placed into a padded Mayo stand. The trochanter is then reattached with a four-wire technique. Two horizontal wires are placed through drill holes in the lesser trochanter and brought out anteriorly and posteriorly. Two vertical wires are placed through drill holes in the proximal femur that exit above the shoulder of the prosthesis. The vertical wires are passed through small drill holes in the greater trochanter. The trochanter is grasped with a clamp by an assistant and reduced in the trochanteric bed (Fig. 14). Occasionally, in cases involving lengthening of the limb, re-

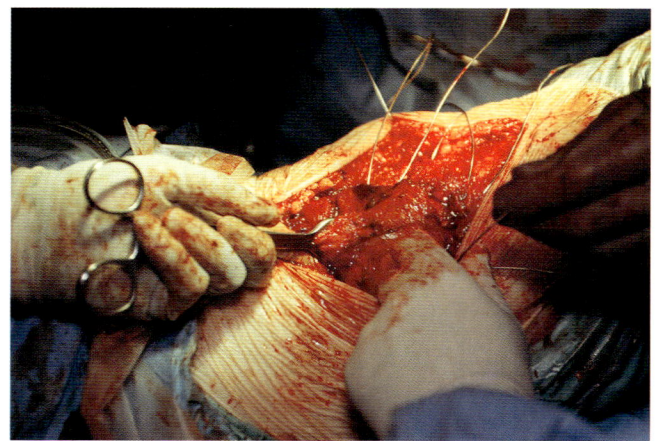
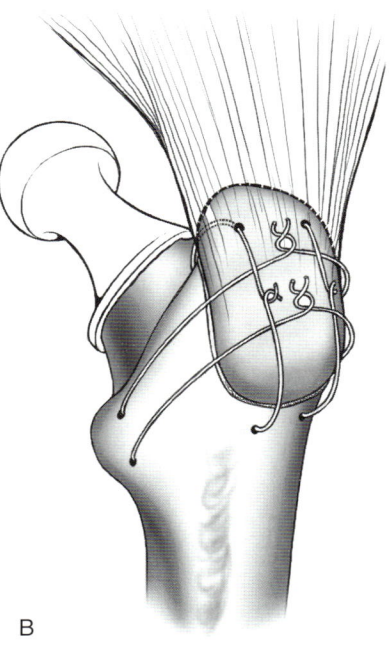

Figure 14. (A) Trochanteric reattachment is facilitated by an assistant with a large bone forceps grasping the trochanter and reducing it back in the trochanteric bed. (B) Trochanteric reattachment is achieved by using the four-wire technique.

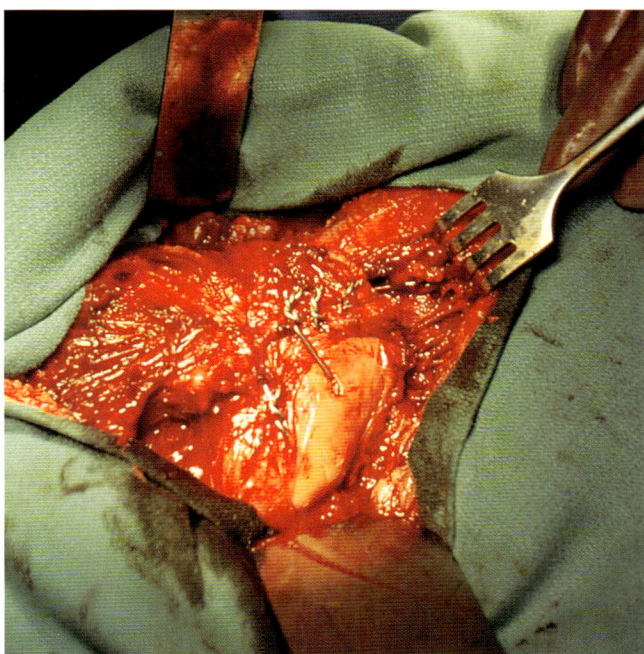

Figure 15. At the conclusion of trochanteric reattachment, a secure trochanter is recreated. Note the rake retractor at the right of the trochanter grasping the origin of the vastus lateralis.

lease of a portion of the abductors from the iliac wing will be necessary to facilitate reduction of the trochanter. Care must be taken to place the trochanter onto a bed of bleeding cancellous bone, rather than onto cement or metal. The trochanter is held in place by the assistant and the vertical wires tightened with a Harris wire-tightener and twisted, but not cut to allow further tightening, if necessary. The horizontal wires are then tightened and, if necessary, the vertical wires are retightened. Then all wire ends are bent back against the lateral femur to prevent trochanteric bursitis. At the conclusion of a trochanteric reattachment, the result should be a well-fixed, secure trochanter (Fig. 15). The vastus lateralis fascia should then be repaired back to the trochanter, using nonabsorbable suture.

POSTOPERATIVE MANAGEMENT

Following surgery, a postoperative anteroposterior and cross-table lateral view radiographs are obtained to check cement technique and trochanteric reattachment and to verify reduction of the prosthesis. The patient is placed in balanced suspension traction in the recovery room, which allows comfort and relative immobilization of the operated limb.

On the first postoperative day, the balanced suspension traction is removed, and the patient is allowed to dangle at bedside with the aid of a physical therapist. Gait training commences the following day. Weight bearing is restricted to no more than 50 pounds on the operated limb with the use of a walker or crutches. Drains, if inserted, are removed on the first postoperative day, and the bolster dressing is changed on the second or third postoperative day.

In cases where stability of the hip or fixation of the greater trochanter is questionable or when patient compliance with postoperative restrictions is doubtful, a 1 1/2 spica or commercial hip abductor brace is applied immediately prior to discharge. The patient is usually discharged to home or to an extended care facility on the fifth to seventh postoperative day.

During the hospitalization, anticoagulation is carried out with low molecular weight heparin or warfarin. The patient is seen back in the office for a postoperative wound check at two weeks following surgery, at which time the staples are removed. Protective weight bearing continues for the next four weeks at which time spica cast immobilization, if present, is removed and the patient is allowed to progress weight bearing. We ask the patients to use crutches or a walker for six weeks following the surgery, followed by a cane for six weeks. They do not begin abductor strengthening exercises until the fourth month.

Complications

Unfortunately, revision total hip replacement is more complex than primary hip reconstruction and, as expected, complications are more common.

Dislocation. Dislocations have been reported to occur in up to 20% of patients following revision total hip replacement (11). Early dislocation is treated by expedient reduction, usually in the operating room, and application of external immobilization, either a spica cast or commercially available brace for six weeks. Trochanteric nonunion commonly leads to postoperative dislocations and, if present, must be rectified by appropriate repair. Component malposition, particularly acetabular retroversion, may lead to early dislocations following surgery and may require repeat revision if dislocations occur.

Infection. The risk of sepsis following revision total hip surgery has been reported to be at least double that encountered in primary total hip replacements. Draining wound hematomas must be aggressively treated by debridement in the operating room to prevent infection (7). Early deep sepsis within two weeks after surgery may be treated successfully by debridement and retention of the components combined with culture-specific intravenous antibiotics for a period of four to six weeks, with an expected cure rate approaching 70% (10). Proper, careful surgical technique and meticulous wound hemostasis combined with prophylactic antibiotics may help decrease the rate of this complication. The role of antibiotic-loaded cement in preventing infections in total hip revisions performed for aseptic loosening is not clear, but at present we prefer antibiotic-loaded cement to provide a "safety factor" in revision total hip arthroplasty.

Neurovascular Injury. Neurovascular injury in revision total hip replacement is more common than in primary total hip replacement, chiefly due to difficulty in exposure and aberrant retractor placement. Care must be taken when placing retractors, particularly anterior and posterior acetabular retractors, to avoid injury to the iliac and femoral vessels and sciatic nerve, respectively. Sciatic and peroneal nerve palsies following revision total hip replacement occur from lengthening, retractor placement, and excessive postoperative bleeding (12). The prognosis for recovery of function in patients with nerve palsies following revision THR, as would be expected, is directly related to the degree of neutral injury. Nerve palsies in patients who recover some motor function immediately following have a better prognosis than those with severe dysesthesias or complete nerve palsies at discharge (9). In most cases, postoperative nerve palsies should be observed and recovery documented using electroconductive studies. Immediate intervention is occasionally necessary, such as in stretch-induced nerve palsies caused by overlengthening of a limb, in which case shortening of the modular femoral neck may be beneficial.

Femoral Fracture. Postoperative femoral shaft fractures can occur when the canal has been violated during cement removal. A defect in the femoral canal is often noted on postoperative radiographs when a bolus of cement is seen in the soft tissue surrounding the proximal femur. If a femoral canal perforation occurs during cement removal, it is best to proceed with insertion of a longer stemmed component to bypass the defect in the femoral canal, which acts as a stress riser by two canal widths to prevent postoperative fractures. Often canal perforation is not recognized until the initial postoperative radiographs. If it can be clearly documented that the perforation is well above the tip of the stem, then no intervention is necessary. However, if a defect is clearly noted extending distal past the tip of the stem, then application of strut allografts may be necessary to prevent late fracture.

ILLUSTRATIVE CASE FOR TECHNIQUE

The patient is an 89-year-old male who underwent cemented total hip replacement on the left side in 1981 and on the right side in 1982. His right hip was subsequently revised for aseptic loosening in 1988 (Fig. 16). The patient presented with severe left-hip pain and radiographic evidence of femoral component loosening. Despite his age, he was medically very fit and a suitable candidate for revision total hip replacement using cement on the femoral side.

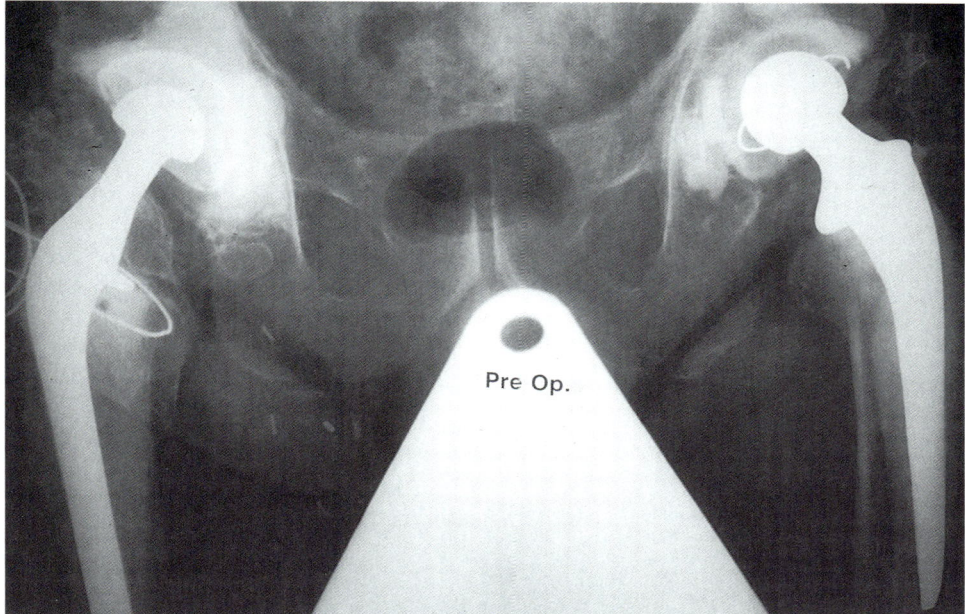

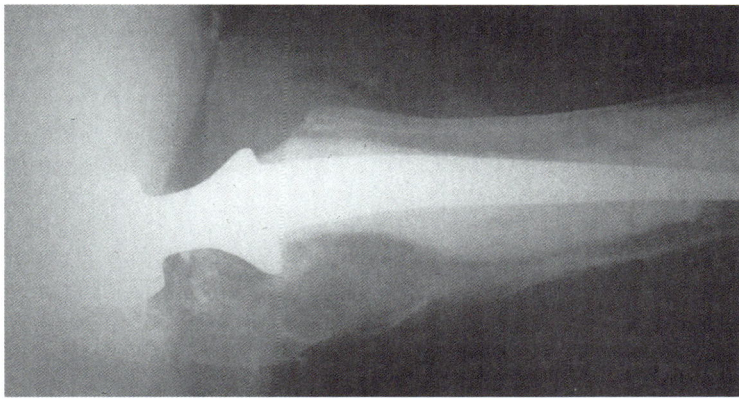

Figure 16 A, B. Preoperative radiographs show, on the left, a cemented THR with obvious loosening of the femoral component.

The patient underwent revision of the left hip, using the hybrid technique, with a cemented long-stem femoral component, using the Grade B cement technique and an uncemented acetabular component (Fig. 17). The patient recovered uneventfully, and at three months postop was walking with a cane.

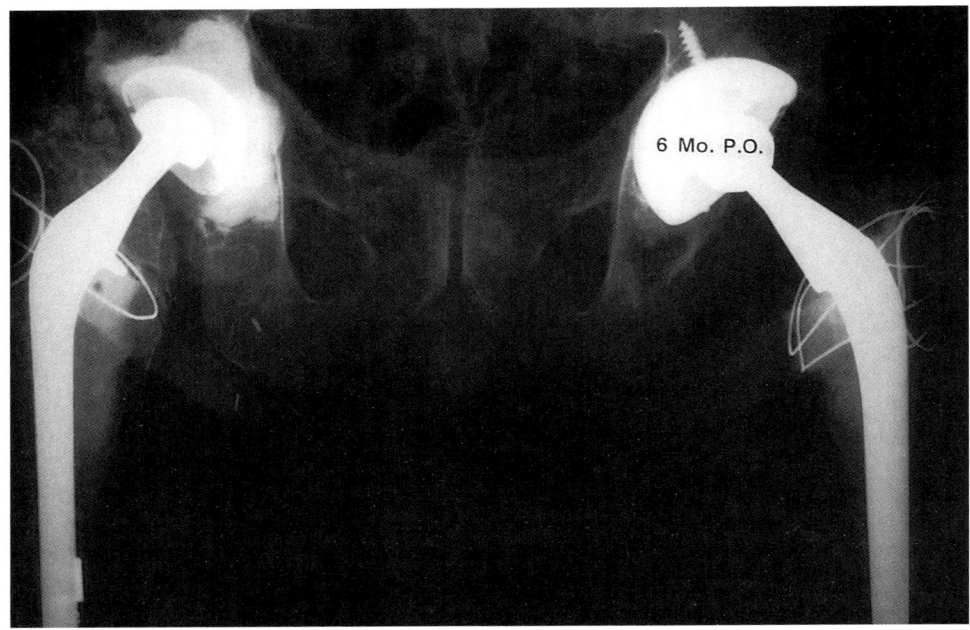
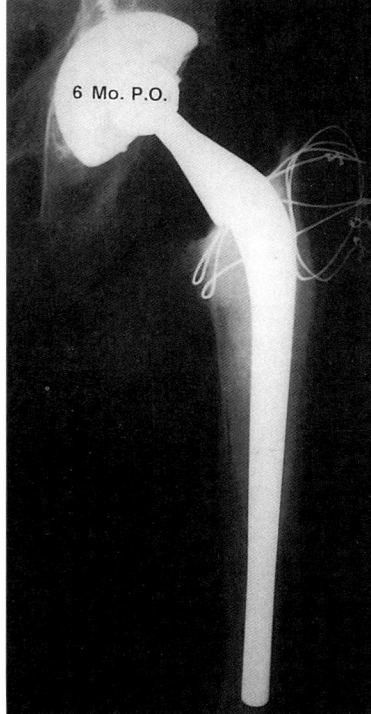
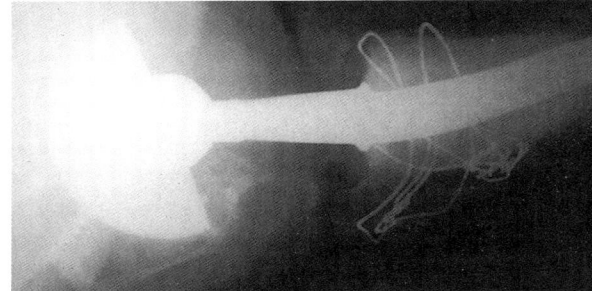

Figure 17 A, B, C. Radiographs taken six months postoperatively show a cemented long-stem femoral component with Grade B cement technique. Note the secure reattachment of the greater trochanter.

RECOMMENDED READING

1. Callaghan, J. J., Salvati, F. A., Pellicci, P. M., Wilson, P. D. and Ranawat, C. S. Results of a revision for mechanical failure after cemented total hip replacement. 1979–1981. *J. Bone Joint Surg.*, 67(A):1074–1085, 1985.
2. Collis, D. K. Revision total hip arthroplasty with cement. *Semin. Arthroplasty*, 4:38–49, 1993.
3. Estok, D. M., and Harris, W. H. Long-term results of cemented femoral revision surgery using second generation techniques. An average 11.7-year follow-up evaluation. *Clin. Orthop.*, 299:190–202, 1994.
4. Katz, R. P., Callaghan, J. J., Solomon, P. M., and Johnston, R. C. Cemented revision total hip arthroplasty using contemporary techniques: A minimum 10-year follow-up study. *J Arthroplasty*, 9:103, 1994.
5. Kavanaugh, B. F., Ilstrup, D. M., and Fitzgerald, R. H. Revision total hip arthroplasty. *J. Bone Joint Surg.*, 67(A):517–526, 1985.
6. Mulroy, W. F., and Harris, W. H. Revision total hip arthroplasty with use of so-called second generation cementing techniques for aseptic loosening of the femoral component. A 15-year average follow-up study. *J. Bone Joint Surg.*, 78(A):325–330, 1996.
7. Nassar, S. A. Prevention and treatment of sepsis in total hip replacement surgery. *Orthop. Clin. N. Am.*, 23:265–277, 1992.
8. Pellicci, P. M. Wilson, P. D., Sledge, C. B., Salvati, E. A., Ranawat, C. S., Poss, R. and Callaghan, J. J. Long-term results of revision total hip replacement. A follow-up report. *J. Bone Joint Surg.*, 67(A):513–516, 1985.
9. Schmalzreid, T. P., Amstutz, H. C., Dorey, F. J. Nerve palsy associated with total hip replacement. *J. Bone Joint Surg.*, 73(A):1074–1080, 1991.
10. Tsukyama, D. T., Estrada, R. and Gustilo, R. B. Infection after total hip arthroplasty. A study of the treatment of 106 infections. *J. Bone Joint Surg.*, 78(A):512–523, 1996.
11. Williams, J. F. Gottesman, M. J., and Mallory, T. H. Dislocation after total hip arthroplasty. Treatment with an above-knee hip spica cast. *Clin. Orthop.*, 171:53–58, 1982.
12. Wasielewski, R. C., Crossett, L. S., and Rubash, H. E. Neural and vascular injury in total hip arthroplasty. *Orthop. Clin. N. Am.*, 23:219–235, 1992.

17B

Revision with Cementless Stem Technique

Mark Barba and Wayne G. Paprosky

INDICATIONS/CONTRAINDICATIONS

Fully coated stems can be used routinely for femoral stem revision. They are applicable in nearly all cases with the exception of those requiring an allograft prosthetic composite due to massive proximal femoral bone loss or those cases with diaphyseal widening so great that an impaction bone grafting technique would be considered, as in femurs with a diaphyses wider than 22 mm.

The extended proximal femoral trochanteric osteotomy can aid in the four main objectives in revision surgery: exposure, implant removal, correction of deformity and revision component implantation. Tissue quality can be poor in revision surgery. In certain cases of acetabular failure, revision of the femur may be indicated as an aid in soft-tissue tensioning. Stability is paramount in revision surgery and should not be compromised in an effort to maintain equal leg lengths. It is important to counsel the patient regarding leg-length issues. We have found that an additional benefit of the extended osteotomy is the ease with which it allows for soft-tissue tensioning.

The following section describes the essential components of revision of a failed femoral stem with a fully porous coated straight stem designed to obtain distal ingrowth fixation.

PREOPERATIVE PLANNING

An (AP) view of the pelvis and an AP and lateral of the proximal two-thirds of the femur are needed for planning.

M. Barba, M.D. and W. G. Paprosky: Central DuPage Hospital, Winfield, Illinois 60190.

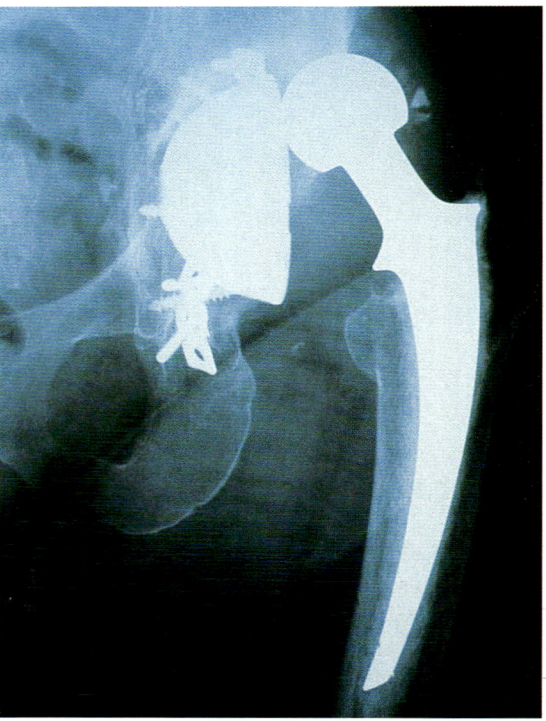 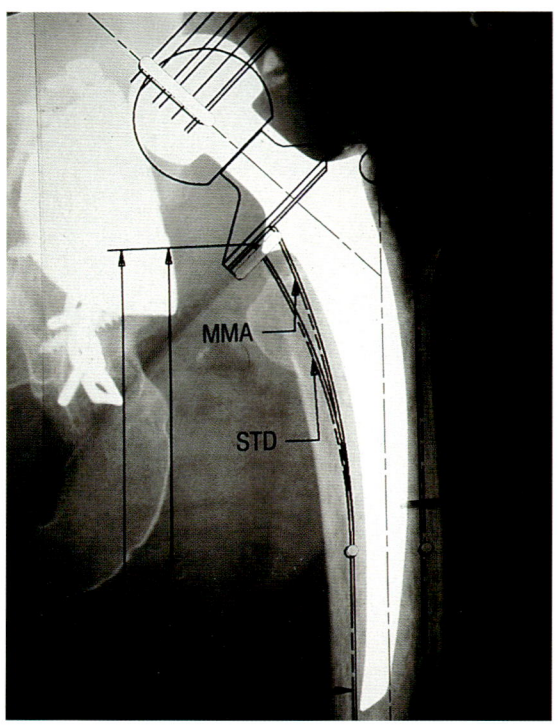

Figure 1. Preoperative view of a total hip reconstruction which failed secondary to instability. In this example, the socket is malpositioned and will require revision. The femoral component also demonstrates a significant radiolucency and will require concomitant revision.

Figure 2. A templated radiograph using a six-inch, fully coated stem. The template is aligned neutrally. Cement is some distance from the osteotomy site; however, note the cement is poorly bonded and should pose no difficulty with removal.

Templates are used to choose the shortest stem possible that will be surrounded by a cylinder of cortical bone for 4 to 5 cm into the isthmus. This is the ultimate goal of the operation. The lateral view is used to determine whether a curved or straight stem is appropriate.

Templating the depth of implantation is now considered (Figs. 1 and 2). First the acetabular reconstruction is templated to determine the center of rotation. This is marked on the film. Next femoral templates are applied by estimating the "anatomic position" of the component within the femoral canal. This is typically 1 cm proximal to the lesser trochanter. Using an intermediate neck length, the center of the head is then marked. By comparing the two marks, conclusions regarding tissue tension and leg lengths can be made. Typically, a combination of prosthetic height and neck length that increases offset and length is chosen, as this is often needed to achieve stability.

The distalmost level of the extended trochanteric osteotomy is determined by the following factors. First, the osteotomy should not jeopardize fixation. The transverse limb of the osteotomy should be at a level that will preserve approximately 4 to 6 cm of tight isthmic fit of the distal portion of the ingrowth stem cement. If the cement plug is more substantial than that seen in Fig. 2, a more distal osteotomy can be selected, but attention must be paid to the planned location of the distal 4 to 6 cm of the implanted stem. This section should not be compromised by the osteotomy. Fortunately, the osteotomy provides unimpeded access to the isthmus. We have noted that a significant number of revision femurs have a preoperative varus deformity. This places the femur at risk for a varus and undersized implantation. Use of the osteotomy helps to avoid this consequence.

The distal osteotomy level is measured from an easily identified landmark such as the vastus tubercle for use as an intraoperative reference.

SURGICAL TECHNIQUE

Exposure

We use a posterior approach. The pseudocapsule and external rotators are raised in a single flap. The gluteus maximus tendon is released. When the hip is encountered, we dislocate the joint, if possible. However, with severe protrusio or heterotopic ossification, dislocation may be difficult to achieve. If the joint cannot be dislocated, we perform the extended osteotomy and remove heterotopic ossification.

Extraction

After thoroughly clearing the introitus of the femur of granuloma, scar, and bone, a loose prosthesis has a chance of being pulled free. Be aware of any impingement of the prosthesis shoulder and the greater trochanter, as this can fracture the trochanter. Use of a barrel-shaped high-speed burr can help open this area. If the prosthesis pulls out readily, we then proceed to the osteotomy. If it does not, we will do the osteotomy with the prosthesis in situ. It is technically easier if the prosthesis is removed prior to osteotomy.

Osteotomy

The hip is extended and internally rotated 15 to 20 degrees to allow for proper positioning of the femur. The vastus lateralis is separated from the posterolateral femur along the linea aspera down to the level of the distal extent of the osteotomy. This is determined from the preoperative templating and can be measured either from the tip of the greater trochanter or by using the removed stem as a guide. The vastus is then elevated anteriorly off the femur only at the distal site of the osteotomy, and a retractor is placed at this site to protect the tissue during completion of the distal osteotomy cut. The osteotomy site is marked along the posterolateral femur just anterior to the linea aspera (Fig. 3).

When the incision is viewed posteriorly (Fig. 4), the sucker is on the tip of the greater trochanter and the gluteus medius muscle is to the right. In this case the prosthesis was eas-

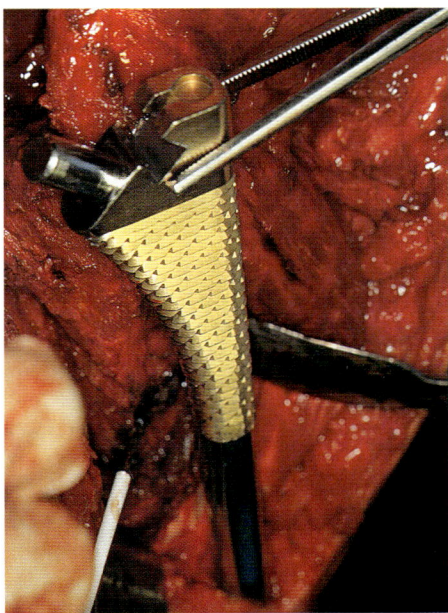

Figure 3. Cautery is used to mark the distal extent of the osteotomy at a level that will provide adequate coverage of the cylindrical distal portion of the fully coated stem.

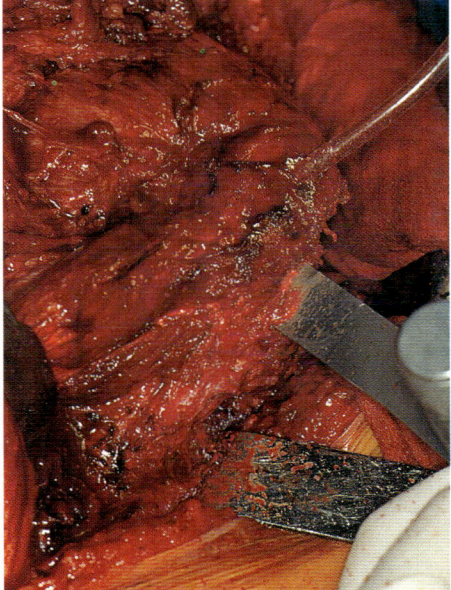

Figure 4. Viewed posteriorly, the sucker is on the tip of the greater trochanter and gluteus medius muscle to the right.

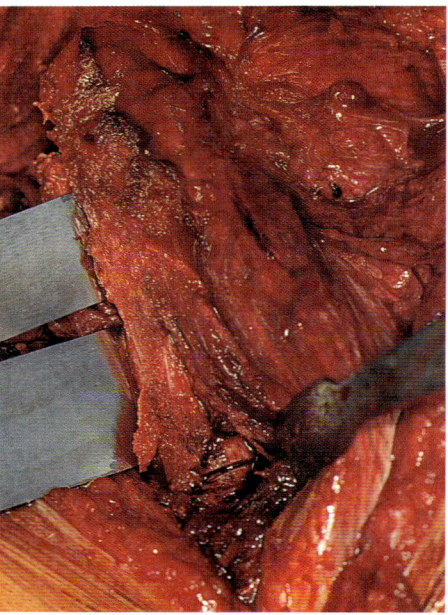

Figure 5. Wide Lambotte osteotomes are passed from posterior to anterior and used to lever open the osteotomy in a controlled fashion.

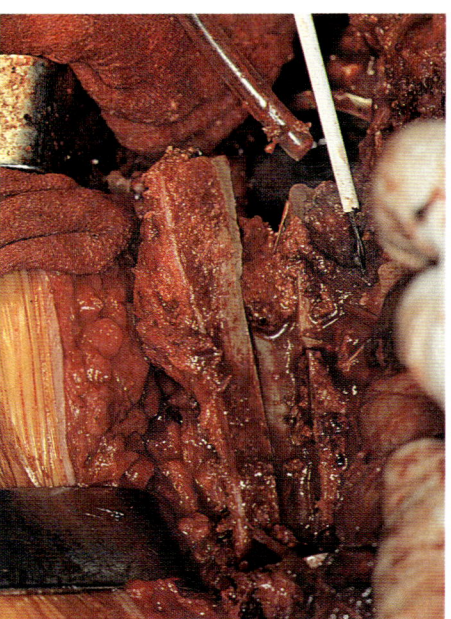

Figure 6. The release of anterior scar tissue with the cautery device is shown.

ily removed after clearing the shoulder area of bone and soft tissue and using a tamp on the collar to facilitate extraction. An oscillating saw is then used to section the proximal femur in half distally to the area where the Hohmann retractor is located in the bottom right corner. The transverse limb of the osteotomy is made with a thin high-speed burr at the level of the Hohmann retractor, which corresponds to the tip of the removed prosthesis.

Wide Lambotte osteotomes are then passed from posterior to anterior (Fig. 5), the multiple osteotomes are used to lever open the osteotomy in a controlled fashion, protecting both the osteotomy fragment and the anterior soft tissue attachments. The gluteus medius, gluteus minimus, and vastus lateralis remain attached to the osteotomized portion of bone.

Release of anterior tissue must be performed carefully prior to reflecting the osteotomized fragment anteriorly. This maneuver prevents fracture of the medial posterior femur or the osteotomized fragment (Fig. 6). The assistant initially holds the trochanteric fragment by hand as the tissue is released. After the fragment is mobilized anteriorly, a Hohmann retractor can be inserted to facilitate exposure.

Pedestal

Often a distal cement plug or bony pedestal remains. Burring the visible area of the canal and making a perforation with a drill or pencil burr will allow the passing of a crochet hook. The bone or cement can then be pulled out. Care must be taken to avoid a perforation, and it is prudent to advance cautiously with the drills or burrs. An alternate style is to drill the distal cement 1 to 2 cm with cement drills and tap the cement plug with cement taps. This is repeated as needed.

Reaming

After all the cement, neocortex, and distal pedestal have been removed, reaming is undertaken. A clear canal will help keep the reamer centered and neutrally aligned in the

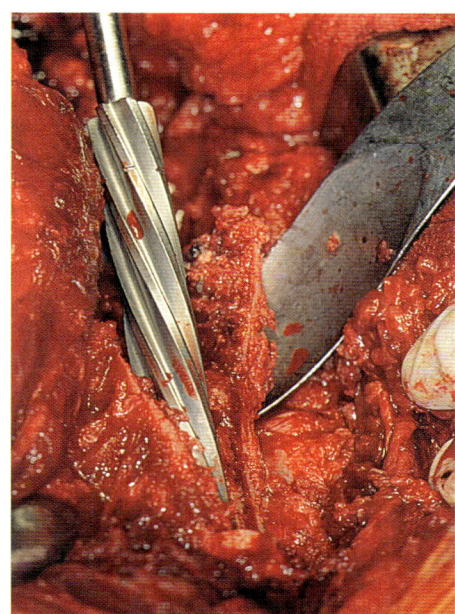

Figure 7. The hash mark on the reamer corresponds to the level of the collar and should be referenced to the templated implantation level. In the case shown, the canal was ultimately reamed up to 16.0 mm, and a 16.5 mm component was implanted. Reaming was begun at 10 mm and increased until there was minimal bite at 13.5 mm. The 15.0/13.5 broach fit line to line and could be used as a trial, but reaming to 14.0 mm provided an extra measure of safety and adjustment. The canal was thus reamed to 14.0 mm and a 15.0/13.5 broach was placed and trial reduced until a stable height and neck length was determined.

femoral canal. With straight stems, solid reamers are utilized, while for curved stems, flexible reamers are used.

The length of reaming is determined from the length of stem necessary achieve fixation. Only the length necessary for fixation is reamed. In general, this is 4 to 6 cm distal to the osteotomy. Reaming is performed in neutral alignment with special attention to avoid varus. Varus orientation of the reamers occurs if the proximal trochanteric region is not osteotomized and the reamer obtains 3 point contact with the diaphysis distally and the trochanter proximally. If the proximal trochanteric region is left intact, reaming must be started laterally enough while avoiding impingement from the greater trochanter. As mentioned, this can be impossible in cases with a preoperative varus deformity and is a specific indication to perform an osteotomy. A Charnley T-handled awl must insert freely into the diaphysis without proximal obstruction to assure neutral reamer positioning.

Sequential reaming is then performed, increasing reamer diameter until good endosteal cortical contact is obtained (Fig. 7). Reaming is stopped 0.5 mm below the size of the prosthesis to be implanted. This point is one of the most crucial in cementless femoral revisions.

Templating is a helpful, albeit inexact, way to size the canal with respect to final reamed diameters. The template is probably accurate to plus or minus one size, but bone quality and magnification must be considered. A patient with healthy cortices will give good feedback during reaming. The reamer will labor through the strong bone and there is little question when to stop. This is not as pronounced in patients with diminished bone quality.

To facilitate the decision of when to stop reaming, we insert a T-handle reamer the same size as the prosthesis to be implanted into the prepared channel. If rotational stability is achieved with 4 to 5 cm of reamer remaining proud, this is the diameter prosthesis chosen. If rotational stability is not obtained, the femur is reamed up. If more than 5 cm of reamer is showing, then the introitus is reamed line to line to prevent fracture on insertion. Under-reaming insures a tight fit, but at the risk of fracturing. In our experience a 4 to 5 cm distance of 0.5 mm underreamed canal is safe. In addition, a prophylactic Luque wire placed 1 cm distal to the osteotomy is a wise precaution.

Broaching

Next, the appropriate broach is inserted. Usually broaching is unnecessary for proximal preparation due to the loss of proximal bone. However, it is useful for trial reduction. The cylindrical distal portion of the broaches is 1.5 mm in diameter less than the actual prosthesis. For example, a 15.0 mm broach has a stem diameter of 13.5 mm (referred to as 15.0/13.5). Solution prostheses are manufactured in 1.5 mm increments beginning at 10.5 mm and ending at 22.5 mm.

Broaching is undertaken chiefly to detemine stem version and neck length, as there is usually adequate space in the proximal femur to accommodate a prosthesis without the broaching procedure (Fig. 8). Additionally, one may select a prosthesis with a more narrow proximal profile. These stems have utility especially when the surgeon is working without an osteotomy, when a tight proximal femur can limit anteversion in the standard body prosthesis.

With a broach implanted, a midrange neck length is chosen, and the hip is reduced. If the hip remains reduced in the 90–90 position (90 degrees flexion-90 degrees internal rotation) (Fig. 9), adequate soft tissue tension has been obtained. We also test the limb in the "sleeping position" lateral decubitus with the operated leg crossed over the nonoperative one.

Trial reduction is one of the most important steps in revision and total hip arthroplasty. It is through the trial reduction, that the component positions can be altered to achieve stability. This is accomplished by modifying neck length, height, and version. The most important consideration is stability. If the hip is unstable, the cause may be simply due to poor tensioning. In that case, either add neck length or implant the stem proudly while maintaining a good fixation.

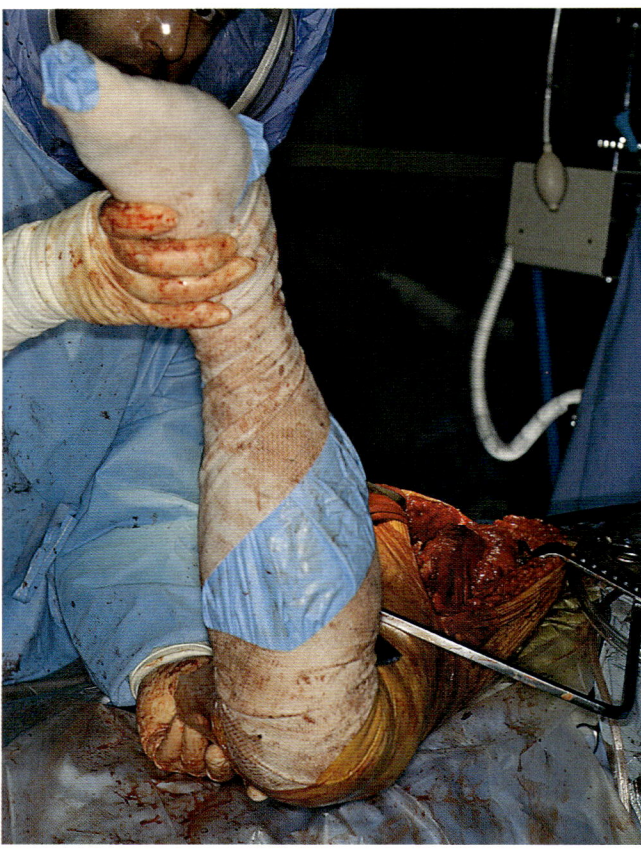

Figure 8. With a trial broach in place, the hip is checked in the 90-90 degree revision. In this example, the hip is placed in 90 degrees of internal rotation and flexed to the limit of the soft tissue. In reality this is often somewhat short of 90 degrees.

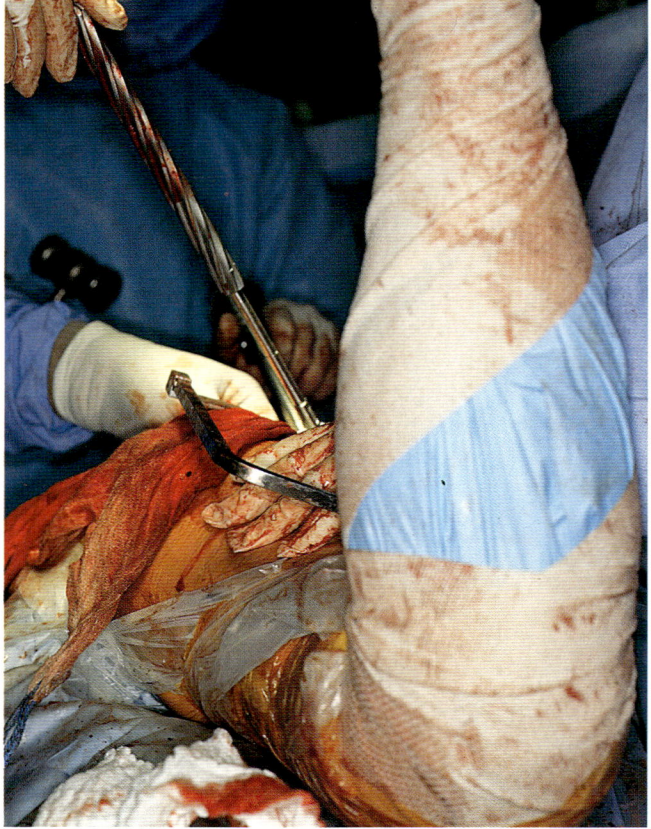

Figure 9. Implantation of the component is shown with a reamer placed to control rotation. The degree of anteversion can be seen clearly by observing the angle of the reamer to the leg.

Management of Impingement

When ranging the hip, attention must be paid to impingement. This can be due to contact of the trunion with the perimeter of the cup. This is easily recognized and can be managed by modifying the component position. However, occasionally the anterior femur at the level of the calcar can act as a fulcrum against the anterior soft tissues, remaining pseudocapsule, and pelvis. Thinning the anterior trochanteric bone with an oscillating saw can manage this problem. Less commonly, the hip can be tight in external rotation and a limited anterior capsulectomy is done until proper tension is achieved.

Implantation

The component is implanted using a reamer placed in the extraction hole to help control rotation (Fig. 10). On average, the angle of the inserted reamer to the leg is 25 degrees and is the femoral anteversion. Initial insertion of the stem may require little force and can usually be accomplished by hand until the stem engages the region of the canal that is relatively undersized by 0.5 mm. Insertion of the femoral stem past this point should require repeated blows from a heavy mallet on the stem impactor. Once the stem begins to engage the under-reamed segment of femur in which fixation will be achieved, it becomes more difficult

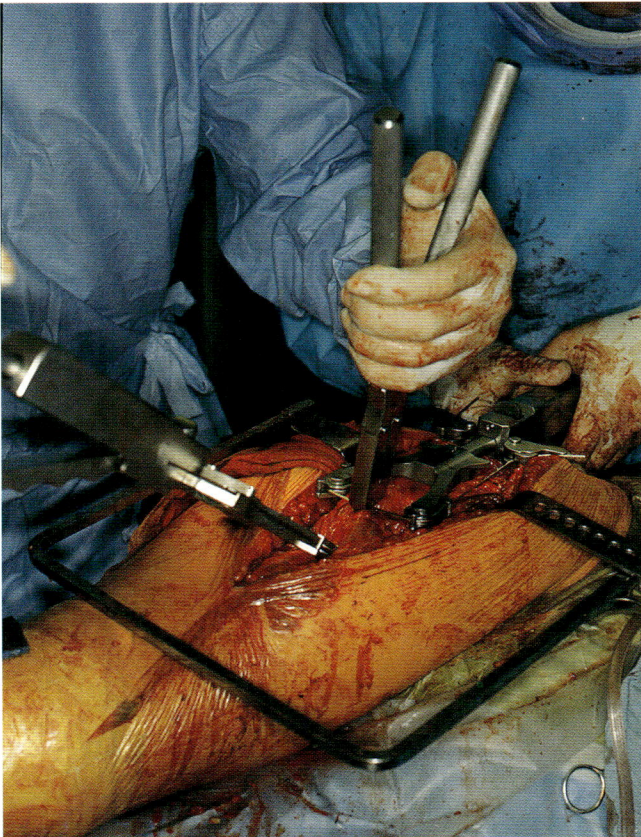

Figure 10. Following cable tightening and prior to crimping, the hip can be tested for shuck and stability. Problems of insufficient abductor tension can be managed by removing bone from the distal segment of the osteotomy fragment and advancing the segment distally on the femur.

to alter the anteversion. Thus the anteversion must be closely monitored during the initial 2 to 3 cm of prosthetic seating into the segment of the canal that will provide fixation.

As the stem engages, the surgeon must determine the depth of insertion based on the trial insertion and on reductions and landmarks chosen to measure the depth of implant insertion. This is most commonly the relationship of the inferior border of calcar with remaining medial bone stock. If the stem stops advancing, a shorter neck length may be employed, and if a more distal insertion is required to obtain good fixation, either a longer neck or advancement of the trochanteric fragment may be needed.

Once the stem has been inserted, trial heads may be used to perform a final trial reduction to assess hip stability and length.

Once the revision prosthesis has been inserted, the osteotomy fragment is shaped with a high-speed burr to shape the fragment to fit over the lateral shoulder of the prosthesis. Multiple are then used to wire the fragment down. Abductor laxity can be addressed by shortening the fragment and advancing it distally (Fig. 11). The limb can be put through a range of motion before the cables are crimped so that and the trochanteric fragment position can be fine tuned.

In cases where the proximal femur is very thin, atrophic, patulous, or porotic, the cables used to hold the osteotomy segment in place may be used to "collapse" the proximal medial bone sleeve to the implant. As all stem stability has been gained from the distal "scratch fit," this maneuver only serves to bring the healthy proximal bone closer to the ingrowth surface of the proximal stem.

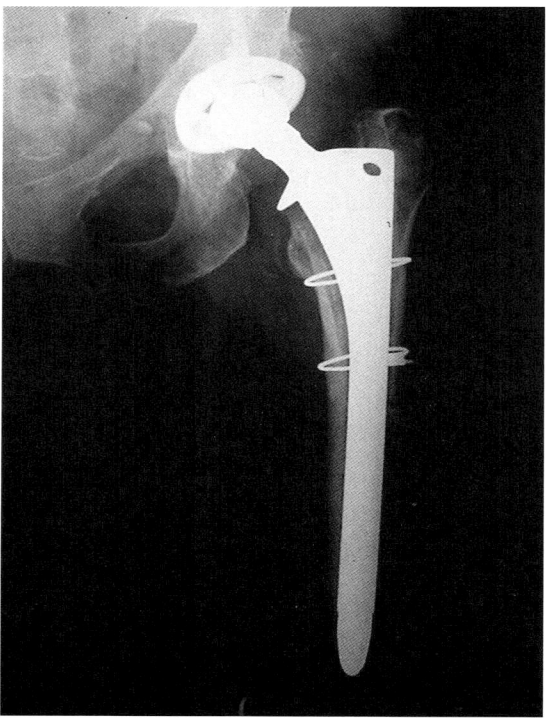

Figure 11. Postoperative view of a 6-in. fully coated stem with osteotomy fixed with two cables. Note that the stem is implanted in neutral alignment and there is greater than 4 cm of canal filling fit. The stem is placed with a collar in anatomic purchase and gains stability from distal purchase.

POSTOPERATIVE MANAGEMENT

All revision patients are placed in an off-the-shelf abduction orthosis. It is set at 30 degrees of abduction with a flexion stop at 70 degrees. This brace is continued for eight weeks. For six weeks the patients are kept at 30% weight bearing with a walker. They are then advanced to full weight bearing by eight weeks and protected as needed with a cane. We use fully coated ingrowth stems widely in our revision practice. We have noted a loosening rate of 2.4% of 311 hip revisions at an average of 8.2 years.

While thigh pain is uncommon and rarely clinically bothersome, it may occur. Patients with thin, osteopenic femurs and large stems seem to be at greater risk. Fortunately, there is clinical evidence that stiffening the femur by placement of allograft bone plates may be useful in managing this complication.

COMPLICATIONS

Specific complications referable to this technique relate specifically to component implantation, and in this regard two alternate complications are worth discussing. Fracture of the femur may occur on insertion of a stem into a canal that has been inadequately prepared for the implant. Alternatively, an undersized stem may fail to obtain rotational and axial stability so that micro motion is present with loading leading to ingrowth failure.

For the experienced surgeon, implantation of the appropriately sized stem is guided by several clues, including visual, auditory and tactile feedback that can be gained only with experience. These clues are obtained by paying careful attention to parameters such as "cortical chatter" during reaming, the quality of bone encountered at various depths of reaming, and the appearance of bone in the reamer flutes from those depths. The feel of reamers on a hand chuck at the final reaming size, rather than a power reamer, can give the surgeon a good sense of the actual quality of the bone at the reamed size chosen. Fracture may be avoided in particularly hard bone by reaming a short transition zone (1 cm) between the open intramedullary cavity above and the interference fit segment below. If there is any question of difficulty at the initial insertion into this zone, a cerclage wire placed at this region may decrease the incidence of fracture at the time of stem insertion. Unfortunately, a stem that is implanted and found to be loose, either by virtue of rotational instability or insufficient resistance encountered during component insertion, should be removed and the femur prepared to accept a larger component.

17C

Impaction Grafting with Cement

W. E. Michael Mikhail and Lars Weidenhielm

INDICATIONS/CONTRAINDICATIONS

The indication is aseptic mechanical failure of cemented and cementless femoral stems, with bone loss of the proximal femur with cortical defects and thinning from stress shielding and wear-induced osteolysis. In these revisions the proximal femur is usually only a thin cortical shell. The prerequisite for the procedure is that an intact "tube" can be reconstructed and the defects covered with strut grafts and/or wire mesh to allow for tight packing of the bone graft and stable fixation of the femoral component in the impacted graft. Osteolytic lesions in the distal part of the femur or around long stems do not contraindicate this procedure. In these cases, however, reinforcement of the femur with cortical strut allograft and a long-stem option to bypass the lytic or defective areas is sometimes advisable. The lytic lesions usually disappear with time, and a "normalization" of the distal femur occurs.

For cases with an infected loose THA, a two-stage exchange is recommended. The infected THA is removed, and the infection is treated. When the infection is cleared, a prosthesis can be implanted with impaction grafting technique, as described below. Active infection is an absolute contraindication for using the aforementioned technique. Additional relative contraindications include significant shaft deformity proximally, lack of sufficient cortical tube diameter to pack the allograft material into the proximal femur and still have room for the cement and stem, and the inability to manage cortical defects as noted above.

PREOPERATIVE PLANNING

In the preoperative planning of THA revision, a proper analysis of the femoral environment including integrity of the bone-cement interface, the presence or absence of cortical defects, and the thickness of the femoral cortex both proximally and distally to the stem

---

W. E. M. Mikhail, M.D.: Department of Orthopedic Surgery, Medical College of Ohio, Toledo, Ohio 43699.

L. Weidenhielm, M.D.: Karolinska Institute, Department of Orthopaedics, St. Goran Hospital, S-11281 Stockholm, Sweden.

should be performed. Many classifications of bone-stock loss exist today. Assessment of bone-stock loss on a four-grade scale according to the Endo-Klinik classification has worked well in our environment (1).

In particular, the proposed reconstruction must be templated, noting the appropriate stem diameter and its corresponding length. A 2-mm mantle and 5 to 6 mm of impacted graft, in addition to the stem, must be allowed for. The management of potential cortical defects must be planned to protect very lytic or thinned cortical bone at the tip of the reconstruction when present. The ability of the chosen stem to reproduce leg length, soft tissue, and hip stability should be calculated.

SURGICAL TECHNIQUE

Exposure of the hip is performed through a modified direct lateral approach with the patient on the contralateral side, or the exposure of the surgeon's choice or preference. It is absolutely essential for the surgeon to recognize that this operation cannot be properly performed through an inadequate exposure. The upper end of the femur must be delivered into the wound so that the proximal end of the canal can be opened up in to the greater trochanter at least 1 cm distal to the midline axis of the canal. Only then can the new medullary canal be correctly orientated, adequately impacted, and properly cemented. The failed femoral component is removed. The femoral canal is cleaned of any old cement, fibrous membrane, or any particulate debris, and thoroughly lavaged using standard techniques.

Defects in the cortex must be "patched" with fine wire mesh and/or strut allograft secured with cerclage wires prior to packing. Prophylactic wiring of the femur before packing is recommended when cortical integrity is tenuous, as vigorous impaction of the graft may fracture the femur. A guide wired is threaded into a stiff medullary plug and placed in the distal canal with the largest cannulated tamp that the femur can accomodate. The wire should be threaded completely through the plug with approximately 5 mm of pin protruding through the bottom of the plug. The plug is driven distal to areas of lytic bone, and a packer, smaller in size than the plug, and is used to confirm seating (Figs. 1–3). It is essential to ensure that the plug does not subside during the later packing/tamping process. A tendency for the plug to subside during impaction can be controlled by driving a small

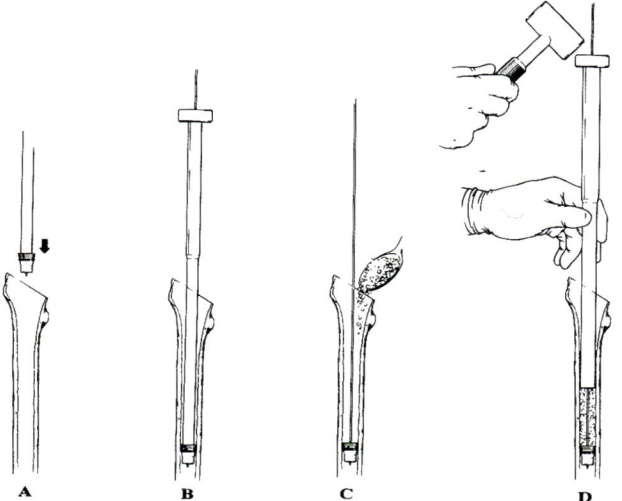

Figure 1. (A) Insertion of distal plug. (B) The plug is driven distal to the areas of lytic bone. (C) Grafting the femoral canal. (D) Packing the distal 1/3 of the canal.

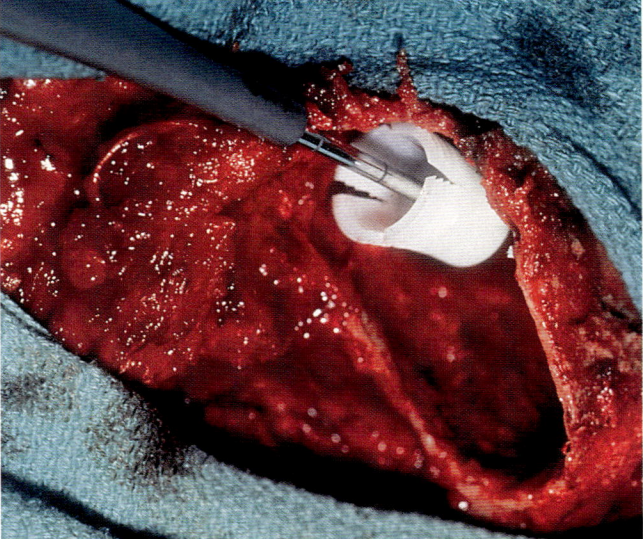

Figure 2. Intraoperative photograph: The distal plug is put on the threaded guide wire.

17C IMPACTION GRAFTING WITH CEMENT

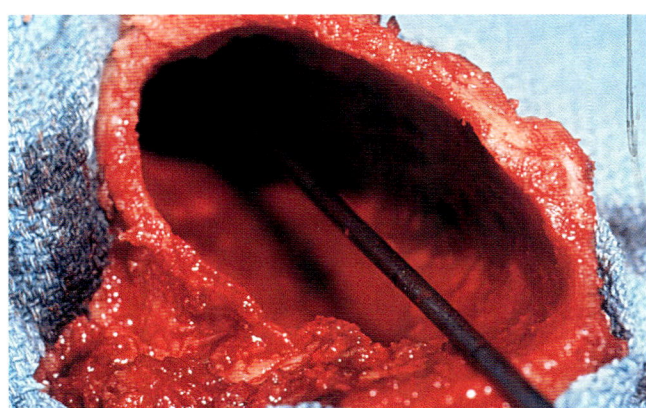

Figure 3. Intraoperative photograph: The plug is introduced into the femoral canal.

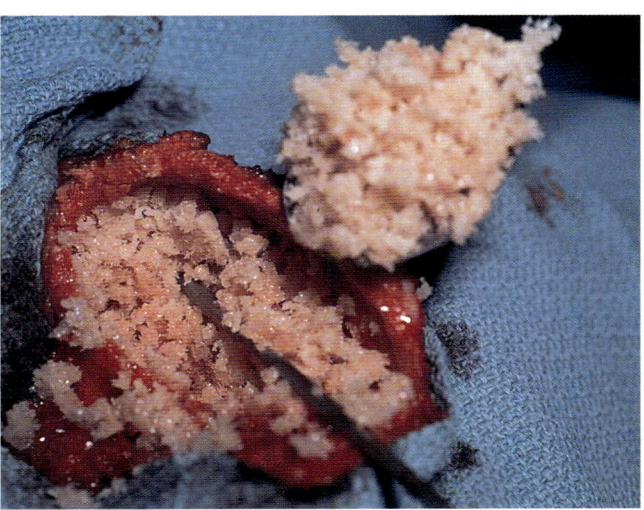

Figure 4. Intraoperative photograph: Morselized bone graft is introduced.

Kirschner wire across the femur and either through the plug or just below it. This wire is removed once impaction has been completed. The guide wire should exit the proximal femur near the lateral endosteal cortex, which is in line with the axis of the center of the femur. The intramedullary plug will center the guide wire in the distal canal. The use of a cannulated system has greatly reduces the incidence of malposition of the stem.

It is preferable to use cancellous allograft obtained from the femoral condyles or the proximal tibiae for packing. Three- to five-millimeter fresh-frozen allograft chips are used (Figs. 2, 4). The allograft is inserted into the femur and packed into the canal with a small diameter cannulated packer. This step is repeated until the distal one-third of the proximal femur has been filled (Fig. 1D). Larger diameter packers are used as the diameter of the canal increases. A cannulated tamp approximately one or two sizes smaller than the final component is introduced over the guide wire. More graft material is introduced and the tamp is impacted until fully seated (Fig. 5 A and B). This process is repeated, progressing up in tamp size, until the planned size is firmly seated. The tamp of the planned size should allow for a uniform layer of bone graft of approximately 5 to 6 mm thickness (Fig. 6). The

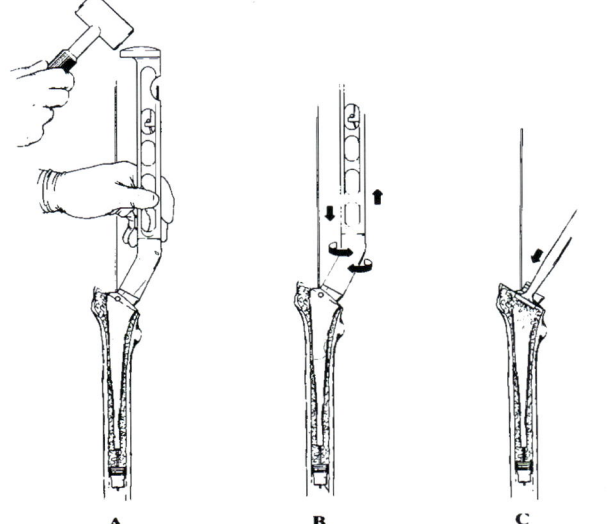

Figure 5. (A) Proximal packing with cannulated tamps. (B) Rotation is applied to ensure adequate seating. (C) Final packing with proximal packers.

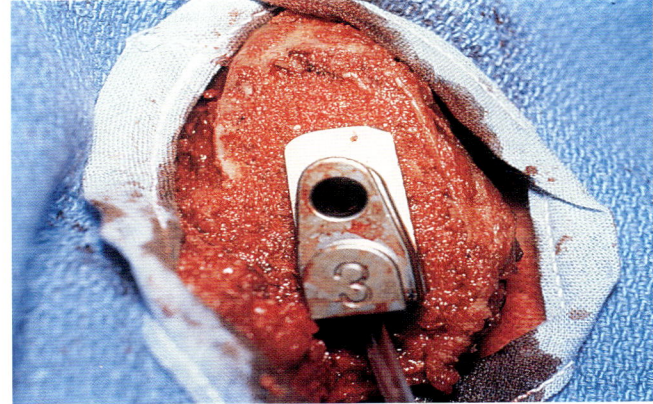

Figure 6. Intraoperative photograph: The tamp of the planned size in place with a uniform layer of bone graft of approximately 5 to 6 mm thickness.

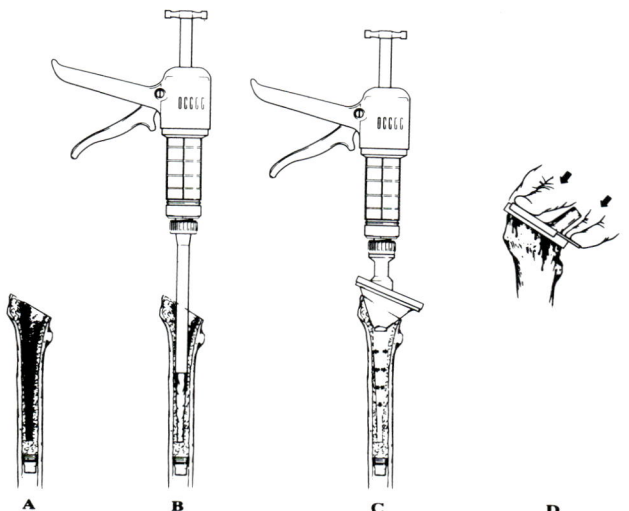

Figure 7. (A) The neomedullary canal. (B) The cement is introduced into the medullary canal. (C) Pressurizing cement with proximal seal. (D) Introducing the stem and final pressurisation with plate.

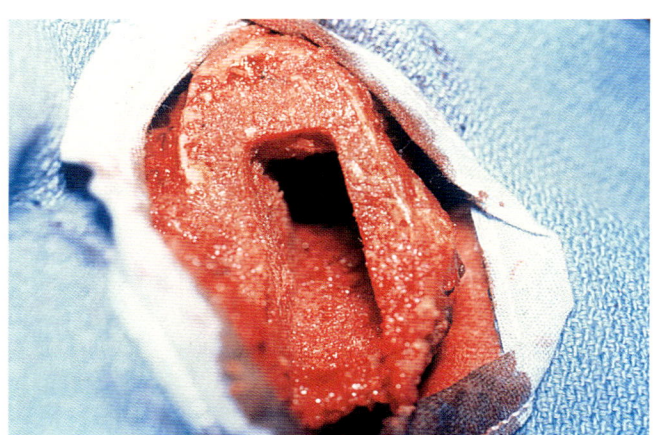

Figure 8. Intraoperative photograph: A complete "neomedullary" canal has been formed.

driving handle is detached, and final packing of the canal is completed with proximal packers around the tamp (Fig. 5C). Pooled blood at the distal end of the stem is extracted through suction applied in the guide wire hole in the tamp. The tamp is left in place until immediately before cement insertion. The tamps are oversized compared to the corresponding stems to allow for a uniform 2- to 3-mm thick cement mantle. A complete "neomedullary" canal has been formed (Figs. 7, 8).

The same amount of cement used for primary total hip arthroplasties is impregnated with antibiotics, vacuum mixed, and introduced into the neomedullary canal in a retrograde fashion. It is important that the cement dough that is introduced into the canal is in a relatively low viscosity state, otherwise, adequate penetration of the graft by cement cannot be achieved. A cement gun with a *small* tapered nozzle, is used to inject cement into the narrow distal stem area (Fig. 7B). A second larger nozzle is used to complete filling of the proximal femur and to pressurize the cement. The femoral pressurizer seal and plate are attached and pressure is applied and held until the cement reaches a doughy consistency (Fig. 7C). The revision hollow centralizer is applied to the distal end of the implant prior to stem insertion. The appropriate size stem is inserted (Fig. 7D). This implant we use is forged from cobalt-chromium alloy, double tapered and polished. Oversizing the stem is a major error and will be at the expense of the thickness of both the graft and the cement mantle. Prophylactic antibiotic treatment and prophylactic anticoagulation are routinely used.

POSTOPERATIVE MANAGEMENT

Usually the patients can be mobilized with weightbearing as tolerated on the operated leg, the first day after surgery. If the bone quality is very poor, we allow partial weightbearing for the first eight weeks. The same restrictions that are applied after primary THR to avoid dislocation, are applied here.

COMPLICATIONS

The major complication is fracture of the femur. It is important to use a precise technique and avoid "short cuts." The need for a full and free exposure of the upper femur together with all diaphyseal defects cannot be overemphasized. An intraoperative femoral fracture is most commonly produced by inadequate soft tissue release. A fracture can also occur during the impaction of the graft. Fractures can usually be fixed with cerclage wires and allograft bone struts or plates, and the impaction grafting procedure can be continued. Late femoral fractures can occur, especially during the first postoperative year. They are best managed by ORIF (open reduction and internal fixation), sometimes with bone grafting of the fracure site. Dislocations are managed by closed reduction in most cases.

ILLUSTRATIVE CASE

A 61-year-old man received a cemented total hip arthroplasty (Dual Lock, DePuy Corp., Warsaw, IN) for osteoarthritis in 1980. Revision arthroplasties were performed in 1984 (to a cemented PCA stem, Howmedica Corp., E. Rutherford, NJ), and 1987 (noncemented long-stem PCA and autogenous bone graft and a PCA acetabular cup). In June of 1991, the uncemented PCA was revised because of aseptic loosening accompanied by gross proximal femoral bone loss (Fig. 9). It is worth mentioning that most of the graft around the PCA stem was resorbed and the remaining part was dead bone and fibrous tissue. A cemented CPT stem (Zimmer Corp. Warsaw, IN) was inserted with impaction grafting technique, using two morselized femoral condyles and two ounces of cancellous allograft bone chips. Additional strut allografts were applied to reinforce the stress shielded proximal femoral cortex (Fig. 10). Cultures obtained at revision surgery were negative. A technetium SPECT scan performed 12 months after revision surgery showed increased uptake in the proximal femur.

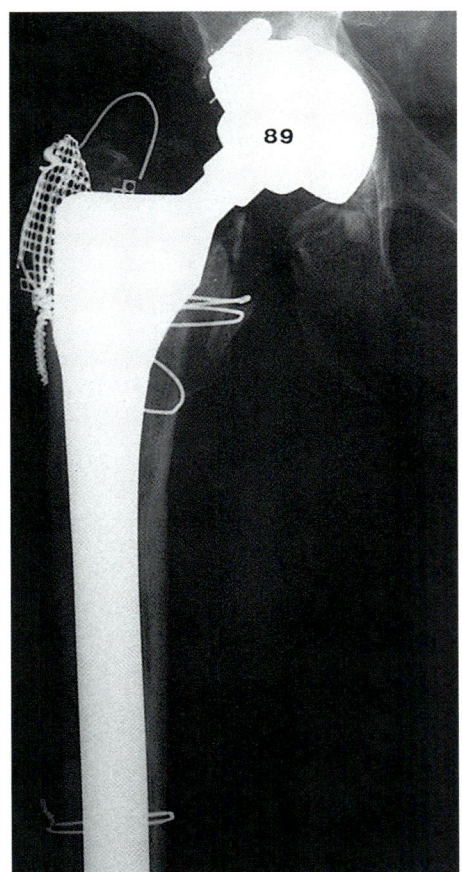

Figure 9. Radiograph: case example at revision arthroplasty showing a noncemented long-stem PCA component and cerclage wires around the femur.

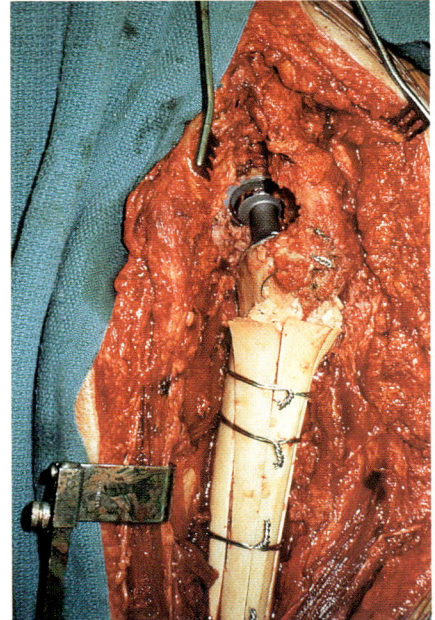

Figure 10. Intraoperative photograph: case example at revision of the reconstructed proximal femur with the new CPT-stem cemented in place.

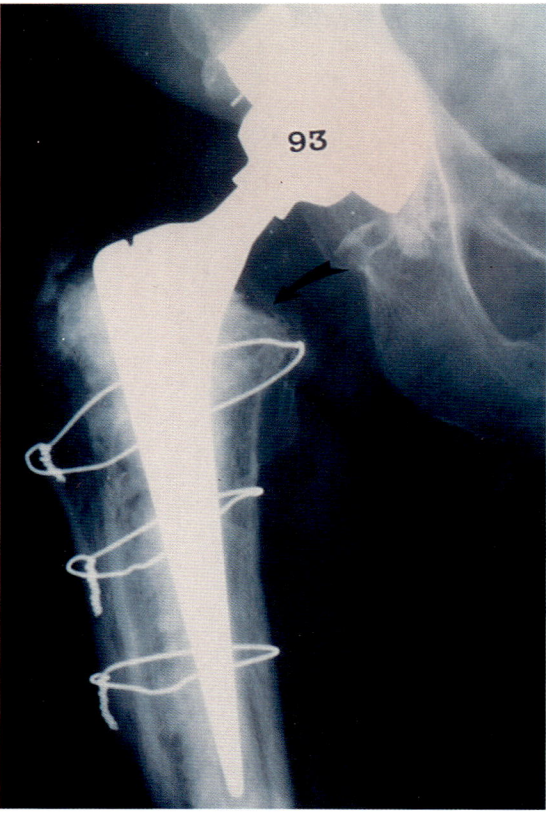

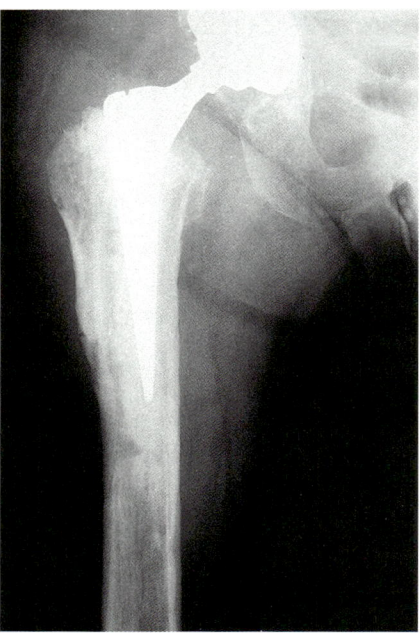

Figure 12. Anteroposterior radiograph showing the incorporation of the strut graft.

Figure 11. Radiograph: case example at time of biopsy showing a well-cemented femoral stem without radiolucent lines around the cement mantle. The stem has subsided 2 mm within the cement mantle. The bone in the proximal femur shows signs of trabecular remodeling especially on the lateral side of the stem. The strut graft is radiologically incorporated.

Postoperatively the patient did well, but developed lateral thigh pain due to the cerclage wires (Fig. 11). The wires were removed twenty-seven months after revision arthroplasty, at which time biopsies were obtained of the proximal femur. The bone in the proximal femur showed signs of trabecular remodelling. The biopsy confirmed presence of newly formed, viable bone (Fig. 12). Radiographs at the time of biopsy showed a well-cemented femoral stem, without radiolucent lines at either interface. The strut graft was radiologically incorporated (Fig. 13).

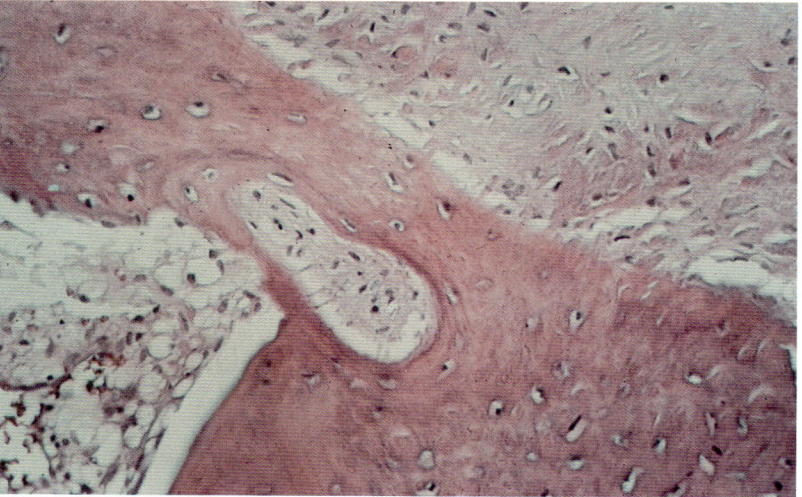

Figure 13. Biopsy showing the presence of newly formed viable bone.

RECOMMENDED READING

1. Engelbrecht, E, and Heinert, K.: Klassifikation und Behandlungsrichtlinien von knockensubstansverlusten bei Revisionsoperationen am huftgelenk—mittelfristige Ergebnisse. Primare und revisionsalloartroplastik Hrgs—Endo-Klinik, Hamburg, Berlin, etc: Springer-Verlag, 1987:189–201.
2. Gie, G. A., Linder, L., Ling, R. S. M., Simon, J. P., Slooff, T. J. J. H., and Timperley, A. J.: Impacted cancellous allografts and cement for revision total hip arthroplasty. *J. Bone Joint Surg*, 75B:14–21, 1993.
3. Gie, G. A., Linder, L., Ling, R. M. S., Simon, J.-P., Sloof, T. J. J. H., and Timperley, A. J.: Contained morselized allograft in revision total hip arthroplasty. Surgical technique. *Orthop. Clin. North Am.*, 24:717–725, 1993.
4. Ling, R. S. M., Timperley, A. J., and Linder, L.: Histology of cancellous impaction grafting in the femur. *J. Bone Joint Surg.*, 75B:693–696, 1993.
5. Nelissen, R. G. H. H., Bauer, T. W., Weidenhielm, L. R. A., LeGolvan, D. P., and Mikhail, W. E. M.: Revision hip arthroplasty with the use of cement and impaction grafting. *J. Bone Joint Surg.*, 77-A:412–422, 1995.
6. Schreurs, B. W.: Reconstructive options in revision surgery of failed total hip arthroplasties. Thesis, Nijmegen, The Netherlands, 1994.
7. Sloof, T. J., Huiskes, R., van Horn, J., and Lemmens, A.: Bone grafting in total hip replacement for acetabular protrusion. *Acta. Orthop. Scand.*, 55:593–596, 1984.
8. Weidenhielm, L. R. A., Nelissen, R. G. H. H., Mikhail, W. E. M., and Bauer, T. W.: Surgical technique and early results in revision THA with a cemented, tapered, collarless, polished stem and contained morselized allograft. *J. Orthopaedic Techniques* 2[3]; 113–122, 1994.
9. Mikhail, W.E.M., Ling, R.S.M., Weidenhielm, L-R.A., Gie, G.A. Revision of the femoral component: impaction grafting. In: Callaghan, J.J., Rosenberg, A.G., Rubash, H.E., editors. *The adult hip*. New York: Lippincott-Raven Publishers, pp. 1527–1536.

17D

Allograft-Prosthetic Composite Reconstruction

Michael J. Hejna

INDICATIONS/CONTRAINDICATIONS

Femoral bone deficiency in revision hip surgery can be addressed with the use of allograft bone in various forms. The allograft-prosthetic composite construct consists of a structural proximal femoral allograft into which a femoral component is cemented. When a long-stem femoral component is used, the protruding distal end of the prosthesis provides intramedullary fixation of the construct to the host femur, while if a short stem is employed, supplementary fixation is generally required. Ultimate stability of the femoral component is achieved after union of the allograft to the host femur.

We have found the allograft-prosthetic composite (APC) construct useful in the treatment of complete segmental cortical defects and combined segmental-cavitary defects of the proximal femur. The primary advantages of the APC reconstruction are in the restoration of proximal femoral bone stock and in allowing for a biologic repair of the abductor mechanism. It is especially useful in relatively young patients where the availability of bone stock for future surgery is a consideration, and it is a particularly appropriate solution

M. J. Hejna, M.D.: Department of Orthopaedic Surgery, Rush Medical College, Chicago, Illinois 60612.

for periprosthetic fractures in situations where internal fixation is undesirable or unlikely to succeed—for example, in patients with loose femoral stems and substantial proximal bone loss. APC reconstruction is commonly used in the management of deficiency of the proximal femur following tumor resection.

Where restoration of bone stock can be accomplished by forms of bone grafting that are less destructive to the host femur—for example, through the use of cortical struts or cancellous impaction grafting—APC reconstruction should not be used. Specialized implants such as calcar-replacement-type implants are more appropriate in smaller segmental defects extending less than 3 cm from the calcar. Debilitated patients with limited expectation for ambulation or inability to perform protected-weight bearing ambulation during the period of healing of the allograft-host junction may be best treated with a modular oncology-type implant. Allograft prosthetic composite surgery is best thought of as a surgery of last resort where other more conservative options are less likely to succeed.

PREOPERATIVE PLANNING

Patient Evaluation

As in all revision hip surgery, general medical evaluation of the patient prior to surgery is important. Assessment of the patient's ability to tolerate an extensive surgical procedure and to protect the allograft through partial weight bearing in the postoperative period is necessary. Infection should be ruled out as a cause of implant failure. If the APC reconstruction is to follow resection of a bone tumor, the need for postoperative chemotherapy or radiation should be established, and patients requiring these adjunctive treatments must be counseled regarding the potential for delayed bone healing. Many of these patients will be better served by modular oncology implants.

Acetabular Exposure

If wide acetabular exposure is necessary, a standard trochanteric osteotomy should be planned. Otherwise, the proximal femur should be split in the manner of the extended trochanteric osteotomy, preserving the continuity of the greater trochanter with the lateral cortex of the femur.

Osteotomy

The nature of the femoral deficiency is adequately assessed with standard radiographs, which should include the full length of the femur. The level of femoral transection will be dictated by the size and location of the bony deficiency, the length of the femoral component to be inserted, and the method of fixation of host to allograft that will be employed. Occasionally, a slightly more distal level of osteotomy can be planned to take advantage of the exposure provided for femoral component and cement removal.

Leg Lengths

Leg length estimation is based on the preoperative radiographs and clinical measurements. Accurate intraoperative assessment of leg length using proximal femoral landmarks is not possible in this form of reconstruction, thus, determination of the post-implantation leg length is based on the resection level and overall length of the allograft construct, including the prosthetic head and neck.

Allograft

Attention must be directed preoperatively to the length and diameter of the allograft available. Adequate allograft length must be available to produce a step cut of at least 4 cm with several centimeters excess to allow for fine tuning during implantation. As noted above, in order to compensate for leg length inequality, the length of the composite implanted may need to be greater than the length of bone resected. If the host femoral canal is particularly ectatic, an invagination technique may be necessary, requiring a substantially longer segment of allograft bone.

For standard noninvagination technique, the allograft diameter should approximate that of the host femur or be slightly smaller to facilitate soft tissue closure. The smallest allograft that will accommodate a stem large enough to be press-fit into the distal femur is most appropriate.

Resection of malignant tumors of the proximal femur with wide surgical margins will generally include transection of the abductor tendons. The allograft proximal femur used in these cases must have a stump of the abductor tendon for soft tissue repair of the abductor mechanism. This should be evident from specimen radiographs of the allograft and should be noted preoperatively. Even in cases where host abductor tendon and trochanter are intact, the allograft abductor may be used to help reconstitute the abductor mechanism.

Radiographs are occasionally mislabelled with respect to the side from which the allograft was harvested. Thus, the surgeon should inspect the specimen radiographs and, if possible, the allograft bone itself prior to the procedure.

Femoral Component

A femoral component of sufficient length should be selected to allow for cement fixation in the allograft and press-fitting of the portion of the stem protruding from the graft into the host canal. Because of the thick cortical bone of the typical tissue donor, the allograft canal is generally narrower than that of the host. Thus the ideal femoral component for this technique is relatively narrow proximally and does not taper; it should be sufficiently long to bypass the host-allograft junction by at least 6 cm. Preoperative templating of the allograft may indicate that the allograft intramedullary canal may need to be widened by removal of endosteal bone. Appropriate reamers and burrs should be available for this purpose.

Fixation for Rotational Stability

Sufficient stability at the host-bone junction is rarely achieved by press-fit of the stem into the host canal alone. Additional stability can be provided by mechanical interlock (step cut), compression plating, distal cementing, or use of a prosthesis with distal interlocking. Stepcut interlocking of the allograft-host junction is preferred because it requires less soft-tissue stripping of the femur, minimizes the number of holes in the allograft, and reduces operating time. The method of fixation should be determined preoperatively by accurate templating, and appropriate instruments and implants should be available.

SURGICAL TECHNIQUE

A lateral longitudinal incision is created, incorporating previous scars where possible. The subcutaneous tissue is divided down to and through the fascia lata, while the fascia is separated from the underlying vastus lateralis. The vastus lateralis is reflected anteriorly from the lateral intermuscular septum to expose the posterolateral aspect of the femur. A standard trochanteric osteotomy is performed if necessary for acetabular exposure. If this

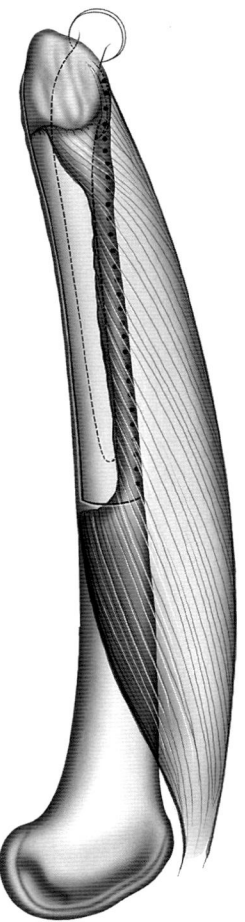 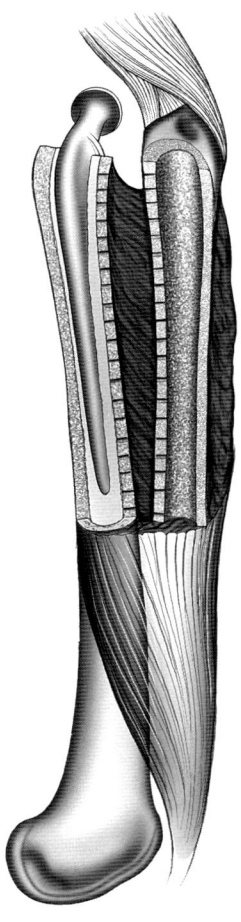

Figure 1. Lateral view of femur showing outline of extended trochanteric osteotomy for removal of stem and cement.

Figure 2. Lateral view of femur after extended trochanteric osteotomy with the lateral portion of the proximal femur reflected anteriorly.

is not necessary, an extended trochanteric osteotomy may be performed (Figs. 1, 2). A longitudinal saw cut is then made along the posterior edge of the trochanteric fragment. The anterior longitudinal osteotomy is performed after splitting the muscle at the appropriate interval. It is created with a series of drill holes connected using an osteotome. This is analogous to the creation of an extended trochanteric osteotomy. After the transverse osteotomies are made, the proximal femur is opened like a book to expose the femoral component and cement. These are removed and acetabular reconstruction is performed if necessary.

If rotational stability is to be achieved by step cut, the lateral and medial portions of the femur will be divided at different levels. This must be carefully outlined on the femur, as the quality of the bone and the site(s) of femoral cortical deficiency may influence the pattern of the step cut. In any case, the surgeon must take into account the level of healthy host bone available, the length of the allograft, and any extension of the femoral osteotomy needed for clearing the medullary canal contents.

The proximal femoral allograft is prepared on the back table. If possible, initial preparation of the allograft should be performed by a second surgeon while the exposure and acetabular reconstruction are being performed. This can substantially reduce operating time. Graft cultures are taken prior to preparation for implantation. The greater trochanter is removed unless a soft tissue abductor repair is necessary, based on the patient's anatomy. Resect the femoral head free-hand, or use cutting templates for the selected femoral component (Fig. 3). Remove cancellous bone from the allograft calcar, and then ream and broach the allograft. Due to the thick cortices typical of the young donor, it is usually necessary to ream a substantial amount of endosteal bone in order for the allograft to accommodate a sufficiently large stem.

Cut the allograft to length based on preoperative templating, leaving the graft one to two centimeters long to allow for fine tuning. Outline the step cut on the allograft with a marking pen. The arc of allograft circumference subtended by the distal portion of the step should be left slightly greater than necessary to allow for rotational fine tuning. The extending tab of the step cut can be carefully trimmed with an oscillating saw until the fit is tight. Take care to ensure that the rotational alignment of the proximal femoral fragment is appropriate following the keying in of the step cut. Cortical match-sticks can be used to create a tighter fit at the step cut if excessive bone has been removed, and, if necessary, the step cut can be shortened. Pay attention to the position of the limb during fine tuning of the allograft to prevent neurological injury and vascular compromise.

Ideally, the protruding portion of the stem of the femoral component is press-fit into the distal fragment. The fit may not be tight if the cortex is thin or the canal is ectatic. Perform a trial reduction, and assess stability and leg length. Trial heads should be available, and attention must be directed to several factors including equalization of leg length, soft tissue tension, component rotation, and hip stability.

When a satisfactory trial reduction has been accomplished, the trial components and allograft are removed. Cement the femoral component into the allograft on the back table. Lavage and dry the canal thoroughly. Pressurize cement into the canal using a fingertip to occlude the distal end of the canal (Fig. 4). Excess cement is removed from the protruding

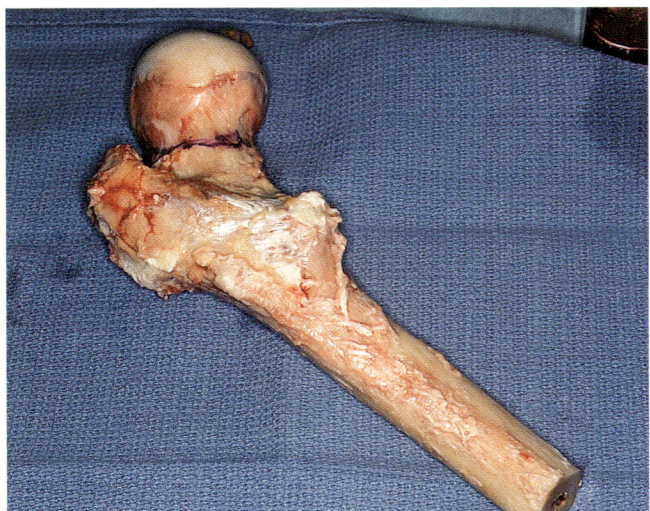

Figure 3. Allograft prior to preparation of the medullary canal. Extension of the femoral head. The canal is cleaned with pulsatile lavage and dried thoroughly.

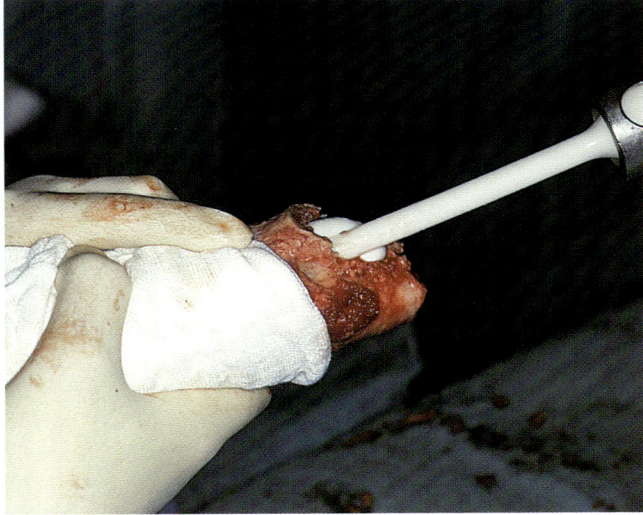

Figure 4. Cement is introduced into the allograft medullary canal. Cement may be pressurized by occluding the canal distally with a fingertip.

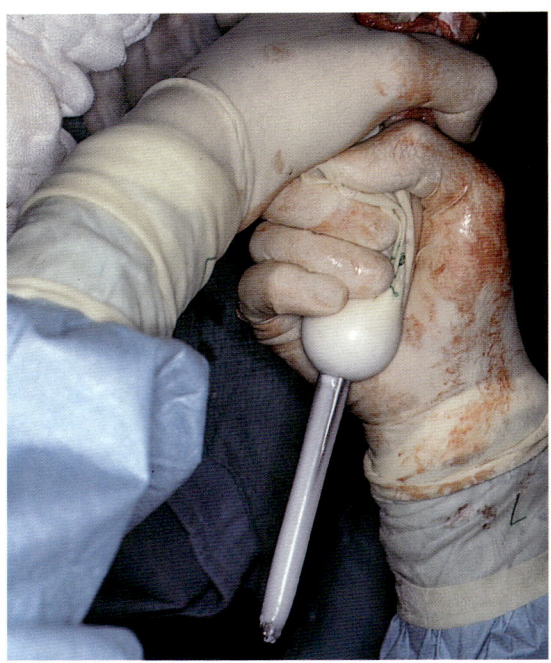

Figure 5. The long-stem femoral component is then inserted into the allograft. The surgical glove over the distal end of the allograft serves as a diaphragm, preventing the stem tip from dragging cement from the canal.

end of the femoral component and from the bone surfaces (Fig. 5). After the cement is cured, the allograft-prosthetic composite is inserted into the distal fragment (Fig. 6). Use 16-gauge Luque wires to cerclage the step cut. Mobilize the previously split proximal femur and apply this bone to the surface of the femur, bridging the host-allograft junction.

Figure 6. (A) The APC stem is then inserted into the host canal. Trial reduction may then be performed. (B) Insertion of the APC into the host femur and fixation with cerclage wires.

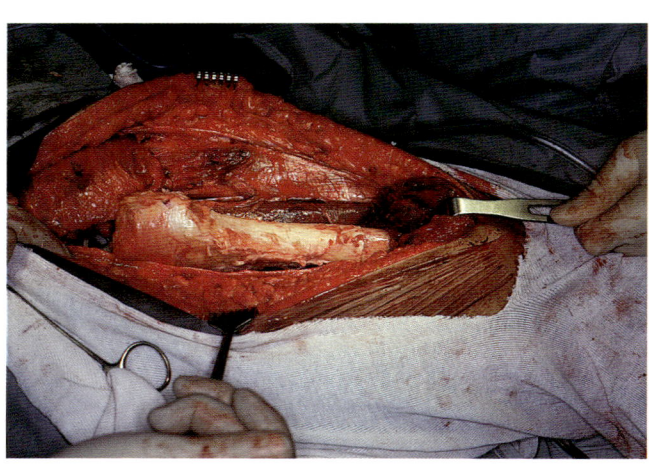
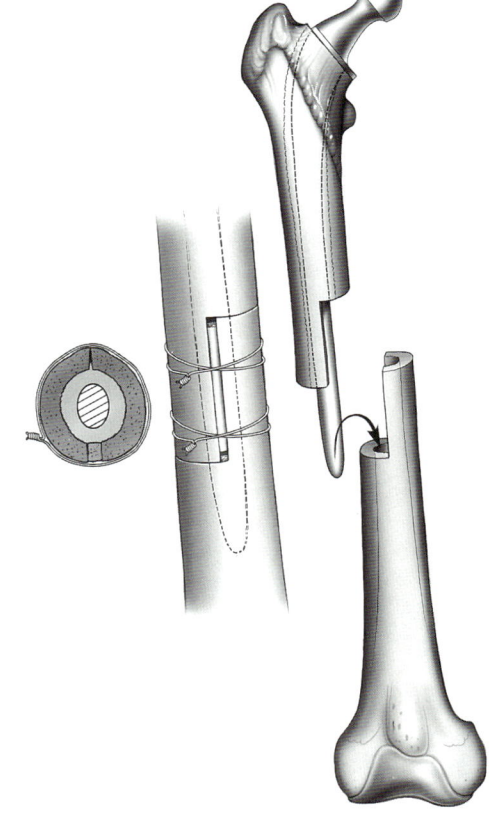

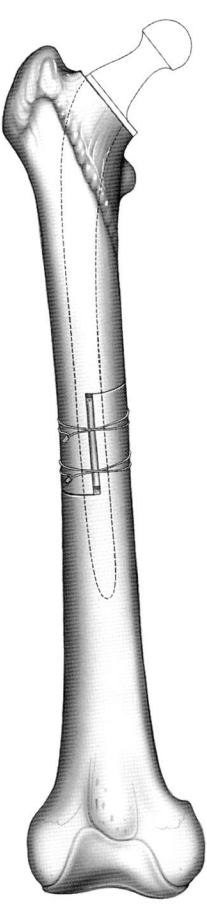

Figure 7. APC after attachment of host greater trochanter and cerclage of remaining host metadiaphyseal bone to the allograft.

This serves as a vascularized cortical strut. The host bone struts are affixed to the reconstructed femur with cerclage wires, and the wires fixing the step cut are buried. The construct can be quite bulky, and a portion of the host proximal femur may need to be removed in order to repair the fascia lata. Alternatively, morsellize this bone, and apply it to the allograft-host junction.

The host greater trochanter is attached to the APC by standard wire technique or a cable-grip system (Fig. 7). Care should be taken to minimize the number of drill holes made in the allograft. Advancement of the trochanter may be necessary for stability. If the tendon of the host abductor is to be repaired to the allograft tendon, this should be done with non-absorbable suture.

Occasionally, the proximal femoral anatomy will not allow for a satisfactory step cut. This may occur when the cortex is extremely thin or ectatic. Alternative methods of distal fixation include press-fit, use of a femoral component that allows for distal interlocking, plate fixation, and distal cementing. In these instances the femur is cut square for a typical butt joint. Experience with distal interlocking type of prosthesis is limited. If cementing the stem into the host is considered, the patient may be better served with a modular oncology-type prosthesis, though the allograft construct allows for more physiologic reconstruction of the abductor mechanism. If the host femur distal intramedullary canal is excessively

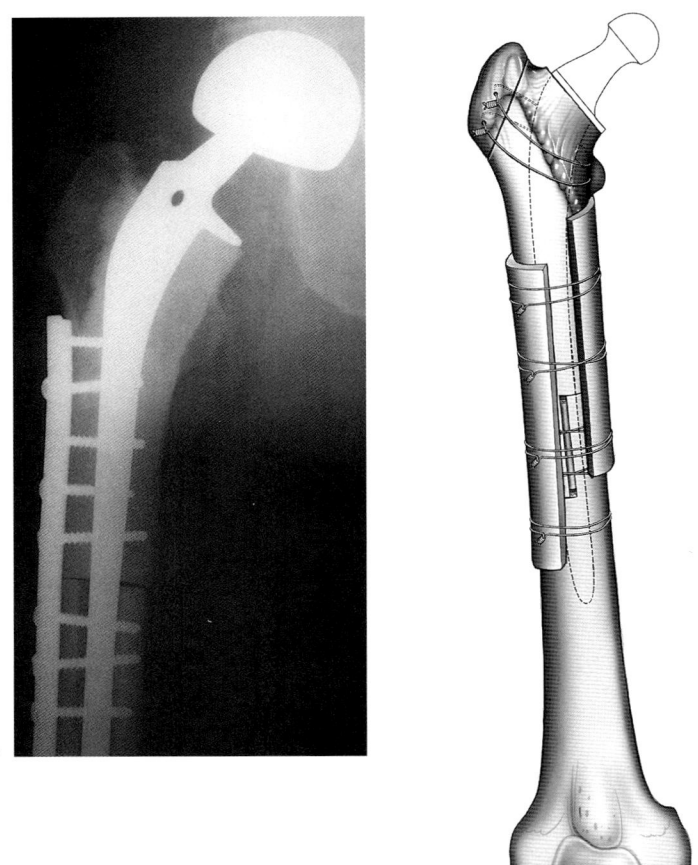

Figure 8. (A) Radiograph demonstrating APC construct. (B) APC after insertion.

wide, a modified step cut may be employed allowing for partial invagination of the allograft into the host. Supplemental fixation will be required in this instance.

For plate fixation, a 4.5 mm, staggered-hole plate can be used (Fig. 8). Screws are angled to avoid the femoral stem. This is difficult in the proximal fragment where the diameter of the bone relative to the stem is small. Drilling through the APC should be done carefully to avoid breaking the drill bit. Do not allow the bit to stop spinning, as it may become stuck in the cement. Use of self-tapping screws reduces the likelihood of breaking a tap within the bone. Placement of screws oblique to the plate, in order to bypass the femoral stem, will result in the screw heads sitting proud. Overtightening, in an effort to seat the screw heads may result in the screw heads shearing off. Screws inaccurately placed in the distal fragment may displace the stem and result in both loss of fit at the host-allograft junction and angular deformity. Care should be taken that the plate does not end at the level of the stem tip, creating a significant stress-riser.

Hemostasis is obtained, and the fascia of the vastus lateralis is repaired with a running absorbable suture. The fascia lata is repaired over suction drains with interrupted nonabsorbable sutures. Skin and subcutaneous tissue are closed in the standard fashion, and sterile dressings are applied.

When the proximal femur is resected for tumor, a cuff of normal tissue is removed to achieve wide surgical margins. The hip capsule is divided at the rim of the acetabulum. The abductor tendon is transected near its insertion at the greater trochanter. The level of femoral osteotomy should be 5 cm from the distal extent of the tumor. Care should be taken to prevent contamination of the allograft with tumor cells. Instruments used in the resection of the tumor should not be used in the preparation of the allograft. The hip is redraped, and instruments are changed prior to implantation of the APC. Soft-tissue coverage of the APC is generally less problematic following tumor resections because of the bulk of tissue removed. A slightly larger allograft may therefore be used. Autogenous bone is generally not available for bone grafting of the host-allograft junction.

POSTOPERATIVE MANAGEMENT

Suction drains are maintained for 48 hr postoperatively, as are prophylactic antibiotics. Cultures of the graft taken prior to implantation should be monitored and infectious disease consultation obtained to assist in the interpretation of any positive cultures. Physical therapy is initiated as the patient's medical condition permits. As the ultimate success of the APC construct depends on healing of the host-allograft junction, typically requiring three to six months, protected weight bearing is necessary during that period. Active abduction is restricted in the early postoperative period to allow healing of the greater trochanter or other abductor mechanism repair.

COMPLICATIONS

The exposure for APC reconstruction is extensive. Substantial bleeding may occur if septal perforator vessels are not controlled. The anesthesia team should be well apprised of the potential for bleeding and autologous blood or a cell-saver should be considered. Care must be taken to avoid injury to nerves and vessels during placement of cerclage wires, and the limb should not be allowed to stretch the remaining soft tissue structures while the allograft is being prepared.

A number of complications related to the allograft and its preparation may occur. Most are preventable. The surgeon must personally check on the availability of the graft and its characteristics. Fractures of the allograft during preparation must be avoided, as biologic healing of the allograft is not possible. The surgeon should be prepared to perform an alternative form of supplemental fixation if the step cut is fractured.

Late complications of allografts include resorption, fracture, and nonunion. Resorption is minimized by preventing revascularization by minimizing the number of holes made in the graft. Late fractures of the body of the graft are uncommon due to the presence of the stem. Nonunion of the greater trochanter is a common complication and even with healing, late fracture may occur. Nonunion at the host-allograft diaphyseal junction is potentially disastrous, as it may result in fatigue failure of the stem. If healing is not radiographically evident by six months, cancellous autografting of the host-allograft junction should be considered.

Dislocation following APC reconstruction may be related to several causes. One should not be misled by the appearance of the neck cut at the time of surgery or on subsequent radiographs, as the allograft does not have soft tissue attachments. The length of the neck relative to the lesser trochanter does not reflect soft-tissue tension. Soft-tissue tension is determined by the overall length of the allograft prosthetic component and by the position of the greater trochanter. Component position is critical to achieving stability.

ILLUSTRATIVE CASE FOR TECHNIQUE

Failed femoral component at 10 years post primary cemented total hip arthroplasty (Fig. 9). As anticipated from the preoperative radiographs, removal of the femoral component and cement resulted in a substantial proximal femoral deficiency (Fig. 10). The patient un-

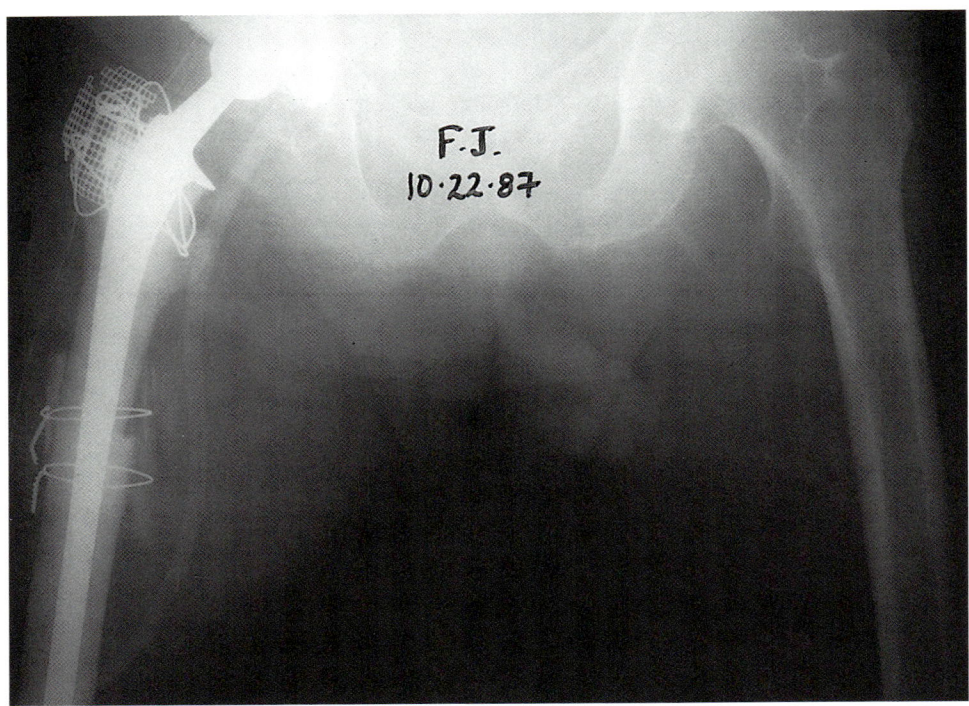

Figure 9. Preoperative radiograph shows failed hardware.

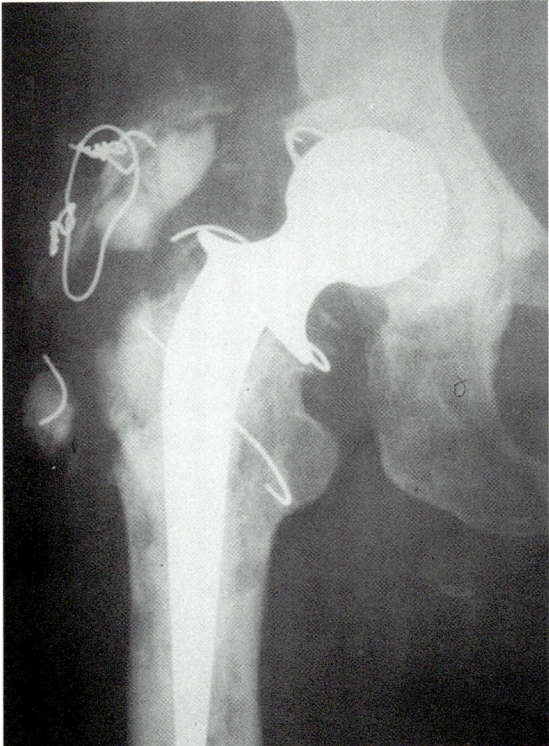

Figure 10. Postoperative radiograph showing revision arthroplasty of the hip using an APC construct.

derwent revision total hip arthroplasty. The proximal femur was replaced with an allograft-prosthetic composite using a long stem femoral component. Rotational stability was provided by step-cut osteotomy.

RECOMMENDED READING

Gross, A.E., "Reconstruction o fhte femur in revision arthroplasty of the hip." in *Total Hip Revision Surgery,* J.O. Galante, A.G. Rosenberg, and J.J. Callaghan, eds., Raven Press, Ltd, New York, 1995.

Head, W. C., Berklacich, F. M., Malinin, T. I., and Emerson, R. H., Jr.: Proximal femoral allografts in revision total hip arthroplasty. *Clin. Orthop. Rel. Res.*, 225:22–36, 1987.

Subject Index

A

abductors, fixation of, after arthroplasty, using direct lateral approach, 37
acetabular cup positioner, for hybrid total hip arthroplasty, 292, 292f
acetabular dysplasia, pelvic osteotomy for, 178–199. *See also* pelvic osteotomy, for acetabular dysplasia
acetabular fractures
    extended iliofemoral approach to, 103f–110f, 103–111
        acetabular exposure in, 108, 110f–111f, 111
        case study of, 120, 121f–122f
        dissection in, 107–108, 108f–110f
        fracture reduction in, 111, 112f–113f, 114
        surgical access in, 105–106, 106f
        for T-type fractures, 111–112, 112f
        wound closure in, 114
    with femoral head fractures, 164, 171
    ilioinguinal approach to, 93f–103f, 93–103
        case study of, 114
        dissection in, 95, 96f–101f, 97, 100
        exposure of acetabulum in, 100, 100f–101f
        fracture reduction in, 102–104, 103f–104f
        incision in, 95, 96f
        screw placement in, 103f, 103–104
        surgical access in, 84–85f
        use of pelvic reconstruction plates in, 102f, 102–103
    Kocher-Langenbeck approach to, 87–94, 88f–93f
        case study of, 116, 117f–118f
        dissection in, 88f, 89–90
        exposure of acetabulum in, 91, 91f
        femoral distraction in, 92, 92f
        incision in, 88f, 89
        pelvic reduction in, 93f, 93–94
        positioning in, 87, 88f, 89
        protection of sciatic nerve in, 90, 91f
        in T-type fractures, 92
        use of spring hook plates in, 93
        wound closure in, 94
    operative fixation of
        case study of, 114
        choice of approach for, 86–87
        complications of, 112
        deep venous thrombosis prophylaxis in, 86, 116
        indications for, 83
        patient preparation in, 87
        postoperative management in, 111–114
        "saw bones" pelvis with, 92f–93f, 104f
acetabular retractors, positioning of, in anterolateral approach, 68, 70f
acetabular revision, 347–357
    acetabular preparation in, 349, 352, 353f–354f
    case study of, 355, 355f–356f, 357
    choice of approach to, 349, 350f–352f
    complications of, 354–355
    contraindications to, 347–348
    exposure of iliac wing in, 352f
    incision in, 350f
    indications for, 347–348, 348f
    postoperative management of, 354
    preoperative planning for, 348–349, 349f
    reinforcement shell for, 353f
acetabulum, exposure of
    in anterolateral approach, 68, 70f–71f
    in cemented total hip arthroplasty, 259–260, 261f
    in direct lateral approach, 32, 33f
    in fixation of acetabular fractures
        using extended iliofemoral approach, 108, 110f–111f, 111
        using ilioinguinal approach, 100, 100f–101f

acetabulum, exposure of, in fixation of acetabular fractures *(contd.)*
    using Kocher-Langenbeck approach, 91, 91*f*
    in hybrid total hip arthroplasty, 289, 289*f*–290*f,* 291
    in posterior approach, 7, 10, 11*f*
    in Vancouver hip arthrodesis, 229, 232*f*–233*f*
allograft
    for impaction grafting, 389, 389*f*
    for revision arthroplasty, femoral stem, 361–362
allograft-prosthetic composite (APC) reconstruction, 375
    allograft preparation in, 376, 387*f*
    case study of, 404*f*–405*f,* 404–405
    cement insertion in, 377
    complications of, 384
    compression plate application in, 377
    contraindications to, 375
    indications for, 375
    postoperative management of, 381
    preoperative planning for, 376
    trial reduction in, 377, 401*f*
    trochanteric osteotomy in, 397, 398*f*
    trochanteric reattachment in, 377
anterolateral approach, 57–80
    acetabular exposure in, 68, 67*f*–68*f*
    assessment of stability in, 74, 75*f*–76*f*
    capsulotomy in, 68, 69*f*
    case example of, 78–80, 79*f*
    closure in, 78, 79*f*
    complications of, 78
    contraindications to, 57
    dissection in, 60, 62*f,* 63–64, 64*f*
    division and removal of femoral neck in, 65, 67*f,* 68, 69*f*
    femoral neck exposure in, 70, 73*f*
    final prosthesis insertion in, 75, 77*f*–78*f,* 78
    incision in, 59*f,* 59, 61*f*
    indications for, 57
    joint capsule exposure in, 64–65, 63*f*–64*f*
    positioning in, 59–61
    positioning of acetabular retractors in, 68, 68*f*
    postoperative management in, 78–79
    preparation of femoral medullary canal in, 74, 75*f*
    rehabilitation after, 78–79
    soft tissue examination in, 69, 70, 72*f*
    trial prosthesis insertion in, 72, 75, 75*f*–76*f*
    Watson-Jones, to femoral head/neck fractures, 170–171
antibiotics, after secondary total hip arthroplasty, 341–342
aorta, thoracic, injury to, with femoral head fractures, 164
arthritis, posttraumatic, intertrochanteric osteotomy for, 212

arthrodesis, Vancouver, 227–241. *See also* Vancouver hip arthrodesis
arthroplasty, dislocation after, with posterior approach, 3
avascular necrosis
    after fixation of acetabular fractures, 116
    after fixation of femoral head fractures, 163

B

balloon device, for cemented total hip arthroplasty, 263*f*–264*f*
Bernese periacetabular osteotomy, 182*f*–183*f*
blade plates, for intertrochanteric osteotomy, 216
bleeding, during allograft-prosthetic composite reconstruction, 403
bone
    ectopic, after fixation of femoral head fractures, 173
    quality of, and results using transtrochanteric approach, 51
bone failure, after fixation of intertrochanteric fractures, 149
bone loss, classification of, in planning for acetabular revision, 348*f*
broaching, in revision total hip arthroplasty, with cementless stem technique, 382–383, 383*f*
Brumback classification, of femoral head fractures, 165, 166*f*

C

capsule tension, in cemented total hip arthroplasty, 267
capsulotomy
    in anterolateral approach, 68, 69*f*
    in cemented total hip arthroplasty, 259
    in direct lateral approach, 21, 23*f*–24*f*
    in hybrid arthroplasty, 283, 284*f*–285*f*
    in intertrochanteric osteotomy, 215*f*
    in posterior approach, 7, 8*f*–9*f*
    in transtrochanteric approach, 45
    in Vancouver hip arthrodesis, 229, 232*f*–233*f*
cemented total hip arthroplasty, 239–263
    acetabular exposure in, 259–260, 261*f*
    anesthesia for, 243
    balloon device for, 263*f*–264*f*
    capsule tension in, 267
    capsulotomy in, 259
    case study of, 274, 275*f*–276*f,* 277
    cement mixing in, 262, 263*f*
    cement placement in, 262, 264*f*–265*f,* 267, 268*f*
    choice of approach in, 258, 258*f*
    complications of, 258–259
    contraindications to, 239–240

SUBJECT INDEX

dissection in, 258–259, 260f
femoral neck osteotomy in, 259–260, 261f
incision in, 244, 245f
indications for, 239
placement of prosthesis in, 249
positioning in, 244, 244f
postoperative management in, 257–258
preoperative planning for, 240–242
reaming in, 261–262, 262f, 264–265, 266f
selection of prosthesis in, 243
socket positioning in, 261, 262f
suturing in, 255f, 266
wound closure in, 270f, 270–271
cementless total hip arthroplasty, 291–315
acetabular component insertion in, 304f–307f, 304–306
case study of, 318
"cheese grater" reamer for, 304f
complications of, 317
contraindications to, 291
expected outcome of, 318
exposure in, 296, 302f, 304
femoral component insertion in, 311, 315f
femoral preparation in, 320–323, 322f–324f
indications for, 291
positioning in, 301f
postoperative management of, 311, 313, 316
preoperative planning in, 291
templating in
femoral, 294
leg length measurement for, 296, 297f–300f
size of acetabular component and, 306, 294f
trial reduction in, 309, 311, 312f–315f
wound closure in, 311
Charnley reamer, for femoral preparation, in hybrid total hip arthroplasty, 279f
"cheese grater" reamer, for cementless total hip arthroplasty, 304f
chisels
for intertrochanteric osteotomy, 206, 207f, 208, 209f, 211, 211f
for spherical acetabular osteotomy, 186f, 189, 189f–190f
complete blood count (CBC), in infected total hip arthroplasty, 322
compression plates, application of
in allograft-prosthetic composite reconstruction, 399, 401, 403f
in Vancouver hip arthrodesis, 234–235, 237f
compression screws, insertion of, in fixation of intertrochanteric fractures, 132–135, 132f–135f
computed tomography (CT), of femoral head fractures, 164–165
cysts, supra-acetabular, 208f

D

deep venous thrombosis (DVT)
after cemented total hip arthroplasty, 259
prophylaxis for
with acetabular fractures, 86, 116
in cementless total hip arthroplasty, 325
developmental dysplasia, intertrochanteric osteotomy for, 201–202
direct lateral approach, 19–36
contraindications to, 19–20
indications for, 19–20
lateral decubitus position for, 24–34, 27f–36f
acetabular exposure in, 32, 33f
complications of, 35
dissection in, 28, 29f–30f, 31
draping in, 26f–28f, 26–27
exposure in, 27, 27f–28f
incision in, 27, 27f
leg length measurement in, 30f, 31
positioning in, 27, 27f–28f
postoperative management in, 35
reduction in, 32, 34f
surgical dislocation in, 31f–32f, 31–32
suturing in, 33, 34f–36f
trochanter drilling in, 32–33, 34f–35f
preoperative planning for, 20
supine position for, 20–25, 21f–26f
capsulotomy in, 21, 22f–24f
deep dissection in, 20–21, 22f–25f
incision in, 20, 21f
positioning in, 20, 21f
superficial dissection in, 20, 21f–22f
surgical dislocation in, 23
suturing in, 26f
dislocation
after arthroplasty
cemented, 259–260
cementless, 317
hybrid, 289
with posterior approach, 3, 14
revision, with cemented femoral component, 355
using direct lateral approach, 35
surgical, in direct lateral approach, 23, 31f–32f, 31–32
DVT. See deep venous thrombosis (DVT)

E

ectopic bone, after fixation of femoral head fractures, 173

F

femoral fractures
after arthroplasty, revision, with cemented femoral component, 360
after impaction grafting, 376–377

femoral fractures *(contd.)*
  intraoperative, in cementless total hip arthroplasty, 330–331
femoral head, dislocation of, complete, trochanteric osteotomy for, 4t, 4–5
femoral head fractures, in young patients
  with acetabular fractures, 164, 171
  case study of, 165f–168f, 164–168
  classification of, 161–163, 162f, 165, 166f
  complications of, 164f, 163
  with concurrent neck fractures, 170–171
  excision of fragments in, 171
  imaging of, 156
  injuries associated with, 156
  isolated, 158, 158f
  postoperative management of, 162–163
  preoperative planning in, 163
  treatment goals in, 161–162
femoral medullary canal, preparation of, in anterolateral approach, 72, 74f
femoral neck
  division and removal of, in anterolateral approach, 65, 67f, 68, 69f
  exposure of, in anterolateral approach, 70, 73f
  fractures of, with femoral head fractures, 170–171
  osteotomy of
    in cemented total hip arthroplasty, 259–260, 261f
    in hybrid total hip arthroplasty, 285, 287, 287f–288f
femoral nerve
  injury to
    after arthroplasty
      using anterolateral approach, 79
      using direct lateral approach, 30f, 37
    after pelvic osteotomy, 196
  lateral cutaneous, protection of, during operative fixation of acetabular fractures, 97
femoral stem, revision total hip arthroplasty using, 345, 360f
femoral templating, in cementless total hip arthroplasty, 294
femur
  drilling of, in transtrochanteric approach, 46, 47f–48f
  exposure of, in revision total hip arthroplasty, with cemented femoral component, 353–358, 355f
  preparation of
    in cementless total hip arthroplasty, 306–308, 308f–310f
    in hybrid total hip arthroplasty, 292, 193f–196f, 197
"figure-of-four" position, for fixation of femoral head fractures, 167f
four-wire technique, in transtrochanteric approach, 39, 39f
fracture, of wires. *See* Wire fracture
fractures. *See under* specific site

G

Gigli saw, use of, in transtrochanteric approach, 43f–44f, 43
gluteal artery, injury to, after fixation of acetabular fractures, 115
gluteal nerve, injury to, after arthroplasty, using direct lateral approach, 29f–30f, 37
gluteal neurovascular bundle, protection of, in fixation of acetabular fractures, using extended iliofemoral approach, 107
gluteus medius tendon, transection of, in fixation of acetabular fractures, using extended iliofemoral approach, 107, 110f
grafting. *See also* allografts
  impaction. *See* impaction grafting
guide wire, position of
  in fixation of intertrochanteric fractures, 135, 135f–138f
  in periacetabular osteotomy, 197f–198f
  in spherical acetabular osteotomy, 188, 188f

H

heterotopic ossification
  after acetabular fracture fixation, prophylaxis for, 114, 116
  after arthroplasty
    cemented, 260
    cementless, 317
    using direct lateral approach, 37
  after pelvic osteotomy, 196
hip
  developmental dysplasia of, intertrochanteric osteotomy for, 201–202
  exposure of, in hybrid arthroplasty, 268, 269f–270f
  surgical approaches to. *See under* specific approaches
hip arthrodesis, Vancouver technique for, 227–241. *See also* Vancouver hip arthrodesis
hip pain, differential diagnosis of, 240–250
hip screws, intramedullary, for fixation of intertrochanteric fractures, 149f–154f, 149–155. *See also* intramedullary hip screw
hockey stick incision, for direct lateral approach, 28, 29f
Hohmann retractors, for periacetabular osteotomy, 195f
hybrid total hip arthroplasty, 265
  capsulotomy in, 269, 270f–271f
  cementing of femoral component in, 297, 284f–288f, 286, 288
  complications of, 289

contraindications to, 279–281
exposure of acetabulum in, 289, 289f–290f, 291
exposure of hip joint in, 282, 283f–284f
femoral neck osteotomy in, 285, 287, 287f–288f
incision in, 281, 282f
indications for, 279–281
insertion of acetabular component in, 291f–292f, 291–292
leg length measurement in, 285, 286f
postoperative management of, 302–303
preoperative planning for, 281
preparation of femur in, 292, 293f–296f, 297
results of, 303

I

iliac wing, exposure of, in acetabular revision, 352f
ilioinguinal approach, to acetabular fractures, 93f–103f, 93–103. *See also* acetabular fractures, ilioinguinal approach to
ilium, osteotomy of, 196f
image intensifier, use of, in intertrochanteric osteotomy, 206, 207f
impaction grafting, with cement, 387–393
case study of, 377, 377f–378f, 379
complications of, 376
contraindications to, 373
exposure in, 374
formation of "neomedullary canal" in, 376, 376f
indications for, 373
insertion of distal plug in, 374, 375f
postoperative management of, 376
preoperative planning in, 374
impaction osteotomy, intertrochanteric, 208
"index line," in templating, for total hip arthroplasty, 234f
infection
after acetabular revision, 340
after arthroplasty, revision, with cemented femoral component, 360
after cemented total hip arthroplasty, 259
after fixation of acetabular fractures, 115
after fixation of intertrochanteric fractures, 149
infracotyloid groove, osteotomy of, 194f
intertrochanteric fractures, 119–152
case study of, 150f–151f, 150
classification of, 125–126, 127f
complications of, 149–150
open reduction and internal fixation of, 147, 148f–149f
operative fixation of
anesthesia in, 122
compression screw insertion in, 141–142, 143f–145f
contraindications to, 119
exposure in, 127–132, 127f–132f
fracture stabilization in, 131–132, 140f–143f, 147, 148f
guide wire position in, 135, 135f–138f
incision in, 136, 137f–138f
indications for, 119
intramedullary hip screw for, 149f–154f, 149–155. *See also* intramedullary hip screw
with irreducible fractures, 131f–136f, 131–132, 135
plate insertion in, 135f–137f, 135–138
positioning in, 128, 129f
preoperative planning in, 119–122, 120f–121f
reduction in, 122, 123f–130f, 131
supplemental, 146–147, 147f
wound closure in, 148, 148f
postoperative management of, 147
intertrochanteric osteotomy, 201–214
blade plates for, 207
case study of, 211f–213f, 210–214
complications of, 209, 210f
exposure in, 214f–215f, 214–215
impaction, 218
indications for, 201
placement of Steinmann pins in, 206, 206f–207f
positioning in, 213f–214f, 213–214
postoperative management of, 209
preoperative planning for, 202–203
reduction of, 210, 210f
use of chisels in, 206, 207f, 208, 209f, 211, 211f
use of image intensifier in, 206, 207f
intra-articular osteotomy, as complication of pelvic osteotomy, 196
intramedullary hip screw, for fixation of intertrochanteric fractures
incision in, 140, 140f
insertion of compression screw in, 151, 152f–154f
positioning in, 149–150
reaming in, 150, 151f

J

joint aspiration, in infected total hip arthroplasty, 322

K

knees, injury to, with femoral head fractures, 164
Kocher-Langenbeck approach, to acetabular fractures, 87–94, 88f–93f. *See also* Acetabular fractures, Kocher-Langenbeck approach to

L

Lambotte osteotomy, in revision total hip arthroplasty, with cementless stem technique, 365, 365f–366f
lateral approach, direct, 19–37. *See also* direct lateral approach
leg length
   discrepancy in, after cemented total hip arthroplasty, 260
   measurement of
      in allograft-prosthetic composite reconstruction, 382
      in cementless arthroplasty, 296, 297f–298f
      in direct lateral approach, 30f, 31
      in hybrid arthroplasty, 271, 272f

M

malalignment, after pelvic osteotomy, 196
malposition, of Vancouver hip arthrodesis, 225
malreduction, of femoral head fractures, 173
malunion, after fixation of intertrochanteric fractures, 149
Milford classification, of femoral head fractures, 165
"monkey trap" defect, 334, 335f

N

"neomedullary canal," formation of, in impaction grafting, 376, 376f
nerve palsy, after cementless total hip arthroplasty, 315
nonunion
   after allograft-prosthetic composite reconstruction, 404
   after fixation of intertrochanteric fractures, 149
   after Vancouver hip arthrodesis, 239

O

obturator nerve, injury to, after pelvic osteotomy, 196
ossification, heterotopic. *See* Heterotopic ossification
osteonecrosis, intertrochanteric osteotomy for, 212
osteotomes
   for hybrid total hip arthroplasty, 294f
   for periacetabular osteotomy, 184f
osteotomy. *See under* specific site

P

pelvic osteotomy, for acetabular dysplasia, 173–199
   contraindications to, 173
   indications for, 173, 174f–175f
   periacetabular. *See* periacetabular osteotomy
   preoperative planning in, 176f, 176–178
   spherical. *See* spherical acetabular osteotomy
pelvic reconstruction plates, for acetabular fractures, in ilioinguinal approach, 102f, 102–103
pelvis, reduction of, in fixation of acetabular fractures, using Kocher-Langenbeck approach, 93f, 93–94
periacetabular osteotomy, 184f, 192–205, 193f–204f
   case study of, 197f, 197
   complications of, 196
   displacement of, 190, 190f
   dissection in, 192, 193f
   fixation of, 193
   Hohmann retractors for, 195f
   osteotomes for, 194f
   placement of Schanz screw in, 184f, 190
   positioning in, 192
   position of guide wire in, 197f–198f
   postoperative management of, 195
   sequence of, 182–192, 184f–194f
   wound closure in, 194f, 195
peroneal nerve, injury to, after hybrid arthroplasty, 303–304
physical examination, preoperative, 254–255
Pipkin classification, of femoral head fractures, 165, 166f
piriformis tendon, release of
   in anterolateral approach, 72f
   in fixation of acetabular fractures, 91
   in posterior approach, 7, 8f
PMMA, for cementing of femoral component, in hybrid total hip arthroplasty, 297, 298f, 302, 302f
positioning. *See under* specific procedure and specific approach
posterior approach, 3–17
   acetabular exposure in, 7, 10, 11f
   capsulotomy in, 7, 8f–9f
   case study of, 16–17, 17f–17f
   complications of, 14, 16
   contraindications to, 3–4
   history of, 4
   incision for, 5f–6f, 7
   indications for, 3–4
   positioning for, 5, 7
   postoperative management in, 14
   preoperative planning for, 4t, 4–5
   release of external rotator tendons in, 7, 7f
   release of piriformis tendon in, 7, 8f
   trochanter suturing in, 12, 13f–15f
posttraumatic arthritis, intertrochanteric osteotomy for, 212
prosthesis
   insertion of, in anterolateral approach, 72, 75, 75f–78f

placement of
in cemented total hip arthroplasty, 262, 264f–265f, 267, 269f
in cementless total hip arthroplasty, 318f–321f, 318–320
removal of, in arthroplasty infection, 338–339
selection of, in cemented total hip arthroplasty, 257
protrusion deformity, cemented total hip arthroplasty for, 255–256
pseudocapsule, excision of, in revision total hip arthroplasty, with cemented femoral component, 366f–367f, 366–367
pubic ramus, osteotomy of, 194, 195f

R

reamers
Charnley, for femoral preparation, in hybrid total hip arthroplasty, 293f
"cheese grater," for cementless total hip arthroplasty, 318f
rectus femoris muscle, retraction of, in direct lateral approach, 30f
reduction, in direct lateral approach, 32, 34f
rehabilitation
after arthroplasty
cemented total hip, 271–272
cementless, 327
using anterolateral approach, 78–79
using direct lateral approach, 34
using posterior approach, 14
using transtrochanteric approach, 55
after fixation of femoral head fractures, 171
after fixation of intertrochanteric fractures, 157
after intertrochanteric osteotomy, 220–221
after pelvic osteotomy, 205
after Vancouver hip arthrodesis, 235
reinforcement shell, for acetabular revision, 353f
revision total hip arthroplasty
with cemented femoral component, 363–376
case study of, 374, 375f–376f
cement removal in, 369
cement replacement in, 369–371, 370f–371f
complications of, 373–374
contraindications to, 363
dissection in, 365f, 366
excision of pseudocapsule in, 366f–367f, 366–367
femoral exposure in, 367–368, 369f
incision in, 364, 365f
indications for, 363
positioning in, 364, 365f
postoperative management of, 373
preoperative planning in, 363–364, 364f
templating for, 364, 364f

trochanteric osteotomy in, 366f–367f, 366–367
trochanteric reattachment in, 372f–373f, 372–373
with cementless stem technique, 377–386
broaching in, 382–383, 383f
complications of, 386
contraindications to, 377
exposure in, 379
extraction in, 379
impingement in, 384
implantation in, 384f–385f, 384–386
incision in, 379, 380f
indications for, 377
osteotomy in, 379–380, 380f–381f
pedestal management in, 380
postoperative management of, 386
preoperative planning in, 377–379, 378f
reaming in, 380–382, 382f
templating for, 378, 378f
femoral stem, 359–362, 360f
impaction grafting for, 387–393. See also impaction grafting
rotator tendons, external, release of, in posterior approach, 7, 7f

S

"saw bones" pelvis, with acetabular fractures, 92f–93f, 104f
Schanz screw, placement of, in periacetabular osteotomy, 187f, 187
sciatic nerve
injury to
after arthroplasty
revision, with cemented femoral component, 374
using posterior approach, 16
after pelvic osteotomy, 196
protection of, during fixation of acetabular fractures, using Kocher-Langenbeck approach, 90, 91f
shear-type fractures, intertrochanteric, operative fixation of, 125, 125f
Smith-Peterson anterior approach, to fixation of femoral head fractures, 166–170, 167f–170f
soft tissue
absence of, after arthroplasty, using posterior approach, 14, 16
examination of, in anterolateral approach, 68, 70, 72f
spherical acetabular osteotomy, 178f
case study of, 206–208, 207f–208f
chisels for, 178f, 178
complications of, 196
displacement of, 181, 181f
dissection in, 186, 187f–188f, 188
fixation of, 183
incision in, 176, 177f
position of guide wire in, 178, 178f

spherical acetabular osteotomy, 179f (contd.)
   postoperative management of, 195
   preoperative planning for, 178f
   surgical approach for, 175, 187f–190f, 178
   wound closure in, 192
spring hook plates, for fixation of acetabular fractures, 93
Steinmann pins, placement of, in intertrochanteric osteotomy, 216, 216f–217f
supra-acetabular cyst, 208f

T

templating
   for revision total hip arthroplasty
      with cemented femoral component, 364, 364f
      with cementless stem technique, 378, 378f
   for total hip arthroplasty
      case study of, 249, 250f–251f
      cemented, 255
      cementless, 306, 306f–314f, 308, 310
         femoral, 308
         size of acetabular component and, 306, 308, 308f
      measurement sites in, 246f–247f, 246–247
      sizing in, 247, 248f–249f
      uses of, 245
thoracic aorta, injury to, with femoral head fractures, 164
three-wire technique, in transtrochanteric approach, 38f, 41, 47f, 49
tonsil clamp, for trochanteric wiring, 50, 50f
total hip arthroplasty (THA)
   cemented, 253–277. *See also* cemented total hip arthroplasty
   cementless, 305–332. *See also* cementless total hip arthroplasty
   hybrid, 279–304. *See also* hybrid total hip arthroplasty
   rehabilitation after. *See* Rehabilitation
   revision. *See* revision total hip arthroplasty
   secondary, after infection, 335–345
      case study of, 343f–344f, 343–345
      complications of, 343
      debridement in, 339, 340f
      exposure in, 338, 338f
      indications for, 335–337, 336f
      joint aspiration in, 336
      positioning in, 338, 339f–340f
      postoperative management of, 341–342
      preoperative planning in, 337–338
      prosthesis removal in, 338–339
      reimplantation procedure in, 342
      wound closure in, 339
   templating for, 245–251. *See also* Templating

transtrochanteric approach, 37–55
   bone quality and, 51
   capsulotomy in, 45
   case study of, 55, 55f
   complications of, 53–54
   contraindications to, 37
   femoral drilling in, 46, 47f–48f
   four-wire technique in, 39, 39f
   incision in, 40, 40f
   indications for, 37–38
   osteotomy in, 42f–43f, 45
   postoperative management in, 53
   preoperative planning for, 38
   suturing in, 52f–53f, 53
   three-wire technique in, 38f, 41, 47f, 49
   trochanteric drilling in, 48f, 49
   trochanteric retraction in, 45, 46f
   trochanteric wiring in, 49f–54f, 49–53
   two-wire technique in, 38f–41f, 41
   use of Gigli saw in, 41f–43f
trochanter
   drilling of
      in direct lateral approach, 32–33, 34f–35f
      in transtrochanteric approach, 48f, 49
   nonunion of, after arthroplasty, using transtrochanteric approach, 55–56
   reattachment of
      in allograft-prosthetic composite reconstruction, 399, 401, 403f
      in revision total hip arthroplasty, with cemented femoral component, 372f–373f, 372–373
   retraction of, in transtrochanteric approach, 45, 46f
   wiring of, in transtrochanteric approach, 49f–54f, 49–53
trochanteric osteotomy
   in allograft-prosthetic composite reconstruction, 397, 398f
   for dislocated femoral head, 4t, 4–5
   in revision total hip arthroplasty, with cemented femoral component, 366f–367f, 366–367
   in Vancouver hip arthrodesis, 231f
T-type acetabular fractures, operative fixation of
   extended iliofemoral approach to, 111–112, 112f
   Kocher-Langenbeck approach to, 94
two-wire technique, in transtrochanteric approach, 38f–41f, 41

V

Vancouver hip arthrodesis, 207–231
   acetabular exposure in, 229, 232f–233f
   application of compression plate in, 234–235, 237f
   capsulotomy in, 229, 232f–233f
   case study of, 239–240, 240f–241f
   complications of, 229

contraindications to, 227
dissection in, 229, 230*f*–231*f*
incision in, 228, 229*f*
indications for, 227
positioning in, 228*f*, 228–229
postoperative management of, 235
preoperative planning in, 227–228
reaming in, 233*f*–236*f*, 234
trochanteric osteotomy in, 231*f*
vascular injury, from pelvic osteotomy, 206

W

Watson-Jones anterolateral approach
    to femoral head/neck fractures, 170–171
    to intertrochanteric osteotomy, 213*f*–214*f*, 213-214
wire fracture, after transtrochanteric osteotomy, 56
wire tighteners, for trochanteric wiring, 54, 55*f*